Atrial Fibrillation: Clinical Cardiology

Atrial Fibrillation: Clinical Cardiology

Editor: Caleb Bell

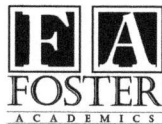

FA FOSTER
ACADEMICS

www.fosteracademics.com

www.fosteracademics.com

FA
FOSTER
ACADEMICS

Cataloging-in-Publication Data

Atrial fibrillation : clinical cardiology / edited by Caleb Bell.
    p. cm.
Includes bibliographical references and index.
ISBN 978-1-63242-599-7
1. Atrial fibrillation. 2. Atrial arrhythmias. 3. Cardiovascular system--Diseases.
4. Cardiology. I. Bell, Caleb.
RC685.A72 A87 2019
616.128--dc23

Foster Academics,
118-35 Queens Blvd., Suite 400,
Forest Hills, NY 11375, USA

ISBN 978-1-63242-599-7 (Hardback)

Contents

Chapter 25

Chapter 26

Chapter 27

Chapter 28

Permissions

Contributors

Index

Preface

Over the recent decade, advancements and applications have progressed exponentially. This has led to the increased interest in this field and projects are being conducted to enhance knowledge. The main objective of this book is to present some of the critical challenges and provide insights into possible solutions. This book will answer the varied questions that arise in the field and also provide an increased scope for furthering studies.

Atrial fibrillation is the abnormal rhythm of the heart, which is characterized by rapid and irregular beating of the atria. It often begins as brief periods of abnormal beating, and gets longer and fairly constant over time. It is associated with an increased risk of dementia, stroke and heart failure. Although symptoms are generally absent, occasionally there may be cases of lightheadedness, chest pain, heart palpitations and shortness of breath. Atrial fibrillation can be diagnosed by an investigation of the complete patient profile, including medical history and physical examination, transthoracic echocardiogram, electrocardiogram, serum thyroid stimulating hormone level, etc. It can be treated with medications that work to slow down the heart rate to acceptable rates or convert the heart rhythm to a normal sinus rhythm. Electrical cardioversion, ablation and anti-clotting medications like direct oral anticoagulants and warfarin may be recommended. This book aims to shed light on some of the unexplored aspects of atrial fibrillation. It includes some of the vital pieces of work being conducted across the world, on atrial fibrillation and clinical cardiology. It is a vital tool for all researching or studying cardiology as it gives incredible insights into emerging trends and concepts.

I hope that this book, with its visionary approach, will be a valuable addition and will promote interest among readers. Each of the authors has provided their extraordinary competence in their specific fields by providing different perspectives as they come from diverse nations and regions. I thank them for their contributions.

Editor

Genome-Wide Identification of Expression Quantitative Trait Loci (eQTLs) in Human Heart

Tamara T. Koopmann[1♦], Michiel E. Adriaens[1♦], Perry D. Moerland[2], Roos F. Marsman[1], Margriet L. Westerveld[1], Sean Lal[3], Taifang Zhang[4], Christine Q. Simmons[5], Istvan Baczko[6], Cristobal dos Remedios[3], Nanette H. Bishopric[4,7], Andras Varro[6], Alfred L. George, Jr.[5], Elisabeth M. Lodder[1], Connie R. Bezzina[1*]

1 Department of Experimental Cardiology, Heart Failure Research Centre, Academic Medical Center, Amsterdam, The Netherlands, 2 Bioinformatics Laboratory, Department of Clinical Epidemiology, Biostatistics and Bioinformatics, Academic Medical Center, Amsterdam, The Netherlands, 3 Muscle Research Unit, Department of Anatomy, Bosch Institute, The University of Sydney, Sydney, Australia, 4 Department of Medicine, University of Miami School of Medicine, Miami, Florida, United States of America, 5 Division of Genetic Medicine, Department of Medicine, Vanderbilt University, Nashville, Tennessee, United States of America, 6 Department of Pharmacology and Pharmacotherapy, Faculty of Medicine, University of Szeged, Szeged, Hungary, 7 Department of Molecular and Cellular Pharmacology, University of Miami School of Medicine, Miami, Florida, United States of America

Abstract

In recent years genome-wide association studies (GWAS) have uncovered numerous chromosomal loci associated with various electrocardiographic traits and cardiac arrhythmia predisposition. A considerable fraction of these loci lie within inter-genic regions. The underlying trait-associated variants likely reside in regulatory regions and exert their effect by modulating gene expression. Hence, the key to unraveling the molecular mechanisms underlying these cardiac traits is to interrogate variants for association with differential transcript abundance by expression quantitative trait locus (eQTL) analysis. In this study we conducted an eQTL analysis of human heart. For a total of 129 left ventricular samples that were collected from non-diseased human donor hearts, genome-wide transcript abundance and genotyping was determined using microarrays. Each of the 18,402 transcripts and 897,683 SNP genotypes that remained after pre-processing and stringent quality control were tested for eQTL effects. We identified 771 eQTLs, regulating 429 unique transcripts. Overlaying these eQTLs with cardiac GWAS loci identified novel candidates for studies aimed at elucidating the functional and transcriptional impact of these loci. Thus, this work provides for the first time a comprehensive eQTL map of human heart: a powerful and unique resource that enables systems genetics approaches for the study of cardiac traits.

Editor: John R.B. Perry, Institute of Metabolic Science, United Kingdom

Funding: The authors acknowledge the support from the Netherlands CardioVascular Research Initiative (CVON PREDICT): the Dutch Heart Foundation, Dutch Federation of University Medical Centres, the Netherlands Organisation for Health Research and Development and the Royal Netherlands Academy of Sciences. Tissue collections performed at Vanderbilt University were supported by NIH grant HL068880 (A.L.G.). The funders had no role in study design, data collection and analysis, decision to publish, or preparation of the manuscript.

Competing Interests: The authors have declared that no competing interests exist.

* E-mail: c.r.bezzina@amc.uva.nl

♦ These authors contributed equally to this work.

Introduction

It is well established that many cardiac traits and susceptibility to heart disease are heritable [1,2,3,4,5,6,7]. Several genome-wide association studies (GWAS) have uncovered common genetic variation, in the form of single nucleotide polymorphisms (SNPs), impacting on cardiac traits such as susceptibility to atrial fibrillation [8], ventricular fibrillation [9], heart rate [10] and electrocardiographic (ECG) indices of cardiac conduction [11,12,13,14] and repolarization [15,16]. There is widespread consensus that functional studies of GWAS-defined loci will advance our understanding of the molecular underpinnings of the associated traits.

SNPs identified by GWAS are considered to impact the respective clinical phenotype, either directly or indirectly by virtue of linkage disequilibrium (LD) with the causal variant(s) in the context of a haplotype. Many trait-associated haplotypes occur in non-coding regions of the genome [17] and are hypothesized to modulate the respective trait through effects on gene expression [18]. Such SNPs are particularly challenging to understand because they may exert effects on the trait either by affecting the expression of a neighbouring gene (cis-effect) or the expression of a gene located elsewhere in the genome (trans-effects). One way of understanding GWAS signals thus entails interrogating trait-associated variants for association with differential transcript abundance by expression quantitative trait locus (eQTL) analysis. Studying gene expression level effects of disease-associated haplotypes has successfully uncovered the molecular mechanisms underlying loci associated with increased risk of myocardial infarction [19], coronary artery disease [20] and colorectal cancer [21]. In recent years, multiple genome-wide eQTL resources have become available for various tissues including brain, liver and adipose tissue [22,23,24,25,26,27,28,29]. Because eQTLs may be

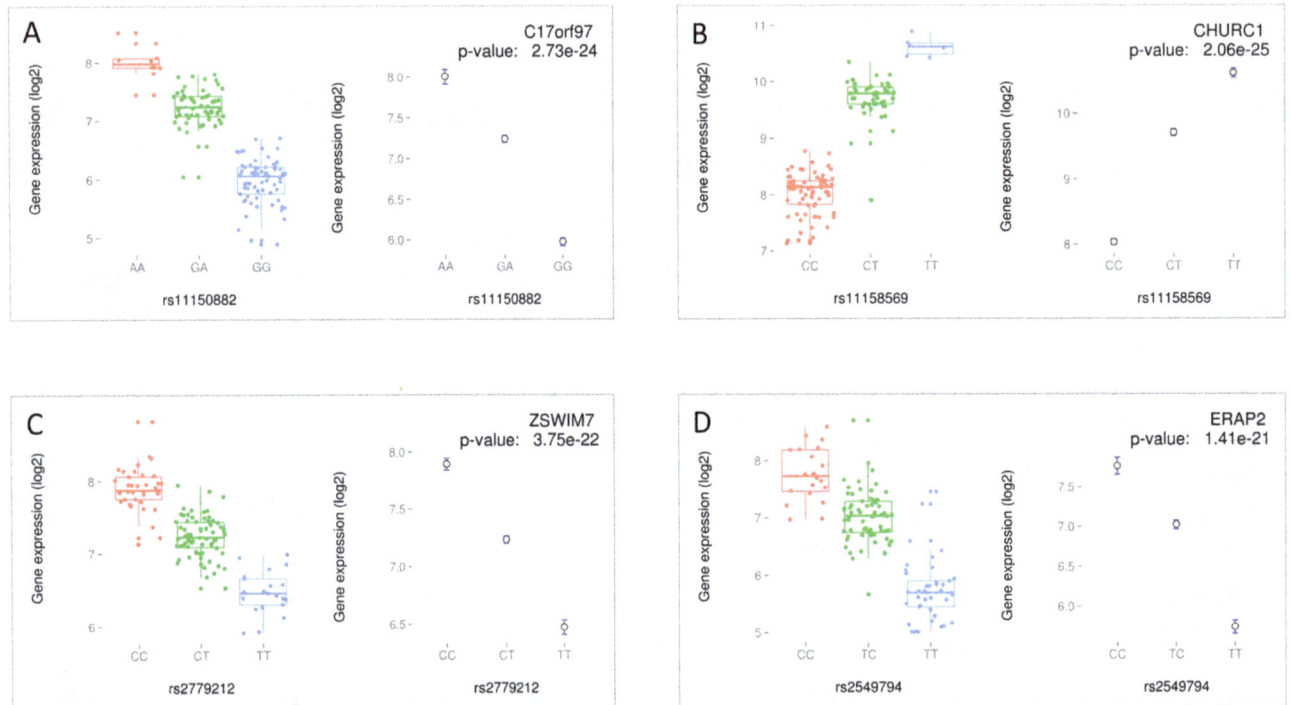

Figure 1. Overview plots for top *cis* eQTLs. An overview of the 4 most significant *cis* eQTLs: rs11150882 with *C17orf97* (panel A), rs11158569 with *CHURC1* (panel B), rs2779212 with *ZSWIM7* (panel C) and rs2549794 with *ERAP2* (panel D). On the left of each panel, box-and-whisker plots of mRNA levels for all genotypes. On the right, mean and standard-error plots of mRNA levels for all genotypes are illustrated. Right upper corner gives the association p-value and the gene name.

tissue-specific, a similar resource for human heart is anticipated to have great value [23,29,30,31].

To this end, we have generated a human heart eQTL resource by genome-wide genotyping and determination of transcript abundance in 129 human donor heart samples. We subsequently overlaid previously identified cardiac trait GWAS signals with the identified eQTLs to identify candidate causal genes for the effects at these GWAS loci. This work provides an eQTL map of human heart, a resource that is likely to play an important role in furthering our understanding of the mechanisms associated with loci identified in GWAS on cardiac traits.

Results

General design of study

We collected left ventricular samples from 180 non-diseased human hearts of unrelated organ donors whose hearts were explanted to obtain pulmonary and aortic valves for transplant surgery or explanted for heart transplantation but not used due to logistical reasons (e.g. no tissue-matched recipient was available). The subjects were assumed to be mainly of Western European descent. mRNA and DNA were isolated according to standard procedures. Transcript abundance was measured using the HumanHT-12 v4.0 whole genome array (Illumina) and genotyping was carried out using the HumanOmniExpress genome-wide SNP arrays (Illumina).

Data preprocessing and normalization

Gene transcript abundance: Of the 47,231 transcripts whose expression levels were measured on the array, only those that were expressed above background level and for which the probe sequence mapped unambiguously to the genome and did not contain common SNPs, were used in further analyses. This procedure left 18,402 transcripts for eQTL analysis. Model-based background correction and normalization across arrays and transcripts was performed to correct for technical variance present in gene expression levels. A total of 162 arrays passed the standardized microarray gene expression quality control.

Genotyping: Manhattan distance clustering and principal component analysis of the genotype data of 154 samples that were successfully genotyped, revealed 13 genetic outliers (**Figure S1**). To ensure a genetically homogenous group for further analysis, samples pertaining to these clusters were removed. An additional 12 samples were removed due to low call rate (<95%), high proportion of alleles identical-by-state (>95%), or extreme heterozygosity (FDR 1%). Only SNPs with a minor allele frequency (MAF) higher than 0.15 were considered in eQTL analysis. This cutoff was chosen to ensure sufficient power to detect eQTLs within a broad range of effect sizes (**Figure S2**). Imputation was performed using the HAPMAP Phase III data (see Materials & Methods for details). This left 129 samples (74 male, 55 female; age 41 ± 14), 18,402 transcripts and 897,683 SNPs for eQTL analysis.

Genome-wide eQTL mapping

Each of the measured transcripts was tested for association with all SNPs using linear modeling, taking age, sex and clinical/university center as covariates. We thus identified 6402 significant eQTLs (FDR $\leq$0.05). To remove redundant signals and identify independent expression-controlling loci, we performed linkage-disequilibrium (LD)-pruning. For this we grouped SNPs exhibiting LD (r^2>0.6) into clusters, revealing 771 independent loci regulating 429 unique transcripts. These results are comparable

Table 1. Overview of the 30 most significant *cis* eQTLs, reported as independent LD-pruned SNP clusters (see Materials & Methods).

LD cluster	Top SNP ID	Chr.	SNP position	Gene TSS position	Gene strand	Gene symbol	eQTL p-value	Minor allele	Major allele	eQTL beta	eQTL MAF	Distance top SNP to gene	Relative top SNP position	Illumina Probe ID
1	rs11158369	14	65400069	65381079	+	CHURC1	2.06E-25	T	C	1.50	0.24	0	inside	ILMN_1798177
2	rs11150882	17	259648	260118	+	C17orf97	2.73E-24	A	G	1.11	0.29	-470	upstream	ILMN_1707137
3	rs2779272	17	15876655	15903006	-	ZSWIM7	3.75E-22	T	C	-0.70	0.44	3220	downstream	ILMN_3298167
4	rs2549794	5	96244549	96211644	+	ERAP2	1.41E-21	C	T	1.06	0.42	0	inside	ILMN_1743145
5	rs335632	5	76728085	76788332	-	WDR41	4.44E-20	G	A	-0.87	0.17	0	inside	ILMN_1778488
6	rs1051470	12	118583232	118573870	+	PEBP1	1.74E-19	T	C	-1.70	0.38	0	inside	ILMN_3285785
7	rs4837796	9	123610288	123605320	+	LOC253039	2.36E-19	G	A	0.69	0.38	0	inside	ILMN_3236498
8	rs12358834	10	29778270	30024730	-	SVIL	2.83E-19	C	A	-1.37	0.16	0	inside	ILMN_3298400
9	rs8413	9	139323311	139934256	-	INPP5E	1.45E-18	G	A	-0.60	0.40	0	inside	ILMN_1811301
10	rs799082	10	16556710	16478942	+	PTER	2.78E-18	A	G	-0.74	0.45	966	downstream	ILMN_1795336
11	rs11586488	1	22348556	22351707	+	HSPC157/LINC00339	8.56E-18	C	T	1.01	0.23	-3151	upstream	ILMN_3272768
12	rs4822466	22	24312204	24384284	-	GSTT1	1.10E-17	G	A	-2.04	0.45	63935	downstream	ILMN_1730054
12	rs5742363	22	24299147	24309026	+	DDTL	3.57E-15	C	T	0.47	0.42	-9879	upstream	ILMN_3244439
12	rs5742363	22	24299147	24236565	+	MIF	9.86E-06	C	T	0.17	0.42	61738	downstream	ILMN_1807074
13	rs7168451	15	41672384	41694658	-	NDUFAF1	1.43E-17	G	A	-0.63	0.28	7163	downstream	ILMN_1754421
14	rs1603117	4	70395945	69962193	+	UGT2B7	7.49E-17	G	A	-1.41	0.37	417240	downstream	ILMN_1679194
14	rs1603117	4	70395945	69434245	-	UGT2B17	2.25E-16	G	A	-1.21	0.37	-961700	upstream	ILMN_1808677
14	rs1603117	4	70395945	70080449	-	UGT2B11	3.64E-14	G	A	-0.98	0.37	-315496	upstream	ILMN_1810233
14	rs1603117	4	70395945	70361626	-	UGT2B4	5.77E-11	G	A	-0.67	0.37	-34319	upstream	ILMN_2206500
15	rs10876864	12	56401085	56435686	+	RPS26/LP10	8.22E-16	G	A	0.46	0.36	-34601	upstream	ILMN_3290019
16	rs720201	2	61376463	61372243	+	C2orf74	1.06E-15	G	A	0.61	0.42	0	inside	ILMN_1754501
17	rs4796398	17	7208197	7210318	+	EIF5A	1.39E-15	G	A	0.34	0.39	-2121	upstream	ILMN_1794522
18	rs1222809	5	79917517	79950800	-	DHFR	2.00E-15	G	A	-0.92	0.22	4528	downstream	ILMN_3232696
19	rs530411	19	39927540	39926618	-	RPS16	4.43E-15	A	G	0.20	0.37	-922	upstream	ILMN_1651850
20	rs10051931	5	94001476	93954391	+	ANKRD32	8.79E-15	G	A	-0.47	0.33	0	inside	ILMN_2214278
21	rs1887547	1	110295772	110283660	-	GSTM3	1.21E-14	A	G	-0.65	0.36	-12112	upstream	ILMN_1736184
22	rs2240147	19	989730	984328	+	WDR18	1.95E-14	A	C	0.42	0.18	0	inside	ILMN_1694479
23	rs10088428	8	28909523	28747911	+	HMBOX1	2.14E-14	A	G	-0.52	0.24	0	inside	ILMN_1720059
24	rs113413	22	24292264	24384284	-	GSTT1	3.05E-14	G	A	-2.25	0.39	83875	downstream	ILMN_1730054
24	rs113413	22	24292264	24309026	+	DDTL	5.74E-12	G	A	0.49	0.39	-16762	upstream	ILMN_3244439
25	rs9568	15	41573612	41694658	-	NDUFAF1	3.71E-14	A	C	-0.59	0.27	105935	downstream	ILMN_1754421
26	rs443140	6	86189520	86388451	-	C6orf160	4.41E-14	T	C	-0.54	0.48	197205	downstream	ILMN_1653794
27	rs11007559	10	29698286	30024730	-	SVIL	6.04E-14	A	C	-1.02	0.21	47991	downstream	ILMN_3298400
28	rs6663	12	109886603	109915155	-	KCTD10	1.00E-13	A	G	0.55	0.26	0	inside	ILMN_1719064

Table 1. Cont.

LD cluster	Top SNP ID	Chr.	SNP position	Gene TSS position	Gene strand	Gene symbol	eQTL p-value	Minor allele	Major allele	eQTL beta	eQTL MAF	Distance top SNP to gene	Relative top SNP position	Illumina Probe ID
29	rs2395943	6	42940673	42946981	−	PEX6	1.05E-13	A	G	−0.66	0.43	0	inside	ILMN_1683279
30	rs11800014	1	22414070	22351707	+	HSPC157/LINC00339	2.04E-13	A	G	0.97	0.16	56355	downstream	ILMN_3272768

The MAF and beta (effect size per copy of the minor allele) for the most significant SNP of each cluster is listed. LD = linkage disequilibrium, TSS = transcription start site, Chr. = chromosome.

to eQTL studies in other non-diseased tissues of similar sample size [22,23,24,28,29].

Of these 771 eQTLs, 770 were *cis*-eQTLs for 428 unique transcripts ($p < 2.82 \times 10^{-5}$; FDR ≤ 0.05), where the associated SNPs lie within 1 Mb of the transcriptional start site (TSS) of the cognate transcript. For the four most significant *cis*-eQTLs, box-and-whisker plots and mean-standard-error plots for the individual genotypes are given in **Figure 1**. An overview of the most significant *cis*-eQTLs is given in **Table 1** and the complete results are given in supplemental **Table S1**.

Of the independent significant eQTLs, one was found to be in *trans* ($p < 2.12 \times 10^{-11}$; FDR ≤ 0.05), with the expression of *LOC644936* located on chromosome 5 being seemingly modulated by an eQTL (rs852423) on chromosome 7. However, as *LOC644936* is a known pseudogene of *ACTB* and rs852423 is located within *ACTB*, we cannot rule out the possibility that rs852423 is in fact a *cis* eQTL for *ACTB* rather than a *trans* eQTL for LOC644936. Using BLAST to align the microarray probe sequence of *LOC644936* to the human transcriptome uncovered a partial match with *ACTB* in addition to a 100% match with *LOC644936*.

Integration of eQTL data with cardiac GWAS loci

In order to provide candidate genes for the reported heart-related GWAS loci, we listed the 102 SNPs previously associated with a cardiac trait at genome-wide statistical significance ($p_{gwas} \leq 5 \times 10^{-8}$), representing 74 independent loci (LD-pruned with $r^2 > 0.6$, see Materials & Methods). These corresponded to loci associated with ventricular fibrillation/sudden cardiac death, atrial fibrillation, heart rate, PR interval, QRS duration and QTc interval. Of these, the 64 SNPs that displayed a MAF of 15% or higher in the eQTL sample were overlaid with the eQTL data to identify transcripts under genetic regulation by these loci. All GWAS SNPs were tested for association with transcript levels of all 18,402 transcripts in this study. We identified a *cis* association between rs9912468, a modulator of QRS duration [12] with the level of expression of the *PRKCA* transcript at genome-wide statistical significance ($p = 2.90 \times 10^{-9}$, see **Figure 2A**). Besides *PRKCA*, no other GWAS SNP displayed an eQTL association p-value that passed the stringent Bonferroni-corrected p-value threshold ($p < 0.05/64$ SNPs $\times 18,402$ transcripts $\sim 4 \times 10^{-8}$). A total of 34 SNPs were associated with the transcript level of a gene at a $p \leq 0.05$ (**Table 2**). Among these, rs8049607, a modulator of QTc-interval [16] was found to be associated in *cis* with the transcript level of *LITAF* ($p < 5 \times 10^{-4}$, **Figure 2C**), and rs7612445 and rs6882776, both associated with heart rate [10] were associated in *cis* with the transcript levels of *GNB4* ($p < 2 \times 10^{-4}$, **Figure 2B**) and *NKX2-5* ($p < 6 \times 10^{-3}$, **Figure 2D**), respectively. The number of nominal associations for the 64 cardiac trait-associated SNPs tested represents a more than 7-fold enrichment ($p < 0.05$, see Materials & Methods) compared to a random selection of 64 variants from the entire set of SNPs used in eQTL analysis.

Discussion

We conducted a genome-wide eQTL analysis in 129 samples of normal human myocardium, identifying genetic variation regulating gene expression in human heart and uncovering 771 genome-wide significant independent eQTLs. This resource, heretofore unavailable in human heart will contribute to advancing our understanding of the genetic mechanisms underlying loci associated with cardiac traits. All but one of the eQTLs identified were *cis* eQTLs. Other eQTL studies have identified only few *trans* eQTLs [22,24,28,29], illustrating the general

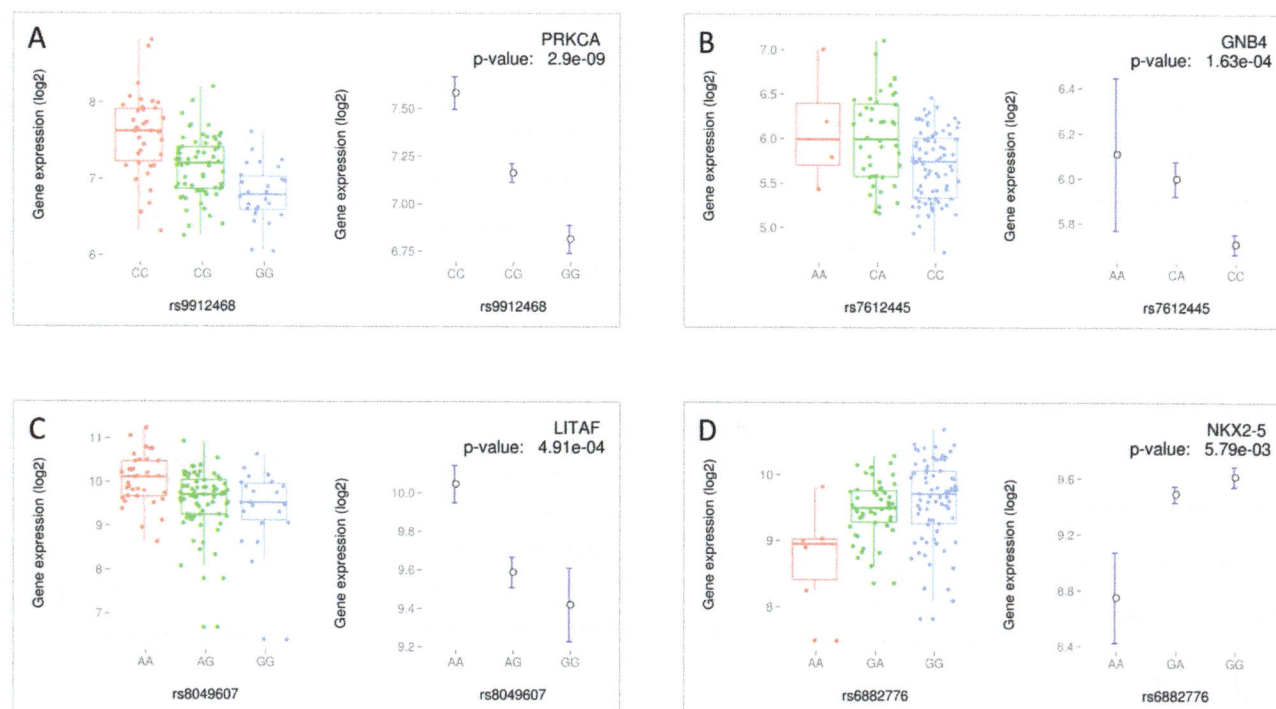

Figure 2. eQTL overview plots for 4 cardiac trait GWAS candidate genes. An overview of 4 GWAS *cis* eQTLs: rs9912468 with *PRKCA* (panel A), rs7912445 with *GNB4* (panel B), rs8049607 with *LITAF* (panel C) and rs6882776 with *NKX2-5* (panel D). On the left of each panel, box-and-whisker plots of mRNA levels for all genotypes. On the right, mean and standard-error plots of mRNA levels for all genotypes are illustrated. Right upper corner gives the association p-value and the gene name.

difficulty of detecting *trans*-regulatory variants in eQTL studies [31,32]. Based on larger eQTL studies in other tissues [22,24,25,26,29] as many as 4000 independent cardiac *cis* eQTLs are expected to be present, hence the results presented here are a subset of this theoretical complete set of cardiac eQTLs.

In recent years, many novel loci associated with a number of cardiac traits, including cardiac arrhythmia and ECG indices, have been discovered. However, the identification of (novel) genes at these loci has lagged behind. The availability of a cardiac eQTL resource is likely to aid in the dissection of these loci by providing a means of prioritizing candidate genes for follow-up functional studies. Indeed, our current findings already provide candidate genes for a number of these loci (**Table 2**). One such example is the *PRKCA* gene for the effect observed on QRS duration for the rs9912468-tagged haplotype on chromosome 9. *PRKCA* encodes protein kinase C alpha, a fundamental regulator of cardiac contractility and Ca^{2+} handling in cardiomyocytes [33]. The mechanism by which it regulates QRS duration is unknown. Other candidates include the *LITAF* gene (encoding lipopolysaccharide-induced TNF factor) for the rs8049607-tagged haplotype associated with QTc-interval and the *GNB4* gene (encoding guanine nucleotide binding protein) for the rs7912445-tagged haplotype associated with heart rate. None of these eQTLs (for *PRKCA*, *LITAF* and *GNB4*) have been previously identified in non-cardiac tissues.

The utility of this approach is further evidenced by the fact that the 64 GWAS SNPs were enriched in nominally significant eSNPs as compared to a random selection of 64 variants from the entire set of SNPs used in eQTL analysis. Such an enrichment was reported before for GWAS loci in general based on eQTLs identified in lymphoblastoid cell lines from HAPMAP samples [18].

The eQTLs we identified represent an enriched set of highly relevant candidates to test in future studies for association with cardiac traits and disease. Among the highly significant eQTLs listed in **Table 1**, at least two SNPs could also be interesting from a pharmacogenetic point of view. One is rs1222809 which was found to be strongly associated with the expression level of the *DHFR* gene encoding dihydrofolate reductase, a putative target of the drug methotrexate. Of note previous studies have provided evidence that rs1650697, which is in complete LD with rs1222809, may be associated with adverse events to methotrexate in patients with rheumatoid arthritis [34,35]. The other potentially interesting eQTL from a pharmacogenetic point of view is rs4822466 which was found to be highly associated with the expression of *GSTT1*, a gene encoding the liver detoxifying enzyme Glutathione S-transferase T1.

The eQTLs we identified are expected to be enriched in the regulatory regions of the genome such as promoter regions, enhancers and transcription factor binding sites [36]. Recent work has begun to uncover these relationships for adult human heart [37]. However, formal testing for enrichment of eQTLs in the known regulatory regions [37] did not provide statistically significant enrichment (data not shown). At least in part, this may be due to the limited number of eQTLs we have identified.

A limitation of the presented study concerns the fact that not all transcripts have been tested for eQTL effects. Transcripts that were expressed below the (array-based) detection level or for which probe design was not optimal could not be tested. Conversely, not all haplotypes in the genome were tested as for instance we only tested SNPs with a MAF higher than 0.15. Furthermore, our sample size and therefore statistical power was limited, preventing the identification of eQTLs of smaller effect and *trans* eQTLs. The interpretation of the data concerning SNPs from GWAS presented

Table 2. Look-up of SNPs from cardiac GWAS in eQTL data.

LD cluster	SNP	Chr.	SNP Position	eQTL gene TSS position	eQTL Gene Symbol	eQTL p-value	eQTL beta	eQTL MAF	GWAS trait	Reported GWAS candidate gene	Candidate gene was measured	References
1	rs9912468	17	64318357	64298926	PRKCA	2.90E-09	−0.37	0.45	QRS duration	PRKCA	Y	[12]
1	rs9912468	17	64318357	65241319	HELZ	1.08E-02	−0.16	0.45	QRS duration	PRKCA	Y	idem
2	rs7612445	3	179172979	179169371	GNB4	1.63E-04	0.28	0.20	Heart rate	GNB4	Y	[10]
2	rs7612445	3	179172979	179280708	ACTL6A	2.69E-02	0.11	0.20	Heart rate	GNB4	Y	idem
2	rs7612445	3	179172979	178866311	PIK3CA	3.77E-02	−0.11	0.20	Heart rate	GNB4	Y	idem
3	rs8049607	16	11691753	11681322	LITAF	4.91E-04	−0.32	0.45	QTc duration	LITAF,CLEC16A, SNN, ZC3H7A, TNFRSF17	Y, N, Y, N	[15,16]
4	rs10824026	10	75421208	75255782	PPP3CB	3.00E-02	−0.10	0.17	Atrial fibrillation	SYNPO2L	Y	[56]
4	rs10824026	10	75421208	74870210	NUDT13	3.94E-02	−0.13	0.17	Atrial fibrillation	SYNPO2L	Y	idem
5	rs2968864	7	150622162	151574316	PRKAG2	1.0E-03	0.13	0.22	QTc duration	KCNH2	N	[15,16]
5	rs2968864	7	150622162	150020758	ACTR3C	1.49E-03	−0.11	0.23	QTc duration	KCNH2	N	[15,16]
5	rs2968864	7	150622162	150026938	C7orf29	3.69E-02	0.09	0.23	QTc duration	KCNH2	N	idem
6	rs223116	14	23977010	24912007	SDR39U1	3.57E-03	0.16	0.26	Heart rate	MYH7, NDNG	N, N	[57]
6	rs223116	14	23977010	24424298	C14orf167	4.06E-03	0.19	0.26	Heart rate	MYH7, NDNG	N, N	idem
6	rs223116	14	23977010	23938898	NGDN	1.45E-02	−0.10	0.26	Heart rate	MYH7, NDNG	N, N	idem
6	rs223116	14	23977010	24912007	C14orf124	1.69E-02	0.23	0.26	Heart rate	MYH7, NDNG	N, N	idem
6	rs223116	14	23977010	24605378	PSME1	3.23E-02	0.09	0.26	Heart rate	MYH7, NDNG	N, N	idem
6	rs223116	14	23977010	24701648	GMPR2	3.37E-02	0.09	0.26	Heart rate	MYH7, NDNG	N, N	idem
7	rs7784776	7	46620145	45927959	IGFBP1	5.71E-03	0.08	0.43	QRS duration	IGFBP3	Y	[12]
8	rs6882776	5	172664163	172662315	NKX2-5	5.79E-03	−0.24	0.24	Heart rate	NKX2-5	Y	[10]
8	rs6882776	5	172664163	172261223	ERGIC1	2.23E-02	−0.14	0.24	Heart rate	NKX2-5	Y	idem
9	rs12143842	1	162033890	161169105	NDUFS2	6.44E-03	0.15	0.28	QTc duration	OLFML2B, NOS1AP	N, Y	[15,16,58]
9	rs12143842	1	162033890	161147758	B4GALT3	2.17E-02	−0.10	0.28	QTc duration	OLFML2B, NOS1AP	N, Y	idem
10	rs6800541	3	38774832	39149130	GORASP1	7.17E-03	0.12	0.41	PR duration	SCN10A	N	[11]
10	rs6801957	3	38767315	39149130	GORASP1	8.17E-03	0.12	0.41	PR duration	-	-	[59]
10	rs6801957	3	38767315	39149130	GORASP1	8.17E-03	0.12	0.41	QRS duration	SCN10A	N	[12]
10	rs6795970	3	38766675	39149130	GORASP1	9.64E-03	0.12	0.40	PR duration	SCN10A	N	[13,14]
10	rs6795970	3	38766675	39149130	GORASP1	9.64E-03	0.12	0.40	QRS duration	SCN10A	N	[14]
10	rs6599250	3	38784029	39149130	GORASP1	1.23E-02	0.12	0.41	PR duration	-	-	[59]
10	rs6599254	3	38795555	39149130	GORASP1	1.23E-02	0.12	0.41	PR duration	-	-	idem
11	rs13030174	2	232271284	231989824	HTR2B	7.78E-03	−0.15	0.22	Heart rate	B3GNT7	Y	[10]
12	rs13165478	5	153869040	153825517	SAP30L	8.72E-03	0.13	0.36	QRS duration	HAND1-SAP30L	N	[12]
12	rs13165478	5	153869040	154317776	GEMIN5	1.47E-02	0.12	0.36	QRS duration	HAND1-SAP30L	N	idem
13	rs2242285	3	66431602	66119285	SLC25A26	8.94E-03	0.19	0.47	QRS duration	LRIG1-SLC25A26	N	idem
14	rs7562790	2	36673555	36582713	LOC100288911	1.04E-02	−0.20	0.40	QRS duration	CRIM1	N	idem

Table 2. Cont.

LD cluster	SNP	Chr.	SNP Position	eQTL gene TSS position	eQTL Gene Symbol	eQTL p-value	eQTL beta	eQTL MAF	GWAS trait	Reported GWAS candidate gene	Candidate gene was measured	References
15	rs2074518	17	33324382	33307517	LIG3	1.1E-03	0.15	0.48	QTc duration	LIG3,RFFL	Y,N	[15]
15	rs2074518	17	33324382	34136459	TAF15	3.6E-02	0.14	0.48	QTc duration	LIG3,RFFL	Y,N	idem
15	rs2074518	17	33324382	33885110	SLFN14	4.2E-02	−0.04	0.48	QTc duration	LIG3,RFFL	Y, N	idem
16	rs13376333	1	154814353	153963239	RPS27	2.66E-02	−0.20	0.31	Atrial fibrillation	KCNN3	Y	[8]
16	rs13376333	1	154814353	153958806	RAB13	4.22E-02	0.09	0.31	Atrial fibrillation	KCNN3	Y	idem
17	rs7433723	3	38784957	39149130	GORASP1	1.18E-02	0.12	0.42	PR duration	-	-	[59]
18	rs3922844	3	38624253	38537763	EXOG	1.34E-02	0.15	0.32	PR duration	SCN5A	Y	idem
19	rs365990	14	23861811	23398661	PRMT5	1.49E-02	−0.09	0.40	Heart rate	MYH6	Y	[10,14]
19	rs452036	14	23865885	23398661	PRMT5	1.49E-02	−0.09	0.40	Heart rate	MYH6	Y	[57]
19	rs365990	14	23861811	24711880	TINF2	1.81E-02	−0.13	0.40	Heart rate	MYH6	Y	[10,14]
19	rs365990	14	23861811	23340960	LRP10	2.22E-02	−0.07	0.40	Heart rate	MYH6	Y	idem
19	rs452036	14	23865885	23340960	LRP10	2.22E-02	−0.07	0.40	Heart rate	MYH6	Y	[57]
19	rs355990	14	23861811	23526747	CDH24	2.70E-02	−0.09	0.40	Heart rate	MYH6	Y	[10,14]
19	rs452036	14	23865885	23526747	CDH24	2.70E-02	−0.09	0.40	Heart rate	MYH6	Y	[57]
20	rs2924292	21	18787176	18985268	BTG3	1.96E-02	−0.19	0.48	Sudden cardiac death	CXADR, BTG3	N, Y	[9]
21	rs13245899	7	100497131	100797686	AP1S1	2.01E-02	−0.15	0.18	Heart rate	ACHE	Y	[10]
21	rs314370	7	100453208	99933688	PILRB	2.40E-02	−0.08	0.17	Heart rate	SLC12A9	Y	[57]
21	rs13245899	7	100497131	99933688	PILRB	2.47E-02	−0.08	0.18	Heart rate	ACHE	Y	[10]
21	rs13245899	7	100497131	99717481	TAF6	4.12E-02	−0.13	0.18	Heart rate	ACHE	Y	idem
21	rs314370	7	100453208	100797686	AP1S1	4.74E-02	−0.13	0.17	Heart rate	SLC12A9	Y	[57]
22	rs1321311	6	36622900	36164550	BRPF3	2.02E-02	0.10	0.28	QRS duration	CDKN1A	N	[14]
23	rs835389	12	131621762	131323819	STX2	1.1E-02	0.09	0.35	Heart rate	GPR133	N	[10]
24	rs4657178	1	162110610	161520413	FCGR3A	2.44E-02	−0.10	0.23	QTc duration	NOS1AP	Y	[60]
25	rs1152591	14	64680848	65569227	MAX	2.50E-02	0.14	0.49	Atrial fibrillation	SYNE2	N	[56]
26	rs7980799	12	33576990	34175216	ALG10	2.63E-02	−0.06	0.43	Heart rate	SYT10	Y	[10]
27	rs4725982	7	150637863	150020296	LRRC61	2.78E-02	−0.07	0.24	QTc duration	KCNH2	N	[15,16]
27	rs4725982	7	150637863	151038847	NUB1	4.88E-02	0.06	0.24	QTc duration	KCNH2	N	idem
28	rs727957	21	35880072	34915198	GART	3.39E-02	0.13	0.17	QTc duration	KCNE1	Y	[14]
29	rs12498374	4	111584419	110481355	CCDC109B	4.54E-02	−0.21	0.23	Atrial fibrillation	-	-	[61]
30	rs7312625	12	114799974	114846000	LOC255480	4.88E-02	−0.05	0.26	PR duration	TBX5	Y	[59]
31	rs826838	12	39106731	39299420	CPNE8	1.3E-02	0.14	0.42	Heart rate	CPNE8	Y	[10]
31	rs826838	12	39106731	39837192	KIF21A	3.8E-02	−0.09	0.422481	Heart rate	CPNE8	Y	idem
32	rs6127471	20	36844038	37434348	PPP1R16B	3.3E-02	0.16	0.46	Heart rate	KIAA1755	N	idem
33	rs2067615	12	107149422	107168399	RIC8B	4.8E-02	0.09	0.47	Heart rate	RFX4	Y	idem

Table 2. Cont.

LD cluster	SNP	Chr.	SNP Position	eQTL gene TSS position	eQTL Gene Symbol	Reported GWAS candidate gene	GWAS trait	eQTL MAF	eQTL beta	eQTL p-value	Candidate gene was measured	References
34	rs4074536	1	116310967	115632121	TSPAN2	CASQ2	QRS duration	0.28	−0.08	1.05E-02	Y	[12]

Overview of eQTL effects of reported cardiac electric trait related GWAS SNPs. Only GWAS SNPs reaching genome-wide significance as stated in the original studies (p-value ≤5×10^{-8}) and with nominal eQTL association (p≤0.05) are reported. This resulted in 34 independent loci. *PRKCA* (rs9912468, QRS duration) reaches genome-wide significance (4×10^{-8}, represented in bold in table). The beta is defined as the effect size per copy of the minor allele. LD = linkage disequilibrium, TSS = transcription start site, Chr. = chromosome, Y = yes, N = no.

in **Table 2** must take these considerations into account. Additionally, the single *trans* eQTL we identified is likely a false discovery and will require further investigation.

Our study was conducted in left ventricular myocardium. However, it is well known that different cardiac compartments such as the atria or the specialized conduction system display different gene expression patterns [38,39,40,41] and eQTL effects might thus differ across cardiac compartments. Furthermore, we have no information relating to cardiac traits such as ECG indices in the 129 individuals from whom the left ventricular samples were obtained; we were therefore unable to correlate gene expression with cardiac traits in these individuals [23,42].

In summary, we here provide the first eQTL map of human left ventricular myocardium that will enable systems genetics approaches in the study of cardiac traits.

Materials and Methods

Ethics statement

Investigations using the human ventricular samples conformed to the principles outlined in the Helsinki Declaration of the World Medical Association. The ethical review boards of University of Szeged (Ethical Review Board of the University of Szeged Medical Center; Szeged, Hungary), Vanderbilt University (Institutional Review Board of Vanderbilt University School of Medicine; Nashville, USA), University of Miami (Institutional Review Board of the University of Miami School of Medicine; Miami, USA), and the University of Sydney (Human Research Ethics Committee (HREC); Sydney, Australia) approved procurement and handling of the human cardiac material. Written informed consent from the donor or the next of kin was obtained for use of this sample in research. All data was analyzed anonymously.

Sample collection

Left ventricular samples were obtained from 180 non-diseased human hearts of unrelated organ donors whose hearts were explanted to obtain pulmonary and aortic valves for transplant or valve replacement surgery or explanted for transplantation but not used due to logistical reasons. The tissues were ascertained at the University of Szeged (Hungary; n = 79), Vanderbilt University (Nashville, USA; n = 46), University of Miami (USA; n = 30), and the University of Sydney (Australia; n = 25) and assumed to consist mainly of subjects of Western European descent based on self-reported ethnicity. The Vanderbilt samples were procured with the assistance of the National Disease Research Interchange (Philadelphia, PA).

Generation and processing of gene expression data

Total RNA was extracted from the human left ventricular heart samples using the *mir*Vana miRNA isolation kit (Ambion) at the AMC, Amsterdam, The Netherlands. Sample processing order was randomized. RNA quality was assessed by Agilent Bioanalyzer (minimum RIN = 7) and spectrophotometry (minimum 260 nm:280 nm = 1.8). The Illumina TotalPrep-96 RNA Amplification Kit was used to generate cRNA starting from 200 ng total RNA. Genome-wide gene expression data was generated using Illumina HumanHT-12 v4 BeadArrays, containing 47,231 probes representing 28,688 RefSeq annotated transcripts (ServiceXS, Leiden, The Netherlands), following the instructions of the manufacturer.

Raw expression data were imported into the Illumina Bead-Studio and summarized at probe-level for each sample without normalization or background correction. The summarized data were subsequently imported into R (version 2.15.3) [43] using the beadarray package [44]. Quality control was performed using the ArrayQualityMetrics package in R [45]. Samples displaying transcriptional stratification using hierarchical clustering were omitted from the analysis. The summarized data of the 162 remaining samples was background corrected and quantile normalized using the *neqc* algorithm [46] across all samples. The *neqc* algorithm is the current standard data-preprocessing method for Illumina gene expression BeadArrays [47], and has been applied in eQTL studies with comparable sample size [29,30].

Probes containing common SNPs (HAPMAP Phase III release 2) [27,29] and probes whose sequence did not align or aligned ambiguously to the human reference genome (HG19), according to up-to-date Illumina HumanHT-12 v4.0 BeadArray annotation available from the Bioconductor project, were left out of the analysis. Additionally, probes with median expression levels below a study specific threshold (the median expression levels of Y chromosome transcripts in the female subjects of the sample population) were not considered for subsequent analyses.

Genotyping and genotype imputation

DNA was extracted for genotyping from 162 heart samples that passed the gene expression analysis quality control criteria (see above) at the AMC, Amsterdam, The Netherlands. Genome-wide SNP genotyping was carried out using Illumina HumanOmniExpress Beadchips interrogating 733,202 genetic markers (Genome Analysis Center, Helmholtz Zentrum München, Germany). A total of 8 samples had sample quality issues (and were not hybridized) or failed hybridization, leaving genotype data for 154 samples. Quality control was performed in the *GenABEL* [48] package in R using default settings. Samples with low call rate ($<$ 95%), extreme heterozygosity (FDR 1%) or high proportion of alleles identical-by-state ($>$95%) were removed. Additionally, any remaining samples showing genetic stratification through Manhattan distance hierarchical clustering (using the *popgen* [49] package in R), and confirmed with principal component analysis [48], were not considered (**Figure S1**).

Power calculations were performed (with a fixed FDR of 0.05) to assess the influence of MAF on power in relation to observed gene expression fold changes. Based on these results, a MAF threshold of 0.15 was chosen to ensure sufficient power to detect *cis* eQTLs within a broad range of effect sizes (**Figure S2**). Additionally, assuming Hardy-Weinberg equilibrium, a MAF of 0.15 or higher yields an expected number of three individuals homozygous for the minor allele, which we considered the minimum for fitting a meaningful additive genetic model.

Imputation was performed using the MACH software [50] and the HAPMAP Phase III data. Only SNPs imputed with sufficient confidence were considered, using the estimate of the squared correlation between imputed and true genotypes. By setting the cut-off at 0.30, most of the poorly imputed SNPs are filtered out, compared to only a small number ($<$1%) of well imputed SNPs [51].

eQTL statistical analysis

After pre-processing and stringent quality control of gene expression and genotypic data as described above, a total of 129 heart samples were used in eQTL analysis. Each transcript was tested for association with SNP genotypes genome-wide using linear modeling (assuming an additive genetic model), taking age, gender and tissue collection center as covariates, using the *GenABEL* package [48] in R. Correction for multiple testing was performed on the complete set of *cis* eQTL p-values in the *qvalue* package in R [52]. A q-value (FDR) $\leq$0.05 was considered significant for *cis* eQTLs, corresponding to a p-value of

2.82×10^{-5}. *Cis* relations were defined as those within 1 Mb of a transcription start site (TSS), in accordance with previous reports demonstrating that over 90% of *cis* SNPs are situated within 100 Kb of a TSS [26,27,29,47,53]. SNPs with an LD R^2 of larger than 0.6 were considered dependent and LD-pruned into clusters (LD clusters), in accordance with previous studies [23,29,30]. For *trans* eQTLs, only results with a p-value $<5\times10^{-8}$ were considered (corresponding to a target α (or p value) of 0.05 with a Bonferroni correction for 1 million independent tests [54,55]). Correction for multiple testing was done by using a step-up Benjamini & Hochberg procedure on all p-values $<5\times10^{-8}$, and a q-value (FDR) $\leq$0.05 was considered genome-wide significant for *trans* eQTLs, corresponding to a p-value of 2.12×10^{-11}.

eQTL biological interpretation and candidate gene prioritization

To prioritize candidate genes for further studies, additional data sources were integrated. Additional trait and disease associated SNPs were extracted from PubMed (www.ncbi.nlm.nih.gov/ pubmed; search terms: 'GWAS' AND 'cardiac', 'atrial fibrillation', 'sudden cardiac death', 'ECG [electrocardiographic]', 'PR interval', 'QRS', 'QT', 'repolarization'), the NHGRI catalog of published GWAS (http://www.genome.gov/gwastudies/), and GWAS central (https://www.gwascentral.org) on January 8, 2013. Analyses were restricted to samples of European ancestry. Results were classified into six categories: sudden cardiac death, atrial fibrillation, heart rate, PR duration, QRS duration and QTc duration. Next, each GWAS SNP passing genome-wide significance in the respective study (5×10^{-8}, a target α of 0.05 with a Bonferroni correction for 1 million independent tests) was tested for association with expression of all 18,402 measured transcripts. To determine the number of independent loci, LD-pruning was performed by merging all GWAS SNPs with LD $r^2>0.6$ (HAPMAP R22 and HAPMAP Phase III). The p-value threshold for significant eQTL effects was set at 4×10^{-8}, a target α of 0.05 with a Bonferroni correction for 1,177,728 tests (64 independent loci $\times$18,402 transcripts).

To quantify the enrichment of eQTLs among the cardiac trait GWAS SNPs, we generated 100,000 randomized independent SNP sets of the same size as the number of independent GWAS loci, and with corresponding MAF distribution and proximity to genes. The number of nominally significant eQTL associations for the original independent GWAS loci is referred to as Q. Next, for each random set S_i, we determined the number of eQTLs at nominal significance (p$\leq$0.05), referred to as Q_i. The simulations yielded a fold-enrichment score, calculated as the average over all random sets of the ratio between Q and Q_i, and an empirical p-value, calculated as the proportion of simulations in which the number of eQTLs exceeds the number of nominally significant eQTL associations in the original independent GWAS loci.

Public access to microarray data

The microarray genotyping and gene expression data of the study have been deposited online at the Gene Expression Omnibus (GEO), with accession number GSE55232.

Supporting Information

Figure S1 Manhattan distance hierarchical clustering dendogram of 154 genotyped subjects. Manhattan distance hierarchical clustering revealed several genotypic outliers. The clustering was repeated using principal component analysis, identifying the same groups of outliers.

Figure S2   Results of eQTL power analyses in relation to MAF and gene expression fold change. eQTL power analyses were performed for different minimum minor allele frequencies (0.05, 0.10, 0.15, 0.20, 0.30 and 0.40). The gene expression fold change is defined as $\log_2$ difference in gene expression observed per copy of the minor allele. In each analysis, for each $\log_2$ fold change X, all eQTLs with an absolute $\log_2$ fold change larger than X were considered, and the power was calculated as the percentage of those eQTLs for which the null hypothesis is rejected at FDR ≤ 0.05.

Table S1   Table of all significant eQTLs. This table contains the complete results for all significant non-diseased human heart eQTLs (FDR ≤ 0.05). It contains for each SNP-transcript pair the SNP ID, gene or transcript IDs (HGNC, Entrez Gene, RefSeq), genomic locations, minor and major allele, minor

allele frequency, beta (effect size per copy of the minor allele), p-value and distance between SNP and gene. The table is sorted on HGNC official gene symbol.

Acknowledgments

The authors are grateful to Michael Tanck for helpful discussion and advice on the statistical analysis of the genotyping data, and to Dr. Jolanda van der Velden for her help in acquisition of cardiac samples.

Author Contributions

Conceived and designed the experiments: TTK MEA CRB. Performed the experiments: TTK MLW. Analyzed the data: MEA PDM. Contributed reagents/materials/analysis tools: SL TZ CQS IB CdR NHB ALG AV RFM. Wrote the paper: TTK MEA CRB EML.

References

1. Jouven X, Desnos M, Guerot C, Ducimetiere P (1999) Predicting sudden death in the population: the Paris Prospective Study I. Circulation 99: 1978–1983.
2. Friedlander Y, Siscovick DS, Weinmann S, Austin MA, Psaty BM, et al. (1998) Family history as a risk factor for primary cardiac arrest. Circulation 97: 155–160.
3. Kolder IC, Tanck MW, Bezzina CR (2012) Common genetic variation modulating cardiac ECG parameters and susceptibility to sudden cardiac death. Journal of molecular and cellular cardiology 52: 620–629.
4. Dekker LRC, Bezzina CR, Henriques JPS, Tanck MW, Koch KT, et al. (2006) Familial sudden death is an important risk factor for primary ventricular fibrillation: a case-control study in acute myocardial infarction patients. Circulation 114: 1140–1145.
5. Lubitz SA, Yin X, Fontes JoD, Magnani JW, Rienstra M, et al. (2010) Association between familial atrial fibrillation and risk of new-onset atrial fibrillation. JAMA : the journal of the American Medical Association 304: 2263–2269.
6. Myers RH, Kiely DK, Cupples LA, Kannel WB (1990) Parental history is an independent risk factor for coronary artery disease: the Framingham Study. American heart journal 120: 963–969.
7. Hawe E, Talmud PJ, Miller GJ, Humphries SE (2003) Family history is a coronary heart disease risk factor in the Second Northwick Park Heart Study. Annals of human genetics 67: 97–106.
8. Ellinor PT, Lunetta KL, Glazer NL, Pfeufer A, Alonso A, et al. (2010) Common variants in KCNN3 are associated with lone atrial fibrillation. Nat Genet 42: 240–244.
9. Bezzina CR, Pazoki R, Bardai A, Marsman RF, de Jong JS, et al. (2010) Genome-wide association study identifies a susceptibility locus at 21q21 for ventricular fibrillation in acute myocardial infarction. Nat Genet 42: 688–691.
10. den Hoed M, Eijgelsheim M, Esko T, Brundel BJ, Peal DS, et al. (2013) Identification of heart rate-associated loci and their effects on cardiac conduction and rhythm disorders. Nat Genet 45: 621–631.
11. Pfeufer A, van Noord C, Marciante KD, Arking DE, Larson MG, et al. (2010) Genome-wide association study of PR interval. Nat Genet 42: 153–159.
12. Sotoodehnia N, Isaacs A, de Bakker PI, Dorr M, Newton-Cheh C, et al. (2010) Common variants in 22 loci are associated with QRS duration and cardiac ventricular conduction. Nat Genet 42: 1068–1076.
13. Chambers JC, Zhao J, Terracciano CM, Bezzina CR, Zhang W, et al. (2010) Genetic variation in SCN10A influences cardiac conduction. Nat Genet 42: 149–152.
14. Holm H, Gudbjartsson DF, Arnar DO, Thorleifsson G, Thorgeirsson G, et al. (2010) Several common variants modulate heart rate, PR interval and QRS duration. Nat Genet 42: 117–122.
15. Newton-Cheh C, Eijgelsheim M, Rice KM, de Bakker PI, Yin X, et al. (2009) Common variants at ten loci influence QT interval duration in the QTGEN Study. Nat Genet 41: 399–406.
16. Pfeufer A, Sanna S, Arking DE, Muller M, Gateva V, et al. (2009) Common variants at ten loci modulate the QT interval duration in the QTSCD Study. Nat Genet 41: 407–414.
17. Cookson W, Liang L, Abecasis G, Moffatt M, Lathrop M (2009) Mapping complex disease traits with global gene expression. Nature reviews Genetics 10: 184–194.
18. Nicolae DL, Gamazon E, Zhang W, Duan S, Dolan ME, et al. (2010) Trait-associated SNPs are more likely to be eQTLs: annotation to enhance discovery from GWAS. PLoS genetics 6: e1000888.
19. Musunuru K, Strong A, Frank-Kamenetsky M, Lee NE, Ahfeldt T, et al. (2010) From noncoding variant to phenotype via SORT1 at the 1p13 cholesterol locus. Nature 466: 714–719.
20. Visel A, Zhu Y, May D, Afzal V, Gong E, et al. (2010) Targeted deletion of the 9p21 non-coding coronary artery disease risk interval in mice. Nature 464: 409–412.
21. Pittman AM, Naranjo S, Jalava SE, Twiss P, Ma Y, et al. (2010) Allelic variation at the 8q23.3 colorectal cancer risk locus functions as a cis-acting regulator of EIF3H. PLoS genetics 6: e1001126.
22. Zou F, Chai HS, Younkin CS, Allen M, Crook J, et al. (2012) Brain expression genome-wide association study (eGWAS) identifies human disease-associated variants. PLoS genetics 8: e1002707.
23. Hernandez DG, Nalls MA, Moore M, Chong S, Dillman A, et al. (2012) Integration of GWAS SNPs and tissue specific expression profiling reveal discrete eQTLs for human traits in blood and brain. Neurobiol Dis 47: 20–28.
24. Fu J, Wolfs MGM, Deelen P, Westra H-J, Fehrmann RSN, et al. (2012) Unraveling the regulatory mechanisms underlying tissue-dependent genetic variation of gene expression. PLoS genetics 8: e1002431.
25. Schadt EE, Molony C, Chudin E, Hao K, Yang X, et al. (2008) Mapping the genetic architecture of gene expression in human liver. PLoS Biol 6: e107.
26. Mehta D, Heim K, Herder C, Carstensen M, Eckstein G, et al. (2013) Impact of common regulatory single-nucleotide variants on gene expression profiles in whole blood. European journal of human genetics : EJHG 21: 48–54.
27. Dubois PCA, Trynka G, Franke L, Hunt KA, Romanos J, et al. (2010) Multiple common variants in the HLA region influence celiac disease susceptibility and influencing immune gene expression. Nature genetics 42: 295–302.
28. Rotival M, Zeller T, Wild PS, Maouche S, Szymczak S, et al. (2011) Integrating genome-wide genetic variations and monocyte expression data reveals trans-regulated gene modules in humans. PLoS genetics 7: e1002367.
29. Grundberg E, Small KS, Hedman ÅsK, Nica AC, Buil A, et al. (2012) Mapping cis- and trans-regulatory effects across multiple tissues in twins. Nature genetics 44: 1084–1089.
30. Nica AC, Parts L, Glass D, Nisbet J, Barrett A, et al. (2011) The architecture of gene regulatory variation across multiple human tissues: the MuTHER study. PLoS genetics 7: e1002003.
31. Petretto E, Mangion J, Dickens NJ, Cook SA, Kumaran MK, et al. (2006) Heritability and tissue specificity of expression quantitative trait loci. PLoS genetics 2: e172.
32. Grundberg E, Kwan T, Ge B, Lam KC, Koka V, et al. (2009) Population genomics in a disease targeted primary cell model. Genome research 19: 1942–1952.
33. Kooij V, Boontje N, Zaremba R, Jaquet K, dos Remedios C, et al. (2010) Protein kinase C alpha and epsilon phosphorylation of troponin and myosin binding protein C reduce Ca2+ sensitivity in human myocardium. Basic research in cardiology 105: 289–300.
34. Owen SA, Hider SL, Martin P, Bruce IN, Barton A, et al. (2013) Genetic polymorphisms in key methotrexate pathway genes are associated with response to treatment in rheumatoid arthritis patients. Pharmacogenomics J 13: 227–234.
35. Wessels JA, de Vries-Bouwstra JK, Heijmans BT, Slagboom PE, Goekoop-Ruiterman YP, et al. (2006) Efficacy and toxicity of methotrexate in early rheumatoid arthritis are associated with single-nucleotide polymorphisms in genes coding for folate pathway enzymes. Arthritis and rheumatism 54: 1087–1095.
36. Brown CD, Mangravite LM, Engelhardt BE (2013) Integrative modeling of eQTLs and cis-regulatory elements suggests mechanisms underlying cell type specificity of eQTLs. PLoS genetics 9: e1003649.
37. May D, Blow MJ, Kaplan T, McCulley DJ, Jensen BC, et al. (2012) Large-scale discovery of enhancers from human heart tissue. Nat Genet 44: 89–93.
38. Gaborit N, Le Bouter S, Szuts V, Varro A, Escande D, et al. (2007) Regional and tissue specific transcript signatures of ion channel genes in the non-diseased human heart. The Journal of physiology 582: 675–693.

39. Sharma S, Razeghi P, Shakir A, Keneson BJ 2nd, Clubb F, et al. (2003) Regional heterogeneity in gene expression profiles: a transcript analysis in human and rat heart. Cardiology 100: 73–79.

40. Nerbonne JM, Guo W (2002) Heterogeneous expression of voltage-gated potassium channels in the heart: roles in normal excitation and arrhythmias. Journal of cardiovascular electrophysiology 13: 406–409.

41. Tsubakihara M, Williams NK, Keogh A, dos Remedios CG (2004) Comparison of gene expression between left atria and left ventricles from non-diseased humans. Proteomics 4: 261–270.

42. Gaunt TR, Shah S, Nelson CP, Drenos F, Braund PS, et al. (2012) Integration of genetics into a systems model of electrocardiographic traits using HumanCVD BeadChip. Circulation Cardiovascular genetics 5: 630–638.

43. R-Core-Team (2012) R: A Language and Environment for Statistical Computing.

44. Dunning MJ, Smith ML, Ritchie ME, Tavare S (2007) beadarray: R classes and methods for Illumina bead-based data. Bioinformatics (Oxford, England) 23: 2183–2184.

45. Kauffmann A, Gentleman R, Huber W (2009) arrayQualityMetrics—a bioconductor package for quality assessment of microarray data. Bioinformatics (Oxford, England) 25: 415–416.

46. Shi W, Oshlack A, Smyth GK (2010) Optimizing the noise versus bias trade-off for Illumina whole genome expression BeadChips. Nucleic acids research 38: e204.

47. Stranger BE, Nica AC, Forrest MS, Dimas A, Bird CP, et al. (2007) Population genomics of human gene expression. Nature genetics 39: 1217–1224.

48. Aulchenko YS, Ripke S, Isaacs A, van Duijn CM (2007) GenABEL: an R library for genome-wide association analysis. Bioinformatics (Oxford, England) 23: 1294–1296.

49. Tibshirani R, Walther G, Hastie T (2001) Estimating the number of clusters in a dataset via the Gap statistic. J R Statist Soc 63: 411–423.

50. Scott LJ, Mohlke KL, Bonnycastle LL, Willer CJ, Li Y, et al. (2007) A genome-wide association study of type 2 diabetes in Finns detects multiple susceptibility variants. Science (New York, NY) 316: 1341–1345.

51. MACH-Development-Team (2013) MACH website.

52. Storey JD, Tibshirani R (2003) Statistical significance for genomewide studies. Proc Natl Acad Sci U S A 100: 9440–9445.

53. Emilsson V, Thorleifsson G, Zhang B, Leonardson AS, Zink F, et al. (2008) Genetics of gene expression and its effect on disease. Nature 452: 423–428.

54. Dudbridge F, Gusnanto A (2008) Estimation of significance thresholds for genomewide association scans. Genetic epidemiology 32: 227–234.

55. Pe'er I, Yelensky R, Altshuler D, Daly MJ (2008) Estimation of the multiple testing burden for genomewide association studies of nearly all common variants. Genetic epidemiology 32: 381–385.

56. Ellinor PT, Lunetta KL, Albert CM, Glazer NL, Ritchie MD, et al. (2012) Meta-analysis identifies six new susceptibility loci for atrial fibrillation. Nat Genet 44: 670–675.

57. Eijgelsheim M, Newton-Cheh C, Sotoodehnia N, de Bakker PI, Muller M, et al. (2010) Genome-wide association analysis identifies multiple loci related to resting heart rate. Hum Mol Genet 19: 3885–3894.

58. Nolte IM, Wallace C, Newhouse SJ, Waggott D, Fu J, et al. (2009) Common genetic variation near the phospholamban gene is associated with cardiac repolarisation: meta-analysis of three genome-wide association studies. PloS one 4: e6138.

59. Smith JG, Magnani JW, Palmer C, Meng YA, Soliman EZ, et al. (2011) Genome-wide association studies of the PR interval in African Americans. PLoS genetics 7: e1001304.

60. Arking DE, Pfeufer A, Post W, Kao WH, Newton-Cheh C, et al. (2006) A common genetic variant in the NOS1 regulator NOS1AP modulates cardiac repolarization. Nat Genet 38: 644–651.

61. Lubitz SA, Sinner MF, Lunetta KL, Makino S, Pfeufer A, et al. (2010) Independent susceptibility markers for atrial fibrillation on chromosome 4q25. Circulation 122: 976–984.

2

Carvedilol for Prevention of Atrial Fibrillation after Cardiac Surgery: A Meta-Analysis

Hui-Shan Wang*, Zeng-Wei Wang, Zong-Tao Yin

Department of Cardiovascular Surgery, Shenyang Northern Hospital, Shenyang, Liaoning Province, China

Abstract

Background: Postoperative atrial fibrillation (POAF) remains the most common complication after cardiac surgery. Current guidelines recommend β-blockers to prevent POAF. Carvedilol is a non-selective β-adrenergic blocker with anti-inflammatory, antioxidant, and multiple cationic channel blocking properties. These unique properties of carvedilol have generated interest in its use as a prophylaxis for POAF.

Objective: To investigate the efficacy of carvedilol in preventing POAF.

Methods: PubMed from the inception to September 2013 was searched for studies assessing the effect of carvedilol on POAF occurrence. Pooled relative risk (RR) with 95% confidence interval (CI) was calculated using random- or fixed-effect models when appropriate. Six comparative trials (three randomized controlled trials and three nonrandomized controlled trials) including 765 participants met the inclusion criteria.

Results: Carvedilol was associated with a significant reduction in POAF (relative risk [RR] 0.49, 95% confidence interval [CI] 0.37 to 0.64, $p < 0.001$). Subgroup analyses yielded similar results. In a subgroup analysis, carvedilol appeared to be superior to metoprolol for the prevention of POAF (RR 0.51, 95% CI 0.37 to 0.70, $p < 0.001$). No evidence of heterogeneity was observed.

Conclusions: In conclusion, carvedilol may effectively reduce the incidence of POAF in patients undergoing cardiac surgery. It appeared to be superior to metoprolol. A large-scale, well-designed randomized controlled trial is needed to conclusively answer the question regarding the utility of carvedilol in the prevention of POAF.

Editor: Rudolf Kirchmair, Medical University Innsbruck, Austria

Funding: The authors have no support or funding to report.

Competing Interests: The authors have declared that no competing interests exist.

* E-mail: wanghuishanCA@126.com

Introduction

Despite significant advances in anesthetic and surgical techniques, postoperative atrial fibrillation (POAF) remains the most common complication after cardiac surgery [1–3]. The incidence of POAF varies from 11% to 40%, depending on the definition and the method of monitoring [1–3]. Although this arrhythmia is usually benign and self-limiting, it may result in hemodynamic instability, a longer hospital stay, and increased health care costs [1–3]. Given the clinical consequences attributable to POAF, its prevention is of great importance. To date, many pharmacologic approaches have been attempted to prevent POAF, for example, β-blockers, amiodarone, and magnesium [4]. Most reviews reflect a growing consensus in favor of the prophylactic administration of β-blockers for cardiac surgery patients [5]. In addition, updated American College of Cardiology/American Heart Association (ACC/AHA) 2006 guidelines recommend β-blockers for the prevention of POAF [6].

Despite the extensive studies, the exact pathophysiology of POAF is for the moment far from being fully elucidated [1–3]. A growing body of evidence suggests that markers of inflammation and oxidative injury are elevated in atrial fibrillation patients [7–10]. Carvedilol, a non-selective β-adrenergic blocking agent approved for use in heart failure cases, has a number of ancillary activities including anti-inflammatory and antioxidant properties [11,12]. Moreover, unlike other beta-blockers, carvedilol antagonizes the rapid-depolarizing sodium channel, the human ether-a-go-go-related gene potassium channel, and the L-type calcium channel [11,12], which suggests a pharmacologic profile similar to amiodarone, a proven anti-arrhythmic agent for the prevention of POAF [13]. Theoretically, this should reduce the incidence of arrhythmia, including POAF. All these properties of carvedilol have generated interest in its use as a prophylactic agent for POAF. Recently, several relevant studies regarding prophylactic carvedilol in preventing POAF have been published [14–19]. However, the role of carvedilol in preventing POAF remains unknown. We therefore undertook a meta-analysis of published studies to the efficacy of carvedilol in preventing POAF for adult patients undergoing cardiac surgery.

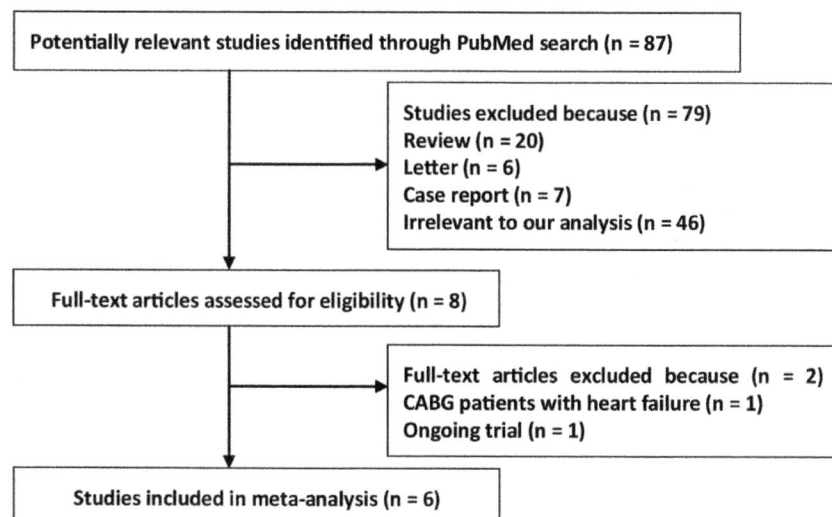

Figure 1. Selection process for clinical trials.

Methods

Literature search and inclusion criteria

Two investigators searched PubMed database for relevant articles published up to September 2013. The initial search terms were carvedilol and atrial fibrillation. No language restriction was imposed. In addition, the reference lists of identified studies were manually checked to include other potentially eligible trials. This process was performed iteratively until no additional articles could be identified.

The following inclusive selection criteria were applied: (i) study design: comparative trial; (ii) study population: adult patients undergoing cardiac surgery; (iii) intervention: carvedilol (no matter what regimen applied); (iv) comparison intervention: control (placebo or other beta-blockers) and (v) outcome measure: the incidence of POAF.

Data extraction and outcome measures

Two investigators independently extracted the following data from each trial: first author, publication year, number of patients (carvedilol/control), patient characteristic, regimen of intervention (carvedilol/control), definition and monitoring of POAF, study design, the incidence of POAF, and length of hospital stay (LOS). Extracted data were entered into a standardized Excel file. The primary outcome was the incidence of POAF. Secondary outcome included LOS.

Statistical analysis

Differences were expressed as relative risks (RRs) with 95% confidence intervals (CIs) for dichotomous outcomes, and weighted mean differences (WMDs) with 95% CIs for continuous outcomes. Heterogeneity across studies was tested by using the I^2 statistic, which was a quantitative measure of inconsistency across studies. Studies with an I^2 statistic of 25% to 50% were considered to have low heterogeneity, those with an I^2 statistic of 50% to 75% were considered to have moderate heterogeneity, and those with an I^2 statistic of >75% were considered to have a high degree of heterogeneity [20]. An I^2 value greater than 50% indicates significant heterogeneity [21]. A fixed-effects model was used ($I^2 \leq 50\%$), and a random-effects model was used in the case of significant heterogeneity ($I^2 > 50\%$). We further conducted subgroup analyses according to type of control, surgery type, and study design. We also investigated the influence of a single study on the overall risk estimate by omitting one study in each turn. We did not assess publication bias [22], because the pooled estimate included fewer than ten trials. A p value <0.05 was considered statistically significant. All statistical analyses were performed using Stata version 11.0 (Stata Corporation, College Station, Texas, USA).

Results

Study identification and selection

The initial search yielded 87 relevant publications of which 79 were excluded for various reasons (review, letter, case report, or irrelevant to the current analysis) based on the titles and abstracts. The remaining eight were then retrieved for full text review, two of them were also excluded because one was focused in patients undergoing coronary bypass graft with heart failure and one was currently ongoing [23,24]. Thus, six studies were included in the final analysis [14–19]. The flowchart of studies included in meta-analysis was shown in Figure 1.

Study characteristics

The basic characteristics of studies included in the meta-analysis are shown in Table 1. These studies were published between 2003 and 2010. The sample size of these studies ranged from 53 to 207 (total 765). Four studies in this meta-analysis enrolled patients undergoing coronary artery bypass grafting (CABG) only [15–18]. The remaining two included patients undergoing CABG and/or valve surgery [14,19]. Carvedilol was administered orally by different regimens and formulations. Timing of initiation for carvedilol prophylaxis was 3–10 days before the surgery in the preoperative prophylaxis studies [15,16,19] and within 24 hours of surgery in the postoperative group [17,18]. Definition of POAF in terms of duration varied among the studies. All the patients were monitored using electrocardiography.

Primary outcome: POAF

The definition and monitoring of POAF in each trial are summarized in Table 2. Overall, six studies including 765 patients were included in this analysis (356 in the carvedilol group and 409

Table 1. Characteristics of studies included in the meta-analysis.

Study (Reference)	Sample size (Carvedilol/Control)	Patient characteristic	Mean age (year)/Male (%)	Regimen of intervention Carvedilol	Regimen of intervention Control	POAF Carvedilol	POAF Control	LOS (days) Carvedilol	LOS (days) Control	Study design
Merritt 2003 [14]	115(26/89)	Adult patients undergoing CABG and/or VS	60.3/NA	NA	Metoprolol/atenolol	2/26	28/89	5.9±1.9	6.9±4.5	Non-RCT
Haghjoo 2007 [15]	120(60/60)	Adult patients undergoing CABG	61/52.5	6.25 mg twice daily, oral, starting from 10 days before surgery, then increasing until to the maximum	Metoprolol 25 mg twice daily, oral, starting from 10 days before surgery, then increasing until to the maximum	9/60	20/60	NA	NA	RCT
Acikel 2008 [16]	110(55/55)	Adult patients undergoing CABG	60/71.8	12.5 mg twice daily, starting on 3 days prior to surgery, lasting to the morning of surgery, then titrating according to hemodynamic responses after CABG	Metoprolol 50 mg twice daily, starting on 3 days prior to surgery, lasting to the morning of surgery, then titrating according to hemodynamic responses after CABG	9/55	20/55	NA	NA	RCT
Tsuboi 2008 [17]	160(80/80)	Adult patients undergoing CABG	66.5/70.6	5 or 10 mg/day, oral, starting on postoperative days 1 or 2, then increasing until to the maximum	Placebo	12/80	27/80	17.0±6.2	22.0±12.3	Non-RCT
Yoshioka 2009 [18]	53(31/22)	Adult patients undergoing CABG	67/68	2.5 mg/day, oral, starting on postoperative days 1 or 2	Placebo	4/31	7/22	NA	NA	Non-RCT
Ozaydin 2013 [19]	207(104/103)	Adult patients undergoing CABG and/or VS	63/72.5	6.25 mg twice daily, starting from 7 days before surgery, if not tolerated, a 3.125 mg twice daily dose was given	Metoprolol 50 mg once daily dose, starting from 7 days before surgery, if not tolerated, a 25 mg twice daily dose was given	25/104	37/103	NA	NA	RCT

CABG, coronary artery bypass grafting; LOS, length of hospital stay; NA, no data available; POAF, postoperative atrial fibrillation; RCT, randomized controlled trial; VS, valve surgery.

Table 2. Definition and monitoring of POAF.

Study (Reference)	Definition of POAF	Monitoring of POAF
Merritt 2003 [14]	NA	NA
Haghjoo 2007 [15]	Absent P wave before the QRS complex together with irregular ventricular rhythm on the rhythm strips, lasting longer than 5 minute.	ECG and 12-lead ECG were need to confirm
Acikel 2008 [16]	An irregular rhythm with no prominent P waves lasting 30 s or more	Automated arrhythmia detectors in cardiac ICU, and simultaneous telemetric display of ECG in the ward
Tsuboi 2008 [17]	Absent consistent P waves before each QRS complex and an irregular ventricular rate and as episodes of atrial fibrillation that persisted for over 10 min.	12-lead ECG
Yoshioka 2009 [18]	Lasted more than 5 minutes or required intervention for angina or hemodynamic compromise, or any episode that required intervention for angina or hemodynamic compromise.	Monitoring system on a rhythm strip or 12-lead ECG
Ozaydin 2013 [19]	An irregular rhythm with the absence of discrete P-waves lasting 5 min during hospitalization	Continuous ECG monitoring and all-day Holter

ECG, electrocardiogram; NA, no data available; POAF, postoperative atrial fibrillation; ICU, intensive care unit.

in the control group). Meta-analysis of six studies using a fixed-effects model suggested that carvedilol significantly reduced the incidence of POAF in patients undergoing cardiac surgery compared with control (RR 0.49, 95% CI 0.37 to 0.64, p<0.001; Figure 2). There was no heterogeneity among the studies ($I^2 = 0\%$, heterogeneity p = 0.645; Figure 2).

Then we further conducted subgroup analyses based on type of control (metoprolol vs. placebo), surgery type (CABG and/or valve surgery vs. CABG only), and study design (randomized trials vs. nonrandomized trials). Table 3 shows the results of subgroup analyses for POAF. The results suggested that carvedilol appeared to be superior to metoprolol for the prevention of POAF (RR 0.51, 95% CI 0.37 to 0.70, p<0.001;

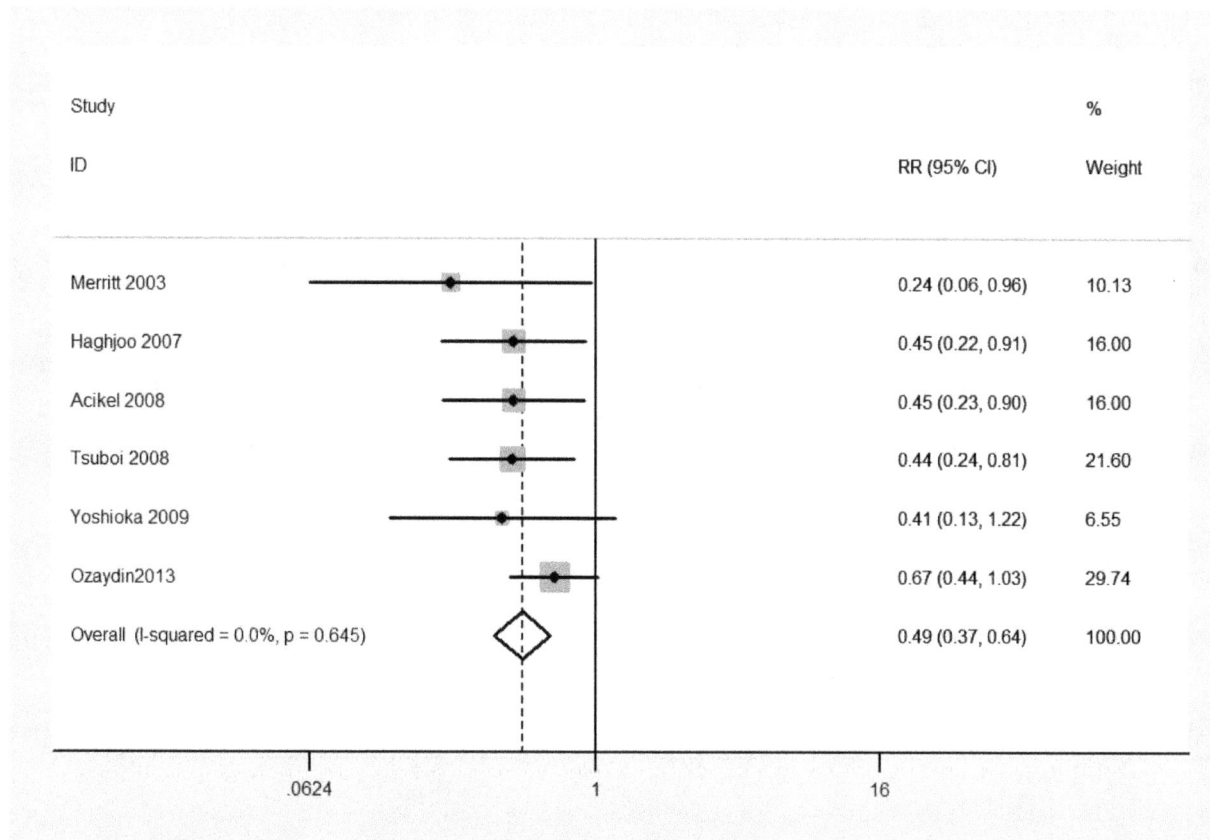

Study ID	RR (95% CI)	% Weight
Merritt 2003	0.24 (0.06, 0.96)	10.13
Haghjoo 2007	0.45 (0.22, 0.91)	16.00
Acikel 2008	0.45 (0.23, 0.90)	16.00
Tsuboi 2008	0.44 (0.24, 0.81)	21.60
Yoshioka 2009	0.41 (0.13, 1.22)	6.55
Ozaydin2013	0.67 (0.44, 1.03)	29.74
Overall (I-squared = 0.0%, p = 0.645)	0.49 (0.37, 0.64)	100.00

.0624   1   16

Figure 2. Effect of carvedilol versus control on the incidence of postoperative atrial fibrillation.

Table 3. Results of subgroup analyses for POAF.

Subgroup analysis	n (N)	Carvedilol	Control	OR (95% CI)	p value	I²(%)	Heterogeneity p
Study design							
RCTs [15,16,19]	3 (437)	43/219	77/218	0.56 (0.40–0.77)	<0.001	0	0.489
Non-RCTs [14,17,18]	3 (328)	18/137	62/191	0.38 (0.23–0.64)	<0.001	0	0.723
Surgery type							
CABG and/or valve surgery [14,19]	2 (322)	27/130	65/192	0.56 (0.37–0.85)	0.007	51.7	0.15
CABG only [15–18]	4 (443)	34/226	74/217	0.44 (0.31–0.64)	<0.001	0	0.999
Type of comparison							
Metoprolol [14–16,19]	4 (552)	45/245	105/307	0.51 (0.37–0.70)	<0.001	0	0.408
Placebo [17,18]	2 (213)	16/111	34/102	0.44 (0.26–0.74)	0.002	0	0.886

CABG, coronary artery bypass grafting; RCT, randomized controlled trial; n, number of patients; N, number of trials.

Figure 3). No evidence of heterogeneity was observed in subgroup analysis. Influence analysis suggested exclusion of any single study did not materially alter the overall combined RR, with a range from 0.41 (0.29 to 0.59) to 0.52 (0.39 to 0.68), which adds robustness to our results.

Secondary outcome: LOS

Two trials reported the effect of carvedilol on LOS and provided available data (expressed as mean ± standard deviation) with a total of 275 patients. The combined analysis using a random-effects model showed that carvedilol did not significantly reduce LOS (WMD −2.75, 95% CI −6.64 to 1.14, p = 0.17), with

a high degree of heterogeneity between the trials (I² = 82.9%, heterogeneity p = 0.016).

Publication bias

Publication bias was not assessed because of the limited number (below 10) of studies included in the analysis.

Discussion

Meta-analysis of all six included studies using a fixed-effects model illustrates that carvedilol may effectively reduce the incidence of POAF in adult patients undergoing cardiac surgery.

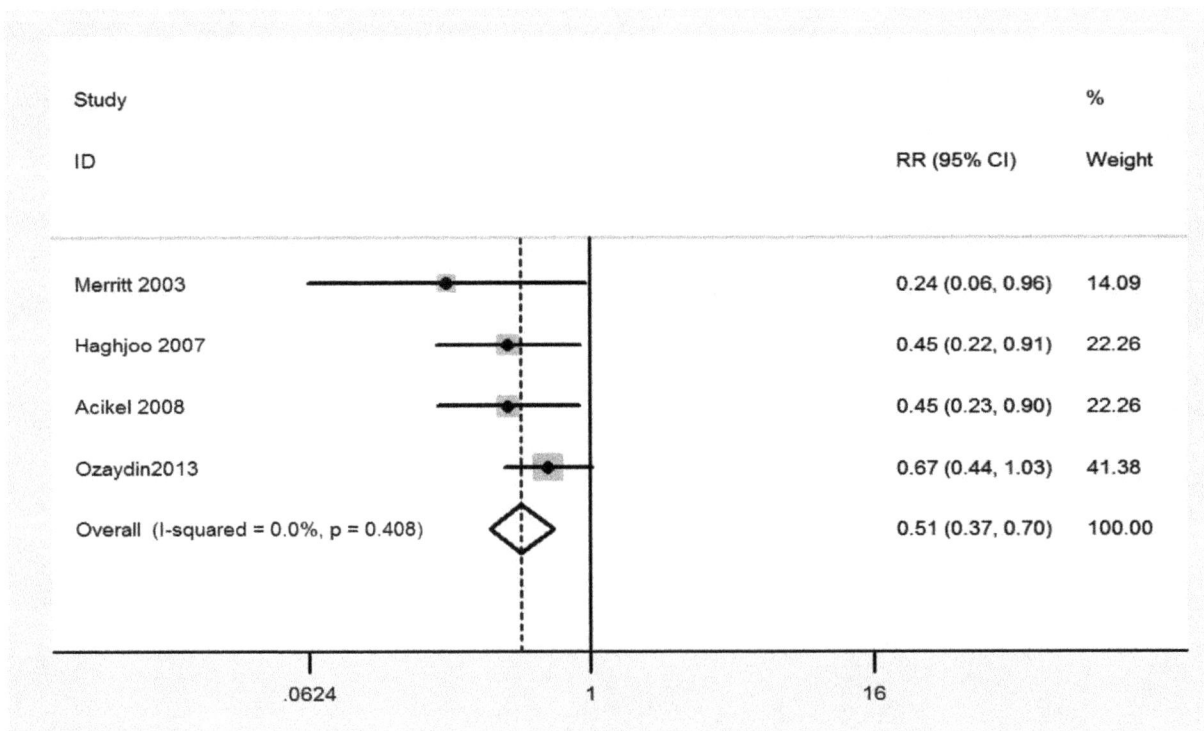

Study ID		RR (95% CI)	% Weight
Merritt 2003		0.24 (0.06, 0.96)	14.09
Haghjoo 2007		0.45 (0.22, 0.91)	22.26
Acikel 2008		0.45 (0.23, 0.90)	22.26
Ozaydin 2013		0.67 (0.44, 1.03)	41.38
Overall (I-squared = 0.0%, p = 0.408)		0.51 (0.37, 0.70)	100.00

.0624   1   16

Figure 3. Effect of carvedilol versus metoprolol on the incidence of postoperative atrial fibrillation.

The mechanisms that carvedilol reduces the incidence of POAF are not entirely known. However, there is now an increasing body of evidences that oxidative stress [25], and inflammation [26,27], and increased sympathetic activation [28] are involved in the pathogenesis of POAF. Carvedilol is a β blocker with antioxidant and anti-inflammatory properties [11,12], and reduces sympathetic activity [29]. From a pathophysiological point of view, it is plausible that the abovementioned properties of carvedilol might result in the favorable effect on the prevention of POAF.

Recently, Khan et al carried out a meta-analysis of randomized controlled trials and confirmed the efficacy of prophylactic beta-blockers against POAF [30]. Both the Khan meta-analysis and our meta-analysis showed that carvedilol appeared to be more effective than metoprolol for the prevention of POAF. Compared with metoprolol, carvedilol has been shown to increase the levels of antioxidant enzymes (superoxide dismutase and glutathione peroxidase). Moreover, carvedilol may have direct antiarrhythmic profile through electrophysiological traits, since it blocks multiple cationic channels (Na^+, K^+, and Ca^{2+}) [11,12]. These properties of carvedilol, which are not equally shared by metoprolol, may partly explained superior efficacy of carvedilol in preventing POAF. In addition, numerous trials indicate that carvedilol is better than conventional β1-selective β blockers on reducing sympathetic activation, a risk factor for atrial fibrillation [28,29].

In this meta-analysis carvedilol did not significantly reduce the LOS. The total incidence of POAF is 26.1% (200 of 765), less than one-third of patients develop POAF and still fewer develop prolonged atrial fibrillation, so the effect of carvedilol on LOS in patients prone to atrial fibrillation would have to be very large to be able to detect an effect of LOS in the total population. In addition, a relatively small number of samples (only two studies) provided available data on LOS, additional studies or data are warranted.

One problem with the use of carvedilol to prevent POAF is that the majority of patients does not develop POAF after cardiac surgery but would still be exposed to possible side effects. In this meta-analysis, two trials reported carvedilol was well tolerated and side effects attributable to carvedilol were detected. And one trial reported complication rates were similar between carvedilol and control groups, including postoperative myocardial infarction and renal dysfunction.

Several potential limitations of this meta-analysis merit consideration. First, our study included only six studies and some of them have a modest sample size. Overestimation of the treatment effect is more likely in smaller studies compared with larger samples. Second, our analysis is based on six clinical studies, and half of them were non-randomized controlled trials. The targeted population, adopted carvedilol protocols, type of control, and study design differed among the included studies. These factors may result in the heterogeneity and have potential impact on our results. Furthermore, these studies lack homogeneity in both the method of postoperative monitoring and in their definition of POAF. This may lead to potential underestimation and/or overestimation of the true incidence of POAF. Finally, it was possible that some missing and unpublished data may lead to bias in effect size.

In conclusion, despite its various limitations, our study is clinically valuable because it revealed that carvedilol leads to lower incidence of POAF than control and appears to be superior to metoprolol as the current study clearly delineated. Carvedilol may effectively reduce the incidence of POAF in patients undergoing cardiac surgery. On the basis of this encouraging finding, we believe that research on the field is promising and should be continued. At least the ongoing COMPACT [24], which is a prospective, multi-center, randomized, open-label, active-controlled trial, will answer the question of whether or not carvedilol is more superior to metoprolol in preventing POAF in patients undergoing CABG.

Author Contributions

Conceived and designed the experiments: HSW ZWW ZTY. Performed the experiments: HSW ZWW ZTY. Analyzed the data: HSW ZWW ZTY. Contributed reagents/materials/analysis tools: HSW ZWW ZTY. Wrote the paper: HSW ZWW ZTY.

References

1. Ommen SR, Odell JA, Stanton MS (1997) Atrial arrhythmias after cardiothoracic surgery. N Engl J Med 336:1429–1434.
2. Aranki SF, Shaw DP, Adams DH, Rizzo RJ, Couper GS, et al. (1996) Predictors of atrial fibrillation after coronary artery surgery. Current trends and impact on hospital resources. Circulation 94:390–397.
3. Mathew JP, Fontes ML, Tudor IC, Ramsay J, Duke P, et al. (2004) A multicenter risk for atrial fibrillation after cardiac surgery. JAMA 291:1720–1729.
4. Burgess DC, Kilborn MJ, Keech AC (2006) Interventions for prevention of postoperative atrial fibrillation and its complications after cardiac surgery: a meta-analysis. Eur Heart J 27:2846–2857.
5. Eagle KA, Guyton RA, Davidoff R, Edwards FH, Ewy GA, et alACC/AHA 2004 guideline update for coronary artery bypass graft surgery: a report of the American College of Cardiology/American Heart Association Task Force on Practice Guidelines (Committee to Update the 1999 Guidelines for Coronary Artery Bypass Graft Surgery). Circulation 110:e340–437.
6. Fuster V, Rydén LE, Cannom DS, Crijns HJ, Curtis AB, et al. (2011) 2011 ACCF/AHA/HRS focused updates incorporated into the ACC/AHA/ESC 2006 Guidelines for the management of patients with atrial fibrillation: a report of the American College of Cardiology Foundation/American Heart Association Task Force on Practice Guidelines developed in partnership with the European Society of Cardiology and in collaboration with the European Heart Rhythm Association and the Heart Rhythm Society. J Am Coll Cardiol 57:e101–198.
7. Aviles RJ, Martin DO, Apperson-Hansen C, Houghtaling PL, Rautaharju P, et al. (2003) Inflammation as a risk factor for atrial fibrillation. Circulation 108:3006–3010.
8. Mihm MJ, Yu F, Carnes CA, Reiser PJ, McCarthy PM, et al. (2011) Impaired myofibrillar energetics and oxidative injury during human atrial fibrillation. Circulation 104:174–180.
9. Gaudino M, Andreotti F, Zamparelli R, Di Castelnuovo A, Nasso G, et al. (2003) The -174G/C interleukin-6 polymorphism influences postoperative interleukin-6 levels and postoperative atrial fibrillation. Is atrial fibrillation an inflammatory complication? Circulation 108 Suppl 1:II195–199.
10. Carnes CA, Chung MK, Nakayama T, Nakayama H, Baliga RS, et al. (2001) Ascorbate attenuates atrial pacing-induced peroxynitrite formation and electrical remodeling and decreases the incidence of postoperative atrial fibrillation. Circ Res 89:E32–38.
11. McBride BF, White CM (2005) Critical differences among beta-adrenoreceptor antagonists in myocardial failure: debating the MERIT of COMET. J Clin Pharmacol 45:6–24.
12. Stroe AF, Gheorghiade M (2004) Carvedilol: beta-blockade and beyond. Rev Cardiovasc Med 5 Suppl 1:S18–27.
13. Daoud EG, Strickberger SA, Man KC, Goyal R, Deeb GM, et al. (1997) Preoperative amiodarone as prophylaxis against atrial fibrillation after heart surgery. N Engl J Med 337:1785–1791.
14. Merritt JC, Niebauer M, Tarakji K, Hammer D, Mills RM (2003) Comparison of effectiveness of carvedilol versus metoprolol or atenolol for atrial fibrillation appearing after coronary artery bypass grafting or cardiac valve operation. Am J Cardiol 92:735–736.
15. Haghjoo M, Saravi M, Hashemi MJ, Hosseini S, Givtaj N, et al. (2007) Optimal beta-blocker for prevention of atrial fibrillation after on-pump coronary artery bypass graft surgery: carvedilol versus metoprolol. Heart Rhythm 4:1170–1174.

16. Acikel S, Bozbas H, Gultekin B, Aydinalp A, Saritas B, et al. (2008) Comparison of the efficacy of metoprolol and carvedilol for preventing atrial fibrillation after coronary bypass surgery. Int J Cardiol 126:108–113.

17. Tsuboi J, Kawazoe K, Izumoto H, Okabayashi H (2008) Postoperative treatment with carvedilol, a beta-adrenergic blocker, prevents paroxysmal atrial fibrillation after coronary artery bypass grafting. Circ J 72:588–591.

18. Yoshioka I, Sakurai M, Namai A, Kawamura T (2009) Postoperative treatment of carvedilol following low dose landiolol has preventive effect for atrial fibrillation after coronary artery bypass grafting. Thorac Cardiovasc Surg 57:464–467.

19. Ozaydin M, Icli A, Yucel H, Akcay S, Peker O, et al. (2013) Metoprolol vs. carvedilol or carvedilol plus N-acetyl cysteine on post-operative atrial fibrillation: a randomized, double-blind, placebo-controlled study. Eur Heart J 34:597–604.

20. Higgins JP, Thompson SG, Deeks JJ, Altman DG (2003) Measuring inconsistency in meta-analyses. BMJ 327:557–560.

21. Armitage P, Berry G, Matthews JNS (2002) Analysing Means and Proportions. Statistical Methods in Medical Research. Oxford, UK: Blackwell Science 83–146.

22. Song F, Eastwood AJ, Gilbody S, Duley L, Sutton AJ (2000) Publication and related biases. Health Technol Assess 4:1–115.

23. Marazzi G, Iellamo F, Volterrani M, Caminiti G, Madonna M, et al. (2011) Comparison of effectiveness of carvedilol versus bisoprolol for prevention of postdischarge atrial fibrillation after coronary artery bypass grafting in patients with heart failure. Am J Cardiol 107:215–219.

24. Kamei M, Morita S, Hayashi Y, Kanmura Y, Kuro M (2006) Carvedilol versus Metoprolol for the prevention of atrial fibrillation after off-pump coronary bypass surgery: rationale and design of the Carvedilol or Metoprolol Post-Revascularization Atrial Fibrillation Controlled Trial (COMPACT). Cardiovasc Drugs Ther 20:219–227.

25. Huang CX, Liu Y, Xia WF, Tang YH, Huang H (2009) Oxidative stress: a possible pathogenesis of atrial fibrillation. Med Hypotheses 72:466–467.

26. Kumagai K, Nakashima H, Saku K (2004) The HMG-CoA reductase inhibitor atorvastatin prevents atrial fibrillation by inhibiting inflammation in a canine sterile pericarditis model. Cardiovasc Res 62:105–111.

27. Ozaydin M, Dogan A, Varol E, Kapan S, Tuzun N, et al. (2007) Statin use before by-pass surgery decreases the incidence and shortens the duration of postoperative atrial fibrillation. Cardiology 107:117–121.

28. Kalman JM, Munawar M, Howes LG, Louis WJ, Buxton BF, et al. (1995) Atrial fibrillation after coronary artery bypass grafting is associated with sympathetic activation. Ann Thorac Surg 60:1709–1715.

29. Miranda SM, Mesquita ET, Dohmann HF, Azevedo JC, Barbirato GB, et al. (2010) Effects of short-term carvedilol on the cardiac sympathetic activity assessed by 123I-MIBG scintigraphy. Arq Bras Cardiol 94: 308–312, 328–332.

30. Khan MF, Wendel CS, Movahed MR (2013) Prevention of post-coronary artery bypass grafting (CABG) atrial fibrillation: efficacy of prophylactic beta-blockers in the modern era: A meta-analysis of latest randomized controlled trials. Ann Noninvasive Electrocardiol 18:58–68.

3

In Vivo Human Left-to-Right Ventricular Differences in Rate Adaptation Transiently Increase Pro-Arrhythmic Risk following Rate Acceleration

Alfonso Bueno-Orovio[1]*, Ben M. Hanson[2], Jaswinder S. Gill[3], Peter Taggart[4], Blanca Rodriguez[1]

1 Department of Computer Science, Computational Biology Group, University of Oxford, Oxford, United Kingdom, **2** Department of Mechanical Engineering, University College London, London, United Kingdom, **3** Guy's and St. Thomas' Hospital, London, United Kingdom, **4** The Neurocardiology Research Unit, University College Hospital, London, United Kingdom

Abstract

Left-to-right ventricular (LV/RV) differences in repolarization have been implicated in lethal arrhythmias in animal models. Our goal is to quantify LV/RV differences in action potential duration (APD) and APD rate adaptation and their contribution to arrhythmogenic substrates in the *in vivo* human heart using combined *in vivo* and *in silico* studies. Electrograms were acquired from 10 LV and 10 RV endocardial sites in 15 patients with normal ventricles. APD and APD adaptation were measured during an increase in heart rate. Analysis of *in vivo* electrograms revealed longer APD in LV than RV (207.8 ± 21.5 vs 196.7 ± 20.1 ms; $P<0.05$), and slower APD adaptation in LV than RV (time constant $\tau^s = 47.0\pm14.3$ vs 35.6 ± 6.5 s; $P<0.05$). Following rate acceleration, LV/RV APD dispersion experienced an increase of up to 91% in 12 patients, showing a strong correlation ($r^2 = 0.90$) with both initial dispersion and LV/RV difference in slow adaptation. Pro-arrhythmic implications of measured LV/RV functional differences were studied using *in silico* simulations. Results show that LV/RV APD and APD adaptation heterogeneities promote unidirectional block following rate acceleration, albeit being insufficient for establishment of reentry in normal hearts. However, in the presence of an ischemic region at the LV/RV junction, LV/RV heterogeneity in APD and APD rate adaptation promotes reentrant activity and its degeneration into fibrillatory activity. Our results suggest that LV/RV heterogeneities in APD adaptation cause a transient increase in APD dispersion in the human ventricles following rate acceleration, which promotes unidirectional block and wave-break at the LV/RV junction, and may potentiate the arrhythmogenic substrate, particularly in patients with ischemic heart disease.

Editor: Rajesh Gopalrao Katare, University of Otago, New Zealand

Funding: This study was financially supported by European Commission preDiCT Grant DG-INFSO-224381; United Kingdom Medical Research Council Career Development award to BR; and Medical Research Council (MRC) grant G0901819 to BH and PT. The funders had no role in study design, data collection and analysis, decision to publish, or preparation of the manuscript.

Competing Interests: The authors have declared that no competing interests exist.

* E-mail: alfonso.bueno@cs.ox.ac.uk

Introduction

Ventricular heterogeneity in repolarization is one of the most important contributors to the electrophysiological substrate leading to the occurrence of lethal arrhythmias such as ventricular fibrillation [1–5]. A large number of studies have demonstrated the complex spatio-temporal mechanisms that modulate ventricular heterogeneity in repolarization and pro-arrhythmic risk. Research using animal models has shown that both functional and structural differences between the left and the right ventricles (LV and RV) determine the spatio-temporal organization of ventricular fibrillation [6,7], the generation of arrhythmias in sudden cardiac death syndromes [8], cardiac vulnerability to electric shocks [9], and epicardial repolarization gradient during global ischemia [10]. Even though LV/RV differences in action potential duration (APD) have been reported in several species, including canine [11,12] and swine hearts [13], data in human are scarce. To the best of our knowledge, only one study by Ramanathan *et al.* [14] provides quantitative evidence of the interventricular differences in epicardial APD in 7 normal human subjects, using non-invasive imaging to reconstruct the repolarization pattern from body-surface signals.

Ventricular heterogeneity in repolarization and arrhythmic risk are known to increase with sudden changes in rate [15–17], due to the highly rate-dependent properties of the APD. *In vivo*, *in vitro* and *in silico* studies have shown that, following a rate increase, the human ventricular APD adapts in two distinct phases, starting with a fast decrease lasting only a few beats, then followed by a slow phase of the order of several minutes [18–20]. The dynamics of APD adaptation underlie the adaptation of the QT interval in the electrocardiogram [20]. Importantly, patients with protracted QT interval rate adaptation were associated with high arrhythmic risk [21,22], supporting the importance of ventricular rate adaptation dynamics in arrhythmogenesis. However, very little is known about LV/RV differences in APD rate adaptation, which, if present, could contribute to increased interventricular dispersion in repolarization and arrhythmic risk following rate changes.

The goal of our study is to quantify LV/RV heterogeneities in APD and APD rate adaptation in the human ventricles using *in vivo* electrophysiological recordings, and to investigate their pro-arrhythmic implications using *in silico* simulations. We hypothesized that the human ventricles exhibit LV/RV heterogeneity in both APD and APD rate adaptation, which result in increased interventricular heterogeneity in APD shortly after heart rate acceleration. In our study, LV/RV differences in APD and APD rate adaptation were quantified from *in vivo* electrograms obtained at 10 LV and 10 RV endocardial locations of 15 patients using two decapolar catheters. Ethical limitations prevent the *in vivo* investigation of the pro-arrhythmic consequences of these LV/RV heterogeneities in the patients. We therefore conducted a simulation study to extend the implications of our *in vivo* findings. A human ventricular tissue model was constructed based on the *in vivo* recordings. Simulations were conducted using different stimulation protocols to systematically investigate the contribution of LV/RV heterogeneity in APD and APD rate adaptation to the pro-arrhythmic substrate following rate changes. Based on the higher incidence of in-hospital complications and post-discharge mortality in patients with ischemic regions near the LV/RV junction [23,24], we hypothesize that LV/RV differences in APD rate adaptation contribute to increase the likelihood of unidirectional block at the LV/RV junction in the human ventricles following rate acceleration, which facilitates the establishment of reentry in the presence of an ischemic region.

Methods

Patients

Fifteen patients (4 females, 11 males; aged 35 to 72, median 61; see Table 1) with healthy ventricles were studied prior to radiofrequency ablation for supraventricular arrhythmias, as it is conventional to consider these patients as a group with normal ventricles [25]. The study, according to the principles expressed in the Declaration of Helsinki, was approved by the Guy's and St. Thomas' Hospital Ethics Committee, and written informed consent was obtained from all patients. Antiarrhythmic drugs were discontinued for 5 days before the study. Intrinsic rate for each patient was computed as the average of RR intervals over 1 minute before initiation of programmed pacing.

Data Acquisition

In-situ unipolar electrograms were recorded using two decapolar electrode catheters to quantify interventricular differences in APD and APD adaptation in the human ventricle. Both catheters were positioned in a base-to-apex orientation, one on the postero-inferior endocardial LV wall and the second on the antero-septal RV wall. Pacing was established from the RV apex at a pulse width of 2 ms and stimulus of strength 2×diastolic threshold. A period of 2 minutes was recorded from each patient following a sustained change in rate from their intrinsic rate (median 723.0 ms) to a faster cycle length (CL) of median 500 ms (see Table 1), in agreement with RR intervals observed clinically in exercise tests [22]. After the stabilization period, a standard restitution curve was constructed for each electrogram as previously reported [25].

Signal Analysis

APDs were quantified as the activation-recovery intervals from each unipolar electrogram using the Wyatt method of analysis (Figure 1A), which has been validated following rigorous experimental and theoretical scrutiny [26–28]. The method was incorporated in an automated system, with manual verification [29]. Postprocessing of the APD series (Figure S1 and Text S1) was performed using custom-written routines in MATLAB (Math-Works, Natick, MA).

Table 1. Details of the patients in the study.

Patient	Diagnosis	Sex	Age	Intrinsic cycle length (ms)	Study cycle length (ms)
1	AF	F	59	634±133	500
2	AF	M	52	844±136	500
3	AF	M	60	866±77	500
4	AF	F	72	679±266	500
5	AF	M	67	812±411	500
6	AF	F	69	945±155	500
7	AF	F	56	1091±311	500
8	AF	M	53	989±209	500
9	AF	M	68	567±28*	450†
10	AF	M	69	542±293	500
11	AF	M	35	855±451	500
12	AF	M	60	693±206	500
13	AF	M	61	723±32	600‡
14	AF	M	62	550±119*	500
15	AF	M	70	571±264	500
Mean	–	–	60.9	757.4	503.3
STD	–	–	9.5	173.0	29.7
Median	–	–	61.0	723.0	500.0

All patients were selected in the basis that they had healthy ventricles. AF = atrial fibrillation. Asterisks indicate patients recovering from a previous interrupted stimulation protocol. †Patient 9 required a shorter cycle length of 450 ms in order to maintain capture, avoiding escape beats. ‡Patient 13 reported slight discomfort at the paced rate of 500 ms and was therefore paced at a longer cycle length of 600 ms.

APD adaptation curves following rate acceleration were used to estimate the time constants of the fast (τ^f) and slow (τ^s) phases of APD adaptation for each electrogram by fitting each curve to a double exponential decay (Figure 1B). A robust least-squares algorithm (nlinfit, MATLAB Statistics Toolbox) was used to minimize the effects of outliers. The algorithm was validated against synthetic APD adaptation curves with different levels of noise-to-signal ratios, yielding satisfactory results in all circumstances (maximum relative τ^s error: 0.014±0.124; see Table S1).

Intraventricular APD dispersion in LV and RV (ΔAPD_{LV} and ΔAPD_{RV}, respectively) was quantified for each patient as the difference between the longest and shortest APD in each ventricle at each time point (Figure 1C, shaded areas). Average differences between LV and RV were used to estimate interventricular APD dispersion (ΔAPD_{LV-RV}), following the approach of Ramanathan *et al.* [14]. Mean LV and RV adaptation curves were computed for each patient as the average of all adaptation curves measured in each ventricle (Figure 1C, solid lines). ΔAPD_{LV-RV} was then quantified at each time point as the difference between these average APD adaptation curves.

Statistical Analysis

Data are presented as mean±SD. The paired Student's *t*-test was used to determine statistical significance in LV/RV properties.

Human Ventricular Tissue Simulations

A computer simulation study was conducted to quantify the contribution of LV/RV differences in APD and APD adaptation

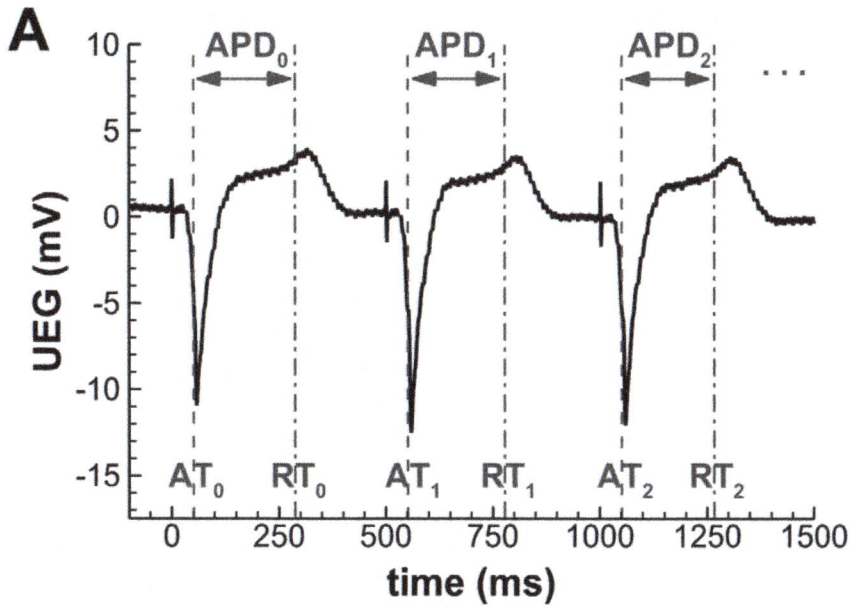

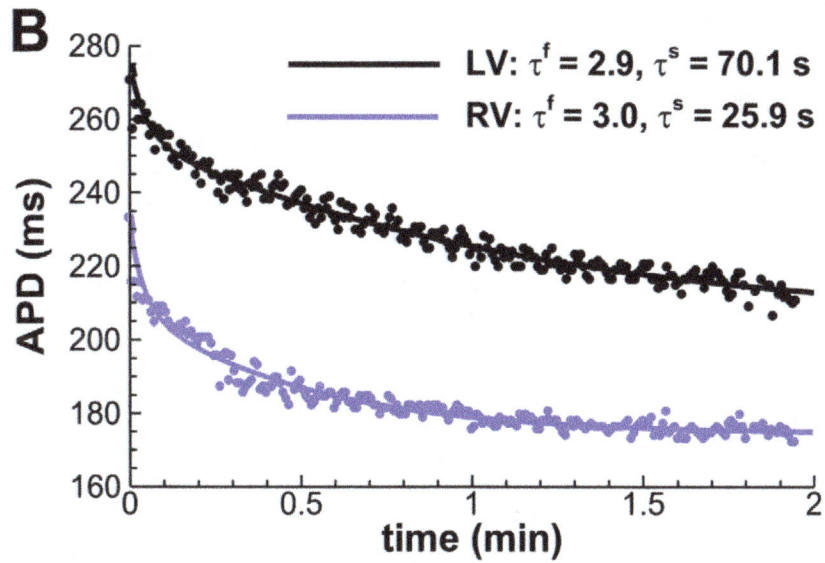

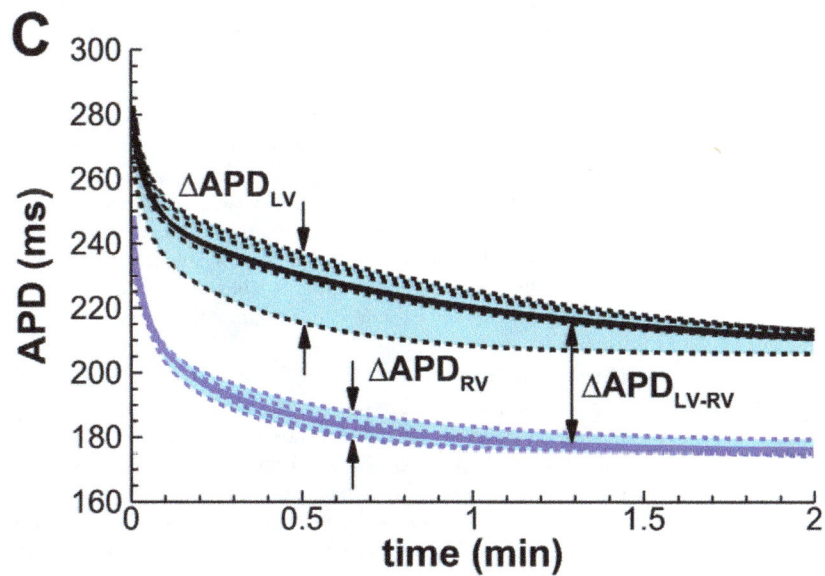

Figure 1. Quantification of intra- and interventricular APD dispersion (ΔAPD) from unipolar electrocardiograms. A: Automatic detection of activation and recovery times (AT/RT), and reconstruction of the APD series. The initiation of programmed pacing coincides here with $t = 0$. **B:** Estimation of fast (τ^f) and slow (τ^s) adaptation time constants by fitting the APD series to a double exponential decay (Patient 3, representative LV/RV mid-ventricular locations). **C:** Intraventricular ΔAPD is measured as the difference between the longest and shortest APD during adaptation (shaded areas). Solid lines indicate average LV/RV adaptations.

characterized in the electrograms to the pro-arrhythmic substrate in the human ventricles following rate acceleration. Simulations of over 1000 beats were conducted using a two-dimensional human ventricular tissue model of 6×6 cm in size incorporating two regions describing RV and LV dynamics (similarly to the approach followed by Pandit *et al.* [10]). The long duration and number of simulations required in our study prevented the use of anatomically-based human ventricular models (real-time estimates based on 100 beats: 6.5 days per 3D simulation on 256 processors using Chaste [30], one of the most efficient and scalable world-wide finite-element solvers for computational cardiac electrophysiology; 3.5 hours per 2D simulation on 4 processors using our specific 2D spectral solver, see "Numerical Techniques").

In all tissue simulations an isotropic monodomain model was used to simulate propagation of electrical excitation, with a diffusion coefficient ($D = 1.171$ cm²/s) specifically calculated for human ventricular tissue [31]. The human virtual tissue was stimulated at the bottom edge perpendicular to the LV/RV junction with CL = 750 ms for 100 beats followed by acceleration to CL = 400 ms. Repolarization patterns were analyzed during rate acceleration occurring both suddenly and progressively during a 1 minute linear CL decay. In order to investigate vulnerability to reentry, ectopic stimulation was applied at the LV/RV junction at the time of maximum APD heterogeneity following rate acceleration. Simulations were conducted in the absence and presence of an inexcitable ischemic region at the LV/RV junction. The ischemic region was considered to be of 1 cm in radius and including non-excitable tissue, as previously described [32–34].

Cellular Model of Human Ventricular Electrophysiology

Testing of our hypotheses requires a human ventricular action potential (AP) model in agreement with our *in vivo* recordings and which allows the independent alteration of APD and its rate dependent properties by varying specific parameters. This is made possible in our study by constructing a new version of the Bueno-Orovio–Cherry–Fenton human AP model [31], modified to capture APD adaptation dynamics as quantified in the electrograms. The model accounts for the sum of all transmembrane currents into three main categories (fast inward, slow inward, and slow outward currents):

$$\partial_t u = -(I_{fi} + I_{si} + I_{so} - I_{stim})$$
$$\partial_t v = (1-m)(1-v)/\tau_v^- - mv/\tau_v^+$$
$$\partial_t w = (1-p)(w^\infty - w)/\tau_w^- - pw/(c\tau_w^+)$$
$$\partial_t s = ((1+\tanh[k_s(u-u_s)]/2) - s)/\tau_s$$
$$\partial_t c = (1-p)(1-c)/\tau_c^- - pc/\tau_c^+$$
$$\partial_t w^\infty = (c^\alpha - w^\infty)/(2\tau^s)$$

where

$$I_{fi} = -vm(u-u_m)(u_u-u)/\tau_{fi}$$
$$I_{si} = -pws/\tau_{si}$$
$$I_{so} = (u-u_0)(1-p)/\tau_0 + p/\tau_{so}$$
$$\tau_v^- = (1-q)\tau_{v1}^- + q\tau_{v2}^-$$
$$\tau_{so} = c\tau_{so1} + (\tau_{so2} - c\tau_{so1})(1 + \tanh[k_{so}(u-u_{so})])/2$$

and

$$m = \begin{cases} 0, u < u_m \\ 1, u \ge u_m \end{cases}, \quad p = \begin{cases} 0, u < u_p \\ 1, u \ge u_p \end{cases}, \quad q = \begin{cases} 0, u < u_q \\ 1, u \ge u_q \end{cases}.$$

The voltage u is rescaled to physiological range by means of the mapping $V_m = 92u - 83$ (mV), with initial conditions given by $u = 0$, $v = 1$, $w = 1$, $s = 0$, $c = 1$, and $w^\infty = 1$. The slow phase of APD adaptation is independently regulated by model parameter τ^s (Figure 2A). APD at sinus rhythm is controlled by the parameter τ_{so1}, therefore allowing for different combinations of APD and APD adaptation to be represented by the human model.

Importantly, model parameters were adapted to reproduce human endocardial AP morphology, and APD and APD restitution properties measured in the *in vivo* unipolar electrograms, using a parameter-fitting algorithm [31]. This yielded the following choice of parameters: $u_0 = 0$, $u_u = 1.4$, $u_m = 0.3$, $u_p = 0.13$, $u_q = 0.2$, $\tau_{v1}^- = 23$, $\tau_{v2}^- = 100$, $\tau_v^+ = 2$, $\tau_w^- = 30$, $\tau_w^+ = 380$, $\tau_c^- = 250$, $\tau_c^+ = 4000$, $\tau_{so1} = 40$, $\tau_{so2} = 1.2$, $\tau_{fi} = 0.115$, $\tau_0 = 6$, $\tau_s = 2$, $\tau_{si} = 2.9013$, $u_s = 0.9087$, $k_s = 2.0994$, $u_{so} = 0.65$, $k_{so} = 2$, $\alpha = 8$.

Resting membrane potential of the model at normal rate (CL = 750 ms) is -83 mV, AP amplitude 130.7 mV, and maximum upstroke velocity 234.3 V/s, all in agreement with previously published physiological data [31]. APD was measured at a fixed threshold of -70 mV, representing 90% of repolarization. APD S_1–S_2 restitution curves were calculated at the center of one-dimensional cables of 2.5 cm length [31]. By varying the S_1 CL used, a family of S_1–S_2 restitution curves was generated (Figure 2B). Comparison with aggregated experimental data obtained from the *in vivo* electrograms is also shown for further model validation. Conduction velocity was measured between neighboring points located at the center of the cable, yielding a maximal value of about 70 cm/s according to experimental results in human [35], and a dispersion of activation times similar to the ones observed experimentally (data not shown).

Numerical Techniques

The simulation software was written in Fortran. The human AP model was integrated using a second-order Euler method in time, with constant time step of 0.025 ms, and a Fourier spectral method in space, allowing a space discretization of 0.03 cm due to the high-order convergence of these methods [36]. The accuracy of the numerical simulations was verified in one-dimensional cables by halving the time and space integration steps and

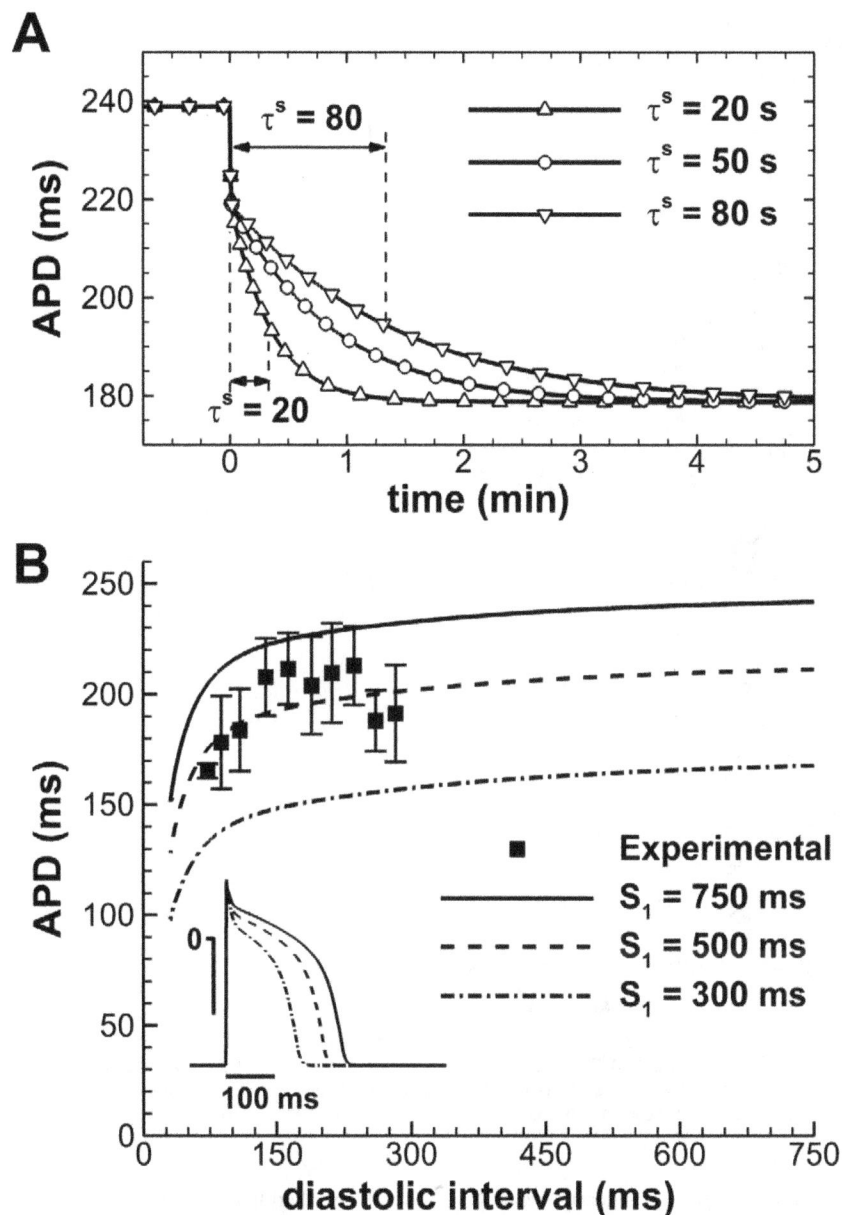

Figure 2. Electrophysiological properties of the human AP model. A: APD adaptation after a sustained change in rate from normal to fast pacing (750 to 400 ms), for different slow APD adaptation time constants. **B:** S_1–S_2 APD restitution at different S_1 cycle lengths. Aggregated experimental restitution data at a CL = 500 ms is shown for comparison. Inset shows steady-state APs at the indicated CLs.

verifying that this resulted in less than 5% change in conduction velocity [31].

Results

In vivo LV/RV Heterogeneity in APD and APD Adaptation Dynamics in Human Ventricles

The analysis of the *in vivo* electrograms revealed significant LV/RV differences in steady-state APD and slow APD adaptation dynamics ($P<0.05$, paired Student's t-test), whereas no statistical LV/RV differences were found for the time constant of the fast phase of APD adaptation ($\tau^f = 3.0 \pm 1.3$ in LV, 2.6 ± 0.8 s in RV). As shown in Figure 3, mean APD is longer in LV than in RV (panel A: 207.8 ± 21.5 and 196.7 ± 20.1 ms, respectively) and time constant of slow phase of APD adaptation is larger in LV than RV

(panel B: $\tau^s = 47.0 \pm 14.3$ and 35.6 ± 6.5 s, respectively). The range of τ^s is also wider in LV than in RV, with $\tau^s = 26.9$–85.2 in LV and $\tau^s = 25.8$–44.0 s in RV. No significant correlations were observed between steady-state APD values and estimated time constants of adaptation (data not shown).

Following rate acceleration, LV/RV differences in APD (ΔAPD_{LV-RV}) experienced an increase of up to 91% (mean±SD: $52.3 \pm 29.4\%$; median: 45.0%) of their initial value in 12 patients, following the pattern illustrated in Figure 3C. Time to peak maximum LV/RV APD dispersion was 26.7 ± 20.1 s (median 24.5 s). Only 3 patients exhibited a monotonic decrease in ΔAPD_{LV-RV} following rate acceleration. The percent of ΔAPD_{LV-RV} increase over their initial value is shown for all patients in Figure 3D. Multiple linear regression analysis of the *in vivo* data showed a strong correlation ($r^2 = 0.90$) of maximum

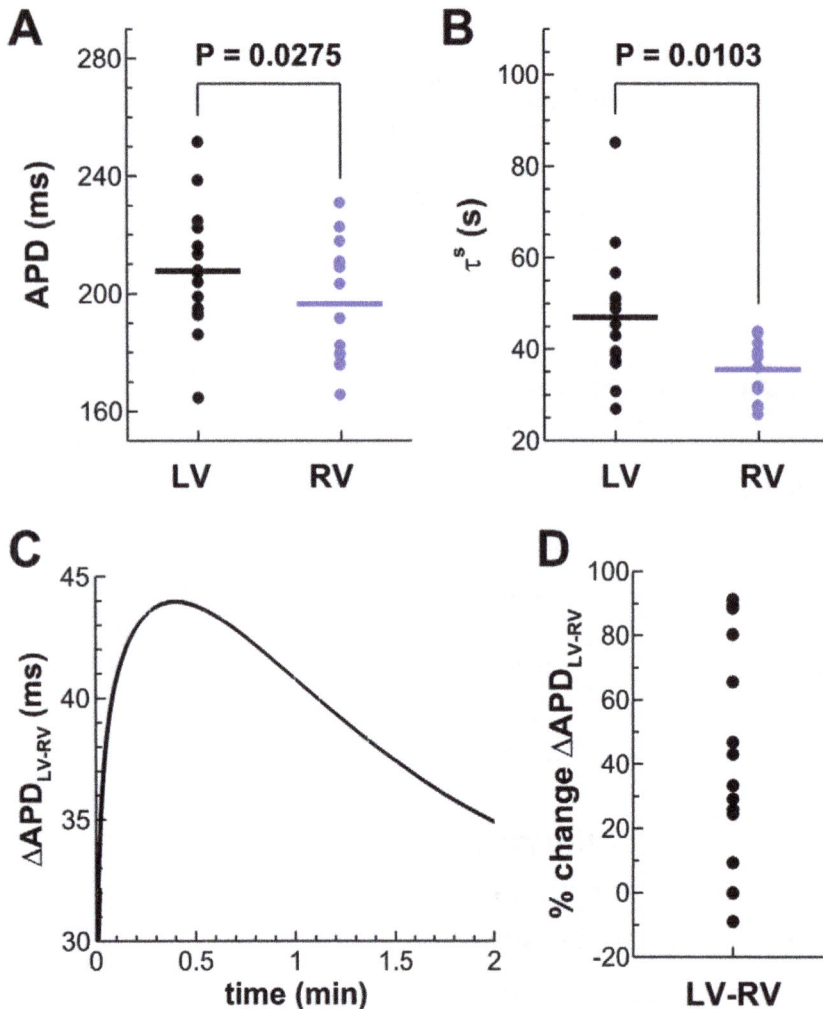

Figure 3. Functional LV/RV differences in the *in vivo* human heart. A,B: Unipolar electrograms revealed longer steady-state APDs at the study CL and slower APD adaptation dynamics in LV compared to RV. **C:** Transient increased LV/RV APD dispersion following rate acceleration in a representative patient (Patient 3). **D:** Percent of ΔAPD_{LV-RV} increase following rate acceleration for all patients of the study.

ΔAPD_{LV-RV} with both initial ΔAPD_{LV-RV} and the LV/RV difference in slow adaptation time constant.

Figure 4 shows a comparison of values of maximum interventricular ΔAPD_{LV-RV} with intraventricular ΔAPD_{LV} and ΔAPD_{RV}. Results show that ΔAPD_{LV-RV} is larger than both ΔAPD_{LV} and ΔAPD_{RV} in 9 patients, highlighting the importance of LV/RV differences in modulating ventricular heterogeneity. In 5 patients, ΔAPD_{LV-RV} is smaller than both ΔAPD_{LV} and ΔAPD_{RV}, and in 1 patient ΔAPD_{LV-RV} is larger than ΔAPD_{RV} but smaller than ΔAPD_{LV}.

In silico Investigation of Pro-arrhythmic Consequences of LV/RV Heterogeneity in APD and APD Rate Adaptation

A simulation study was conducted to further investigate the implications of LV/RV heterogeneity in APD and APD adaptation shown in the *in vivo* recordings. Figure 5 shows the temporal evolution of ΔAPD_{LV-RV} between two points respectively located in the center of the RV and LV areas of the simulation domain, for different magnitudes of interventricular APD dispersion at normal heart rate and combinations of LV/RV adaptation time constants. Stimulation rate was increased from normal rate (CL = 750 ms) to fast pacing (CL = 400 ms) and either suddenly (solid lines) or

linearly over a period of 60 s (dashed lines), the latter replicating rate changes occurring gradually. ΔAPD_{LV-RV} at normal and fast pacing in all scenarios was in range with the one reported in our *in vivo* electrograms, and also in agreement with the average ΔAPD_{LV-RV} of 32 ms reported at normal heart rate by Ramanathan *et al* [14].

In all the considered scenarios, sudden rate acceleration results in a sudden decrease in ΔAPD_{LV-RV} during the fast phase of APD adaptation, followed by a transient increase in ΔAPD_{LV-RV} before a gradual decrease towards the final ΔAPD_{LV-RV} value. For human tissue exhibiting moderate interventricular APD dispersion at normal heart rate ($\Delta APD_{LV-RV} = 22$ ms), and slow APD adaptation time constants of $\tau^s = 30$ and 50 s in RV and LV (Figure 5A), maximum ΔAPD_{LV-RV} however remains very similar to its 22 ms value at normal rhythm. The introduction of larger LV/RV differences in APD adaptation dynamics ($\tau^s = 30$ and 100 s in RV and LV; Figure 5B) results in a significant increase in maximum ΔAPD_{LV-RV} to 33 ms and also in a prolonged time window of increased ΔAPD_{LV-RV} of over 400 beats. An additional increase of interventricular APD dispersion at normal heart rate to $\Delta APD_{LV-RV} = 32$ ms (Figure 5C) results in similar qualitative patterns than in Figure 5B, but exhibiting a larger maximum

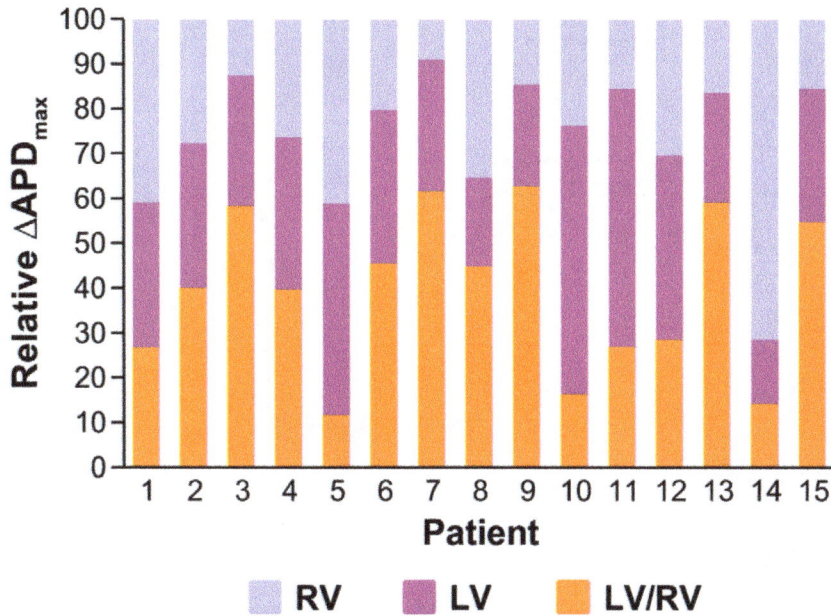

Figure 4. Comparison of maximum interventricular ΔAPD_{LV-RV} with intraventricular ΔAPD_{LV} and ΔAPD_{RV} for all patients in the study.

ΔAPD_{LV-RV} reaching 40 ms. Furthermore, in the three cases, the transient initial decrease in ΔAPD_{LV-RV} following a sudden rate change, and attributed to the fast phase of adaptation, was not observed during progressive rate changes (dashed lines).

Simulations were conducted to test the hypothesis that a transient increase in ΔAPD_{LV-RV} following rate acceleration increases the likelihood of unidirectional block and reentry in human ventricular tissue. An ectopic stimulus was applied near the LV/RV border at the time of maximum ΔAPD_{LV-RV}, and subsequent dynamics were investigated. As shown in Figure 6A for scenario A, the maximum ΔAPD_{LV-RV} generated by moderate LV/RV heterogeneity in the slow phase of APD adaptation is not able to produce conduction block following the ectopic excitation ($t = 20$). The ectopic wavefront propagates as an almost circular pattern with its curvature only affected in a small region of the LV ($t = 30$ to 60).

In Figure 6B, however, the increased LV/RV heterogeneity in APD adaptation (scenario B) results in a larger transient dispersion of repolarization, which provides the substrate for the development of effective conduction block in the tissue ($t = 20$, asterisk), setting the stage for initiation of reentry ($t = 30$). However, the two wave fronts eventually merge, producing an excitation pattern similar to the one displayed in Figure 6A, with no wave-break or sustained reentry present in the tissue. Similar behavior was observed for conditions of increased ΔAPD_{LV-RV} at normal heart rate as considered in scenario C (data not shown). Therefore, our results suggest that heterogeneous APD adaptation dynamics between LV and RV, as reported in the *in vivo* electrograms, favor unidirectional block of propagation. However, additional conditions are required for the establishment of reentrant circuits. Our simulation results are therefore consistent with the lack of ventricular arrhythmias in the patients considered in this study, even considering larger LV/RV differences in rate adaptation than the ones reported experimentally (Figure 3B).

Given the high incidence of arrhythmic events in the presence of ischemic regions at the LV/RV junction [23,24], we introduced the presence of an inexcitable region in our 2D model as shown in

Figure 7 (dashed line). Ectopic stimulation was applied close to the ischemic border [37]. Figure 7A shows that, for modest LV/RV heterogeneity in APD adaptation (scenario A), a small dispersion of repolarization is again unable to produce conduction block ($t = 20$), and the ectopic stimulus circumvents the injured region with a normal excitation pattern ($t = 60$ to 160). However, as shown in Figure 7B, increasing LV/RV heterogeneity in rate adaptation (scenario B) results in effective unidirectional block in the LV following ectopic stimulation ($t = 20$), with the establishment of a reentrant circuit facilitated by the scar region ($t = 60$). Importantly, this irregular excitation pattern self-perpetuates in the tissue, eventually finding new areas of conduction block ($t = 110$), and ultimately producing wave-break and fibrillatory-like activity ($t = 220$).

An appropriate timing of the extra stimulus depending on ectopic location was required in our computer simulations in order to yield establishment of reentry. This is in line with previous studies highlighting the existence of a vulnerable window for reentry following ectopic stimulation [38,39]. Hence, multiple combinations of ectopic timing and location could potentially produce similar dynamics as those reported in Figure 7 (data not shown). These findings are also in agreement with previous experimental results [40], highlighting the role of the time of arrival of the premature wavefront at the distal side of the line of block in determining the occurrence of reentry.

Our results therefore show that LV/RV heterogeneity in rate adaptation facilitates unidirectional block and initiation of reentry at the interventricular junction. Previous studies have suggested a possible role of the slow phase of APD adaptation in the transition from ventricular tachycardia to ventricular fibrillation, by modulating wave-break [41,42]. We conducted further investigations to determine whether fast or protracted slow APD adaptation per se (rather than LV/RV differences) modulates the stability of reentrant rotors and wave-break. Over 200 tissue simulations were conducted under different scenarios, including homogeneous and linear gradients in APD adaptation and varying restitution slope steepness, as described in further detail in the

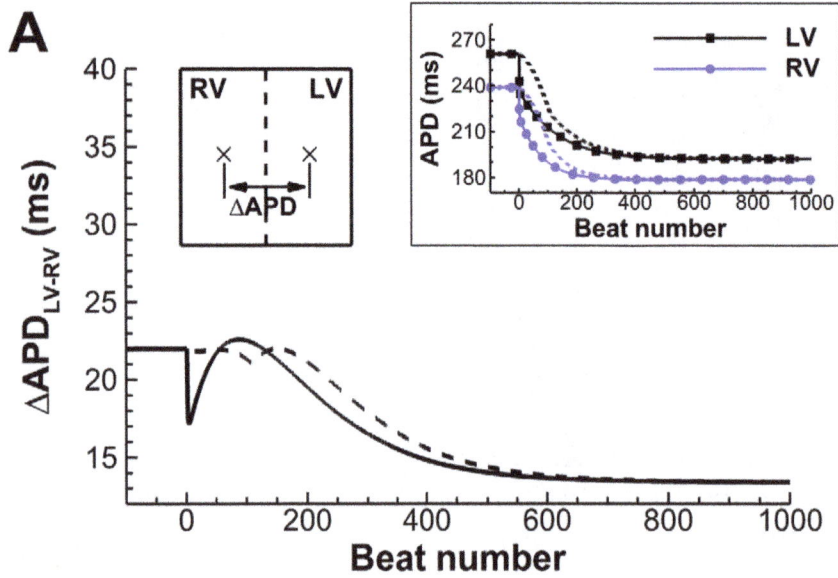

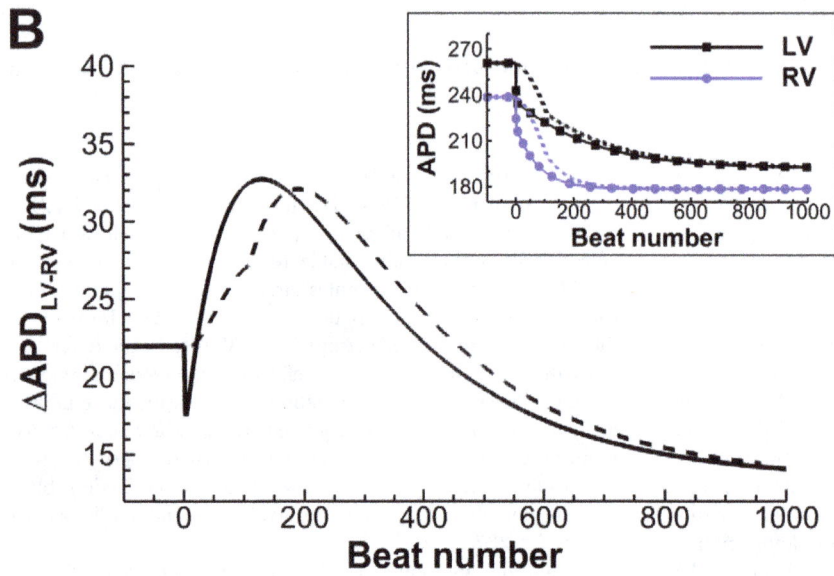

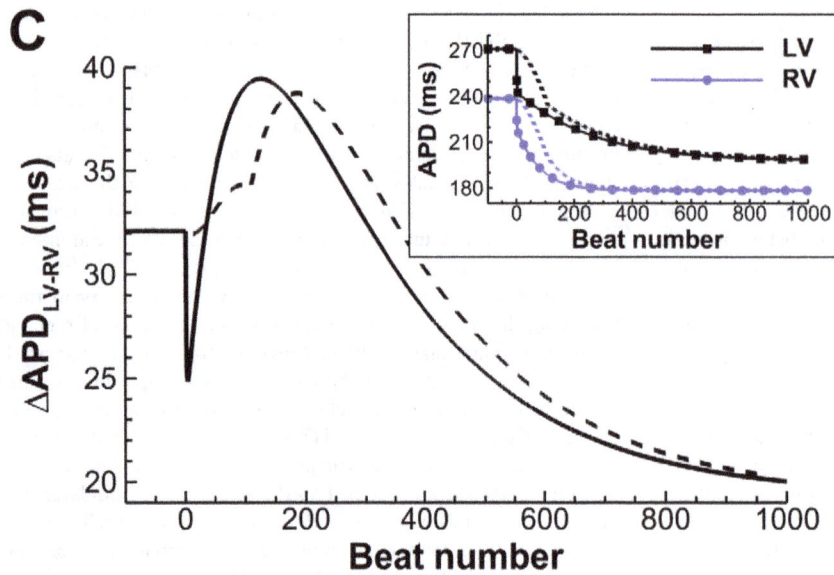

Figure 5. Time evolution of ΔAPD_{LV-RV} due to LV/RV differences in APD adaptation, after a sustained (solid) or a gradual (dashed) change in pacing rate (750 to 400 ms). A: Transient patterns of small ΔAPD_{LV-RV} develop under average conditions of slow APD adaptation. **B:** Conditions of protracted slow APD adaptation increase maximum amplitude and time window of the transient ΔAPD_{LV-RV} pattern. **C:** Conditions of larger ΔAPD_{LV-RV} at normal rate translate into a vertical shift of the transient pattern. Insets show LV/RV APD adaptation in each of the cases, for both stimulation protocols.

Supplemental Material. In summary, our results show that the dynamics of the slow phase of APD adaptation do not modulate wave-break during reentry, but in contrast, this is primarily regulated by the steepness of APD restitution (Figure S2). Therefore, our simulation study identifies LV/RV heterogeneity in APD adaptation, rather than the dynamics of the slow phase of APD adaptation per se, as an important contributor to the substrate of reentrant arrhythmias in the human ventricles following rate acceleration.

Discussion

In the clinical scenario, reentrant arrhythmias are generally considered to be multifactorial in origin, whereby a number of factors combine to generate an appropriate trigger and substrate at a given moment. In order to achieve as complete a mechanistic picture as possible, it is important to identify all the potential individual components.

Electrophysiological recordings from multiple LV and RV endocardial sites, acquired *in vivo* from humans with normal ventricles, exhibit significant LV/RV heterogeneity in APD and APD rate adaptation dynamics. In most patients, LV/RV APD heterogeneity transiently increases following rate acceleration due to LV/RV heterogeneity in rate adaptation. Computer simulations further demonstrate the importance of LV/RV heterogeneity in APD rate adaptation in increasing ventricular dispersion of repolarization following changes in rate and facilitating unidirectional block at the LV/RV junction. In structurally-normal ventricles, the transient increase in LV/RV APD heterogeneity following rate acceleration is insufficient for the establishment of a reentrant circuit. However, in the presence of an ischemic region at the LV/RV junction, LV/RV heterogeneity in APD and APD

rate adaptation promotes initiation and establishment of reentrant circuits and their degeneration into fibrillatory activity, due to unidirectional block at the LV/RV junction.

Our *in vivo* study reports longer APDs in LV than in RV in the human ventricles (Figure 3A), in agreement with previous studies in canine [11,12] and in non-invasive imaging of the human ventricles [14]. Our data also report for the first time slower APD adaptation dynamics in LV than in RV in the human ventricles (Figure 3B). Only a limited number of animal studies have previously suggested the existence of spatial heterogeneities in the slow phase of APD adaptation [43,44]. Our data are thus in agreement with the reported slower APD adaptation in LV compared to RV on the epicardial surface of rabbit hearts [43].

Importantly, our *in vivo* data also show that LV/RV APD heterogeneity transiently increases following rate acceleration in most of the patients (Figures 3C–D). Maximum LV/RV heterogeneity in APD is correlated with both LV/RV heterogeneity in baseline APD and APD rate adaptation, supporting the importance of heterogeneity in APD rate adaptation dynamics in modulating dispersion of repolarization in the human ventricles. This finding is further supported by our simulation results, which show that the transient increase in LV/RV APD heterogeneity also occurs when rate acceleration occurs gradually rather than suddenly (Figure 5).

According to our simulation study, a transient increase in LV/RV APD heterogeneity following rate acceleration promotes unidirectional block, but it is insufficient for the establishment of reentrant circuits (Figure 6). This is consistent with the lack of arrhythmic events in the group of patients evaluated. However, our simulations suggest that the transient increase in LV/RV APD dispersion caused by heterogeneous APD adaptation can act in synergy with a pro-arrhythmic substrate (such as an ischemic

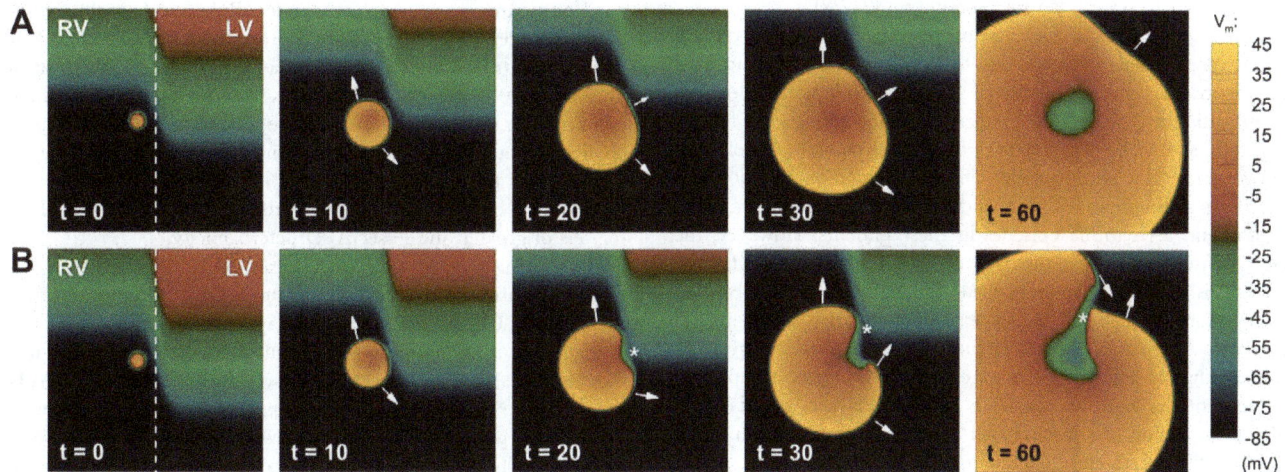

Figure 6. Development of unidirectional block due to transient patterns of interventricular APD dispersion. A: Under average conditions of slow APD adaptation (scenario A), the transient APD dispersion between both ventricles only affects wavefront propagation partially, and the ectopic stimulation excites the whole tissue as a regular beat. **B:** For conditions of protracted slow APD adaptation (scenario B), a larger interventricular APD dispersion is able to produce unidirectional block ($t = 20$, marked by an asterisk), leading to the initiation of reentry ($t = 30$), that subsequently develops in the tissue ($t = 60$). Colorbar denotes transmembrane potential (mV); times indicated since initiation of ectopic stimulation (ms).

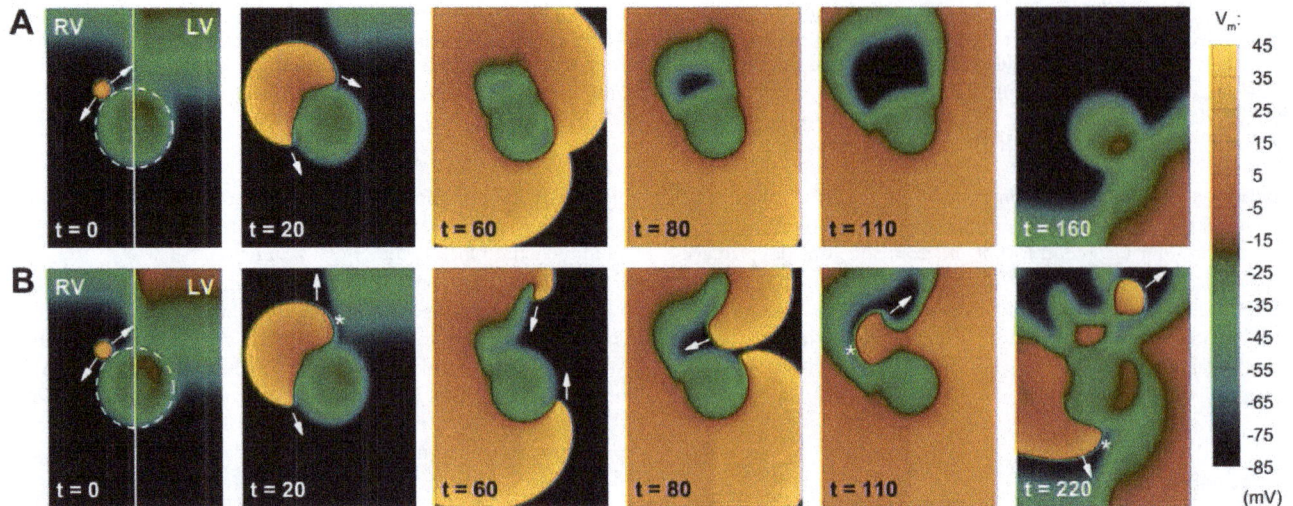

Figure 7. Interaction of transient patterns of interventricular APD dispersion with structural defects of the tissue. The dashed line indicates an inexcitable region in the LV/RV junction. **A:** Under average conditions of slow APD adaptation (scenario A), interventricular APD dispersion is not able to produce conduction block, and the extra-stimulus proceeds circumventing the inexcitable area. **B:** For conditions of protracted slow APD adaptation (scenario B), the top part of the extra activation now finds a region of unidirectional block due to a larger APD dispersion ($t = 20$, marked by an asterisk). The wavefront therefore moves upwards, eventually developing into a reentrant wave ($t = 60$). Since the bottom part of the excitation has been circumventing the obstacle, the top reentrant wave can now proceed in the tissue ($t = 80$), finding new areas of conduction block ($t = 110$), and finally producing wave-break ($t = 220$). Figure annotation as in Figure 6.

region) to promote conduction block, reentrant activity and wave-break, potentially leading to the initiation of ventricular fibrillation (Figure 7B). Based on the high incidence of arrhythmic events and post-discharge mortality in patients with ischemic regions at the LV/RV junction [23,24], the location of the infarcted area was prescribed in our computational study at the interventricular interface. Although different mechanisms than LV/RV differences might be involved in the establishment of reentrant arrhythmias for ischemic regions located outside this functional boundary, our findings provide supporting evidence of the important role of these interventricular differences in promoting the occurrence of arrhythmic events following rate acceleration [15–17], particularly in patients with protracted rate adaptation [21,22].

Our investigations suggest the need to conduct further clinical and experimental investigations to confirm the importance of interventricular heterogeneity in APD rate adaptation for risk stratification in post-infarcted patients. Ideally, a long term follow-up study should be performed to determine possible correlations between LV/RV heterogeneities in slow adaptation, location and extension of the infarcted area, and the number of sudden cardiac deaths and arrhythmic episodes in these patients. However, the electrophysiological examination of ischemic or post-infarcted patients is usually challenging, due to the high risk of inducibility of ventricular fibrillation during examination in this group of patients. A possible way to circumvent these limitations is the use of clinical effort tests, and estimate APD rate adaptation heterogeneities from body surface ECG biomarkers associated to global dispersion of repolarization and its adaptation, such a QT or T-wave peak-to-end adaptation [21,45].

The ionic mechanisms responsible for LV/RV heterogeneity in APD and APD rate adaptation were not investigated in our study due to the impossibility of conducting the recordings *in vivo*. Previous studies have shown that whereas the human ventricular APD is modulated by a number of repolarization currents [46,47], the slow phase of APD adaptation is primarily determined by Na^+ dynamics, and the Na^+/K^+ pump in particular [20]. It is therefore

likely that the LV/RV differences reported in our study could be caused by heterogeneity in a number of ionic currents such as the I_{to} and I_{Ks} currents as reported in the canine ventricle [8,11], and importantly heterogeneity in Na^+/K^+ pump activity as experimentally reported in the rat ventricles [48]. Further experiments in human using Western immunoblots could be used to quantify expressions of Na^+/K^+ pump and other proteins in the LV and RV to shed light into the ionic mechanisms underlying the LV/RV differences in APD and APD adaptation, characterized in our *in vivo* electrograms.

Study Limitations

Electrograms were acquired under RV apical pacing from patients undergoing interventional procedures for atrial arrhythmias, the intrinsic rhythm in the majority of cases being atrial fibrillation. We can not therefore exclude an influence of these conditions in our results. Furthermore, due to associated practical challenges, our recording sites did only cover a reasonably-sized area within the ventricles. Hence, it would be reasonable to assume that over the whole endocardial surface there would be regions of greater and lesser APD heterogeneity.

Due to ethical constraints, electrograms were recorded following rate acceleration from intrinsic rhythm to CL = 500 ms, and thus the role of CL in determining adaptation dynamics was not investigated in the patients. Studies in isolated rabbit and guinea pig myocytes showed time constants of the slow phase of APD adaptation to decrease linearly with decreasing CL [49]. However, this linear dependence may not be present in tissue with intact cell-to-cell coupling, where adaptation time constants were found to be approximately constant for both large and small changes in CL [43].

In our computer simulations, a 2D model of human ventricular tissue with an idealized inexcitable region was used to test our hypothesis, taking into account the high computational cost associated with the simulations. Therefore, when rendered possible by improvements in computational power, further studies should evaluate the role of LV/RV heterogeneity in modulating the pro-arrhythmic substrate, where additional factors such as 3D structure of the human ventricles are taken into account.

Conclusions

We report for the first time *in vivo* LV/RV heterogeneity in APD and, in particular, APD adaptation dynamics in the human ventricle, which are responsible for a transient increase in APD dispersion following rate acceleration. Our *in silico* investigations suggest that patients with LV/RV heterogeneous APD adaptation dynamics might be at higher risk of developing arrhythmias (particularly following an ischemic event), due to a higher likelihood of conduction block, reentry and wave-break which could degenerate to ventricular fibrillation. Our combined *in vivo* and *in silico* study provides new insights that offer a mechanistic explanation of the increased risk of cardiac arrhythmias and sudden cardiac death in patients exhibiting protracted QT adaptation, emphasizing the importance of this biomarker in arrhythmic risk stratification.

Supporting Information

Figure S1 Unipolar electrocardiogram (UEG) postprocessing flowchart.

Figure S2 The slow phase of APD adaptation does not facilitate reentrant wave-break. A: Sustained wave-break when reentry is initiated in a steep APD restitution region, with homogeneous slow time constant of APD adaptation ($\tau^s = 50$ s). B: Stable reentry pattern after reentry initiation in a flatter APD restitution region, with linear apico-basal gradient in the slow time constant of APD adaptation ($\tau^s = 20$–80 s). Times indicated since initiation of reentry (ms); colorbar denotes transmembrane potential (mV).

Table S1 Calibration of the methodology for estimation of slow time constants of APD adaptation. Top: Parameter sets used to generate the synthetic APD series. **Bottom:** Estimated slow time constants of APD adaptation (mean±SD) for different noise instantiations ($n = 100$). Compare results with the last row of the top part of the table.

Text S1 Expanded methods and results.

Author Contributions

Conceived and designed the experiments: PT JG. Performed the experiments: JG. Analyzed the data: ABO BH. Contributed reagents/materials/analysis tools: ABO BH. Wrote the paper: ABO BH JG PT BR.

References

1. Kuo CS, Munakata K, Reddy CP, Surawicz B (1983) Characteristics and possible mechanisms of ventricular arrhythmia dependent on the dispersion of action potential durations. Circulation 67: 1356–1357.
2. Morgan JM, Cunningham D, Rowland E (1992) Dispersion of monophasic action potential duration: demonstrable in humans after premature ventricular extrastimulation but not in steady state. J Am Coll Cardiol 19: 1244–1253.
3. Yuan S, Wohlfart B, Olsson SB, Blomstrom-Lundqvist C (1995) The dispersion of repolarization in patients with ventricular tachycardia. A study using simultaneous monophasic action potential recordings from two sites in the right ventricle. Eur Heart J 16: 68–76.
4. Clayton RH, Taggart P (2005) Regional differences in APD restitution can initiate wavebreak and re-entry in cardiac tissue: a computational study. Biomed Eng Online 20: 4–54.
5. Nash MP, Bradley CP, Sutton PM, Clayton RH, Kallis P, et al. (2006) Whole heart action potential duration restitution properties in cardiac patients: a combined clinical and modelling study. Exp Physiol 91: 339–354.
6. Samie FH, Berenfeld O, Anumonwo J, Mironov SF, Udassi S, et al. (2001) Rectification of the background potassium current: a determinant of rotor dynamics in ventricular fibrillation. Circ Res 89: 1216–1223.
7. Warren M, Guha PK, Berenfeld O, Zaitsev A, Anumonwo JM, et al. (2003) Blockade of the inward rectifying potassium current terminates ventricular fibrillation in the guinea pig heart. J Cardiovasc Electrophysiol 14: 621–631.
8. Di Diego JM, Sun ZQ, Antzelevitch C (1996) I(to) and action potential notch are smaller in left vs. right canine ventricular epicardium. Am J Physiol 271: H548–H561.
9. Rodriguez B, Li L, Eason JC, Efimov JR, Trayanova NA (2005) Differences between left and right ventricular chamber geometry affect cardiac vulnerability to electric shocks. Circ Res 97: 168–175.
10. Pandit SV, Kaur K, Zlochiver S, Noujaim SF, Furspan P, et al. (2011) Left-to-right ventricular differences in I_{KATP} underlie epicardial repolarization gradient during global ischemia. Heart Rhythm 8: 1732–1739.
11. Volders PG, Sipido KR, Carmeliet E, Spätjens RL, Wellens HJ, et al. (1999) Repolarizing K+ currents I_{TO1} and I_{Ks} are larger in right than left canine ventricular myocardium. Circulation 99: 206–210.
12. Ghanem RJ, Burnes JE, Waldo AL, Rudy Y (2001) Imaging dispersion of myocardial repolarization, II: Noninvasive reconstruction of epicardial measures. Circulation 104: 1306–1312.
13. Yuan S, Kongstad O, Hertervig E, Holm M, Grins E, et al. (2001) Global repolarization sequence of the ventricular endocardium: monophasic action potential mapping in swine and humans. Pacing Clin Electrophysiol 24: 1479–1488.
14. Ramanathan C, Jia P, Ganem R, Ryu K, Rudy Y (2006) Activation and repolarization of the normal heart under complete physiological conditions. Proc Natl Acad Sci USA 103: 6309–6314.
15. Eisenberg SJ, Scheinman MM, Dullet NK, Finkbeiner WE, Griffin JC, et al. (1995) Sudden cardiac death and polymorphous ventricular tachycardia in patients with normal QT intervals and normal systolic cardiac function. Am J Cardiol 75: 687–692.
16. Kop WJ, Verdino RJ, Gottdiener JS, O'Leary ST, Bairey Merz CN, et al. (2001) Changes in heart rate and heart rate variability before ambulatory ischemic events. J Am Coll Cardiol 38: 742–749.
17. Lerma C, Wessel N, Schirdewan A, Kurths J, Glass L (2008) Ventricular arrhythmias and changes in heart rate preceding ventricular tachycardia in patients with an implantable cardioverter defibrillator. Med Biol Eng Comput 46: 715–727.
18. Arnold L, Page J, Attwell D, Cannell MB, Eisner DA (1982) The dependence on heart rate of the human ventricular action potential duration. Cardiovasc Res 16: 547–551.
19. Franz MR, Swerdlow CD, Liem LB, Schaefer J (1988) Cycle length dependence of human action potential duration in vivo. Effects of single extrastimuli, sudden sustained rate acceleration and deceleration, and different steady-state frequencies. J Clin Invest 82: 972–979.
20. Pueyo E, Husti Z, Hornyik T, Baczkó I, Laguna P, et al. (2010) Mechanisms of ventricular rate adaptation as a predictor of arrhythmic risk. Am J Physiol Heart Circ Physiol 298: H1577–H1587.
21. Pueyo E, Smetana P, Caminal P, de Luna AB, Malik M, et al. (2004) Characterization of QT interval adaptation to RR interval changes and its use as a risk-stratifier of arrhythmic mortality in amiodarone-treated survivors of acute myocardial infarction. IEEE Trans Biomed Eng 51: 1511–1520.
22. Gill JS, Baszko A, Xia R, Ward DE, Camm AJ (1993) Dynamics of the QT interval in patients with exercise-induced ventricular tachycardia in normal and abnormal hearts. Am Heart J 126: 1357–1363.
23. Lee KL, Woodlief LH, Topol EJ, Weaver WD, Betriu A, et al. (1995) Predictors of 30-day mortality in the era of reperfusion for acute myocardial infarction. Results from an international trial of 41,021 patients. GUSTO-I Investigators. Circulation 91: 1659–1668.
24. Haim M, Hod H, Reisin L, Kornowski R, Reicher-Reiss H, et al. (1997) Comparison of short- and long-term prognosis in patients with anterior wall versus inferior or lateral wall non-Q-wave acute myocardial infarction. Secondary Prevention Reinfarction Israeli Nifedipine Trial (SPRINT) Study Group. Am J Cardiol 79: 717–721.
25. Hanson BH, Sutton P, Elameri N, Gray M, Critchley H, et al. (2009) Interaction of activation-repolarization coupling and restitution properties in humans. Circ Arrhythm Electrophysiol 2: 162–170.
26. Coronel R, de Bakker JMT, Wilms-Schopman FJG, Opthof T, Linnenbank AC, et al. (2006) Monophasic action potentials and activation recovery intervals as measures of action potential duration: experimental evidence to resolve some controversies. Heart Rhythm 3: 1043–1050.
27. Steinbaus BM (1989) Estimating cardiac transmembrane activation and recovery times from unipolar and bipolar extracellular electrograms: a simulation study. Circ Res 64: 449–462.
28. Yue AM, Paisey JR, Robinson S, Betts TR, Roberts PR, et al. (2004) Determination of human ventricular repolarization by noncontact mapping. Validation with monophasic action potential recordings. Circulation 110: 1343–1350.

29. Western DG, Taggart P, Hanson BM (2010) Real-time feedback of dynamic cardiac repolarization properties. Ann Intl Conf IEEE EMBS 114–117.

30. Pitt-Francis J, Pathmanathan P, Bernabeu MO, Bordas R, Cooper J, et al. (2009) Chaste: a test-driven approach to software development for biological modelling. Comp Phys Comm 180: 2452–2471.

31. Bueno-Orovio A, Cherry EM, Fenton FH (2008) Minimal model for human ventricular action potentials in tissue. J Theor Biol 253: 544–560.

32. Udelnov MG (1961) The role of necrosis in the origin of electrocardiographic alterations characteristic of myocardial infarction. Circulation 24: 110–122.

33. Jiang Y, Qian C, Hanna R, Farina D, Dössel O (2009) Optimization of electrode positions of a wearable ECG monitoring system for efficient and effective detection of acute myocardial infarction. Comput Cardiol 36: 293–296.

34. Lysaker M, Nielsen BJ (2006) Towards a level set framework for infarction modeling: An inverse problem. Int J Numer Anal Model 3: 377–394.

35. Taggart P, Sutton PM, Opthof T, Coronel R, Trimlett R, et al. (2000) Inhomogeneous transmural conduction during early ischemia in patients with coronary artery disease. J Mol Cell Cardiol 32: 621–639.

36. Bueno-Orovio A, Pérez-García VM, Fenton FH (2006) Spectral methods for partial differential equations in irregular domains: The spectral smoothed boundary method. SIAM J Sci Comput 28: 886–900.

37. Taggart P, Sutton PM (1999) Cardiac mechano-electric feedback in man: clinical relevance. Prog Biophys Mol Biol 71: 139–154.

38. Qu Z, Garfinkel A, Weiss JN (2006) Vulnerable window for conduction block in a one-dimensional cable of cardiac cells, 1: single extrasystoles. Biophys J 91: 793–804.

39. Qu Z, Garfinkel A, Weiss JN (2006) Vulnerable window for conduction block in a one-dimensional cable of cardiac cells, 1: multiple extrasystoles. Biophys J 91: 805–815.

40. Coronel R, Wilms-Schopman FJG, Opthop T, Janse MJ (2009) Dispersion of repolarization and arrhythmogenesis. Heart Rhythm 6: 537–543.

41. Fenton FH, Evans SJ, Hastings HM (1999) Memory in an excitable medium: a mechanism for spiral wave breakup in the low-excitability limit. Phys Rev Lett 83: 3964–3967.

42. Baher A, Qu Z, Hayatdavoudi A, Lamp ST, Yang MJ, et al. (2007) Short-term cardiac memory and mother rotor fibrillation. Am J Physiol Heart Circ Physiol 292: H180–H189.

43. Mironov S, Jalife J, Tolkacheva EG (2008) Role of conduction velocity restitution and short-term memory in the development of action potential duration alternans in isolated rabbit hearts. Circulation 118: 17–25.

44. Pitruzzello AM, Krassowska W, Idriss SF (2007) Spatial heterogeneity of the restitution portrait in rabbit epicardium. Am J Physiol Heart Circ Physiol 292: H1568–H1578.

45. Mincholé A, Pueyo E, Rodríguez JF, Zacur E, Doblaré M, et al. (2011) Quantification of restitution dispersion from the dynamic changes of the T-wave peak to end, measured at the surface ECG. IEEE Trans Biomed Eng 58: 1172–1182.

46. Romero L, Pueyo E, Fink M, Rodriguez B (2009) Impact of biological variability on human ventricular cellular electrophysiology. Am J Physiol Heart Circ Physiol 297: H1436–H1445.

47. Szentadrassy N, Banyasz T, Biro T, Szabo G, Toth BI, et al. (2005) Apico-basal inhomogeneity in distribution of ion channels in canine and human ventricular myocardium. Cardiovasc Res 65: 851–860.

48. Komniski MS, Yakushev S, Bogdanov N, Gassmann M, Bogdanova A (2011) Interventricular heterogeneity in rat heart response to hypoxia: the tuning of glucose metabolism, ion gradients, and function. Am J Physiol Heart Circ Physiol 300: H1645–H1652.

49. Tolkacheva EG, Anumonwo JMB, Jalife J (2006) Action potential duration restitution portraits of mammalian ventricular myocytes: role of calcium current. Biophys J 91: 2735–2745.

4

How Often Should We Monitor for Reliable Detection of Atrial Fibrillation Recurrence? Efficiency Considerations and Implications for Study Design

Efstratios I. Charitos[1]*, **Paul D. Ziegler**[2], **Ulrich Stierle**[1], **Derek R. Robinson**[3], **Bernhard Graf**[1], **Hans-Hinrich Sievers**[1], **Thorsten Hanke**[1]

1 Department of Cardiac and Thoracic Vascular Surgery, University of Luebeck, Luebeck, Germany, **2** Medtronic Inc., Minneapolis, Minnesota, United States of America, **3** Department of Mathematics, School of Mathematical and Physical Sciences, University of Sussex, Brighton, United Kingdom

Abstract

Objective: Although atrial fibrillation (AF) recurrence is unpredictable in terms of onset and duration, current intermittent rhythm monitoring (IRM) diagnostic modalities are short-termed and discontinuous. The aim of the present study was to investigate the necessary IRM frequency required to reliably detect recurrence of various AF recurrence patterns.

Methods: The rhythm histories of 647 patients (mean AF burden: 12±22% of monitored time; 687 patient-years) with implantable continuous monitoring devices were reconstructed and analyzed. With the use of computationally intensive simulation, we evaluated the necessary IRM frequency to reliably detect AF recurrence of various AF phenotypes using IRM of various durations.

Results: The IRM frequency required for reliable AF detection depends on the amount and temporal aggregation of the AF recurrence (p<0.0001) as well as the duration of the IRM (p<0.001). Reliable detection (>95% sensitivity) of AF recurrence required higher IRM frequencies (>12 24-hour; >6 7-day; >4 14-day; >3 30-day IRM per year; p<0.0001) than currently recommended. Lower IRM frequencies will under-detect AF recurrence and introduce significant bias in the evaluation of therapeutic interventions. More frequent but of shorter duration, IRMs (24-hour) are significantly more time effective (sensitivity per monitored time) than a fewer number of longer IRM durations (p<0.0001).

Conclusions: Reliable AF recurrence detection requires higher IRM frequencies than currently recommended. Current IRM frequency recommendations will fail to diagnose a significant proportion of patients. Shorter duration but more frequent IRM strategies are significantly more efficient than longer IRM durations.

Editor: Alena Talkachova, University of Minnesota, United States of America

Funding: The computational resources for this work were kindly provided by AWS WA, USA (Education Coursework Grant Award: EDU_Charitos_ULuebeckResearch_Fall2012). The grant donor had no role in study design, data collection and analysis, decision to publish, or preparation of the manuscript.

Competing Interests: Drs Charitos, Stierle, Graf, Robinson, and Sievers have no conflict of interest to disclose. Dr. Hanke has received modest lecture honoraria from Medtronic (<10.000 USD). Mr. Ziegler is an employee and stockholder of Medtronic (>10.000 USD).

* E-mail: efstratios.charitos@gmail.com

Introduction

The diagnosis of atrial fibrillation (AF) and the detection of its recurrence after therapeutic interventions are typically performed by electrocardiographic documentation. Reliable and accurate detection of AF recurrence is challenging since its rhythm documentation is discontinuous, whereas the recurrence of AF is often unpredictable [1] and may or may not be accompanied by symptoms [2,3]. Accurate AF recurrence detection is of importance not only for patient management, but also for the scientific, evidence-based evaluation of therapeutic interventions targeting AF recurrence. Under-detection of AF recurrence introduces a significant external bias, distorts the success rates, and thus affects the scientific evaluation of therapeutic interventions.

Implantable, subcutaneous, leadless as well as intra-cardiac continuous monitoring (CM) devices can reliably detect AF [4–8]. However, due to cost considerations and invasiveness of CM, intermittent rhythm monitoring strategies (IRM) of various durations and frequencies are still the most widely used diagnostic modalities for patient monitoring and reporting outcomes. Several groups have compared the efficiency of various IRM strategies with CM devices [5,6,9–11]. It is now a general consensus that IRM will fail to detect AF recurrence, albeit in a percentage of patients that is unknown and difficult to prospectively estimate [5,6,12,13]. The sensitivity of IRM has been reported to range between 30% and 70% for patients with paroxysmal AF [5,6,12,13]. Our group has previously shown that the success rate of any IRM strategy depends on four factors: the quantitative and temporal characteristics of atrial fibrillation recurrence as well as the frequency and duration of the IRMs performed to detect AF recurrence [5].

The aim of the present manuscript is to investigate the IRM frequencies required to reliably (at least 80% or 95% probability) detect AF recurrence of various AF phenotypes and with various IRM durations. We discuss efficiency considerations as well as implications for clinical trial design.

Methods

Data acquired from 647 patients monitored with a CM device (Reveal XT cardiac monitor, n = 73; AT500 pacemaker, n = 574; Medtronic, Inc., Minneapolis, MN, USA) were analyzed. Demographics and detailed patient characteristics are displayed in **Table 1**. All patients provided written informed consent for data collection and use. The study has been approved by the local (University of Lübeck) ethics committee (**Clinical Trial Registration URL**: http://www.clinicaltrials.gov **unique identifier**: NCT00806689). The complete rhythm history of each patient was reconstructed from the CM data. AF burden was defined as the proportion of the total monitored time that a patient was in AF. For example, a patient that spends 50% of the time in AF, has an AF burden of 0.5. However, the AF burden alone cannot describe the temporal characteristics of AF recurrence. For example in **Figure 1A and 1B**, the patients A and B have the same overall amount of AF (AF burden = 0.173) but this AF burden is distributed differently throughout the observation period. To describe the distribution pattern of the AF recurrence we previously proposed the AF density [5,14], as a quantitative measure of the temporal aggregation of the AF burden consisting of values between 0 (AF burden evenly spread over the observation time) and 1 (maximum possible AF burden aggregation, i.e. the complete AF burden occurs as one continuous episode of AF). Details on the calculation of the AF density have been presented in detail previously [5,14]. In brief, for each patient, the time course of the AF burden development was analyzed throughout the monitored period (**Figure 1A and 1B, for patients A and B respectively**) and the *minimum contiguous monitored time* required for the development of each proportion of the patient's total observed AF burden throughout the monitored period was calculated and evaluated for the overall observation period (blue or red dotted line, **Figure 1E and 1F**, respectively). Patient A (**Figure 1A**) develops 10%, 30%, 50%, 70% and 90% of his total observed burden in 2%, 5%, 9%, 13% and 21% of the total monitored time, respectively (blue dotted line, **Figure 1E**), and most of the AF recurrence and burden development occurs between days 30 and 80. This information on the temporal burden development of patient A is displayed in **Figure 1E**. In contrast, patient B (**Figure 1B**) develops 10%, 30%, 50%, 70% and 90% of his total observed burden in 6%, 24%, 48%, 71% and 89% of the total monitored time respectively, since the total burden is spread over more days and as such each day contributes less to the total burden development. This information on the temporal burden development of patient B is displayed in **Figure 1F**. The black diagonal line (**Figure 1E and 1F**) represent the hypothetical development of the patient's AF burden if this burden had been uniformly distributed over the monitored time (same AF duration every day throughout the observation period, uniform burden, **Figure 1C and 1G**). The green dotted line (**Figure 1H**) represents the burden development of a hypothetical patient in which the AF burden (equal in amount to that of patient A and B) occurs as one single continuous episode (maximum density, **Figure 1D**).

For the calculation of the AF density as a measure of temporal AF burden aggregation, the patient's complete rhythm history is scanned and the *minimum contiguous time* required to develop each proportion p of the patients total burden b is calculated (red and blue dotted line, **Figure 1E and 1F**). We define as *AF density*, the ratio of the cumulative deviation of the patient's actual burden development (blue or red area, **Figure 1E and 1F**, respectively) from the hypothetical uniform burden development (black diagonal line, **Figure 1E and 1F**), to that of the hypothetical maximum possible burden aggregation for that level of burden from the hypothetical uniform burden development (the complete burden as one continuous episode, green area, **Figure 1H**). The black diagonal (**Figures 1E, 1F, 1G, 1H**) represents a hypothetical uniform burden aggregation (**Figure 1C**).

For the numerical evaluation of the AF density we define: For a patient with a total AF burden b (expressed as the proportion of the observation time the patient is in AF), who is monitored for time T, we denote the *minimum* contiguous monitored time throughout the monitored period T required for the development of a proportion p of the patient's total observed burden (b) as $T(p; b)$. This time, expressed as the proportion of the total observed time T, is

$$F(p; b) = \frac{T(p; b)}{T}.$$

Figures such as **1E** and **1F** are plots of p against $F(p;b)$ for $0 \leq p \leq 1$.

The cumulative deviation of the patient's actual burden development from the hypothetical uniform burden development (black diagonal line, **Figure 1E, 1F, 1G, 1H**) can be evaluated as

$$\int_0^1 |F(p; b) - p| dp$$

and is equal to the shaded area (**blue shaded area for patient A, Figure 1E; red shaded area for patient B; Figure 1F**). For the hypothetical patient with maximum temporal aggregation of burden b (the complete burden as one continuous AF episode) the cumulative deviation of this patient's burden development (green line, **Figure 1H**) from the hypothetical uniform burden development (black diagonal line, **Figure 1G**) is evaluated as

$$\frac{1 - b}{2}$$

and is equal to the green shaded area (**Figure 1H**). AF density for patients A and B is then the ratio of the blue or red areas respectively, to the green shaded area and is defined as:

$$AF density = 2 * \frac{\int_0^1 |F(p; b) - p| dp}{1 - b}.$$

The AF density as the ratio of the above mentioned areas is therefore a dimensionless quantity and assumes values between 0 and 1, with values close to 0 denoting low burden aggregation (AF burden evenly spread throughout the monitored period, **Figure 1B & 1F** as well as **Figure 1C & 1G**), whereas values close to 1 denote maximal burden temporal aggregation (the complete AF burden occurring as a single continuous episode or "a block of AF", **Figure 1A & 1E** as well as **Figure 1D & 1H**).

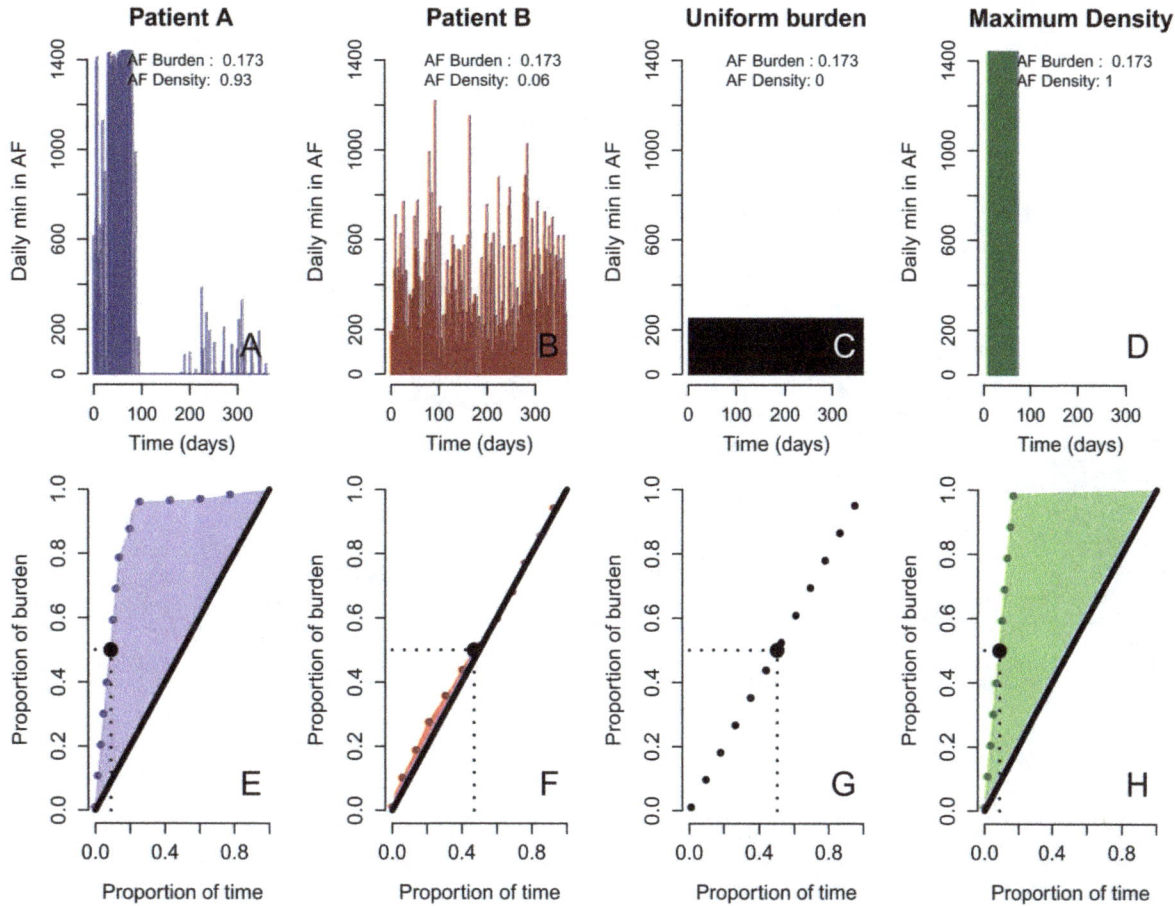

Figure 1. Four examples of different temporal aggregation for the same AF burden (0.173). After reconstruction of the rhythm history (upper panels), the minimum time required for the development of each proportion of the patient's total observed AF burden throughout the monitored period is evaluated (lower panels, dotted lines). AF density is defined as the ratio of the cumulative deviation of the patient's actual burden development (blue or red area) from the uniform burden development (black diagonal line, lower panels and Uniform Burden), to that of the maximum possible burden aggregation for that level of burden (the complete burden as one continuous episode, green area). The black diagonal (lower panels) represents a hypothetical uniform burden aggregation (Uniform Burden). Adapted from [14].

After reconstruction of each patient's complete rhythm history, we used computationally intensive simulation to repeatedly simulate IRM of various durations (1, 7, 14, 30 days) and frequencies (1, 2, 3, ...,12 as appropriate) in every patient. The stochastic process of the simulation procedure was the following: After reconstructing the rhythm history of every patient j, monitored for a total of g days, we defined the sample space $\Omega_{kj} = \{1, 2, ..., g-k+1\}$ to be the set of possible days that a k-day intermittent monitoring session could be started (for $k = 1, 2, 3, ..., 30$). A k-day monitoring session starting on day $i \in \Omega_{kj}$ therefore included the following associated monitored days: $\{i, i+1, ..., i+k-1\}$. To simulate a strategy of n independent k-day monitorings of patient j, n elements were selected at random from Ω_{kj}, except that elements were rejected if their monitored days intersected with the monitored days of previously selected elements. This was performed for all patients of the study population, for monitoring durations of $k = \{1,2,3...,30\}$ days, and for strategies of $n = \{1, 2, 3, ..., 12\}$ monitorings per year, where appropriate. In every simulated IRM, AF was deemed to have been successfully identified if it was observed on at least one of the monitored days. The simulations were performed in all patients, for every IRM strategy (all IRM frequencies and IRM

durations) sufficient times ($>10^5$) to allow stabilization of the inferred probability of AF burden recurrence.

In order to mimic the typical timely follow-up strategy employed in clinical trials, the simulation worked as follows: First, the "first day" of the first monitoring period (IRM) was chosen at random, and then the subsequent k-1 days were counted to make a k day monitoring period (IRM). An example is illustrated in **Figure 2** for the simulation of 7-day monitoring. The first sampled day happened to be on day 179, therefore the 7-day IRM would be on days 179–185. Any future sampling that includes days 173–191 will be rejected (i.e., any 7-day IRM starting on these days would intersect with the sampled IRM on days 179–185).

Second, the simulation procedure then scans the total observation period of the patient and at even intervals (based on the pre-specified IRM frequency) attaches weights at the following days: first sampled day$\pm$k*(365/sampling strategy frequency), where $k = \{1,2,3,4, ..., $ sampling strategy frequency$\}$. In the example shown in **Figure 2**, the algorithm attaches higher sampling weights at days 9, 99, 279 and 370. Gaussian smoothing was used to construct a smoothed sampling weight curve (**Figure 2**) such that the zeniths have about 3 times higher probability to be sampled than the nadirs. Attaching higher sampling probability weights at even intervals mimics the follow-up strategy of clinical

Table 1.

	Total	%
Male	376	58.1
Age	68.9±12.3	
Follow up (mean ± sd, range; years)	1.1±0.4, 0.1–3.7	
History of Atrial Arrhythmia		
Atrial Tachycardia	114	17.6
Atrial Flutter	176	27.2
Paroxysmal AF	475	73.4
Persistent AF	32	4.9
Long lasting persistent AF	35	5.4
History of Cardioversion	18	2.8
Cardiovascular History		
Ischemic Heart Disease	99	15.3
Coronary Artery Disease	220	34.0
Cardiomyopathy	64	9.9
Hypertension	405	62.6
History of ablation for AF		
Cox-Maze III	17	2.6
Left sided only	53	8.2
AV Node Ablation	28	4.3
Other	71	11.0
History of Cardiac Surgery		
CABG	113	17.5
MVR	45	7.0
AVR	41	6.3
TVR	7	1.1
Asc. Aorta Replacement	9	1.4
PVR	1	0.2
NYHA Class		
I	331	51.2
II	234	36.2
III	67	10.4
IV	3	0.5
Pacing Indication		
AV-Block	85	13.1
Sinus node dysfunction	397	61.4
Other	41	6.3
Arrhythmia related medication		
Class I	89	13.8
Class III	251	38.8
Beta-Blocker	212	32.8
Calcium Channel Blocker	56	8.7
Digoxin	144	22.3

Patient demographics: AF: atrial fibrillation; AV: atrioventricular; CABG: coronary artery bypass grafting; MVR: mitral valve replacement/repair; AVR: aortic valve replacement/repair; TVR: tricuspid valve replacement/repair; PVR: pulmonary valve replacement; NYHA: New York Heart Association.

trials, while also simultaneously allowing some randomness (just as in real life follow-up examinations, patients often are seen slightly before or after their nominal follow-update). Thereafter the

simulation proceeds with sampling from the weighted sample space. For every patient and for every IRM duration and frequency, sufficient simulations were carried out ($>10^5$) to estimate the probability of AF detection accurately. The required IRM frequency to achieve at least 80% ($f_{80\%}$) and at least 95% ($f_{95\%}$) probability of AF detection, could then be determined for each patient and IRM duration. All simulated IRM was of the continuous recording type and patient compliance was assumed to be 100%.

Response surface models were used to evaluate the dependency of the probability of AF detection ($f_{95\%}, f_{80\%}$) on AF burden and density. These models are of the form:

$$y = \beta_0 + \sum_i \beta_i x_i + \sum_i \beta_{ii} x_i^2 + \sum_i \sum_{j<i} \beta_{ij} x_i x_j + \varepsilon$$

In modeling $f_{95\%}$ and $f_{80\%}$ it was found appropriate to use its natural logarithm, so that $y = \ln(f_{95\%}$ or $f_{80\%})$, $x_1 =$ AF burden, $x_2 =$ AF density. Separate models were used for the most commonly used IRM durations (24 hours, 7 days, 14 days and 30 days). Backwards stepwise elimination was used to derive the final models which are presented in **Table 2**.

All simulations were performed on multiple parallel AWS (Amazon Web Services, WA, USA) Elastic Cloud Computing high performance compute clusters (cc8.xlarge) running Ubuntu Server Linux 12.04.01 LTS (AWS Cluster Instances). A primer on the infrastructure and use of high performance cloud computing for biomedical research and simulation studies has been published elsewhere [15,16]. The statistical analyses and simulations were performed with R version 2.15.3 [17]. The P values of 2-sided tests are reported.

Results

Estimation of the probability of AF detection with an intermittent monitoring strategy

For a single IRM of n-days duration and for any given AF burden b, observed during any sufficiently large time frame t $(t>>n)$, the probability of successful AF detection ranges between $\cong b$ and 1. Its exact value within the range $[\cong b, 1]$ depends on the temporal aggregation of the AF recurrence [5]. If the AF occurs as one episode, the probability of AF detection is $\cong b$ (**Figure 3, Patient B**), whereas if the AF recurrence is uniformly distributed throughout the observation time the probability of AF recurrence detection is 1 (**Figure 3, Patient A**). We have shown previously that the AF density can efficiently describe the temporal aggregation and thus the recurrence pattern of the AF burden [5,14]. For the IRM durations examined in the present work, AF burden and AF density had a significant effect in determining the probability of successful AF detection with a single random IRM (for all IRM durations: p<0.0001 for AF burden and AF density, R^2 >85%). Using computationally intensive simulation, similar graphs and relationships can be obtained with IRMs of any duration and/or frequency.

Figure 3 left panel shows the effect of AF burden and density on the probability of AF detection of a single 24 hour IRM. Both Patient A and B have been continuously monitored for 364 days and both have an AF burden of 0.2, however the temporal AF burden distribution differs (**Figure 3 right panel**). Patient A has a low temporal AF aggregation (AF spread throughout the observation period with an AF density of 0.28), whereas patient B has the majority of the AF burden developed only between day 50 and 114 (AF density = 0.98). Due to the high temporal aggregation

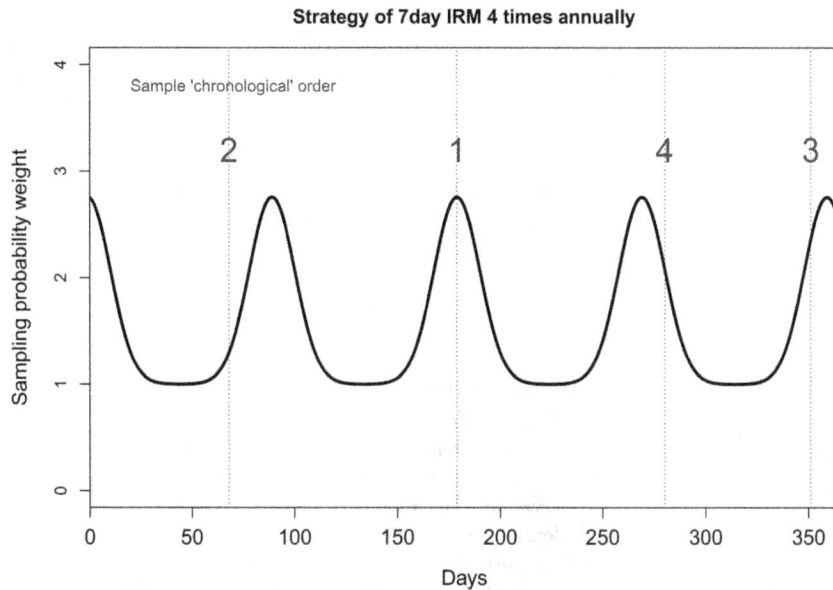

Figure 2. Illustration of the simulation procedure: Initially, the "first day" of the first monitoring period (IRM) was chosen at random, and then the subsequent k-1 days were counted to make a k day monitoring period (IRM). In this example the 7-day IRM would be on days 179–185. Any future sampling that includes days 173–191 will be rejected (any 7 day IRM starting on these days would intersect with the sampled IRM on days 179–185). Second, the simulation procedure scans the total observation period of the patient and at even intervals (based on the pre-specified IRM frequency) attaches weights at the following days: first sampled day±k*(365/sampling strategy frequency), where k={1,2,3,4, ..., sampling strategy frequency}. In this example, the algorithm attaches higher sampling weights at days 9, 99, 279, 370. Gaussian smoothing was used to construct a smoothed sampling weight curve such that the zeniths have about 3 times higher probability to be sampled than the nadirs. Attaching higher sampling probability weights at even intervals mimics the follow-up strategy of clinical trials, while also simultaneously allowing some randomness (just as in real life follow-up examinations, patients often are seen slightly before or after their nominal follow-updatee). Thereafter the simulation proceeds with sampling from the weighted sample space.

(increased AF density), the probability that a random 24-hour IRM will detect AF recurrence in patient B is 0.23. In contrast, in patient A, AF recurrences are distributed over almost every day of the entire monitored time and thus the probability of AF recurrence detection is much higher, 0.9.

Frequency of IRM required to reliably detect AF recurrence according to AF burden and AF density

Since the probability of successful AF identification depends on the AF characteristics (AF burden and AF density), inferences can be drawn regarding how many times IRM should be performed in order to reliably (probability >95%) detect AF recurrence. **Table 2** presents the results of the regression analyses, of the AF characteristics on the required IRM frequency to achieve >95% probability for AF detection. These results are more clearly visualized in **Figures 4–7** which present the frequency of IRM required to detect AF recurrence with 80% and 95% probability as a function of the AF characteristics (AF burden and AF density). For all IRM durations, the IRM frequency required to detect AF recurrence with a 95% probability increases as the AF burden decreases and as the AF density increases (AF burden less spread throughout the observation time) (**Table 2**).

Figures 4–7 indicate that strategies of twelve 24-hour, six 7-day, four 14-day and three 30-day per year will be able to detect on average 96%, 95%, 91%, 90% of all AF recurrence phenotypes (AF burden/AF density combinations) with a probability of 95% (area below the respective IRM frequency dotted lines, **Figure 4–7**). In our patient population, which had a mean burden of 0.12±0.22, the above mentioned IRM strategies would succeed in diagnosing AF recurrence in 83%, 77%, 70%, 68% of these patients (dots below the respective IRM frequency lines, **Figure 4–7**). Patients with even

lower burdens and/or higher densities (dots above the respective IRM frequency lines, **Figure 4–7**) will require more aggressive monitoring strategies which increases the likelihood of poor compliance.

Time efficiency as a function of AF burden and AF density

The time efficiency (sensitivity obtained per day of IRM) was dependent on both AF characteristics (AF burden and AF density) and IRM characteristics (IRM duration and IRM frequency; p<0.001 for all). For the same overall IRM duration, the 24-hour IRM results in higher sensitivity per unit of monitored time than prolonged IRM durations (**Figure 8**). As **Figures 4–7** show, strategies of twelve 24-hour, six 7-day, four 14-day and three 30-day per year will be able to detect on average 96%, 95%, 91% and 90% of all AF recurrence phenotypes (AF burden/AF density combinations) with a probability of 95%, or 83%, 77%, 70% and 68% of our patient population, respectively. However to obtain these sensitivities, these strategies would require a total monitoring time of 12, 42, 56, and 90 days for the 24-hour, 7-day, 14-day and 30-day IRM, respectively.

Discussion

Currently the most widely used diagnostic modality for the detection of AF recurrence is IRM. However, in contrast to other diagnostic examinations in medicine which are required to have the highest possible sensitivity and specificity, the absence of non-invasive and cost efficient alternatives has made IRM a standard for AF recurrence detection and rhythm follow-up even though its sensitivity as a diagnostic test is strikingly low [5,6,11–13,18].

Table 2. Regression (response surface models) of the AF characteristics (AF burden, AF density) on the IRM frequencies required to achieve 95% probability of AF recurrence detection.

Factor	Coefficient (mean±SE)	p
24h IRM model (R² = 70.4%)		
Intercept	−2.01±0.08	<0.001
AF Burden	−4.82±0.40	<0.001
AF Density	1.3±0.11	<0.001
AF Burden²	2.13±0.42	<0.001
7d IRM model (R² = 70.2%)		
Intercept	0.88±0.07	<0.001
AF Burden	−5.09±0.35	<0.001
AF Density	1.90±0.10	<0.001
AF Burden²	3.03±0.39	<0.001
14d IRM model (R² = 69.4%)		
Intercept	0.52±0.06	<0.001
AF Burden	−4.40±0.32	<0.001
AF Density	1.89±0.10	<0.001
AF Burden²	2.67±0.37	<0.001
30d IRM model (R² = 60.4%)		
Intercept	0.22±0.10	0.03
AF Burden	−2.52±0.27	<0.001
AF Density	1.11±0.39	<0.001
AF Burden²	1.32±0.31	<0.001

To restore normality, the natural logarithm of the required IRM frequency was regressed. Separate models were fit for the four IRM modalities (24-hour, 7-day, 14-day, and 30-day). *SE: standard error, IRM: intermittent rhythm monitor, AF: atrial fibrillation.*

Since the identification of AF recurrence is seminal importance for accurate patient management and for the scientific evaluation of therapeutic AF interventions, we sought to determine the frequency of IRMs required to identify AF recurrence with 80% and 95% probability.

Determining the probability of AF detection

Our results indicate that the quantitative AF characteristics (AF burden and AF density) as well as the IRM strategy characteristics (IRM frequency and IRM duration) can determine the probability of successful AF identification using IRM. **Figure 3 Left Panel** shows the interrelation between AF burden and AF density in determining the probability of AF identification with a single random 24-hour IRM. Similar relationships can be obtained for other IRM durations as well as IRM frequencies. Our analyses show that the probability of AF identification increases as the AF density decreases (AF recurrence spread more evenly throughout the observation time) and/or AF burden increases. The influence of AF density on the AF detection probability for any IRM is of critical importance at lower burdens (<0.5) and diminishes progressively at higher (>0.5) AF burdens (**Figure 3 Left Panel**).

Current guidelines and consensus statements address the need for intermittent monitoring for the detection of AF recurrence [12,13,18]. Although most recommendations suggest an IRM monitoring strategy between two and four 24-hour IRM per year for the detection of AF recurrence, most statements simultaneously note that these strategies have a limited sensitivity and a significant proportion of patients with AF recurrence will not be detected. A speculative estimate is that IRM strategies may detect up to 70% of patients with AF recurrence and may have a negative predictive value of up to 50% [12,13,18]. However these estimates, which stem from published studies, cannot be reliably transferred to other studies or other prospectively recruited populations. Our results point out that the sensitivity and thus the required frequency to reliably detect AF recurrence, depends largely on the AF and IRM characteristics and may deviate from the above

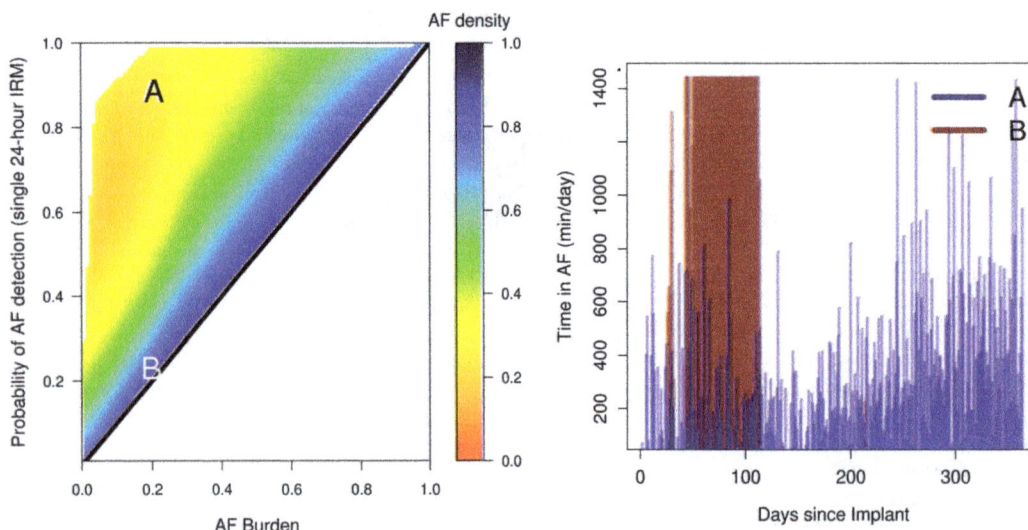

Figure 3. The effect of AF burden and AF density on the probability of AF detection with a single 24-hour IRM (left panel) for the AF recurrence pattern of two example patients (right panel). For any given AF burden b, observed during any time frame, the probability of successful identification using a given IRM duration ranges between ≅b and 1. The range [≅b,1] depends on the temporal aggregation of the AF recurrences (AF density). If the AF occurs as one episode, the probability of AF detection is ≅b (**Patient B**), whereas if the AF recurrence is uniformly spread throughout the observation time the probability of AF recurrence detection is 1 (**Patient A**). *IRM: intermittent rhythm monitor, AF: atrial fibrillation.*

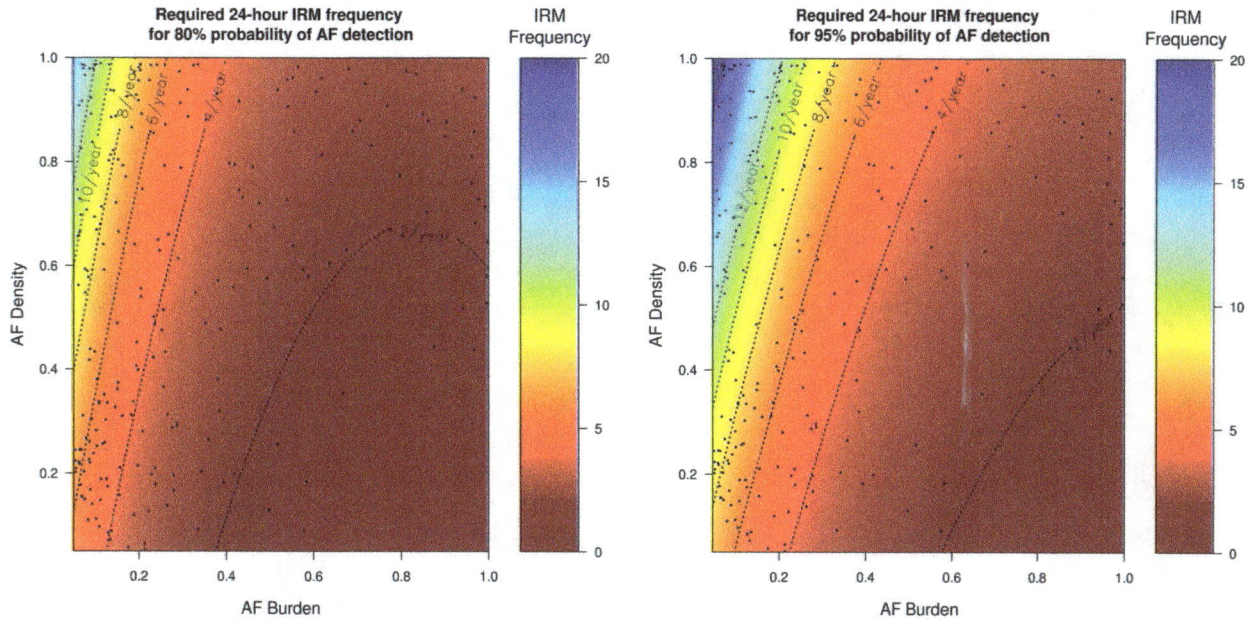

Figure 4. Required 24-hour IRM frequency to achieve 80% (left) and 95% (right) probability of AF detection. The black dots represent our patient population. *IRM: intermittent rhythm monitor, AF: atrial fibrillation.*

estimates. For example, as **Figure 4** illustrates, a strategy of four 24-hour IRMs would fail to identify 75% of our patient population with otherwise proven AF recurrence (**Figure 4**, percentage of black dots being above and to the left of the 4/year dotted line).

Do longer IRM durations lead to increased AF detection?

In light of the limitation of short duration IRM, longer IRM durations have been proposed for more accurate AF recurrence detection. We and others have previously seen that on average, longer duration IRM indeed results in more accurate AF

recurrence detection [5,6]. However, longer IRM pose two distinct disadvantages:

First, the benefit of longer IRM is not linear with respect to the monitoring time. Especially in patients with high density AF, longer IRM may result in little or no practical benefit in terms of the probability of AF recurrence detection [5,14]. The efficiency of longer IRMs diminishes as the monitoring time increases. This is presented in **Figure 8**. When considering the monitored days (the number of days the patient wears the IRM), the 24-hour IRM achieves higher sensitivities, with less monitoring days than all

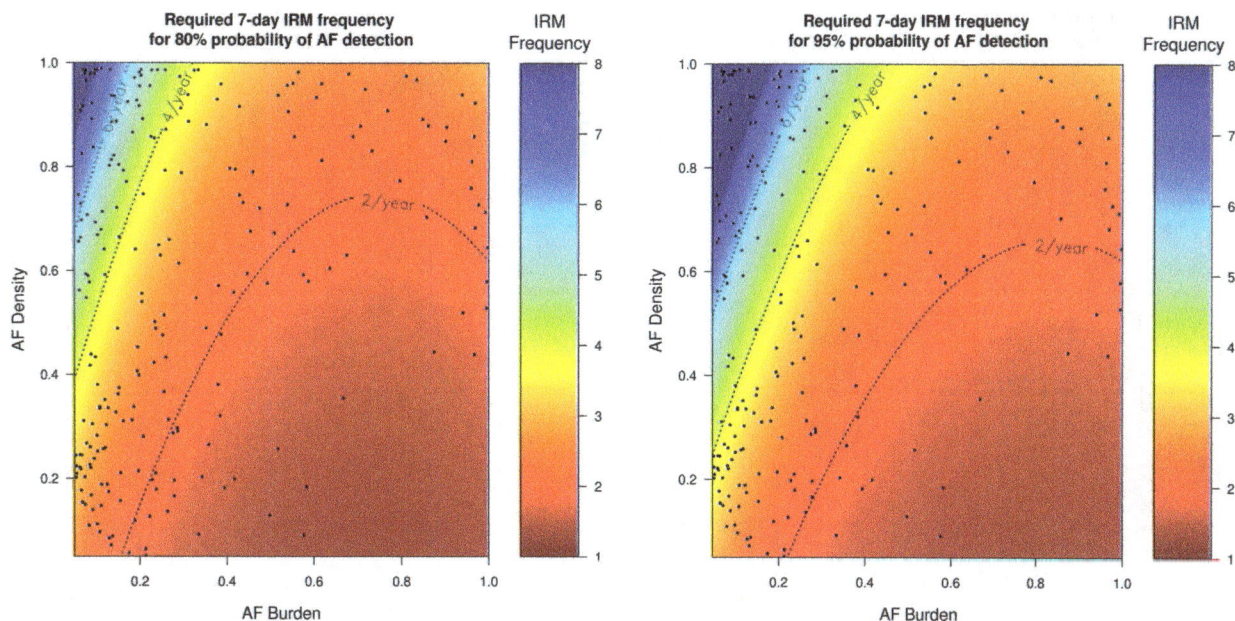

Figure 5. Required 7-day IRM frequency to achieve 80% (left) and 95% (right) probability of AF detection. The black dots represent our patient population. *IRM: intermittent rhythm monitor, AF: atrial fibrillation.*

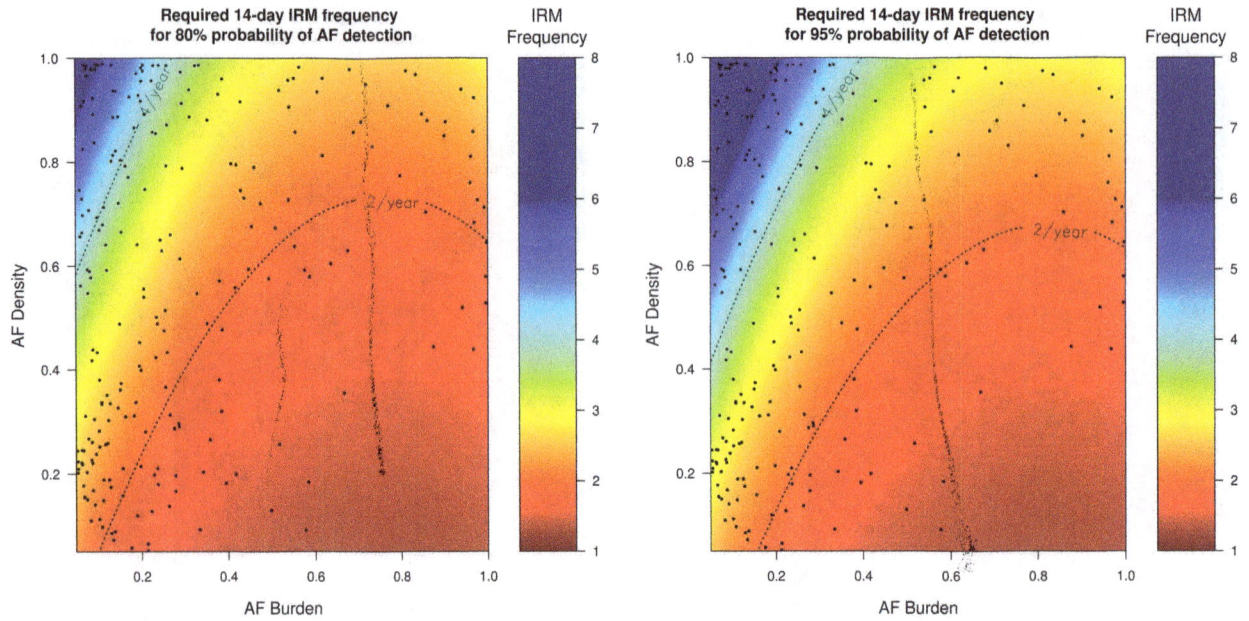

Figure 6. Required 14-day IRM frequency to achieve 80% (left) and 95% (right) probability of AF detection. The black dots represent our patient population. *IRM: intermittent rhythm monitor, AF: atrial fibrillation.*

other prolonged IRM durations. This stems from the fact that an *n*-day IRM will only be able to detect AF recurrence taking place within the *n* consecutive days from the start of the IRM, whereas, 24-hour IRMs are performed *n* times at *n* different time points during the follow-up period and thus will be able on average to detect AF recurrence with greater probability. This is especially important for patients with paroxysmal AF as it has been shown that paroxysmal AF frequently recurs in clusters (higher AF density, low AF burdens) [1] thus monitoring for AF at *n* different

time points is more advantageous than monitoring *n* consecutive days.

Second, there is now significant evidence that longer IRM durations adversely affect patient compliance[12]. Reported causes of patient non-compliance with scheduled monitoring include skin irritation, interference with showering or exercise, and feelings of self-consciousness when wearing the monitoring equipment in public[19]. A recent study with an external arrhythmia monitoring patch reported that the device fell off in 22% of patients and resulted in a mean wear time of 7.9 ± 1.8 days

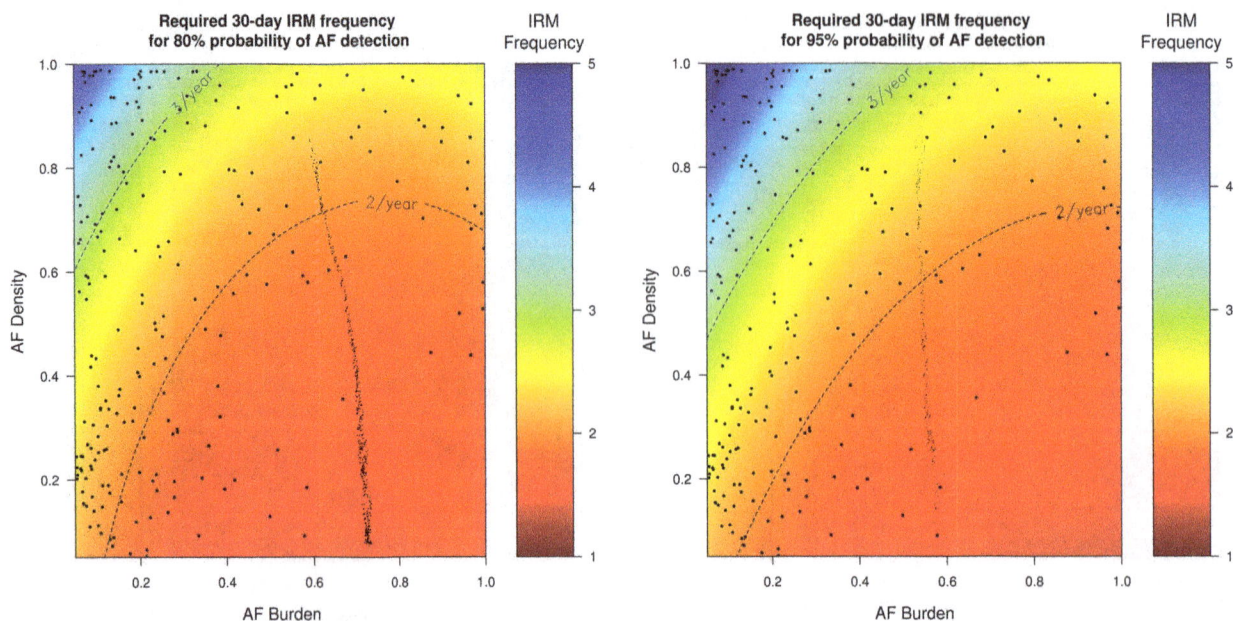

Figure 7. Required 30-day IRM frequency to achieve 80% (left) and 95% (right) probability of AF detection. The black dots represent our patient population. *IRM: intermittent rhythm monitor, AF: atrial fibrillation.*

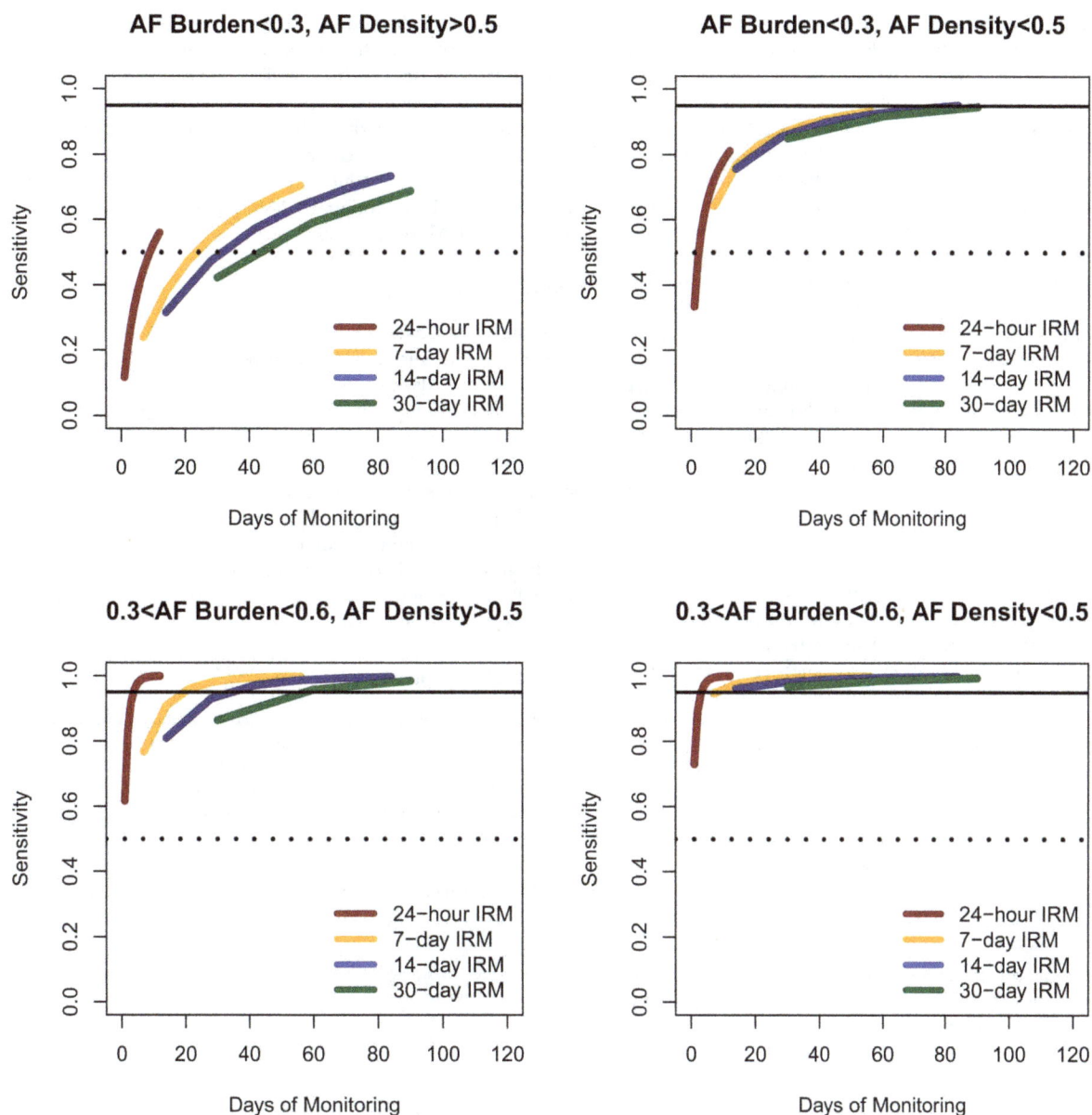

Figure 8. Time efficiency (sensitivity obtained per monitored day) of IRM strategies. For the same amount of total monitored time, shorter IRM durations result in higher sensitivities. The dotted and solid horizontal line represents sensitivities of 0.5 and 0.95 respectively. *IRM: intermittent rhythm monitor, AF: atrial fibrillation.*

instead of the planned 14 days[20]. Kamel at al. reported that patients randomized to monitoring via mobile cardiac outpatient telemetry wore the monitors for 64% of the assigned days and that 25% of patients were not compliant at all with the scheduled monitoring [21]. In another study which utilized the same monitoring technology in 19 patients who recently underwent catheter ablation for AF, only 53% of patients complied with the scheduled monitoring[22]. Shorter, but more frequent IRMs tend to have much higher patient compliance and may result in better AF recurrence detection under real life conditions. Additionally, shorter IRMs performed more frequently may lead to less patient discomfort and disruption of daily activities.

Intermittent rhythm monitoring in the era of continuous monitoring

Although an aggressive monitoring strategy of twelve 24-hour IRM per year may reliably detect the great majority of patients (83.4% of our patient population, 96.0% of the AF burden/AF density plane, **Figure 3**), it should be noted that there is still an element of chance in this process (80% or 95% probability of AF detection) and some patients may be misclassified. This seems to be of importance when designing clinical studies, especially when the outcome of interest is of low incidence. Furthermore, such aggressive strategies still require considerable amount of resources as well as patient compliance and physician commitment.

Continuous monitoring is an attractive alternative to IRM. Indeed, several studies lately have recently surfaced in which follow-up of patients usually after therapeutic interventions for AF is being performed using implantable subcutaneous monitoring devices or using the readings of intra-cardiac devices capable of detecting and recording AF recurrence. A great advantage of this approach is that these devices not only allow much more accurate AF recurrence detection but also can provide the calculation of quantitative AF indices (e.g. AF burden) and may allow better understanding of the AF recurrence dynamics. However, the implantation of leadless CM requires a minor surgical procedure which may carry a small risk of infection or patient discomfort. CM has a higher initial cost, however rhythm disclosure and reporting can be reported remotely via telemetry and patient visits can be scheduled on an "as needed" basis [23]. Additionally, the current generation of implantable leadless CM devices can provide rhythm disclosure for at least 3 years after implantation, a fact which may increase the cost efficiency of CM over that period. Although intra-cardiac and leadless rhythm monitors may fail to detect or may misclassify a small number of AF episodes, these erroneous episodes tend to be very brief in duration and therefore have minimal impact on the overall AF burden measurement. Several studies have shown that these devices can quantify AF burden with ≥98.5% accuracy [4,8].

Nevertheless there is currently no evidence that in patients with AF, continuous rhythm monitoring can improve patient specific outcomes compared to IRM. More data are required to evaluate the impact of CM on patient specific outcomes. However, in the setting of clinical trials, the complete and accurate rhythm disclosure that CM devices provide can lead to a more accurate understanding and scientific evaluation of treatments for AF.

Limitations

Our methodology does not allow and does not take into consideration patient symptoms which may help guide the AF follow-up. However, numerous studies have shown that symptoms have a low sensitivity and specificity [3], which may or may not lead to better and more reliable AF recurrence detection. Moreover, for the scientific evaluation of AF treatments even with the presence of symptoms, and because of their low sensitivity and specificity, AF recurrence still should be electrocardiograph-ically documented. Additionally, recent evidence shows that after invasive AF treatments the ratio of asymptomatic to symptomatic AF episodes increases [2,12]. Therefore, although a limitation, we believe that not accounting for patient symptoms does not limit the validity and applicability of our findings. Additionally, our analysis assumed 100% patient compliance with all simulated IRM strategies. In reality, reduced patient compliance with more intensive external monitoring would further diminish the ability of IRM to detect AF recurrences.

Conclusion

Reliable AF recurrence detection requires higher IRM frequencies than currently recommended, especially for patients with low (<0.5) AF burdens. Current IRM frequency recommendations will fail to identify AF recurrences in a significant – albeit difficult to prospectively estimate - proportion of patients. Shorter duration IRM performed more frequently during the follow-up period are significantly more efficient with respect to time and probably patient compliance than longer duration IRMs for the same amount of monitored time. For the scientific evaluation of AF treatments and confident detection of AF recurrence, especially in the setting of clinical trials, continuous monitoring should be considered.

Acknowledgments

We remain thankful to Katrin Meyer and Martina Schröder for the documentation support. The computational resources were kindly provided by AWS (Amazon Web Services WA, USA, Education Coursework Grant Award: EDU_Charitos_ULuebeckResearch_Fall2012). The grant donor had no role in study design, data collection and analysis, decision to publish, or preparation of the manuscript.

Author Contributions

Conceived and designed the experiments: EC PZ TH. Performed the experiments: EC PZ. Analyzed the data: EC PZ DR. Contributed reagents/materials/analysis tools: EC PZ US DR BG HS TH. Wrote the paper: EC PZ TH.

References

1. Kaemmerer WF, Rose MS, Mehra R (2001) Distribution of patients' paroxysmal atrial tachyarrhythmia episodes: implications for detection of treatment efficacy. J Cardiovasc Electrophysiol 12: 121–130.

2. Verma A, Champagne J, Sapp J, Essebag V, Novak P, et al. (2013) Discerning the incidence of symptomatic and asymptomatic episodes of atrial fibrillation before and after catheter ablation (DISCERN AF): a prospective, multicenter study. JAMA Intern Med 173: 149–156. doi:10.1001/jamainternmed.2013.1561.

3. Strickberger SA, Ip J, Saksena S, Curry K, Bahnson TD, et al. (2005) Relationship between atrial tachyarrhythmias and symptoms. Heart Rhythm 2: 125–131. doi:10.1016/j.hrthm.2004.10.042.

4. Hindricks G, Pokushalov E, Urban L, Taborsky M, Kuck K-H, et al. (2010) Performance of a new leadless implantable cardiac monitor in detecting and quantifying atrial fibrillation: Results of the XPECT trial. Circ Arrhythm Electrophysiol 3: 141–147. doi:10.1161/CIRCEP.109.877852.

5. Charitos EI, Stierle U, Ziegler PD, Baldewig M, Robinson DR, et al. (2012) A comprehensive evaluation of rhythm monitoring strategies for the detection of atrial fibrillation recurrence: insights from 647 continuously monitored patients and implications for monitoring after therapeutic interventions. Circulation 126: 806–814. doi:10.1161/CIRCULATIONAHA.112.098079.

6. Ziegler PD, Koehler JL, Mehra R (2006) Comparison of continuous versus intermittent monitoring of atrial arrhythmias. Heart Rhythm 3: 1445–1452. doi:10.1016/j.hrthm.2006.07.030.

7. Purerfellner H, Gillis AM, Holbrook R, Hettrick DA (2004) Accuracy of atrial tachyarrhythmia detection in implantable devices with arrhythmia therapies. Pacing Clin Electrophysiol 27: 983–992. doi:10.1111/j.1540-8159.2004.00569.x.

8. Passman RS, Weinberg KM, Freher M, Denes P, Schaechter A, et al. (2004) Accuracy of mode switch algorithms for detection of atrial tachyarrhythmias. J Cardiovasc Electrophysiol 15: 773–777. doi:10.1046/j.1540-8167.2004.03537.x.

9. Kottkamp H, Tanner H, Kobza R, Schirdewahn P, Dorszewski A, et al. (2004) Time courses and quantitative analysis of atrial fibrillation episode number and duration after circular plus linear left atrial lesions: trigger elimination or substrate modification: early or delayed cure? J Am Coll Cardiol 44: 869–877. doi:10.1016/j.jacc.2004.04.049.

10. Senatore G, Stabile G, Bertaglia E, Donnici G, De Simone A, et al. (2005) Role of transtelephonic electrocardiographic monitoring in detecting short-term arrhythmia recurrences after radiofrequency ablation in patients with atrial fibrillation. J Am Coll Cardiol 45: 873–876. doi:10.1016/j.jacc.2004.11.050.

11. Hanke T, Charitos EI, Stierle U, Karluss A, Kraatz E, et al. (2009) Twenty-four-hour holter monitor follow-up does not provide accurate heart rhythm status after surgical atrial fibrillation ablation therapy: up to 12 months experience with a novel permanently implantable heart rhythm monitor device. Circulation 120: S177–84.

12. Calkins H, Kuck KH, Cappato R, Brugada J, Camm AJ, et al. (2012) 2012 HRS/EHRA/ECAS expert consensus statement on catheter and surgical ablation of atrial fibrillation: recommendations for patient selection, procedural techniques, patient management and follow-up, definitions, endpoints, and research trial design. J Interv Card Electrophysiol 33: 171–257. doi:10.1007/s10840-012-9672-7.

13. Camm AJ, Kirchhof P, Lip GYH, Schotten U, Savelieva I, et al. (2010) Guidelines for the management of atrial fibrillation: the Task Force for the Management of Atrial Fibrillation of the European Society of Cardiology (ESC). Eur Heart J 31: 2369–2429. doi:10.1093/eurheartj/ehq278.

14. Charitos EI, Ziegler PD, Stierle U, Sievers H-H, Paarmann H, et al. (2013) Atrial fibrillation density: A novel measure of atrial fibrillation temporal aggregation for the characterization of atrial fibrillation recurrence pattern. Applied Cardiopulmonary Pathophysiology 17: 3–10.

15. Fusaro VA, Patil P, Gafni E, Wall DP, Tonellato PJ (2011) Biomedical cloud computing with Amazon Web Services. PLoS Comput Biol 7: e1002147. doi:10.1371/journal.pcbi.1002147.

16. Fusaro VA, Patil P, Chi C-L, Contant CF, Tonellato PJ (2013) A systems approach to designing effective clinical trials using simulations. Circulation 127: 517–526. doi:10.1161/CIRCULATIONAHA.112.123034.

17. R: A Language and Environment for Statistical Computing (2013). Vienna, Austria. Available: http://www.R-project.org/.

18. Kirchhof P, Auricchio A, Bax J, Crijns H, Camm J, et al. (2007) Outcome parameters for trials in atrial fibrillation: executive summary. Eur Heart J 28: 2803–2817. doi:10.1093/eurheartj/ehm358.

19. Henry L, Ad N (2010) Long-term monitoring for patients after surgical ablation of atrial fibrillation: are all devices the same? Innovations (Phila) 5: 259–264. doi:10.1097/IMI.0b013e3181ee5b42.

20. Rosenberg MA, Samuel M, Thosani A, Zimetbaum PJ (2013) Use of a noninvasive continuous monitoring device in the management of atrial fibrillation: a pilot study. Pacing Clin Electrophysiol 36: 328–333. doi:10.1111/pace.12053.

21. Kamel H, Navi BB, Elijovich L, Josephson SA, Yee AH, et al. (2013) Pilot randomized trial of outpatient cardiac monitoring after cryptogenic stroke. Stroke 44: 528–530. doi:10.1161/STROKEAHA.112.679100.

22. Vasamreddy CR, Dalal D, Dong J, Cheng A, Spragg D, et al. (2006) Symptomatic and asymptomatic atrial fibrillation in patients undergoing radiofrequency catheter ablation. J Cardiovasc Electrophysiol 17: 134–139. doi:10.1111/j.1540-8167.2006.00359.x.

23. Crossley GH, Boyle A, Vitense H, Chang Y, Mead RH (2011) The CONNECT (Clinical Evaluation of Remote Notification to Reduce Time to Clinical Decision) trial: the value of wireless remote monitoring with automatic clinician alerts. J Am Coll Cardiol 57: 1181–1189. doi:10.1016/j.jacc.2010.12.012.

5

Is Cryoballoon Ablation Preferable to Radiofrequency Ablation for Treatment of Atrial Fibrillation by Pulmonary Vein Isolation? A Meta-Analysis

Junxia Xu[1,2]*, Yingqun Huang[3], Hongbin Cai[3], Yue Qi[4], Nan Jia[5], Weifeng Shen[6], Jinxiu Lin[3], Feng Peng[3]*, Wenquan Niu[7,8,9]*

1 Department of Geratology, Fuzhou General Hospital of Nanjing Command, PLA, Fuzhou, Fujian, China, 2 Department of Geratology, Fozhou General Hospital, Fujian Medical University, Fuzhou, Fujian, China, 3 Department of Cardiology, The First Affiliated Hospital of Fujian Medical University, Fuzhou, Fujian, China, 4 Department of Epidemiology, Capital Medical University Affiliated Beijing An Zhen Hospital, Beijing Institute of Heart, Lung and Blood Vessel Diseases, Beijing, China, 5 Department of Cardiology, The Fourth People's Hospital of Shenzhen, Shenzhen, Guangdong, China, 6 Department of Cardiology, Ruijin Hospital, Shanghai Jiao Tong University School of Medicine, Shanghai, China, 7 Department of Human Genetics and Biostatistics, Institute of Cardiovascular Disease, Dalian Medical University, Dalian, Liaoning, China, 8 Center for Evidence-Based Medicine, Institute of Cardiovascular Disease, Dalian Medical University, Dalian, Liaoning, China, 9 State Key Laboratory of Medical Genomics, Ruijin Hospital, Shanghai Jiao Tong University School of Medicine, Shanghai, China

Abstract

Objective: Currently radiofrequency and cryoballoon ablations are the two standard ablation systems used for catheter ablation of atrial fibrillation; however, there is no universal consensus on which ablation is the optimal choice. We therefore sought to undertake a meta-analysis with special emphases on comparing the efficacy and safety between cryoballoon and radiofrequency ablations by synthesizing published clinical trials.

Methods and Results: Articles were identified by searching the MEDLINE and EMBASE databases before September 2013, by reviewing the bibliographies of eligible reports, and by consulting with experts in this field. Data were extracted independently and in duplicate. There were respectively 469 and 635 patients referred for cryoballoon and radiofrequency ablations from 14 qualified clinical trials. Overall analyses indicated that cryoballoon ablation significantly reduced fluoroscopic time and total procedure time by a weighted mean of 14.13 (95% confidence interval [95% CI]: 2.82 to 25.45; $P = 0.014$) minutes and 29.65 (95% CI: 8.54 to 50.77; $P = 0.006$) minutes compared with radiofrequency ablation, respectively, whereas ablation time in cryoballoon ablation was nonsignificantly elongated by a weighted mean of 11.66 (95% CI: -10.71 to 34.04; $P = 0.307$) minutes. Patients referred for cryoballoon ablation had a high yet nonsignificant success rate of catheter ablation compared with cryoballoon ablation (odds ratio; 95% CI; P: 1.34; 0.53 to 3.36; 0.538), and cryoballoon ablation was also found to be associated with the relatively low risk of having recurrent atrial fibrillation (0.75; 0.3 to 1.88; 0.538) and major complications (0.46; 0.11 to 1.83; 0.269). There was strong evidence of heterogeneity and low probability of publication bias.

Conclusion: Our findings demonstrate greater improvement in fluoroscopic time and total procedure duration for atrial fibrillation patients referred for cryoballoon ablation than those for radiofrequency ablation.

Editor: Thomas Berger, Medical University Innsbruck, Austria

Funding: The authors have no support or funding to report.

Competing Interests: The authors have declared that no competing interests exist.

* E-mail: fengpengfuzhou@yeah.net (FP); xujunxia1970@aliyun.com (JX); niuwenquan_shcn@163.com (WN)

Introduction

Pulmonary vein isolation (PVI) via catheter ablation has become the recommended choice of treatment for patients with drug-refractory paroxysmal or persistent atrial fibrillation [1]. Conventionally radiofrequency is the preferred source of energy for ablation procedures, whereas its application has been limited by disrupting tissues due to excess heating or generation of inhomogeneous lesions [2,3]. An alternative energy source, cryothermal energy, has recently been developed to overcome this limitation [4]. The cryoballoon catheter is composed of an inner and an outer balloon, and liquid nitrous oxide is delivered into the inner lumen of the balloon and changed into gas, thereby cooling the surrounding tissues to interrupt cellular metabolism and electrical activity. However, the potential benefits of cryoballoon ablation over radiofrequency ablation at present are still subject to an ongoing debate. For example, Linhart et al reported a similar success rate between cryoballoon and radiofrequency ablations [5], whereas the success rate for cryoballoon ablation was obviously high in a clinical trial by Kojodjojo et al [6]. It is worth noting that the majority of published trials on this topic are seriously underpowered, and most are even nonrandomized clinical trials. Given the accumulation of data, we therefore sought to undertake a meta-analysis of clinical trials that compared

Table 1. Baseline characteristics of study patients of all qualified trials in this meta-analysis.

Author (year)	Country	Cryo type	Manufacturer	RF type	Design	Matched	Number	Age (yrs)	Gender (Males)
Linhart M et al (2009)	Germany	23 or 28 mm	Arctic Front	Irrigated RF	Nonrandomized	age, sex	20/20	59.9/58.5	0.75/0.75
Sauren LD et al (2009)	Netherlands	28 mm	Arctic Front	Irrigated RF	Nonrandomized	NA	10/10	58/53	0.7/1
Chierchia GB et al (2010)	Belgium	28 mm	Arctic Front	Irrigated RF	Nonrandomized	NA	46/87	56/56	0.78/0.79
Kojodjojo P et al (2010)	UK	28 mm	Arctic Front	Irrigated RF	Nonrandomized	NA	90/53	57.3/59.3	0.75/0.77
Kuhne M et al (2010)	Switzerland	28 mm	NA	Irrigated RF	Nonrandomized	age, sex	18/25	58/59	0.88/0.84
Sorgente A et al (2010)	Belgium	28 mm	Arctic Front	Irrigated RF	Nonrandomized	NA	30/29	56/56.1	0.74/0.9
Gaita F et al (2011)	Italy	23 or 28 mm	Arctic Front	Irrigated RF	Nonrandomized	NA	36/36	55/57	0.69/0.67
Herrera SC et al (2011)	Germany	23 or 28 mm	Arctic Front	Irrigated RF	Nonrandomized	NA	23/27	61/61	0.65/0.74
Neumann T et al (2011)	Germany	NA	Arctic Front	Irrigated RF	Nonrandomized	NA	45/44	56/58	0.53/0.73
Herrera SC et al (2012)	Germany	23 or 28 mm	Arctic Front	Irrigated RF	Randomized	NA	30/30	57/56	0.83/0.77
Schmidt M et al (2012)	Germany	23 or 28 mm	Arctic Front	Irrigated RF	Nonrandomized	NA	37/178	60/63	0.76/0.84
Betts TR et al (2013)	UK	28 mm	Arctic Front	Irrigated RF	Nonrandomized	age, sex	21/21	54/55	0.67/0.81
Maagh P et al (2013)	Germany	28 mm	Arctic Front	Irrigated RF	Nonrandomized	NA	30/42	59.9/60.6	0.633/0.69
Schmidt B et al (2013)	Germany	28 mm	NA	Irrigated RF	Randomized	NA	33/33	66/63	NA/NA

Abbreviations: Cryo type, type of cryoballoon; RF type, type of radiofrequency ablation; NA, not available. Digital data were expressed as counting or percentages between cryoballoon/radiofrequency techniques unless otherwise indicated.

cryoballoon ablation with radiofrequency ablation in terms of the efficacy and safety for electrical isolation of pulmonary veins.

Methods

This meta-analysis of clinical trials was carried out in accordance with the guidelines set forth by the Preferred Reporting Items for Systematic Reviews and Meta-analyses (PRISMA) statement (Supplementary Checklist S1) [7].

Search strategy

Articles were identified by searching MEDLINE and EMBASE electronic databases from the earliest possible year to September 2013, by reviewing the bibliographies of original eligible reports, and by consulting with experts in this field. The key terms included 'pulmonary vein', 'ablation', 'radiofrequency', 'cryothermal', or 'cryoballoon', together with 'atrial fibrillation' or 'arrhythmias'. Searching results were restricted to 'clinical trials' published in 'English' language.

Table 2. Baseline characteristics of study patients of all qualified trials in this meta-analysis.

Author (year)	AF-d (yrs)	LA-d (mm)	PAF	LVEF (%)	CAD	Hypertens	Diabetes	Success rate	Recurrence rate	Complications
Linhart M et al (2009)	7/7	NA/NA	1/1	59.5/62.5	0.1/0	0.6/0.25	0/0.05	0.5/0.45	0.5/0.55	NA/NA
Sauren LD et al (2009)	NA/NA	NA/NA	1/0.9	NA/NA	NA/NA	NA/NA	NA/NA	NA/NA	NA/NA	NA/NA
Chierchia GB et al (2010)	3.3/3.2	41/42	NA/NA	64/64	0.086/0.05	0.24/0.23	NA/NA	NA/NA	NA/NA	NA/NA
Kojodjojo P et al (2010)	5.6/6	39.6/41.6	1/1	65/60.3	0.06/0.06	0.47/0.26	NA/NA	0.79/0.42	0.21/0.58	NA/NA
Kuhne M et al (2010)	5/3.25	41/42	1/1	60/58	0.16/0.16	NA/NA	NA/NA	NA/NA	NA/NA	NA/NA
Sorgente A et al (2010)	2.8/3.4	40.8/42.4	0.89/0.69	63.9/64.2	0.11/0.07	0.29/0.59	0/0.03	0.66/0.66	0.34/0.35	NA/NA
Gaita F et al (2011)	5.08/6.66	41/43	NA/NA	63/64	NA/NA	0.36/0.31	NA/NA	NA/NA	NA/NA	NA/NA
Herrera SC et al (2011)	NA/NA	40/42	0.65/0.48	NA/NA	NA/NA	0.61/0.59	NA/NA	NA/NA	NA/NA	0.96/0.93
Neumann T et al (2011)	NA/NA	51/53	1/0.614	62/58	0.13/0.07	0.51/0.59	0/0.09	NA/NA	NA/NA	NA/NA
Herrera SC et al (2012)	4.2/5.6	41.4/40	0.7/0.567	NA/NA	NA/NA	0.43/0.47	NA/NA	0.63/0.8	0.37/0.2	0.867/1
Schmidt M et al (2012)	0.83/0.92	46/46	1/0.54	60/58	0.2/0.2	0.58/0.61	0.13/0.11	NA/NA	NA/NA	0.95/0.98
Betts TR et al (2013)	NA/NA	42/45	0.67/0.48	NA/NA	NA/NA	NA/NA	NA/NA	NA/NA	NA/NA	NA/NA
Maagh P et al (2013)	1.04/0.64	38.9/37.5	0.7/0.64	NA/NA	0.13/0.17	0.2/0.095	NA/NA	0.73/0.72	0.27/0.28	NA/NA
Schmidt B et al (2013)	NA/NA	40/41	NA/NA	59/58	0.21/0.18	0.76/0.7	0.06/0.06	NA/NA	NA/NA	1/1

Abbreviations: AF-d, atrial fibrillation duration; LA-d, left atrium diameter; PAF, paroxysmal atrial fibrillation; LVEF, left ventricular ejection fraction; CAD, coronary artery disease; Hypertens, hypertension; NA, not available. Digital data were expressed as counting or percentages between cryoballoon/radiofrequency techniques unless otherwise indicated.

Trial selection

The titles and abstracts of 140 potentially relevant articles were evaluated independently by two investigators (F.P. and W.N.) and the full texts of 54 articles were obtained for further evaluation in duplicate. To avoid double counting of study patients, the corresponding authors were contacted for inquiries if necessary. For trials that produced more than one publication using the same study, data from the most recent or most complete publication were extracted.

Inclusion/exclusion criteria

For inclusion, eligible trials should fulfill the following criteria (all must be satisfied): (1) to involve patients refractory to antiarrhythmic drugs and then referred for PVI by catheter ablation; (2) under treatment of either radiofrequency (including irrigated radiofrequency) or cryoballoon ablation for the first time; (3) to compare either of fluoroscopic time, total procedure time, ablation time, success rate of PVI, and the percentages of recurrent atrial fibrillation and major complications between cryoballoon or radiofrequency ablations. Trials were excluded (one was sufficient for exclusion) if they were cross-over trials or if they were conference abstracts, case reports, case series, editorials, review articles, or non-English articles.

Data extraction

The primary outcome was the success rate of PVI, fluoroscopic time, total procedure time and ablation time. Secondary outcomes consisted of freedom from atrial fibrillation at the end of follow-up and major complications including cardiac tamponade, stroke or transient ischemic attack, pulmonary edema, phrenic nerve palsy, pulmonary vein stenosis, atrioesophageal fistula or death.

From each qualified article, two investigators (F.P. and W.N.) independently extracted the following data if available and entered them into a standard Excel template (Microsoft Corp, Redmond, WA): the first author's surname, publication year, ethnicity, study design, the manufacturer and type of cryoballoon, radiofrequency type, matched information, sample size, fluoroscopic time, total procedure time, ablation time, success rate of PVI, recurrence of atrial fibrillation and major complications, as well as the characteristics of trial patients including age, gender, atrial fibrillation duration, left atrium diameter, previous percutaneous ablation, paroxysmal atrial fibrillation, left ventricular ejection fraction (LVEF), the percentages of coronary artery disease (CAD), hypertension and diabetes between the two arms.

Paroxysmal atrial fibrillation was defined as self-terminating episodes lasting <7 days, persistent atrial fibrillation as episodes between ≥7 days, or requiring a cardioversion to terminate. A distinction between persistent and long-lasting persistent atrial fibrillation was not made. The success of PVI was defined as

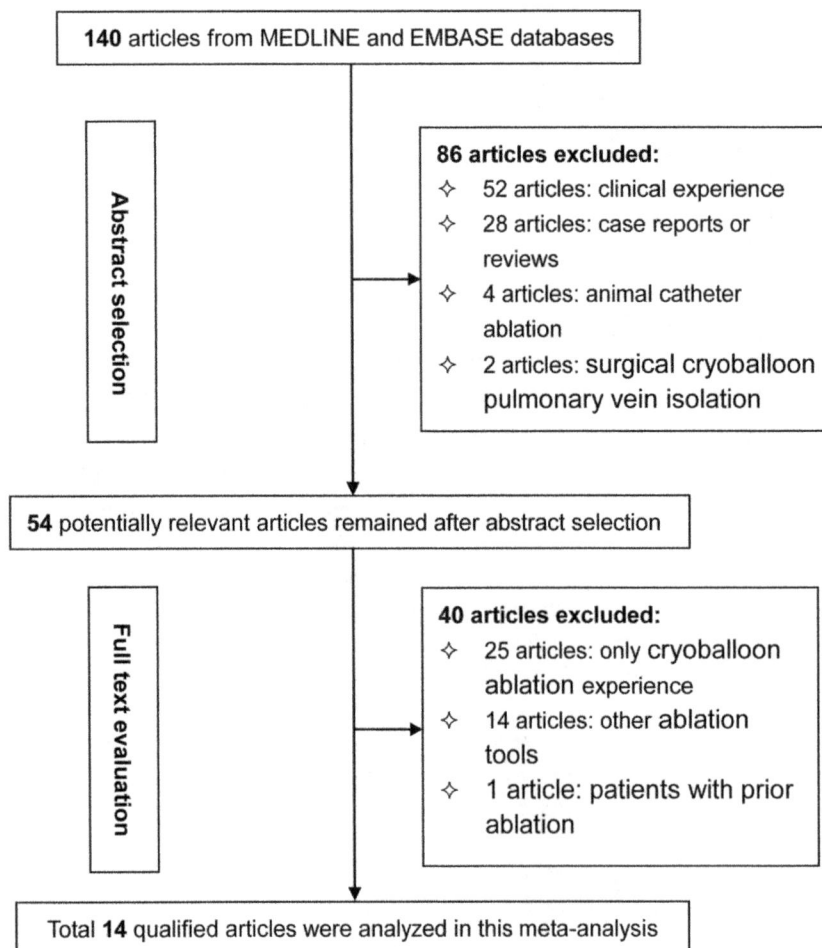

Figure 1. Flow diagram of search strategy and study selection.

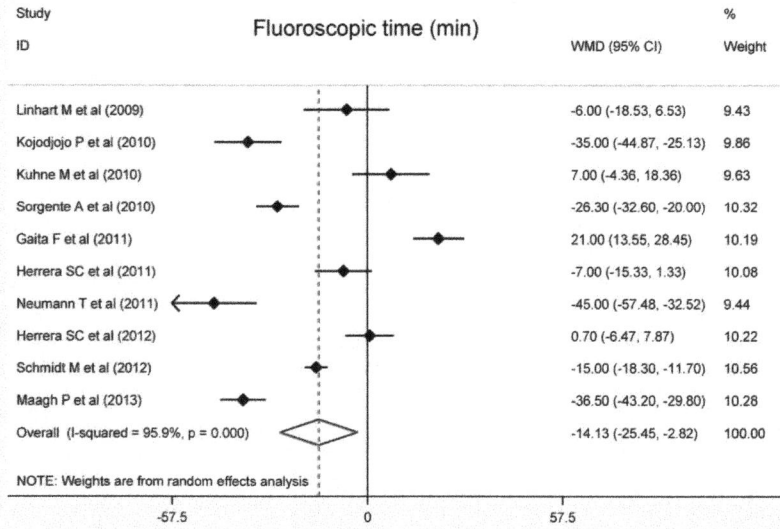

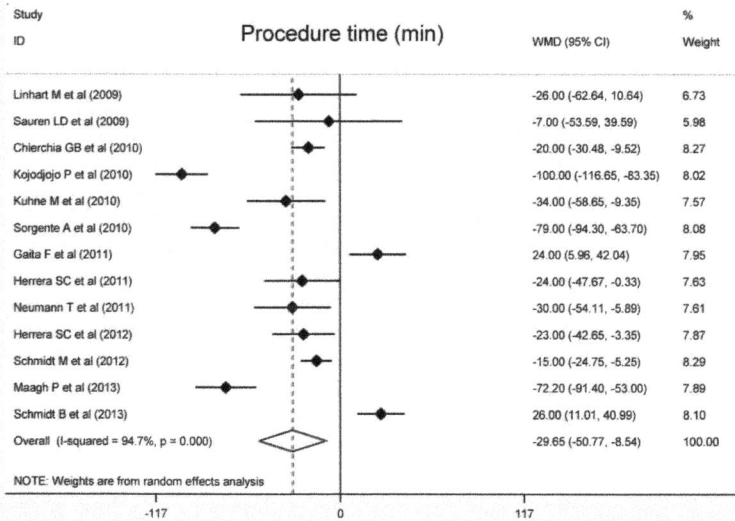

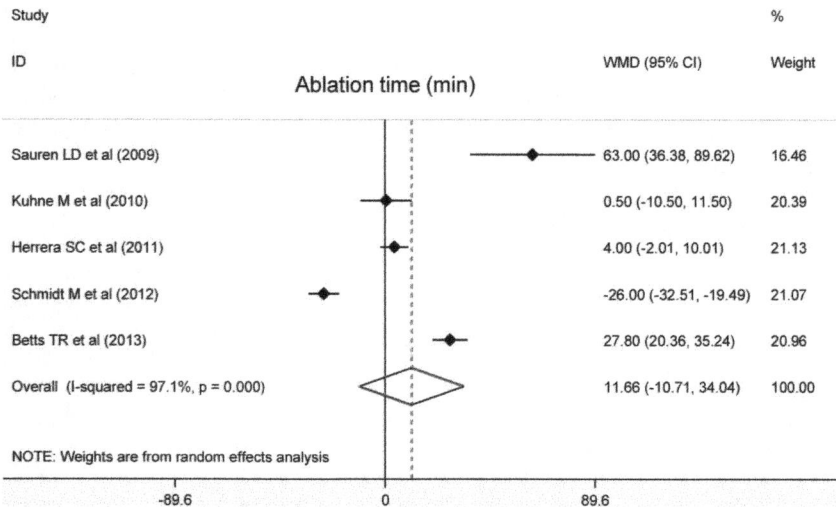

Figure 2. Forest plots of changes of fluoroscopy time, total procedure time and ablation time for cryoballoon ablation versus radiofrequency ablation.

complete PVI, which was confirmed by the disappearance of all pulmonary vein potentials or the dissociation of pulmonary vein potentials from left atrial activity.

Hypertension was diagnosed as the presence of elevated systolic (≥140 mmHg) and/or diastolic (≥90 mmHg) blood pressure, or current use of antihypertensive medications. Diabetes was defined as fasting plasma glucose levels ≥7.0 mmol/L or non-fasting plasma glucose levels ≥11.0 mmol/L, or taking hypoglycemic drugs or receiving parenteral insulin therapy. Data were compared and disagreements regarding whether to include or exclude a trial were resolved by consensus between all authors.

Statistical analysis

Quantitative outcomes were compared by weighted mean difference (WMD) and its 95% confidence interval (95% CI) between cryoballoon and radiofrequency ablation procedures. Categorical variables were evaluated by weighted odds ratio (OR) and the corresponding 95% CI, which were calculated by the Mantel-Haenszel method. The pooled effect estimates were calculated using the inverse-variance weighting under both fixed-effects and DerSimonian & Laird [8] random-effects models.

Heterogeneity was assessed by χ^2 test and quantified using the inconsistency index (I^2) statistic, which ranges from 0% to 100% and is defined as the percentage of the observed between-trial variability that is due to heterogeneity rather than chance. Given that the fixed- and random-effects models produced similar results in the absence of heterogeneity, the random-effects model is thereby adopted.

Sensitivity analysis was performed to assess the contribution of each individual trial to pooled effect estimate by sequentially removing each trial in turn. Meta-regression analysis was used to evaluate the extent to which different trial-level variables explained the heterogeneity of effect estimates between cryoballoon and radiofrequency ablation procedures.

Publication bias was assessed by the Begg's and Egger's tests. The trim-and-fill method was adopted to estimate the number and outcomes of potentially missing trials due to publication bias. P<0.05 was considered statistically significant except for the I^2, Begg's and Egger's statistics where a significance level was set as P<0.10 [9]. The statistical analyses described above were completed using the STATA software (StataCorp, College Station, TX, version 11.2 for Windows).

Results

Eligible trials

Baseline characteristics of all study patients and a flow diagram schematizing the process of excluding articles with specific reasons are summarized in Tables 1 and 2 and Figure 1, respectively. Of 140 potentially relevant articles identified in initial literature search, 14 qualified articles involving 1104 patients referred for catheter ablation were analyzed [5,6,10–21].

All clinical trials were conducted in Caucasians from European countries and published between 2009 and 2013. Eight of 14 trials adopted 28 mm cryoballoon [6,10–13,19–21], and five adopted mixed cryoballoon of 23 mm and 28 mm [5,14,15,17,18]. All trials adopted the irrigated radiofrequency. All but two trials with missing information [12,21] used cryoablation catheter from the Arctic Front (Medtronic, USA). Two of 14 trials had a randomized study design [17,21], and three trials had patients matched on age

and gender between cryoballoon and radiofrequency ablations [5,12,19].

There were respectively 469 and 635 patients referred for cryoballoon and radiofrequency ablation procedures in PVI for the treatment of atrial fibrillation. Distributions of age, atrial fibrillation duration, LVEF, previous percutaneous ablation, CAD, hypertension and diabetes were comparable between patients referred for cryoballoon and radiofrequency ablations (P>0.05). There were more males for radiofrequency ablation (79.2%) than cryoballoon ablation (72.0%) (P = 0.0284). Left atrium diameter was slightly elevated for radiofrequency ablation (42.96% versus 41.89% for cryoballoon ablation, P = 0.0212). By contrast, there were more patients with paroxysmal atrial fibrillation referred for cryoballoon ablation (87.36%) than radiofrequency ablation (71.91%) (P = 0.0076).

Efficacy

Pooling the results of all qualified trials observed that cryoballoon ablation significantly reduced fluoroscopic time and total procedure time by a weighted mean of 14.13 (95% confidence interval [95% CI]: 2.82 to 25.45; P = 0.014) minutes and 29.65 (95% CI: 8.54 to 50.77; P = 0.006) minutes compared with radiofrequency ablation, respectively (Figure 2). In contrast, cryoballoon ablation had longer yet nonsignificant ablation time than radiofrequency ablation (WMD = 11.66 minutes; 95% CI: −10.71 to 34.04; P = 0.307). It is worth noting that the wide confidence intervals generated might result from the small sample sizes of clinical trials involved and the sharply divergent results of the very few trials from overall estimates.

The I^2 values, which quantified heterogeneity between trails, were 95.9%, 94.7% and 97.1% for fluoroscopic time, total procedure time and ablation time, respectively, suggesting strong evidence of between-trial heterogeneity (all P<0.001). As reflected by the Begg's and Egger's tests (Figure 3), there were low probabilities of publication bias for all comparisons. Further adopting the trim-and-fill adjustment method yielded no material changes in pooled effects estimates, and as estimated only two missing trials were required for ablation time to make the funnel plot symmetrical (Figure 3).

Success rate

Success rate of catheter ablation was relatively higher in patients referred for cryoballoon ablation than radiofrequency ablation, the difference exhibiting no statistical significance (OR; 95% CI; P: 1.34; 0.53 to 3.36; 0.538) (Figure 4). There was evident heterogeneity (I^2 = 74.8%; P = 0.003) and no publication bias (Figure S1).

Recurrence and complications

Cryoballoon ablation was also found to be associated with relatively low risk of having recurrent atrial fibrillation (0.75; 0.3 to 1.88; 0.538) and major complications (0.46; 0.11 to 1.83; 0.269) (Figure 4). As indicated by the I^2 statistic, heterogeneity was significant for recurrence rate (I^2 = 74.8%; P = 0.003) but not for complication rate (I^2 = 11.6%; P = 0.323).

Sensitivity analysis

There was not an individual trial influencing the overall effect estimate significantly for all examined comparisons. After removing

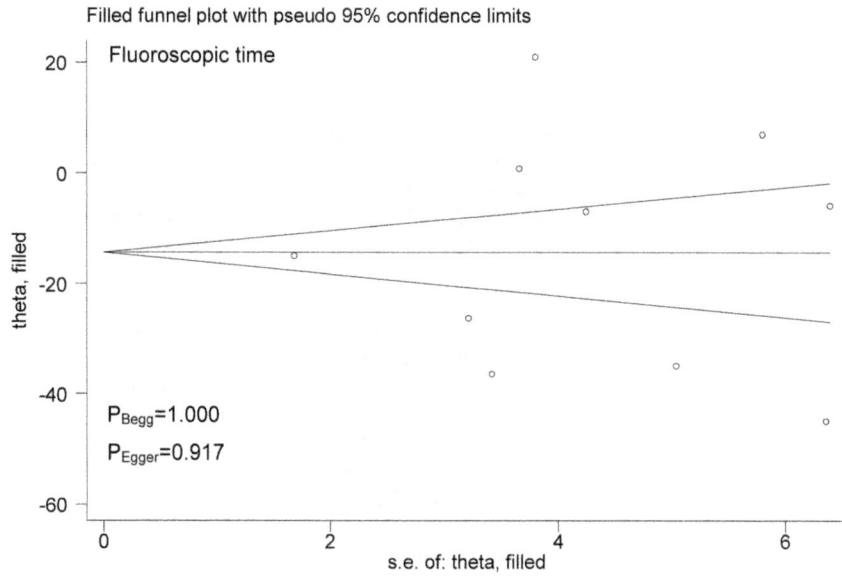

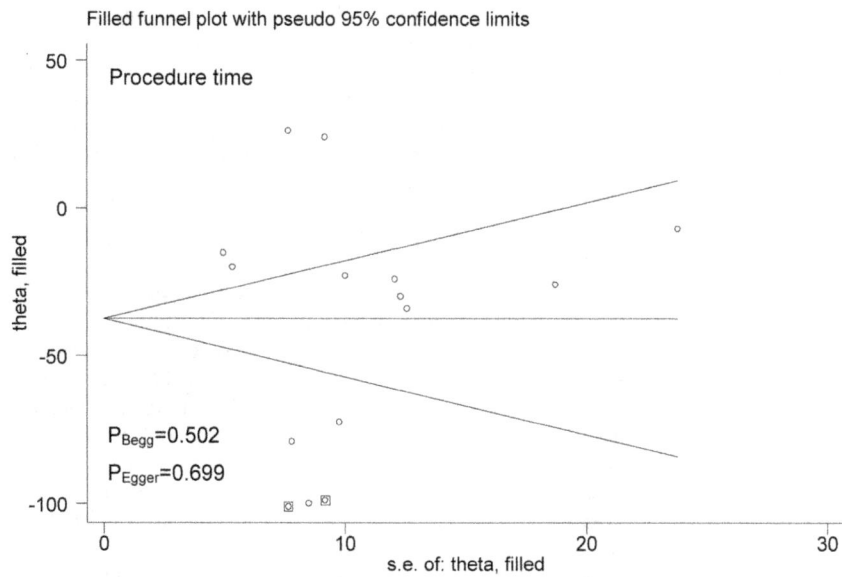

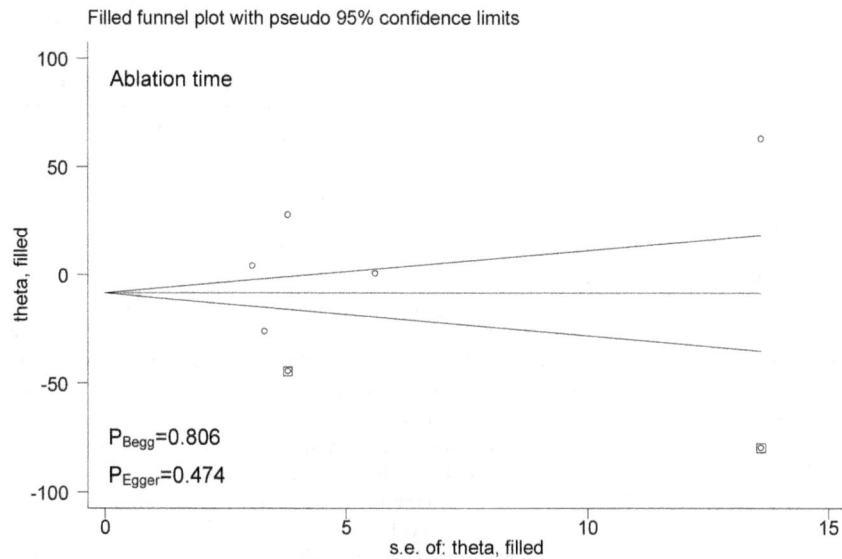

Figure 3. Trim-and-fill funnel plots of fluoroscopy time, total procedure time and ablation time for cryoballoon ablation versus radiofrequency ablation.

each trial and calculating the overall estimate for the remaining trials, the significance of the WMD or OR remained materially unchanged (Figure S2).

Meta-regression analysis

To explore the extent to which trial-level variables account for heterogeneity, a panel of meta-regression analyses were conducted. None of examined variables including age, gender, study design, type of cryoballoon, matched information on age and gender, atrial fibrillation duration, left atrium diameter, previous percutaneous ablation, paroxysmal atrial fibrillation, LVEF, CAD, hypertension and diabetes, contributed significantly to the variation of effect estimates between cryoballoon and radiofrequency ablation procedures (P<0.05 for all) (data not shown).

Discussion

The most noteworthy of this study was that there was greater improvement in fluoroscopic time and total procedure duration in patients referred for cryoballoon ablation than those for radiofrequency ablation in PVI of atrial fibrillation. Moreover, success rate of PVI, the percentages of recurrence of atrial fibrillation and major complications were comparable between the two procedures. To our knowledge, this is so far the first comprehensive meta-analysis comparing cryoballoon ablation with radiofrequency ablation in terms of the efficacy and safety for electrical isolation of pulmonary veins.

Currently radiofrequency and cryoballoon ablations are the two standard ablation systems used for catheter ablation of atrial fibrillation. As an alternative approach to conventional radiofrequency ablation, cryoballoon ablation has been recently developed for PVI. From a technologic viewpoint, a closer match between the cryoballoon size and the size of pulmonary vein ostium would allow for better balloon occlusion, which in turn produces more effective lesions [22]. It has been demonstrated that the catheter point-by-point cryoballoon is an effective approach to generate PVI with clinically satisfactory consequences [23]. Even more remarkably, compared with the first generation cryoballoon that was widely adopted in the majority of included trials in this meta-analysis, the second generation cryoballoon equipped with a modified refrigerant injection system has recently been introduced, and this novel balloon can provide a more homogeneous and effective cooling [24]. There is also evidence that the learning curve for cryoballoon ablation was much shorter than for radiofrequency ablation [25]. All these favorite characteristics will endow cryoballoon ablation with higher procedure efficiency and long-term success rate after cryoballoon ablation.

As reflected in our overall analyses, fluoroscopic time and total procedure duration were greatly improved by using cryoballoon ablation compared with radiofrequency ablation, consistent with the trends of most clinical trials [6,16,18,20]. Contrastingly, there was longer ablation time in cryoballoon technique in this meta-analysis, likely due to the need for pre-procedural computerized tomography imaging, which can further increase the cumulative radiation dose received by the patients and overall costs. Although the success rate of catheter ablation was higher in patients referred for cryoballoon ablation than radiofrequency ablation, there was no observable statistical difference, possibly due to methodological limitations, including inadequate sample size, patient section, and lack of adjustment for confounders. Here, we cannot overlook the

fact that in some clinical centers, selection of cryoballoon or radiofrequency ablation is largely based on the patient's anatomy, that is, patients with unfavorable anatomy on computed tomography may be referred for radiofrequency ablation rather than cryoballoon ablation [22]. Moreover in clinical routine, the patients with high-risk features were more likely to have undergone the procedure with radiofrequency relative to cryoballoon ablation. Nevertheless, we believe that with the accumulation of operational experience, cryoballoon ablation's advantage over radiofrequency ablation will become more and more obvious in clinical practice.

However, a note of caution should be added because heterogeneity might potentially limit the interpretation of our pooled effect estimates. In this meta-analysis, to account for the potential sources of heterogeneity between trials, we undertook a penal of meta-regression analyses, whereas we failed to identify any contributory confounders. The meta-regression analysis, albeit enabling both categorical and continuous variables to be considered, by itself does not have the methodological rigor of a properly designed study that is intended to test the effect of these confounders formally. On the other hand, we must recognize that our meta-regression analysis involved limited trials of insufficient sample sizes, rendering it incapable of performing subgroup analyses and detecting a small or moderate effect estimate. Our results, therefore, might underestimate the virtual changes between cryoballoon and radiofrequency ablations, and definitively there is a need for further large, randomized clinical trials to confirm or refute our findings.

Despite the clear strengths of this meta-analysis including low probabilities of publication bias and the robustness of statistical analyses, interpretation of our findings, however, should be viewed in light of several limitations. First, only two of 14 qualified trials were performed in a randomized design, raising the potential existence of potential biases and/or unmeasured confounders. Although randomized trials can minimize bias and are regarded as the gold standard for quantifying effect estimates, they may not be reflective of patients treated in general clinical practice [26]. Second, our total sample size of 1104 patients was not large enough to draw a firm conclusion, and there were more patients referred for radiofrequency ablation relative to cryoballoon ablation. Third, the left atrium size and percentage of paroxysmal atrial fibrillation were not proportional between the two ablation procedures in this meta-analysis, which might bias our findings, however, our further meta-regression analyses failed to detect their contributory influence on the effect estimates. Fourth, data on major complications were limited in this meta-analysis, and some complications such as phrenic nerve paralysis are typical complications in cryoballoon ablation but rare in radiofrequency ablation. Fifth, the fact that study patients were all Caucasians from European countries limited the generalizability of our findings, reinforcing the future validation in other ethnics. Last but not the least, as with all meta-analyses, despite a low probability of publication bias in this meta-analysis, selection bias cannot be completely excluded, since we merely identified articles from the English journals and published trials.

In conclusion, this study confirms and extends the findings of most clinical trials by demonstrating greater improvement in fluoroscopic time and total procedure duration in atrial fibrillation patients referred for cryoballoon ablation relative to those referred for radiofrequency ablation in PVI. However, it should be noted

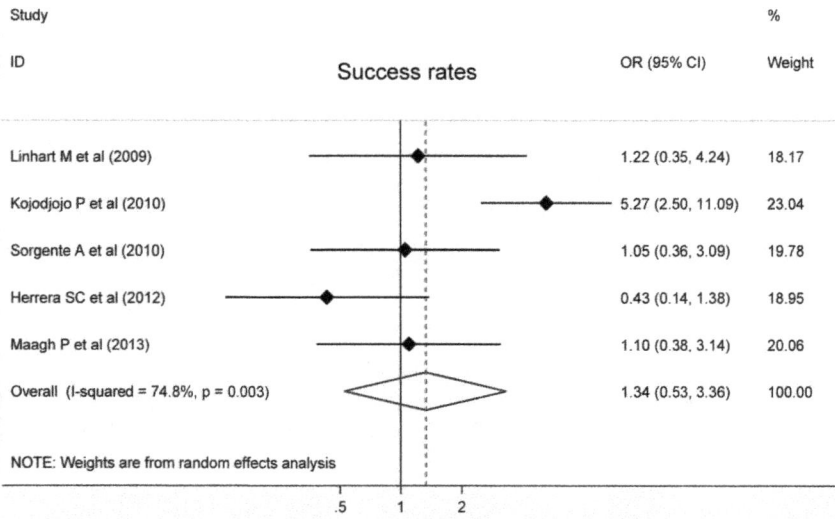

Study ID		OR (95% CI)	% Weight
Success rates			
Linhart M et al (2009)		1.22 (0.35, 4.24)	18.17
Kojodjojo P et al (2010)		5.27 (2.50, 11.09)	23.04
Sorgente A et al (2010)		1.05 (0.36, 3.09)	19.78
Herrera SC et al (2012)		0.43 (0.14, 1.38)	18.95
Maagh P et al (2013)		1.10 (0.38, 3.14)	20.06
Overall (I-squared = 74.8%, p = 0.003)		1.34 (0.53, 3.36)	100.00

NOTE: Weights are from random effects analysis

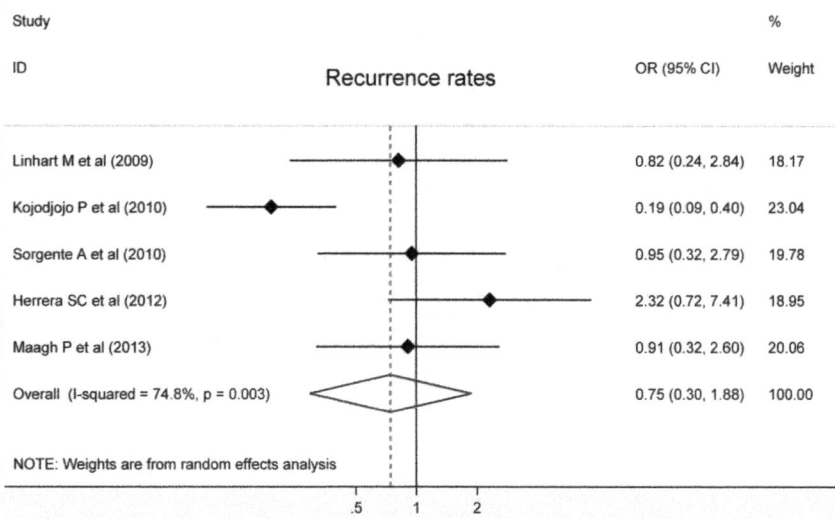

Study ID		OR (95% CI)	% Weight
Recurrence rates			
Linhart M et al (2009)		0.82 (0.24, 2.84)	18.17
Kojodjojo P et al (2010)		0.19 (0.09, 0.40)	23.04
Sorgente A et al (2010)		0.95 (0.32, 2.79)	19.78
Herrera SC et al (2012)		2.32 (0.72, 7.41)	18.95
Maagh P et al (2013)		0.91 (0.32, 2.60)	20.06
Overall (I-squared = 74.8%, p = 0.003)		0.75 (0.30, 1.88)	100.00

NOTE: Weights are from random effects analysis

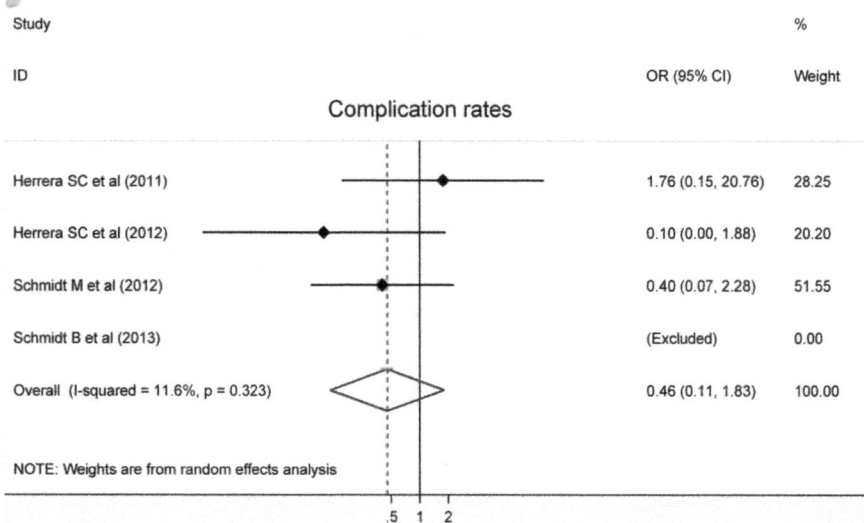

Study ID		OR (95% CI)	% Weight
Complication rates			
Herrera SC et al (2011)		1.76 (0.15, 20.76)	28.25
Herrera SC et al (2012)		0.10 (0.00, 1.88)	20.20
Schmidt M et al (2012)		0.40 (0.07, 2.28)	51.55
Schmidt B et al (2013)		(Excluded)	0.00
Overall (I-squared = 11.6%, p = 0.323)		0.46 (0.11, 1.83)	100.00

NOTE: Weights are from random effects analysis

Figure 4. Forest plots of success rate, recurrence of atrial fibrillation, complication rate for cryoballoon ablation versus radiofrequency ablation.

that success rate of PVI, the percentages of recurrent atrial fibrillation and major complications were comparable between the two procedures. For practical reasons, with the accumulation of data from large randomized clinical trials, successful validation of the present results will revolutionize the current clinical practice and healthcare system by bringing great benefits to doctors and patients alike in the near future.

Supporting Information

Figure S1   Trim-and-fill funnel plot of the success rate of pulmonary vein isolation for cryoballoon ablation versus radiofrequency ablation.

Figure S2   Sensitivity analyses of fluoroscopic time (A), total procedure time (B), ablation time (C) and success rate of pulmonary vein isolation (D) for cryoballoon ablation versus radiofrequency ablation.

Checklist S1   The PRISMA Checklist.

Author Contributions

Conceived and designed the experiments: WN FP. Performed the experiments: JX YH YQ. Analyzed the data: WN FP. Contributed reagents/materials/analysis tools: HC NJ WS JL. Wrote the paper: WN FP.

References

1. Calkins H, Kuck KH, Cappato R, Brugada J, Camm AJ, et al. (2012) 2012 HRS/EHRA/ECAS expert consensus statement on catheter and surgical ablation of atrial fibrillation: recommendations for patient selection, procedural techniques, patient management and follow-up, definitions, endpoints, and research trial design. J Interv Card Electrophysiol 33: 171−257.
2. Pokushalov E, Romanov A, Artyomenko S, Baranova V, Losik D, et al. (2013) Cryoballoon versus radiofrequency for pulmonary vein re-isolation after a failed initial ablation procedure in patients with paroxysmal atrial fibrillation. J Cardiovasc Electrophysiol 24: 274−279.
3. Calkins H, Kuck KH, Cappato R, Brugada J, Camm AJ, et al. (2012) 2012 HRS/EHRA/ECAS Expert Consensus Statement on Catheter and Surgical Ablation of Atrial Fibrillation: recommendations for patient selection, procedural techniques, patient management and follow-up, definitions, endpoints, and research trial design. Europace 14: 528−606.
4. Packer DL, Kowal RC, Wheelan KR, Irwin JM, Champagne J, et al. (2013) Cryoballoon Ablation of Pulmonary Veins for Paroxysmal Atrial Fibrillation: First Results of the North American Arctic Front (STOP AF) Pivotal Trial. J Am Coll Cardiol 61: 1713−1723.
5. Linhart M, Bellmann B, Mittmann-Braun E, Schrickel JW, Bitzen A, et al. (2009) Comparison of cryoballoon and radiofrequency ablation of pulmonary veins in 40 patients with paroxysmal atrial fibrillation: a case-control study. J Cardiovasc Electrophysiol 20: 1343−1348.
6. Kojodjojo P, O'Neill MD, Lim PB, Malcolm-Lawes L, Whinnett ZI, et al. (2010) Pulmonary venous isolation by antral ablation with a large cryoballoon for treatment of paroxysmal and persistent atrial fibrillation: medium-term outcomes and non-randomised comparison with pulmonary venous isolation by radiofrequency ablation. Heart 96: 1379−1384.
7. Moher D, Liberati A, Tetzlaff J, Altman DG (2009) Preferred reporting items for systematic reviews and meta-analyses: the PRISMA statement. Ann Intern Med 151: 264−269, W264.
8. DerSimonian R, Kacker R (2007) Random-effects model for meta-analysis of clinical trials: an update. Contemp Clin Trials 28: 105−114.
9. Bowden J, Tierney JF, Copas AJ, Burdett S (2011) Quantifying, displaying and accounting for heterogeneity in the meta-analysis of RCTs using standard and generalised Q statistics. BMC Med Res Methodol 11: 41.
10. Sauren LD, Y VANB, L DER, Pison L, M LAM, et al. (2009) Transcranial measurement of cerebral microembolic signals during endocardial pulmonary vein isolation: comparison of three different ablation techniques. J Cardiovasc Electrophysiol 20: 1102−1107.
11. Chierchia GB, Capulzini L, Droogmans S, Sorgente A, Sarkozy A, et al. (2010) Pericardial effusion in atrial fibrillation ablation: a comparison between cryoballoon and radiofrequency pulmonary vein isolation. Europace 12: 337−341.
12. Kuhne M, Suter Y, Altmann D, Ammann P, Schaer B, et al. (2010) Cryoballoon versus radiofrequency catheter ablation of paroxysmal atrial fibrillation: biomarkers of myocardial injury, recurrence rates, and pulmonary vein reconnection patterns. Heart Rhythm 7: 1770−1776.
13. Sorgente A, Chierchia GB, Capulzini L, Yazaki Y, Muller-Burri A, et al. (2010) Atrial fibrillation ablation: a single center comparison between remote magnetic navigation, cryoballoon and conventional manual pulmonary vein isolation. Indian Pacing Electrophysiol J 10: 486−495.
14. Gaita F, Leclercq JF, Schumacher B, Scaglione M, Toso E, et al. (2011) Incidence of silent cerebral thromboembolic lesions after atrial fibrillation ablation may change according to technology used: comparison of irrigated radiofrequency, multipolar nonirrigated catheter and cryoballoon. J Cardiovasc Electrophysiol 22: 961−968.
15. Herrera Siklody C, Deneke T, Hocini M, Lehrmann H, Shin DI, et al. (2011) Incidence of asymptomatic intracranial embolic events after pulmonary vein isolation: comparison of different atrial fibrillation ablation technologies in a multicenter study. J Am Coll Cardiol 58: 681−688.
16. Neumann T, Kuniss M, Conradi G, Janin S, Berkowitsch A, et al. (2011) MEDAFI-Trial (Micro-embolization during ablation of atrial fibrillation): comparison of pulmonary vein isolation using cryoballoon technique vs. radiofrequency energy. Europace 13: 37−44.
17. Herrera Siklody C, Arentz T, Minners J, Jesel L, Stratz C, et al. (2012) Cellular damage, platelet activation, and inflammatory response after pulmonary vein isolation: a randomized study comparing radiofrequency ablation with cryoablation. Heart Rhythm 9: 189−196.
18. Schmidt M, Marschang H, Clifford S, Harald R, Guido R, et al. (2012) Trends in inflammatory biomarkers during atrial fibrillation ablation across different catheter ablation strategies. Int J Cardiol 158: 33−38.
19. Betts TR, Jones M, Wong KC, Qureshi N, Rajappan K, et al. (2013) Feasibility of Mitral Isthmus and Left Atrial Roof Linear Lesions Using an 8 mm Tip Cryoablation Catheter. J Cardiovasc Electrophysiol 24: 775−780.
20. Maagh P, Butz T, Plehn G, Christoph A, Meissner A (2013) Pulmonary vein isolation in 2012: is it necessary to perform a time consuming electrophysiological mapping or should we focus on rapid and safe therapies? A retrospective analysis of different ablation tools. Int J Med Sci 10: 24−33.
21. Schmidt B, Gunawardene M, Krieg D, Bordignon S, Furnkranz A, et al. (2013) A Prospective Randomized Single-Center Study on the Risk of Asymptomatic Cerebral Lesions Comparing Irrigated Radiofrequency Current Ablation with the Cryoballoon and the Laser Balloon. J Cardiovasc Electrophysiol.
22. Knecht S, Kuhne M, Altmann D, Ammann P, Schaer B, et al. (2013) Anatomical predictors for acute and mid-term success of cryoballoon ablation of atrial fibrillation using the 28 mm balloon. J Cardiovasc Electrophysiol 24: 132−138.
23. Tse HF, Reek S, Timmermans C, Lee KL, Geller JC, et al. (2003) Pulmonary vein isolation using transvenous catheter cryoablation for treatment of atrial fibrillation without risk of pulmonary vein stenosis. J Am Coll Cardiol 42: 752−758.
24. Li XP, Metzner A, Kuck KH, Ouyang F (2013) Atrial fibrillation in Europe. Chin Med J (Engl) 126: 2747−2752.
25. Klein G, Gardiwal A, Oswald H (2008) Catheter-based cryoablation of atrial fibrillation: state of the art. Minerva Cardioangiol 56: 623−633.
26. Piccini JP, Berger JS, O'Connor CM (2009) Amiodarone for the prevention of sudden cardiac death: a meta-analysis of randomized controlled trials. Eur Heart J 30: 1245−1253.

6

Edoxaban in the Evolving Scenario of Non Vitamin K Antagonist Oral Anticoagulants Imputed Placebo Analysis and Multiple Treatment Comparisons

Paolo Verdecchia[1]*[9], **Fabio Angeli**[2], **Gregory Y. H. Lip**[3], **Gianpaolo Reboldi**[4][9]

1 Department of Medicine, Hospital of Assisi, Assisi, Italy, 2 Cardiology and Cardiovascular Pathophysiology, University Hospital of Perugia, Perugia, Italy, 3 University of Birmingham Centre for Cardiovascular Sciences, City Hospital, Birmingham, United Kingdom, 4 Department of Medicine, University of Perugia, Perugia, Italy

Abstract

Background: Edoxaban recently proved non-inferior to warfarin for prevention of thromboembolism in patients with non-valvular atrial fibrillation (AF). We conducted an imputed-placebo analysis with estimates of the proportion of warfarin effect preserved by each non vitamin K antagonist oral anticoagulant (NOAC) and indirect comparisons between edoxaban and different NOACs.

Methods and Findings: We performed a literature search (up to January 2014), clinical trials registers, conference proceedings, and websites of regulatory agencies. We selected non-inferiority randomised controlled phase III trials of dabigatran, rivaroxaban, apixaban and edoxaban compared with adjusted-dose warfarin in non-valvular AF. Compared to imputed placebo, all NOACs reduced the risk of stroke (ORs between 0.24 and 0.42, all p<0.001) and all-cause mortality (ORs between 0.55 and 0.59, all p<0.05). Edoxaban 30 mg and 60 mg preserved 87% and 112%, respectively, of the protective effect of warfarin on stroke, and 133% and 121%, respectively, of the protective effect of warfarin on all-cause mortality. The risk of primary outcome (stroke/systemic embolism), all strokes and ischemic strokes was significantly higher with edoxaban 30 mg than dabigatran 150 mg and apixaban. There were no significant differences between edoxaban 60 mg and other NOACs for all efficacy outcomes except stroke, which was higher with edoxaban 60 mg than dabigatran 150 mg. The risk of major bleedings was lower with edoxaban 30 mg than any other NOAC, odds ratios (ORs) ranging between 0.45 and 0.67 (all p<0.001).

Conclusions: This study suggests that all NOACs preserve a substantial or even larger proportion of the protective warfarin effect on stroke and all-cause mortality. Edoxaban 30 mg is associated with a definitely lower risk of major bleedings than other NOACs. This is counterbalanced by a lower efficacy in the prevention of thromboembolism, although with a final benefit on all-cause mortality.

Editor: Adrian V. Hernandez, Universidad Peruana de Ciencias Aplicadas (UPC), Peru

Funding: The authors have no support or funding to report.

Competing Interests: This work has not been supported from any Pharmaceutical Company. PV has no conflict of interest to declare; FA has no conflict of interest to declare; GHL has served as a consultant for Bayer, Astellas, Merck, AstraZeneca, Sanofi, BMS/Pfizer, Biotronik, Portola and Boehringer Ingelheim and has been on the speakers bureau for Bayer, BMS/Pfizer, Boehringer Ingelheim, and Sanofi-Aventis; GR has no conflict of interest to declare.

* Email: verdec@tin.it

[9] These authors contributed equally to this work.

Introduction

Vitamin K antagonists (VKA) have long been the only oral anticoagulant agents available for effective thromboprophylaxis in patients with atrial fibrillation (AF). In a landmark meta-analysis of trials conducted in AF patients randomized to either adjusted-dose warfarin versus placebo or control for a mean exposure time of 1.6 years per patient, warfarin reduced the risk of stroke by 64% (95% confidence interval (CI): 49% to 74%), and that of ischemic stroke by 67% (CI: 54% to 77%), as well as a reduction in all-cause mortality by 26% (CI 3% to 43%) [1].

This impressive benefit made it unethical to compare any non vitamin K antagonist oral anticoagulant (NOAC) [2] with placebo in subsequent outcome trials. Consequently, the major studies

published over the past few years with the direct thrombin inhibitor dabigatran [3] and the factor Xa inhibitors rivaroxaban [4], apixaban [5] and, lastly, edoxaban [6], were well-designed non-inferiority trials of each single NOAC versus adjusted-dose warfarin. Notably, any inference about the efficacy of NOACs from these studies assumes that the benefit of warfarin in preventing stroke and systemic embolism approaches that found in prior trials vs placebo or control, as summarized in the above mentioned meta-analysis [1].

After these studies, dabigatran, rivaroxaban and apixaban gained regulatory approval in many countries for prevention of stroke in patients with non valvular AF. The dose of dabigatran 110 mg b.i.d. has not been approved in the Unites States by the Food and Drug Administration (FDA), that approved the 75 mg

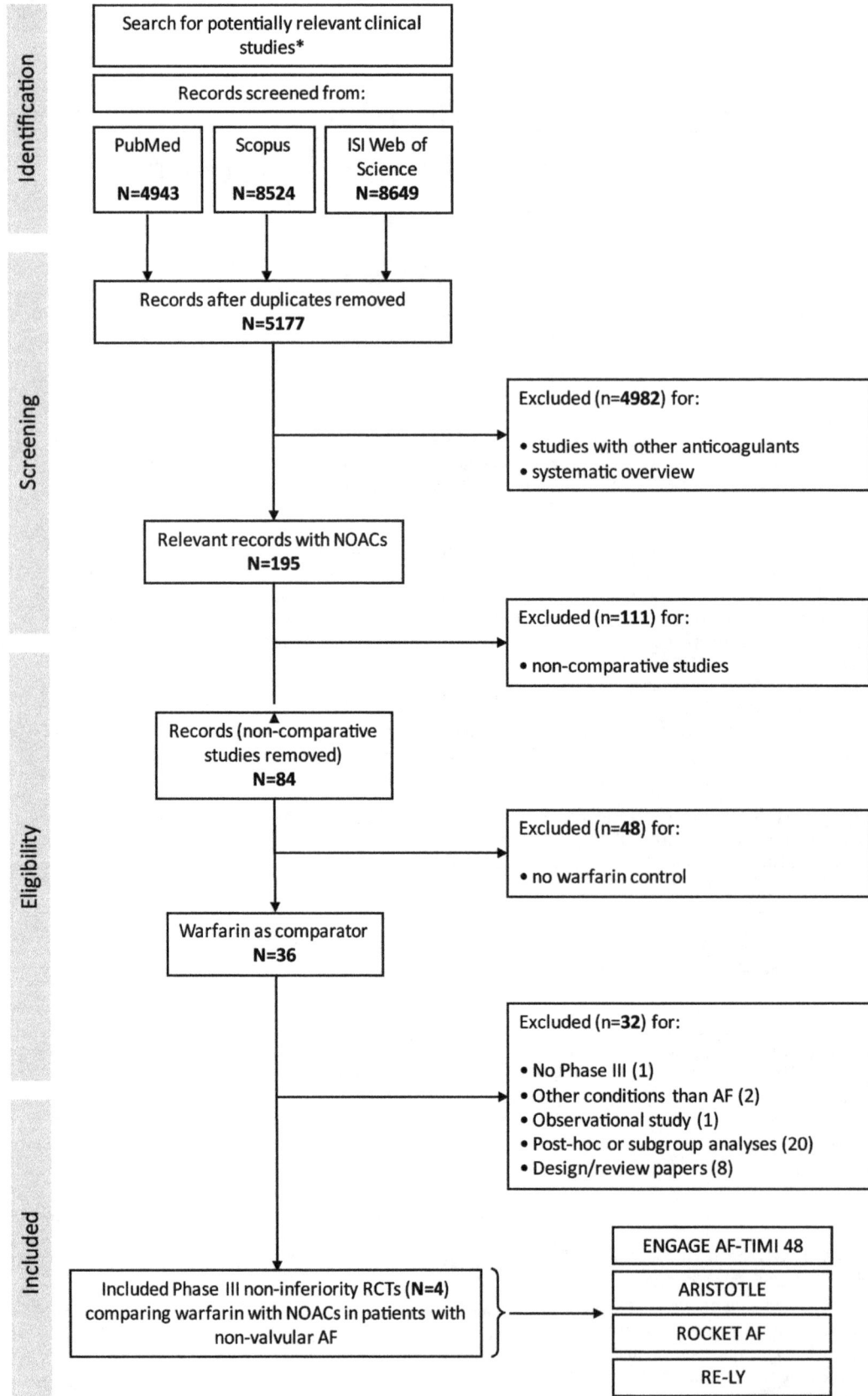

*terms included: "anticoagulants", "oral thrombin inhibitors", "oral factor Xa inhibitors", "dabigatran", "dabigatran etexilate", "dabigatran ethyl ester", "apixaban", "rivaroxaban", "edoxaban", "clinical trial", "atrial fibrillation"

Figure 1. Search strategy and selection of clinical trial according to the PRISMA (Preferred Reporting Items for Systematic reviews and Meta-Analyses) statement for reporting systematic reviews and meta-analyses.

b.i.d. dose in patients with glomerular filtration rate between 15 and 29 ml/min [7].

Although these drugs are valuable alternative to warfarin [8,9], the physician has few arguments to direct his/her choice to one over the other in the absence of direct head-to-head comparisons. Several indirect comparisons have been conducted between dabigatran, rivaroxaban and apixaban [10–15]. In the context of limitations of indirect comparisons [16,17], these analyses suggest a lower risk of stroke/systemic embolism with dabigatran 150 mg bid versus dabigatran 110 mg bid and rivaroxaban, and a lower risk of major bleedings with dabigatran 110 mg bid and apixaban versus dabigatran 150 mg bid and rivaroxaban [18,19].

More recently, edoxaban emerged as the fourth NOAC in its class. In the *Effective Anticoagulation with Factor Xa Next Generation in Atrial Fibrillation–Thrombolysis in Myocardial Infarction 48* (ENGAGE AF-TIMI 48) trial, 21,105 patients with non valvular AF were randomized to adjusted-dose warfarin or two doses (30 mg q.d., 60 mg q.d.) of edoxaban [6]. The primary efficacy endpoint was a composite of stroke and systemic embolism and the main safety end-point was major bleeding [6]. Both doses of edoxaban were non inferior to warfarin for the prevention of stroke and systemic embolism [6]. Thus far, edoxaban has not yet gained approval by FDA and other regulatory Agencies.

The ENGAGE-AF trial [6] expanded the horizon of available alternatives to VKA and offered the opportunity of a more comprehensive evaluation of this class of drugs. In the light of this new trial, the present study has three goals: (1) to estimate the proportion of warfarin effect preserved by each of the NOACs and their efficacy versus a putative placebo on the risk of stroke and all-cause mortality; (2) to update the previous estimates of benefits and harms of NOACs as a whole versus warfarin; (3) to estimate, through indirect comparisons, the relative efficacy and safety of either dose of edoxaban versus different NOACs.

Methods

Study selection

We used the PRISMA (Preferred Reporting Items for Systematic reviews and Meta-Analyses) statement for reporting systematic reviews and meta-analyses of randomized controlled trials (RCTs)

Table 1. Main Characteristics of Trials Evaluating New Oral Anticoagulants for Stroke Prevention in Patients with Nonvalvular Atrial Fibrillation.

Characteristics	RE-LY Dabigatran	ROCKET AF Rivaroxaban	ARISTOTLE Apixaban	ENGAGE AF Edoxaban
Randomized patients, N	18,113	14,264	18,201	21,105
Countries	44 (951 Centers)	45 (1178 Centers)	39 (1034 Centers)	46 (1393 Centers)
Allocation	D 110 mg b.i.d.: N = 6,015	R 20 mg q.d.: N = 7,131 Warfarin: N = 7,133	A 5 mg q.d.: N = 9,120 Warfarin: N = 9,081	E 30 mg q.d.: N = 7,034
	D 150 mg b.i.d.: N = 6,076			E 60 mg q.d.: N = 7,035
	Warfarin: N = 6,022			Warfarin: N = 7,036
Study design	Open label vs. warfarin	Double-blind	Double-blind	Double-blind
	Double-blind D 150 vs. D 110			
Patients lost to follow-up	20	32	69	1
Median duration of follow-up, years	2.0	1.9	1.9	2.8
Age, years	71 (mean)	73 (median)	70 (median)	72 (median)
Female, N	6,599	5,663	6,416	8,040
CHADS$_2$, mean	2.2	3.5	2.1	2.8
Creatinine clearance ≤50 ml/min	19.3	20.7	16.6	19.3
Paroxysmal AF, %	32.8	17.6	15.3	25.4
Prior stroke, TIA or systemic thromboembolism, %	20.0*	54.8	19.4	28.3*
Heart failure, %	32.0	62.5	35.4	57.4
Diabetes mellitus, %	23.3	40.0	25.0	36.1
Hypertension, %	78.9	90.5	87.5	93.5
Drugs at baseline				
Aspirin, %	39.8	36.5	30.9	29.2
Vitamin K antagonist, %	49.6	62.4	57.2	58.9
Average TTR in the warfarin group	64	55	62	65

D, Dabigatran; R, Rivaroxaban; A, Apixaban; E, Edoxaban; N, number of patients; AF, atrial fibrillation; TIA, transient ischemic attack, TTR = time in therapeutic range (International normalized ratio 2.0 to 3.0); CHF, congestive heart failure; DM, diabetes mellitus; HTN, hypertension; CHADS$_2$ indicates CHF, hypertension, age, diabetes mellitus, stroke.
* = Stroke or TIA only.

as a guide for this study (PRISMA checklist S1) [20], including the preparation of a protocol and analysis plan (Protocol S2). Following a literature search (up to January 2014), to perform indirect comparisons and imputed placebo analyses in the non-inferiority setting, we identified four large phase III studies (Figure 1): *Randomized Evaluation of Long-Term Anticoagulation Therapy* (RE-LY) [3], *Rivaroxaban Once Daily Oral Direct Factor Xa Inhibition Compared with Vitamin K Antagonism for Prevention of Stroke and Embolism Trial in Atrial Fibrillation* (ROCKET-AF) [4], *Apixaban for Reduction in Stroke and Other Thromboembolic Events in Atrial Fibrillation* (ARIS-TOTLE) [5], and ENGAGE AF-TIMI 48 [6] (see table 1 for the complete summary of trials'characteristics). For RE-LY [3], we integrated the original data with the update published in 2010 [21]. As shown in figure 1, we excluded systematic overviews or studies with different anticoagulants (n = 4748), non comparative studies (n = 111), studies without warfarin control (n = 48) and other 32 studies for a variety of reasons reported in the table. We included only active control phase III non-inferiority studies because our aim was to provide estimates of the proportion of warfarin effect preserved by NOACs and their efficacy versus an imputed placebo as a measure of assay sensitivity. Active controlled trials might be uninformative as they can neither demonstrate the effectiveness of a new agent nor provide a valid comparison to control therapy unless assay sensitivity can be assured [22,23].

We extracted data on both efficacy and safety outcomes as detailed below and in the study protocol (Protocol S2). Additional data on outcomes, not available in the main papers of included studies, were retrieved from the FDA website (http://www.fda.gov/Drugs/InformationOnDrugs/).

The authors of this study independently extracted all outcome data using a pre-specified form and disagreements were resolved through discussion.

Data synthesis and statistical analysis

Efficacy outcomes included the composite of stroke and systemic embolism (i.e., the primary efficacy outcome event in each of the four trials [3–6]), stroke (i.e., all strokes), hemorrhagic stroke, ischemic or uncertain type of stroke and systemic embolism. For safety, we considered major bleeding, intracranial bleeding, gastrointestinal bleeding, myocardial infarction and all-cause death.

In keeping with previous studies [10,18] the expected effect of NOACs as a class versus warfarin, was calculated as a weighted average using the inverse of the variance of the log(odds ratio (OR)) as weights. For this analysis, the higher doses of dabigatran (150 mg b.i.d. arm of RE-LY [3]) and edoxaban (60 mg q.d. arm of ENGAGE AF-TIMI 48 [6]) were analyzed with data from ROCKET-AF [4] and ARISTOTLE [5]. In a separate analysis, we analyzed the lower doses of dabigatran (110 mg b.i.d. arm of RE-LY [3]) and edoxaban (30 mg q.d. arm of ENGAGE AF-TIMI 48 [6]) with data from the other two trials.

We used the methodology introduced by Hasselblad and Kong to estimate the effects of NOACs versus imputed placebo [24]. Such approach assumes that previous trials tested warfarin versus placebo using the same outcome event as in the trials of NOACs versus warfarin, and that the populations exposed to trials of warfarin vs placebo and warfarin versus NOACs are similar [24]. The imputed placebo approach also relies on the assumption of "constancy" of the beneficial effect of warfarin versus placebo as observed in previous controlled trials [25]. This last assumption, however, is conditioned by the differences in patient characteristics, concomitant medications, intensity of treatment, and other trial design features [22,24,26,27]. In addition, stroke rate seems to be declining over time both in the general population [28] and in AF patients treated with warfarin [29]. An effective way to "discount" for this limitation is to estimate the proportion of the warfarin treatment effect retained by each NOAC [25,30,31]. This is accomplished by determining the ratio of the effect of the new treatment versus putative placebo relative to the effect of the standard treatment versus placebo along with its estimated variance and CI [22,24,26,27]. To prevent further limitations due to the use of a composite outcome (stroke and systemic embolism) in new trials as opposed to older ones, we restricted the imputed placebo analysis to stroke and all-cause mortality, as unequivocal and comparable outcome events in the trials of warfarin vs. placebo [1,32] and NOACs versus warfarin [3–6]. For this purpose, the warfarin treatment effect was derived from a random-effects meta-analysis of 6 historical placebo-controlled trials [33–38] using the OR as the analysis metric.

We made multiple treatment comparisons between edoxaban and other NOACs using the Bucher method [39,40] with warfarin used as common comparator. Because of the limited number of trials and in the absence of head-to-head comparisons between different NOACs, we did not make a formal network or mixed treatment comparison meta-analysis, in line with the recommendations and caveats outlined by the International Society for Pharmacoeconomics and Outcomes Research [41,42]. In brief, we estimated the OR of an event with a given NOAC ($NOAC_1$) versus another NOAC ($NOAC_2$) ($OR_{NOAC1/NOAC2}$) by dividing the OR of $NOAC_1$ versus warfarin ($OR_{NOAC1/warfarin}$) by the OR of $NOAC_2$ versus warfarin ($OR_{NOAC2/warfarin}$). We estimated the OR of selected events for each dose of edoxaban versus dabigatran (each dose), rivaroxaban and apixaban. The Bucher method assumes that the differences between a given NOAC and warfarin in terms of efficacy and safety would have been analogous if tested in different trial populations exposed to different NOACs versus warfarin [16]. However, since different studies were not fully comparable for some features including the thromboembolic risk, reflected by the $CHADS_2$ score, the time in therapeutic range and other methodological aspects (open-label versus double-blind), indirect comparisons should be interpreted prudently [16,17].

We used the R software version 3 (R Foundation for Statistical Computing, Vienna, Austria. URL http://www.R-project.org) for the analyses, with pre-specified efficacy and safety outcomes.

Results

In aggregate, the four trials [3–6] accrued 71,683 patients. Table 1 shows the main features of the four studies [3–6]. The sample size was larger (N = 21,105), and the median duration of follow-up longer (2.8 years) in the ENGAGE AF-TIMI 48 [6] than in the other studies. Similar to ROCKET-AF [4] and ARIS-TOTLE [5], ENGAGE AF-TIMI 48 [6] was a double-blind trial vs warfarin [6], whereas RE-LY [3] was an open-label study of dabigatran versus warfarin with a double-blind comparison between the two different dabigatran doses [3]. Based on the $CHADS_2$ score [43], the risk of stroke in the ENGAGE AF-TIMI 48 trial [6] was intermediate (2.8 points) between ROCKET-AF [4] (3.5 points) on a side, and RE-LY [3] (2.2 points) and ARISTOTLE [5] (2.1 points) on the other side. In terms of prevalence of heart failure, diabetes and hypertension at baseline, the ENGAGE AF-TIMI 48 [6]was more similar to ROCKET-AF [4] than to the other two studies. The average time in therapeutic range was 64.9% (median time 68%) in ENGAGE AF-TIMI 48 [6], as opposed to 64% in RE-LY [3], 55% in ROCKET AF [4] and 62% in ARISTOTLE [5].

Table 2. Weighted Average Effects of New Oral Anticoagulants Versus Warfarin.

| | Any NOAC (Dabigatran 150 mg BID, Apixaban 5 mg BID, Rivaroxaban 20 mg OD, Edoxaban 60 mg OD) vs. Warfarin | | | | Any NOAC (Dabigatran 110 mg BID, Apixaban 5 mg BID, Rivaroxaban 20 mg OD, Edoxaban 30 mg OD) vs. Warfarin | | | |
	Weighted Average Effect OR	95% CI Lower	95% CI Upper	p-value	Weighted Average Effect OR	95% CI Lower	95% CI Upper	p-value
Stroke or Systemic Embolism	0.786	0.715	0.864	<0.001	0.909	0.830	0.996	0.041
Stroke	0.801	0.728	0.881	<0.001	0.937	0.855	1.027	0.166
Hemorrhagic stroke	0.497	0.402	0.615	<0.001	0.433	0.346	0.540	<0.001
Ischemic or uncertain type of stroke	0.919	0.825	1.023	0.123	1.128	1.018	1.250	0.021
Systemic Embolism	0.600	0.417	0.863	0.006	0.811	0.578	1.138	0.225
Major Bleeding	0.848	0.791	0.910	<0.001	0.727	0.676	0.783	<0.001
Intracranial Bleeding	0.479	0.405	0.566	<0.001	0.412	0.345	0.493	<0.001
Gastrointestinal Bleeding	1.287	1.150	1.440	<0.001	1.025	0.910	1.155	0.688
Myocardial Infarction	0.945	0.826	1.082	0.413	1.032	0.904	1.178	0.640
Death from any cause	0.904	0.853	0.958	0.001	0.894	0.844	0.948	<0.001

Only endpoints available in all studies are reported. NOAC = new oral anticoagulant drug; BID = twice daily; OD = once daily; CI = confidence interval; OR = odds ratio.

Weighted average effect versus warfarin

When the higher doses of dabigatran and edoxaban were used for the estimates versus warfarin (Table 2, left side), NOACs as a whole reduced the risk of stroke/systemic embolism (by 21%; p< 0.001), stroke (by 20%; p<0.001), hemorrhagic stroke (by 50%; p<0.001) and systemic embolism (by 40%; p = 0.006). On the safety side, NOACs reduced the risk of major bleedings (by 15%; p<0.001), intracranial bleedings (by 52%; p<0.001) and death from any cause (by 10%; p = 0.001). Ischemic (or uncertain) stroke and myocardial infarction did not differ significantly between NOACs and warfarin, whereas gastrointestinal bleeding were more common with NOACS than with warfarin (by 29%; p< 0.001).When using the lower doses of dabigatran and edoxaban (Table 2, right side), NOACs reduced stroke/systemic embolism (by 9%; p = 0.041) and hemorrhagic stroke (by 37%; p<0.001). All strokes (p = 0.166) and systemic embolism (p = 0.225) did not differ, while the ischemic (or uncertain) type of stroke was more frequent with NOACs than with warfarin (by 13%; p = 0.021). On the safety side, NOACs reduced the risk of major bleedings (by 27%; p<0.001), intracranial bleedings (by 59%; p<0.001) and all-cause death (by 91%; p<0.001), whereas gastrointestinal bleedings (p = 0.688) and myocardial infarction (p = 0.640) did not differ between NOACs and warfarin.

Imputed placebo analysis and proportion of warfarin effect preserved

The comparison of each NOAC versus an imputed placebo on the risk of stroke is shown in figure 2. All NOACs effectively reduced the risk of stroke (all p<0.001). OR ranged between 0.236 for dabigatran 150 mg, and 0.417 for edoxaban 30 mg.

All NOACs reduced the risk of all-cause mortality (figure 3) to a similar extent, with ORs ranging between 0.552 and 0.591 (all p< 0.05). Overall, risk reductions were somewhat larger with NOACs than with warfarin (OR 0.639, 95% CI: 0.414 to 0.987, p = 0.044) but not formally significant.

The estimated proportion of warfarin benefit retained on stroke is shown in figure 4. In increasing order, edoxaban 30 mg preserved 87% (95% CI 71–103) of the protective effect of warfarin, followed by dabigatran 110 mg (108%; 95% CI: 87–129), edoxaban 60 mg (112%; 95% CI: 96–129), rivaroxaban (119%; 95% CI: 98–139), apixaban (124%; 95% CI: 103–144) and dabigatran 150 mg (143%; 95% CI: 116–170). The estimated proportion of warfarin benefit retained on all-cause mortality is shown in figure 5. In increasing order, rivaroxaban preserved 118% (95% CI 87–148) of the protective effect of warfarin, followed by dabigatran 110 mg (121%; 95% CI: 85–157), edoxaban 60 mg (121%; 95% CI: 90–151), apixaban (126%; 95% CI: 90–162), dabigatran 150 mg (128%; 95% CI: 87–168) and edoxaban 30 mg (133%; 95% CI 93–172).

Adjusted indirect comparisons between edoxaban and other agents

OR and 95% CI are reported in tables 3 (efficacy outcomes) and 4 (safety outcomes). The risk of stroke/systemic embolism was significantly higher with edoxaban 30 mg than with dabigatran 150 mg orapixaban. The risk of total stroke and ischemic (or uncertain) stroke was also significantly higher with edoxaban 30 mg than with dabigatran 150 mg, rivaroxaban or apixaban. Apart from systemic embolism and myocardial infarction, which were higher with edoxaban 30 mg than with rivaroxaban, none of the other outcomes showed statistically significant differences between edoxaban 30 mg and any other NOAC. There were no significant differences between the higher dose of edoxaban

Study / Arm		Odds Ratio	95%-CI	p-value
ARISTOTLE - Apixaban 5 mg		0.288	[0.196; 0.422]	<0.001
RE-LY - Dabigatran 150 mg		0.236	[0.157; 0.354]	<0.001
RE-LY - Dabigatran 110 mg		0.337	[0.227; 0.500]	<0.001
ROCKET - Rivaroxaban 20 mg		0.303	[0.205; 0.446]	<0.001
ENGAGE - Edoxaban 60 mg		0.322	[0.222; 0.467]	<0.001
ENGAGE - Edoxaban 30 mg		0.417	[0.289; 0.602]	<0.001
Warfarin Meta-Analysis		0.365	[0.262; 0.509]	<0.001

0.1   0.25 0.5   1 1.5

Anticoagulation Better   Placebo Better

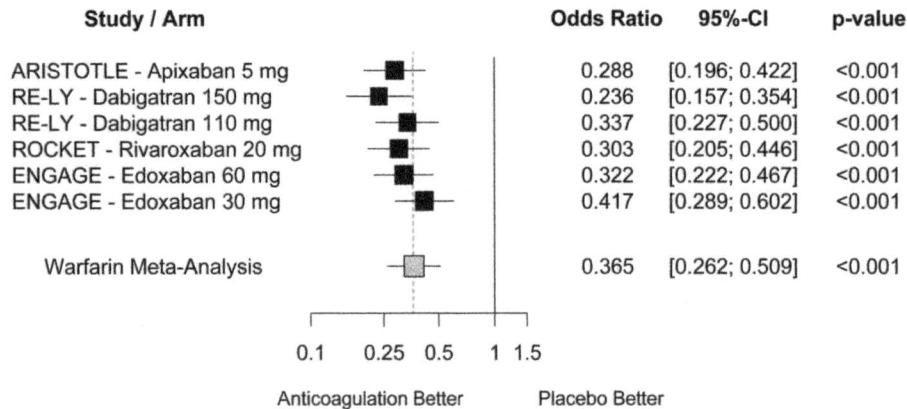

Figure 2. Imputed placebo analysis. Comparison of new oral anticoagulants versus imputed placebo on the risk of stroke.

(60 mg) and any other NOAC in the efficacy outcomes, apart from a slightly higher risk of stroke with edoxaban than rivaroxaban (p = 0.032). The risk of all-cause death did not differ between either dose of edoxaban and other NOACs. The risk of major bleedings (table 4) was significantly lower with edoxaban 30 mg than any other NOAC, and that of gastrointestinal bleedings was lower with edoxaban 30 mg compared with rivaroxaban and both doses of dabigatran. The risk of intracranial bleeding was lower with edoxaban 30 mg versus rivaroxaban. The higher dose of edoxaban did not differ significantly from any other NOAC in terms of safety outcomes, apart from a lower risk of major bleeding compared to rivaroxaban and higher risk of gastrointestinal bleedings compared to apixaban.

Discussion

The main novel finding of the present study is the estimate, obtained through an imputed placebo analysis, of the proportion of warfarin effect preserved by all NOACs on stroke and all-cause mortality in patients with non valvular AF. We based our estimate on a landmark meta-analysis of randomized trials that compared adjusted-dose warfarin versus placebo [1] and four pivotal non-inferiority trials in which 71,683 patients were randomized to adjusted-dose warfarin or NOACs [3–6].

Imputed placebo analysis

This kind of analysis is increasingly performed to estimate how might be the effect of a new treatment if compared versus placebo in the case that a placebo-controlled trial with the new agent would be unethical or unfeasible. Although there is always concern about the value of historic control data, imputed placebo analyses are required by drug regulatory Agencies. For example, the Food and Drug Administration (FDA) approved the use of enoxaparin in the treatment of acute coronary syndrome on the basis of an imputed placebo analysis that included a meta-analysis of randomized trials of unfractionated heparin plus aspirin versus aspirin alone [44], and one randomized comparison of enoxaparin versus unfractionated heparin [45]. Crucial for FDA approval was the demonstration of the high probability that enoxaparin retained at least 80% of the therapeutic effect of unfractionated heparin [23].

In the case of NOACs, placebo controlled trials in patients with non valvular AF would be unethical because warfarin is highly effective in preventing stroke in these patients [1]. When conducting an imputed placebo analysis, two main conditions

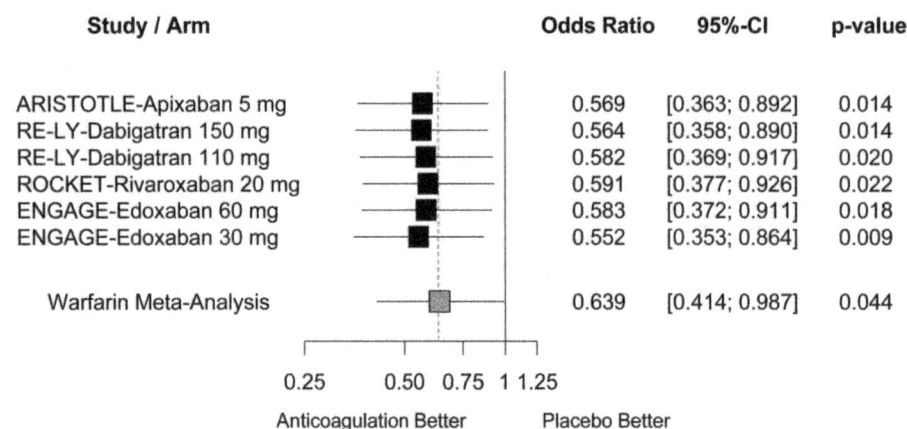

Study / Arm		Odds Ratio	95%-CI	p-value
ARISTOTLE-Apixaban 5 mg		0.569	[0.363; 0.892]	0.014
RE-LY-Dabigatran 150 mg		0.564	[0.358; 0.890]	0.014
RE-LY-Dabigatran 110 mg		0.582	[0.369; 0.917]	0.020
ROCKET-Rivaroxaban 20 mg		0.591	[0.377; 0.926]	0.022
ENGAGE-Edoxaban 60 mg		0.583	[0.372; 0.911]	0.018
ENGAGE-Edoxaban 30 mg		0.552	[0.353; 0.864]	0.009
Warfarin Meta-Analysis		0.639	[0.414; 0.987]	0.044

0.25   0.50   0.75 1 1.25

Anticoagulation Better   Placebo Better

Figure 3. Imputed placebo analysis. Comparison of new oral anticoagulants versus imputed placebo on the risk of all-cause mortality.

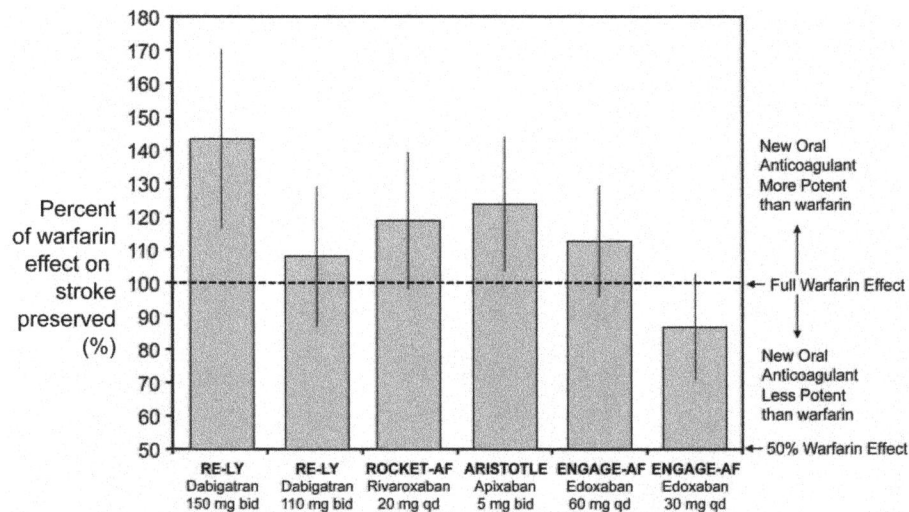

Figure 4. Estimated proportion of warfarin benefit by new oral anticoagulants on the risk of stroke.

are required: (a) there is unequivocal historical evidence, that may or may not be obtained through a meta-analysis, of the comparator's superior efficacy versus placebo; (b) the patients enrolled in the trials of active comparator versus placebo and new treatment versus active comparator share common clinical features.

In the present analysis, all NOACs significantly lowered the risk of stroke versus imputed placebo, with reductions ranging between 71% with the higher dose of dabigatran and 38% with the lower dose of edoxaban (all p<0.001). Consequently, all NOACs retained more that 100% of the benefit of warfarin with the exception of edoxaban 30% that, however, retained 87% of its benefit. The higher dose of dabigatran, apixaban and the lower dose of edoxaban were the sole NOACs that significantly reduces all-cause mortality versus imputed placebo.

Our findings confirmed the results of a recent meta-analysis [46] in showing that NOACs, as a whole, are superior to warfarin in

reducing the primary composite outcome of stroke/systemic embolism and the secondary outcomes of death and hemorrhagic stroke. While intracranial bleedings were less frequent with NOACs than warfarin, gastrointestinal bleedings were more frequent with NOACs, but only with the higher dose regimens.

In the present analysis we focused on edoxaban as the latest entry in the available scenario of NOACs. In the ENGAGE-AF TIMI 48 trial [6], edoxaban 30 mg was non-inferior to adjusted dose warfarin on the primary composite outcome of stroke/systemic embolism and reduced by 13% the risk of all-cause death (p = 0.006) and by 15% the risk of cardiovascular death (p = 0.008). Also, the composite of death or disabling stroke was by 10% lower (p = 0.02) with edoxaban 30 mg than it was with warfarin. In the ENGAGE AF-TIMI 48 trial, edoxaban 30 mg was also associated with a 53% lower risk of major bleeding, and a 33% lower risk of gastrointestinal bleedings versus warfarin.

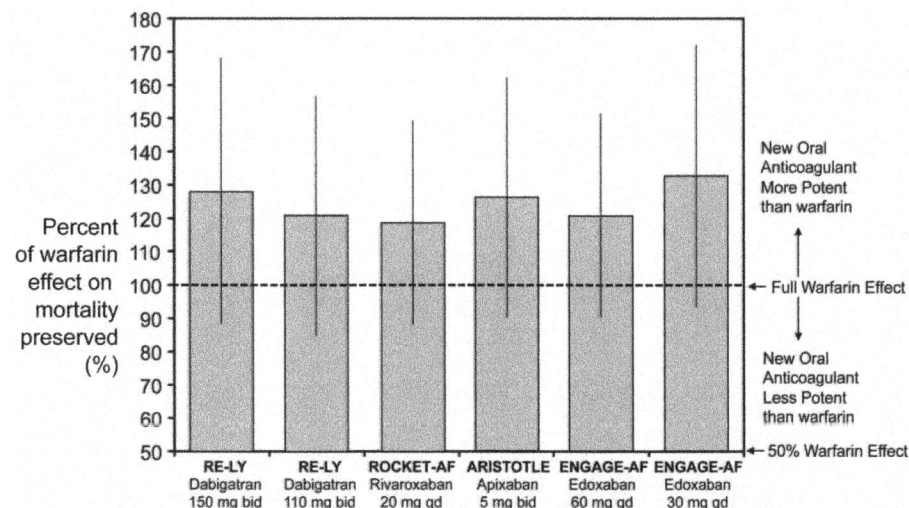

Figure 5. Estimated proportion of warfarin benefit by new oral anticoagulants on the risk of all-cause mortality.

Table 3. Odds ratio (with 95% confidence interval) of indirect comparisons of edoxaban versus dabigatran, rivaroxaban and apixaban. Efficacy end-points. Significant comparisons are printed in bold.

		Stroke or Systemic Embolism	Stroke	Hemorragic Stroke	Ischemic oruncertain stroke	Systemic Embolism	Myocardial Infarction	All-cause Death
Edoxaban 30 mg vs.	Dabigatran 110 mg bid	1.210 (0.922–1.589) p=0.17	1.238 (0.953–1.609) p=0.109	1.067 (0.514–2.214) p=0.862	1.279 (0.961–1.702) p=0.091	1.767 (0.747–4.179) p=0.195	0.917 (0.628–1.338) p=0.652	0.95 (0.801–1.126) p=0.552
	Dabigatran 150 mg bid	**1.684 (1.265–2.242) p<0.001**	**1.767 (1.337–2.334) p<0.001**	1.258 (0.588–2.691) p=0.555	**1.866 (1.378–2.528) p<0.001**	2.060 (0.852–4.983) p=0.109	0.936 (0.641–1.366) p=0.731	0.979 (0.826–1.161) p=0.808
	Rivaroxaban 20 mg qd	1.250 (0.977–1.599) p=0.076	**1.379 (1.072–1.773) p=0.012**	0.571 (0.308–1.059) p=0.076	**1.555 (1.172–2.062) p=0.002**	**5.560 (1.822–16.967) p=0.003**	**1.503 (1.062–2.127) p=0.022**	0.935 (0.801–1.093) p=0.400
	Apixaban 5 mg qd	**1.382 (1.068–1.788) p=0.014**	**1.451 (1.137–1.851) p=0.003**	0.650 (0.37–1.143) p=0.134	**1.563 (1.187–2.057) p=0.001**	1.437 (0.593–3.483) p=0.422	1.372 (0.954–1.974) p=0.088	0.971 (0.832–1.134) p=0.711
Edoxaban 60 mg vs.	Dabigatran 110 mg bid	0.862 (0.649–1.143) p=0.302	0.956 (0.732–1.248) p=0.739	1.747 (0.872–3.501) p=0.116	0.893 (0.666–1.199) p=0.452	0.912 (0.36–2.311) p=0.846	0.718 (0.488–1.055) p=0.092	1.002 (0.846–1.187) p=0.984
	Dabigatran 150 mg bid	1.199 (0.891–1.612) p=0.23	**1.363 (1.026–1.811) p=0.032**	2.060 (0.995–4.262) p=0.052	1.304 (0.955–1.779) p=0.095	1.063 (0.411–2.752) p=0.899	0.733 (0.498–1.078) p=0.114	1.033 (0.871–1.224) p=0.711
	Rivaroxaban 20 mg qd	0.890 (0.687–1.152) p=0.375	1.064 (0.822–1.376) p=0.637	0.935 (0.525–1.664) p=0.819	1.086 (0.812–1.452) p=0.578	2.870 (0.891–9.244) p=0.077	1.176 (0.824–1.679) p=0.372	0.987 (0.845–1.152) p=0.864
	Apixaban 5 mg qd	0.984 (0.752–1.287) p=0.905	1.119 (0.872–1.437) p=0.376	1.065 (0.634–1.787) p=0.813	1.091 (0.822–1.449) p=0.545	0.742 (0.286–1.923) p=0.539	1.074 (0.74–1.558) p=0.707	1.024 (0.878–1.195) p=0.761

Table 4. Odds ratio (with 95% confidence interval) of indirect comparisons of edoxaban versus dabigatran, rivaroxaban and apixaban.

		Major Bleeding	Intracranial Bleeding	Gastrointestinal Bleeding
Edoxaban 30 mg vs.	Dabigatran 110 mg bid	**0.581 (0.47–0.719) p<0.001**	1.033 (0.592–1.803) p=0.909	**0.626 (0.443–0.884) p=0.008**
	Dabigatran 150 mg bid	**0.498 (0.404–0.614) p<0.001**	0.740 (0.441–1.243) p=0.255	**0.465 (0.334–0.649) p<0.001**
	Rivaroxaban 20 mg qd	**0.454 (0.368–0.56) p<0.001**	**0.47 (0.288–0.767) p=0.003**	**0.421 (0.308–0.575) p<0.001**
	Apixaban 5 mg qd	**0.672 (0.544–0.829) p<0.001**	0.729 (0.451–1.177) p=0.196	0.768 (0.543–1.087) p=0.137
Edoxaban 60 mg vs.	Dabigatran 110 mg bid	0.979 (0.802–1.194) p=0.831	1.539 (0.907–2.611) p=0.11	1.142 (0.824–1.581) p=0.426
	Dabigatran 150 mg bid	0.839 (0.691–1.02) p=0.078	1.103 (0.677–1.797)p=0.695	0.849 (0.621–1.16) p=0.303
	Rivaroxaban 20 mg qd	**0.764 (0.628–0.93) p=0.007**	0.700 (0.443–1.107) p=0.127	0.768 (0.575–1.026) p=0.074
	Apixaban 5 mg qd	1.131 (0.929–1.377) p=0.22	1.086 (0.695–1.697) p=0.718	**1.400 (1.009–1.944) p=0.044**

Safety end-points. Significant comparisons are printed in bold.

Skjøth and coworkers recently published an indirect comparison analysis between different NOACs, including edoxaban [47]. Such analysis, however, did not estimate the benefits of each agent versus imputed placebo and the proportion of the warfarin effect preserved. The present study and that by Skjøth and coworkers share the conclusion that edoxaban 60 mg is comparable to apixaban, rivaroxaban and the lower dose of dabigatran, but inferior to the higher dose of dabigatran, for prevention of stroke. In terms of bleeding end-points, the higher dose of edoxaban is comparable to both doses of dabigatran, and associated with less major bleedings than rivaroxaban and more gastrointestinal bleedings than apixaban [47]. Conversely, the lower dose of edoxaban is comparable to the lower dose of dabigatran, but inferior to all other NOACs for prevention of stroke. The poorer efficacy of the lower dose of edoxaban appears to be outweighed by a higher safety, as reflected by a less risk of major bleedings versus all other NOACs and a less risk of gastrointestinal bleedings versus rivaroxaban and both doses of dabigatran.

Our study extends the conclusions by Skjøth and coworkers in showing that, despite its less antithrombotic efficacy, the lower dose of edoxaban significantly reduces the risk of any stroke (by 58%) and all-cause mortality (by 30%) when compared with a putative placebo. At the point estimate, the lower dose of edoxaban preserved 87% of the benefit of warfarin on stroke and 133% of the benefit of warfarin on all-cause mortality. Notably, the 95% CI of the estimated proportion of the warfarin benefit on stroke preserved by edoxaban 30 mg ranged between 69% in the worst case (i.e., the lower limit of the 95% CI) and 103% in the best case (i.e., the upper limit of the 95% CI). For all-cause mortality, it ranged between 93% in the worst case and 172% in the best case.

The preservation of a pre-specified fraction of the benefit of the control drug by the test drug is a concept that is applied routinely in non-inferiority trials [30]. FDA suggests that non-inferiority trials can be considered statistically persuasive when the test drug preserves at least 60% of the effect of the control treatment [48]. Thus, both doses of edoxaban were significantly more effective than imputed placebo in reducing the risk of stroke and preserved a substantial proportion of the benefit of warfarin, in line with the FDA guidance [48].

Limitations of the study

The indirect comparison analysis is used to estimate efficacy or safety differences between treatments in the absence of direct head-to-head comparisons [39,40]. It is unlikely that direct comparisons between different NOACs will be ever undertaken. However, the indirect comparison analysis has well recognized inherent limitations [16,17]. It assumes that the differences tested in the analysis between any NOAC and the common comparator (warfarin in our case) would have been similar ('similarity assumption') also in the context of a different trial population exposed to a different NOAC. The stability of relative treatment effects across trials would make warfarin a credible common comparator. The methods assumes, for example, that the efficacy and safety differences between dabigatran and warfarin found in the RE-LY [3] study would have been the same in the context of the patient population and trial methodology of ROCKET AF [4] or ENGAGE-AF TIMI 48 [6]. By contrast, some differences exist between the four major trials versus warfarin [3–6] that could limit the validity of the similarity assumption by making unclear whether the different effects versus warfarin would be attributable to the NOAC alone. Of utmost importance, the risk of thromboembolic complications, reflected by the CHADS$_2$ score, was higher in the ROCKET AF [4] and ENGAGE AF-TIMI 48 [6] than in the other trials (table 1). However, none of the subgroups analyses of any NOAC versus warfarin on the primary outcome was statistically significant for interaction by CHADS$_2$ score [3–6]. Other confounding factors that may limit the validity of indirect comparison analysis in our setting include the open (RE-LY [3]) versus double blind (other trials) design of warfarin administration, the average time in therapeutic range and the concomitant use of aspirin and other drugs.

Conclusions

In the present study, we tried to put the results of ENGAGE AF-TIMI 48 trial [6] in the scenario of available outcome data on NOACs. Notwithstanding the known caveats of indirect comparisons, while the higher dose of edoxaban did not show important differences from other NOACs in terms of efficacy and safety, the 30 mg dose showed some distinctive features. The better safety profile in terms of major bleedings compared to all other NOACs, and of gastrointestinal bleedings compared to dabigatran and rivaroxaban, would make the lower dose of edoxaban a reasonable option in patients with high or very high risk of bleeding [36]. The lower relative antithrombotic efficacy versus all other NOACs, except the lower dose of dabigatran, should be considered in the light of two findings: 1) the reduction of all-cause mortality in the head-to-head comparison versus warfarin; 2) the significant protective effect on stroke and all-cause mortality in the imputed-placebo analysis and the preservation of a substantial proportion of the protective benefit of warfarin on both outcome measures.

Author Contributions

Conceived and designed the experiments: PV FA GYHL GR. Analyzed the data: PV FA GYHL GR. Contributed reagents/materials/analysis tools: PV FA GYHL GR. Wrote the paper: PV FA GYHL GR.

References

1. Hart RG, Pearce LA, Aguilar MI (2007) Adjusted-dose warfarin versus aspirin for preventing stroke in patients with atrial fibrillation. Ann Intern Med 147: 590–592.
2. Husted S, De Caterina R, Andreotti F, Arnesen H, Bachmann F, et al. (2014) Non-vitamin K antagonist oral anticoagulants (NOACs): No longer new or novel. Thromb Haemost 111:781–782.
3. Connolly SJ, Ezekowitz MD, Yusuf S, Eikelboom J, Oldgren J, et al. (2009) Dabigatran versus warfarin in patients with atrial fibrillation. N Engl J Med 361: 1139–1151.
4. Patel MR, Mahaffey KW, Garg J, Pan G, Singer DE, et al. (2011) Rivaroxaban versus warfarin in nonvalvular atrial fibrillation. N Engl J Med 365: 883–891.
5. Granger CB, Alexander JH, McMurray JJ, Lopes RD, Hylek EM, et al. (2011) Apixaban versus warfarin in patients with atrial fibrillation. N Engl J Med 365: 981–992.
6. Giugliano RP, Ruff CT, Braunwald E, Murphy SA, Wiviott SD, et al. (2013) Edoxaban versus warfarin in patients with atrial fibrillation. N Engl J Med 369: 2093–2104.
7. Beasley BN, Unger EF, Temple R (2011) Anticoagulant options—why the FDA approved a higher but not a lower dose of dabigatran. N Engl J Med 364: 1788–1790.
8. Camm AJ, Lip GY, De Caterina R, Savelieva I, Atar D, et al. (2012) 2012 focused update of the ESC Guidelines for the management of atrial fibrillation: an update of the 2010 ESC Guidelines for the management of atrial fibrillation. Developed with the special contribution of the European Heart Rhythm Association. Eur Heart J 33: 2719–2747.
9. You JJ, Singer DE, Howard PA, Lane DA, Eckman MH, et al. (2012) Antithrombotic therapy for atrial fibrillation: Antithrombotic Therapy and Prevention of Thrombosis, 9th ed: American College of Chest Physicians Evidence-Based Clinical Practice Guidelines. Chest 141: e531S–575S.
10. Lip GY, Larsen TB, Skjoth F, Rasmussen LH (2012) Indirect comparisons of new oral anticoagulant drugs for efficacy and safety when used for stroke prevention in atrial fibrillation. J Am Coll Cardiol 60: 738–746.
11. Rasmussen LH, Larsen TB, Graungaard T, Skjoth F, Lip GY (2012) Primary and secondary prevention with new oral anticoagulant drugs for stroke prevention in atrial fibrillation: indirect comparison analysis. BMJ 345: e7097.
12. Baker WL, Phung OJ (2012) Systematic review and adjusted indirect comparison meta-analysis of oral anticoagulants in atrial fibrillation. Circ Cardiovasc Qual Outcomes 5: 711–719.
13. Mantha S, Ansell J (2012) An indirect comparison of dabigatran, rivaroxaban and apixaban for atrial fibrillation. Thromb Haemost 108: 476–484.
14. Harenberg J, Marx S, Diener HC, Lip GY, Marder VJ, et al. (2012) Comparison of efficacy and safety of dabigatran, rivaroxaban and apixaban in patients with atrial fibrillation using network meta-analysis. Int Angiol 31: 330–339.
15. Sardar P, Chatterjee S, Wu WC, Lichstein E, Ghosh J, et al. (2013) New oral anticoagulants are not superior to warfarin in secondary prevention of stroke or transient ischemic attacks, but lower the risk of intracranial bleeding: insights from a meta-analysis and indirect treatment comparisons. PLoS One 8: e77694.
16. Song F, Loke YK, Walsh T, Glenny AM, Eastwood AJ, et al. (2009) Methodological problems in the use of indirect comparisons for evaluating healthcare interventions: survey of published systematic reviews. BMJ 338: b1147.
17. Cannon CP, Kohli P (2012) Danger ahead: watch out for indirect comparisons! J Am Coll Cardiol 60: 747–748.
18. Harenberg J, Marx S, Wehling M (2012) Head-to-head or indirect comparisons of the novel oral anticoagulants in atrial fibrillation: what's next? Thromb Haemost 108: 407–409.
19. Skjoth F, Larsen TB, Rasmussen LH (2012) Indirect comparison studies—are they useful? Insights from the novel oral anticoagulants for stroke prevention in atrial fibrillation. Thromb Haemost 108: 405–406.
20. Liberati A, Altman DG, Tetzlaff J, Mulrow C, Gotzsche PC, et al. (2009) The PRISMA statement for reporting systematic reviews and meta-analyses of studies that evaluate health care interventions: explanation and elaboration. PLoS Med 6: e1000100.
21. Connolly SJ, Ezekowitz MD, Yusuf S, Reilly PA, Wallentin L (2010) Newly identified events in the RE-LY trial. N Engl J Med 363: 1875–1876.
22. D'Agostino RB Sr, Massaro JM, Sullivan LM (2003) Non-inferiority trials: design concepts and issues - the encounters of academic consultants in statistics. Stat Med 22: 169–186.
23. Durrleman S, Chaikin P (2003) The use of putative placebo in active control trials: two applications in a regulatory setting. Stat Med 22: 941–952.
24. Hasselblad V, Kong DF (2001) Statistical methods for comparison to placebo in active-control trials. Drug Info J 35: 435–439.
25. Kaul S, Diamond GA, Weintraub WS (2005) Trials and tribulations of non-inferiority: the ximelagatran experience. J Am Coll Cardiol 46: 1986–1995.
26. James Hung HM, Wang SJ, Tsong Y, Lawrence J, O'Neil RT (2003) Some fundamental issues with non-inferiority testing in active controlled trials. Stat Med 22: 213–225.
27. Snapinn SM (2004) Alternatives for discounting in the analysis of noninferiority trials. J Biopharm Stat 14: 263–273.
28. Lee S, Shafe AC, Cowie MR (2011) UK stroke incidence, mortality and cardiovascular risk management 1999–2008: time-trend analysis from the General Practice Research Database. BMJ Open 1: e000269.
29. Connolly SJ, Eikelboom J, O'Donnell M, Pogue J, Yusuf S (2007) Challenges of establishing new antithrombotic therapies in atrial fibrillation. Circulation 116: 449–455.
30. Snapinn S, Jiang Q (2011) Indirect comparisons in the comparative efficacy and non-inferiority settings. Pharm Stat 10: 420–426.
31. Snapinn S, Jiang Q (2008) Preservation of effect and the regulatory approval of new treatments on the basis of non-inferiority trials. Stat Med 27: 382–391.
32. Lip GY, Edwards SJ (2006) Stroke prevention with aspirin, warfarin and ximelagatran in patients with non-valvular atrial fibrillation: a systematic review and meta-analysis. Thromb Res 118: 321–333.
33. Kistler JP (1990) The effect of low-dose warfarin on the risk of stroke in patients with nonrheumatic atrial fibrillation. The Boston Area Anticoagulation Trial for Atrial Fibrillation Investigators. N Engl J Med 323: 1505–1511.
34. Koudstaal PJ (1993) Secondary prevention in non-rheumatic atrial fibrillation after transient ischaemic attack or minor stroke. EAFT (European Atrial Fibrillation Trial) Study Group. Lancet 342: 1255–1262.
35. Connolly SJ, Laupacis A, Gent M, Roberts RS, Cairns JA, et al. (1991) Canadian Atrial Fibrillation Anticoagulation (CAFA) Study. J Am Coll Cardiol 18: 349–355.
36. McBride R (1991) Stroke Prevention in Atrial Fibrillation Study. Final results. Circulation 84: 527–539.
37. Petersen P, Boysen G, Godtfredsen J, Andersen ED, Andersen B (1989) Placebo-controlled, randomised trial of warfarin and aspirin for prevention of thromboembolic complications in chronic atrial fibrillation. The Copenhagen AFASAK study. Lancet 1: 175–179.
38. Ezekowitz MD, Bridgers SL, James KE, Carliner NH, Colling CL, et al. (1992) Warfarin in the prevention of stroke associated with nonrheumatic atrial fibrillation. Veterans Affairs Stroke Prevention in Nonrheumatic Atrial Fibrillation Investigators. N Engl J Med 327: 1406–1412.
39. Bucher HC, Guyatt GH, Griffith LE, Walter SD (1997) The results of direct and indirect treatment comparisons in meta-analysis of randomized controlled trials. J Clin Epidemiol 50: 683–691.
40. Edwards SJ, Clarke MJ, Wordsworth S, Borrill J (2009) Indirect comparisons of treatments based on systematic reviews of randomised controlled trials. Int J Clin Pract 63: 841–854.
41. Hoaglin DC, Hawkins N, Jansen JP, Scott DA, Itzler R, et al. (2011) Conducting indirect-treatment-comparison and network-meta-analysis studies: report of the ISPOR Task Force on Indirect Treatment Comparisons Good Research Practices: part 2. Value Health 14: 429–437.
42. Jansen JP, Fleurence R, Devine B, Itzler R, Barrett A, et al. (2011) Interpreting indirect treatment comparisons and network meta-analysis for health-care decision making: report of the ISPOR Task Force on Indirect Treatment Comparisons Good Research Practices: part 1. Value Health 14: 417–428.

43. Gage BF, Waterman AD, Shannon W, Boechler M, Rich MW, et al. (2001) Validation of clinical classification schemes for predicting stroke: results from the National Registry of Atrial Fibrillation. JAMA 285: 2864–2870.

44. Oler A, Whooley MA, Oler J, Grady D (1996) Adding heparin to aspirin reduces the incidence of myocardial infarction and death in patients with unstable angina. A meta-analysis. JAMA 276: 811–815.

45. Antman EM, McCabe CH, Gurfinkel EP, Turpie AG, Bernink PJ, et al. (1999) Enoxaparin prevents death and cardiac ischemic events in unstable angina/non-Q-wave myocardial infarction. Results of the thrombolysis in myocardial infarction (TIMI) 11B trial. Circulation 100: 1593–1601.

46. Ruff CT, Giugliano RP, Braunwald E, Hoffman EB, Deenadayalu N, et al. (2014) Comparison of the efficacy and safety of new oral anticoagulants with warfarin in patients with atrial fibrillation: a meta-analysis of randomised trials. Lancet 383: 955–962.

47. Skjoth F, Larsen TB, Rasmussen LH, Lip GY (2014) Efficacy and safety of edoxaban in comparison with dabigatran, rivaroxaban and apixaban for stroke prevention in atrial fibrillation. An indirect comparison analysis. Thromb Haemost 111. Epub ahead of print.

48. Food and Drug Administration (2010) Guidance for Industry: Non-Inferiority Clinical Trials. Available: http://www.fda.gov/downloads/Drugs/GuidanceComplianceRegulatoryInformation/Guidances/UCM202140.pdf. Accessed 2 January 2014.

7

Efficacy and Safety of Vitamin K-Antagonists (VKA) for Atrial Fibrillation in Non-Dialysis Dependent Chronic Kidney Disease

Judith Kooiman[1]*, Nienke van Rein[1,2], Bas Spaans[1], Koen A. J. van Beers[1], Jonna R. Bank[1], Wilke R. van de Peppel[1], Antonio Iglesias del Sol[3], Suzanne C. Cannegieter[4], Ton J. Rabelink[5], Gregory Y. H. Lip[6], Frederikus A. Klok[1], Menno V. Huisman[1]

1 Department of Thrombosis and Hemostasis, Leiden University Medical Center, Leiden, The Netherlands, 2 Einthoven Laboratory of Experimental Vascular Medicine, Leiden University Medical Center, Leiden, The Netherlands, 3 Department of Internal Medicine, Rijnland Hospital, Leiderdorp, The Netherlands, 4 Department of Clinical Epidemiology, Leiden University Medical Center, Leiden, The Netherlands, 5 Department of Nephrology, Leiden University Medical Center, Leiden, The Netherlands, 6 Haemostasis, Thrombosis, and Vascular Biology Unit, University of Birmingham Centre for Cardiovascular Sciences, City Hospital, Birmingham, United Kingdom

Abstract

Background: Essential information regarding efficacy and safety of vitamin K-antagonists (VKA) treatment for atrial fibrillation (AF) in non-dialysis dependent chronic kidney disease (CKD) is still lacking in current literature. The aim of our study was to compare the risks of stroke or transient ischemic attack (TIA) and major bleeds between patients without CKD (eGFR >60 ml/min), and those with moderate (eGFR 30–60 ml/min), or severe non-dialysis dependent CKD (eGFR <30 ml/min).

Methods: We included 300 patients without CKD, 294 with moderate, and 130 with severe non-dialysis dependent CKD, who were matched for age and sex. Uni- and multivariate Cox regression analyses were performed reporting hazard ratios (HRs) for the endpoint of stroke or TIA and the endpoint of major bleeds as crude values and adjusted for comorbidity and platelet-inhibitor use.

Results: Overall, 6.2% (45/724, 1.7/100 patient years) of patients developed stroke or TIA and 15.6% (113/724, 4.8/100 patient years) a major bleeding event. Patients with severe CKD were at high risk of stroke or TIA and major bleeds during VKA treatment compared with those without renal impairment, HR 2.75 (95%CI 1.25–6.05) and 1.66 (95%CI 0.97–2.86), or with moderate CKD, HR 3.93(1.71–9.00) and 1.86 (95%CI 1.08–3.21), respectively. These risks were similar for patients without and with moderate CKD. Importantly, both less time spent within therapeutic range and high INR-variability were associated with increased risks of stroke or TIA and major bleeds in severe CKD patients.

Conclusions: VKA treatment for AF in patients with severe CKD has a poor safety and efficacy profile, likely related to suboptimal anticoagulation control. Our study findings stress the need for better tailored individualised anticoagulant treatment approaches for patients with AF and severe CKD.

Editor: Kathrin Eller, Medical University of Graz, Austria

Funding: The authors have no support or funding to report.

Competing Interests: The authors have declared that no competing interests exist.

* E-mail: j.kooiman@lumc.nl

Introduction

About one-third of atrial fibrillation (AF) patients suffer from chronic kidney disease (CKD) [1–3], a condition that by itself increases the risk of stroke, even in the absence of AF. Inversely, AF in CKD patients is associated with progression of CKD, cardiovascular morbidity and mortality [4–6].

Antithrombotic treatment is very effective in preventing stroke or a transient ischemic attack (TIA) in patients with AF, both in patients with normal renal function and in those with CKD in terms of a relative risk reduction [7–9]. However, CKD increases a patient's risk of major bleeding complications during antithrombotic treatment [8,10]. The extent to which non-dialysis depen-

dent CKD increases the risk of stroke and major bleeds in AF patients during VKA treatment is understudied, as the main focus in research in this area has been on patients with end-stage-renal disease requiring dialysis. However, these patients comprise less than 1% of the AF population [8,11]. The few studies that have focussed on risks of stroke and/or major bleeding in AF patients with non-dialysis dependent CKD were limited by their small sample size [10,12,13], the absence of information on eGFR levels [8], exclusion of patients with severe CKD [7], or a divergent patient cohort with various indications for VKA treatment [14]. Knowledge about these risks would most certainly provide relevant insights into treatment outcomes in a patient group that frequently attends both cardiology and internal medicine practices. Moreover, with the emergence of novel oral anticoagulants, understanding the risks of stroke and major bleeding events in AF patients with various stages of CKD is essential when evaluating whether these new agents would provide a more favourable risk-benefit ratio than the traditional vitamin K-antagonists (VKA) for this specific patient population [11].

Therefore, the aim of our study was to compare risks of stroke or TIA and major bleeds in patients with moderate or severe CKD and AF treated with VKAs with patients without renal impairment. Second, we assessed the influence of quality of anticoagulation control on the risks of stroke or TIA and major bleeds.

Methods

Patients diagnosed with new onset valvular or non-valvular AF starting VKA treatment between 1997 and 2005 at the Leiden anticoagulation clinic were included in a previously described study cohort [3]. This anticoagulation clinic serves one academic (Leiden University Medical Center, Leiden) and two non-academic teaching hospitals (Diaconessenhuis, Leiden, and Rijnland Hospital, Leiderdorp). Within this cohort of 5039 AF patients, 3316 had no CKD (eGFR >60 ml/min), 1557 (eGFR 30–60 ml/min) had moderate CKD, and 166 patients severe CKD (eGFR <30 ml/min), as measured at start of VKA therapy. For the current analysis, we excluded fourteen patients from the severe CKD group who had acute kidney injury at time of VKA therapy initiation, after which renal function recovered to a less critical CKD stage, thus leaving 152 patients with severe CKD. Since reviewing medical records of all 1557 moderate and 3316 non-CKD patients would be an effort not offsetting the statistical gain, we sampled 300 patients without CKD and 294 patients with moderate CKD for inclusion, matched for age and gender to those with severe CKD. Patients treated with VKA via the Leiden anticoagulation clinic for <7 days were excluded from the study cohort and replaced by others of the same age, gender, and level of renal impairment. Patients on dialysis at start of VKA therapy were also excluded, but were not replaced. Patients were treated with either phenprocoumon (Marcoumar) or acenocoumarol. The study was approved by the ethics committee of the three participating hospitals (ethics committee Leiden University Medical Center, Leiden, the Netherlands) that waived the need for informed consent.

Chart review

Medical records from two sources (i.e. the participating hospitals and the Leiden anticoagulation clinic) were searched for information on patient characteristics at baseline, comorbidity, use of platelet-inhibitors, International Normalized Ratios (INRs) and study outcomes. Renal function was assessed using the abbreviated modification of diet in renal disease (MDRD) formula, as it accurately estimates renal function in elderly patients and the mean age of our study population was high [15,16].

Study outcomes and definitions

Primary outcomes of this study were the combined endpoint of stroke or TIA and the occurrence of major bleeding events. Major bleeding was defined by the International Society of Thrombosis and Hemostasis criteria (i.e. fatal bleeding, any bleeding causing a drop in hemoglobin level ≥1.24 mmol/L and/or requiring transfusion of ≥2 units of whole blood or red cells and/or a symptomatic bleeding in a critical area/organ (intracranial, intraspinal, intraocular, pericardial, or intramuscular with compartment syndrome)) [17]. Secondary endpoints were major adverse cardiovascular events (MACE), fatal MACE and fatal

bleeding. MACE was defined as stroke or TIA, myocardial infarction, intermittent claudication, unstable angina, carotid endarterectomy, coronary artery bypass graft, peripheral arterial bypass or angioplasty [18]. Other variables of interest were time within therapeutic range (TTR) and INR-variability; both established risk factors for MACE and major bleeding complications during VKA treatment [19–23]. INR-values were measured using HepatoQuick (Roche Diagnostics, Mannheim, Germany) and serum creatinine values by using Roche Diagnostics Analyzers (Mannheim, Germany).

Follow- up

Duration of follow-up was defined as time elapsed between the day of initiation and permanent discontinuation of VKA treatment, occurrence of the endpoint of interest, or death, or December 31, 2010. Only the first stroke or TIA, MACE or major bleeding event that occurred was recorded in the database, although some patients had more than one episode of the endpoints. For non-acute MACE such as intermittent claudication, carotid endarterectomy, coronary artery bypass graft, peripheral arterial bypass or angioplasty, the day of diagnosis or intervention was recorded as the date of MACE occurrence.

Statistical analysis

Incidence rates (i.e. events/100 patient years (py)) of primary outcomes were reported with corresponding 95% confidence intervals (CI). As patients with moderate or without CKD were matched for age and gender to those with severe CKD, incidence rates of our study endpoints in the first two patient groups reflect the incidences of these endpoints for the population with this age and sex distribution, rather than that of the overall AF population. Nonetheless, this design allowed us to study relative risks of stroke or TIA and major bleeds between patients with severe or moderate CKD and those without renal impairment, which was our main research question. This analysis was performed using uni- and multivariate Cox regression analyses reporting hazard ratios (HRs) as crude values and as values corrected for age, gender, concomitant use of platelet-inhibitors or non-steroidal anti-inflammatory drugs, hypertension, diabetes mellitus, and congestive heart failure. As for secondary analysis, TTR and INR-variability were calculated using the *Rosendaal* method and the formula by *Cannegieter*, respectively [23,24]. INR-variability and TTR were compared between patients with moderate or severe CKD and non-CKD patients, using first a Kruskal Wallis and second a Mann Whitney U-test, as these values had a non-parametric distribution among the population.

Mediation analysis

A mediation analysis was performed to assess whether the expected increased risks of stroke or TIA, major bleeds and MACE in patients with moderate and severe CKD compared with non-CKD patients were mediated via TTR or INR-variability. This analysis was performed for the three endpoints and the combined endpoint of MACE and major bleeds in a nested case-control study [24]. We chose this design as the duration of follow-up needed to be matched for cases and controls. Cases were patients developing the endpoint of interest. For each case, a maximum of four controls was selected from the total study population of 724 patients who were treated during the same period with VKA while not developing this specific endpoint at the time that the case did (incidence density sampling). A control could be selected for more than one case. INR-variability and TTR were calculated over the entire treatment period, for the last six and the last three months prior to the outcome of interest. For each time frame, only patients with sufficient follow-up were selected for that specific analysis [24]. Crude odds ratios (OR) were then computed for the risks of the four outcomes comparing severe and moderate CKD with non-CKD patients. Next, these ORs were first adjusted for comorbidity, and second for either INR-variability, TTR, or both for each individual time frame.

All statistical analyses were performed in SPSS 20.0 (IBM SPSS statistics, IBM Corp, Somers, NY).

Results

Serum creatinine values were available in 5039 out of 6933 patients with new onset AF at start of VKA therapy. Of those, 733 matched subjects were selected for inclusion for this present study, comprising all patients with non-dialysis depended severe CKD, and a sample of those with moderate or without CKD. Registered duration of VKA treatment in the Leiden anticoagulation clinic was less than seven days in 52 patients who were excluded and replaced by 43 patients of similar gender, age, and level of renal impairment. The remaining nine severe CKD patients could not be replaced (Figure 1). Thus, 724 patients were included in this study, 300 without CKD (eGFR >60 ml/min), 294 with moderate (eGFR 30–60 ml/min) and 130 with severe CKD (eGFR < 30 ml/min). Patient characteristics at baseline are reported in Table 1. Compared with patients without CKD, those with moderate or severe CKD were more likely to have congestive heart failure, hypertension, diabetes mellitus, or a previous episode of major bleeds before initiation of VKA therapy. Median follow-up time was 2.1 years (2.5–97.5percentile 0.0–10.0) for the

endpoint of stroke or TIA and 2.3 years (2.5–97.5percentiles 0.0–10.0) for major bleeding events.

Stroke or TIA and MACE

During follow-up for the primary endpoint, 6.2% (45/724, 1.67/100 py) of patients developed a stroke (29 patients) or TIA (16 patients). The risk of stroke or TIA was increased in those with severe CKD compared with patients without renal dysfunction (HR 2.75, 95%CI 1.25–6.05) or those with moderate CKD (HR 3.93, 95%CI 1.71–9.00, Table 2). The risk of stroke or TIA was similar for patients with moderate and without CKD.

Overall, 14.8% (107/724) of patients developed MACE of whom 28 patients had a stroke, 15 a TIA, 28 a myocardial infarction, 17 an unstable angina pectoris, 11 patients underwent coronary artery bypass grafting, and 8 patients had developed peripheral artery disease (one patient developed a stroke and another patient a TIA after the occurrence of an earlier MACE). Patients with severe CKD were at increased risk of MACE compared with non-CKD patients (adjusted HR 3.57, 95%CI 2.10–6.06) and those with moderate CKD (adjusted HR 3.40, 95%CI 2.05–5.64). MACE risk was similar for those without and with moderate CKD. Twenty-three of 724 patients had a fatal MACE, of whom 14 (60.9%) developed a myocardial infarction and 9 (39.1%) a stroke. Although non-significant, moderate and severe CKD were associated with a 60–90% increased risk of fatal MACE compared with non-CKD patients, respectively.

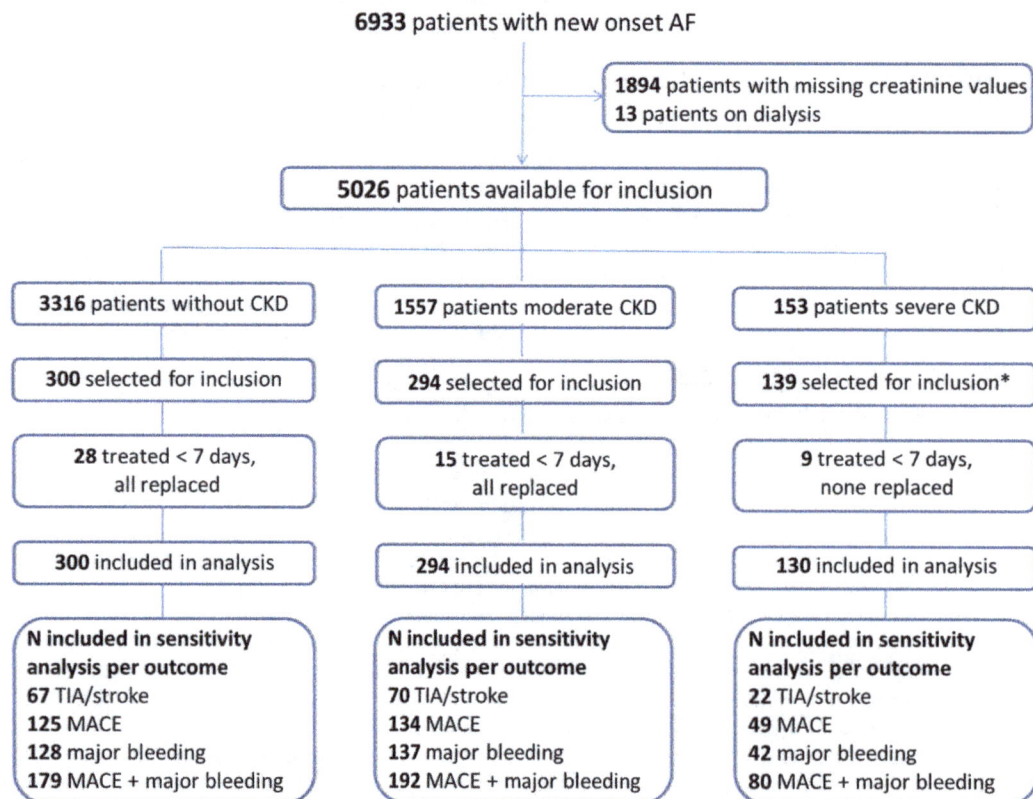

Figure 1. Flow chart. Abbreviations: CKD = Chronic kidney disease, TIA = transient ischemic attack, MACE = major adverse cardiovascular event. * Fourteen patients from the severe CKD group had acute kidney injury at time of VKA therapy initiation, after which renal function recovered to a less critical CKD stage.

Table 1. Patient characteristics at baseline of the total population.

	No CKD eGFR>60 ml/min	Moderate CKD eGFR 30–60 ml/min	Severe CKD eGFR<30 ml/min
N	**300**	**294**	**130**
Mean age (SD)	74(10)	75(10)	76(9)
Gender, m/f	171/129	165/129	73/57
Mean eGFR (SD)	92(37)	46(8)	21(7)
Diabetes Mellitus	35(11.7)	50(17.0)	38(29.2)
Hypertension	138(46.0)	181(61.6)	80(61.5)
Concomitant use of platelet inhibitors	26(8.7)	35(11.9)	7(5.4)
Previous stroke or TIA	47(15.7)	59(20.1)	21(16.2)
Previous major bleeding	14(4.7)	21(7.1)	10(7.7)
Congestive heart failure	50(17.0)	105(35.7)	54(41.5)
INR target range*			
2.0–3.0	1(0.3)	0(0.0)	1(0.8)
2.5–3.5	287(98.6)	280(97.9)	116(97.5)
3.0–4.0	3(1.0)	6(2.1)	2(1.7)
Acenocoumarol**	13(4.3)	15(5.1)	9(7.0)
Phenprocoumon	287(95.7)	278(94.6)	120(93.0)

Data is presented as n, % unless stated otherwise.
CKD = chronic kidney disease, eGFR = estimated glomerular filtration rate, SD = standard deviation, TIA = transient ischemic attack.
* Lacking in 30 patients, ** lacking in one patient.

Major bleeding complications

Major bleeding complications occurred in 15.6% of patients (113/724, 4.8/100 py). Although non-significant, severe CKD was associated with an increased risk of major bleeds compared with patients without renal impairment (adjusted HR 1.66, 95%CI0.97–2.86), and those with moderate CKD (HR 1.86, 95%CI1.08–3.21). Major bleeding risks were similar for those without and with moderate CKD. The most frequent locations of major bleeding were gastrointestinal (34.5%) and intracranial (27.4%) in the total population. Patients with severe CKD were more likely to develop gastrointestinal bleeding (63.6%), yet less frequently developed intracranial haemorrhages (13.6%).

Fatal bleeding occurred in 2.9% of patients (21/724). Severe CKD might be associated with an increased risk of fatal bleeding events compared with non-CKD patients (HR 1.52, 95%CI0.46–5.02, Table 2), and those with moderate CKD (HR 1.90, 95%CI0.57–6.41).

TTR and INR variability

Compared with patients without CKD, TTR was higher in those with moderate CKD (75.1%, p<0.01) whereas TTR was similar in patients with severe CKD (70.3%, p = 0.41, Table 3). The proportion of time spent above target range was higher for all CKD stages compared with patients without renal impairment, and higher for those with severe compared with moderate CKD. Median INR-variability during the entire treatment period significantly increased with each stage of CKD, with median values of 0.5 in patients without CKD, 0.7 (p = 0.03) in those with moderate, and 0.9 (p<0.001) in those with severe CKD. For all three groups, the degree of INR variability can be regarded as below average or unstable anticoagulant control according to previous research [25].

Mediation analysis

Mediation analyses were performed on the influence of TTR and INR-variability on the increased risks of stroke or TIA, MACE and major bleeding complications in severe CKD compared with non-CKD patients. TTR and INR-variability were analysed as continuous and categorical variables (based on 33rd and 66th percentiles) in separate models demonstrating similar results. For all four outcomes, the results demonstrated a decrease in the odds ratio towards unity in severe CKD compared with non-CKD patients, when corrected for either INR-variability or TTR (Table 4 and 5). However, the effect of INR-variability and TTR in the three months prior to combined endpoint of stroke or TIA and to the endpoint of MACE was less pronounced. This might be the result of the low number of INR measurements during this short timeframe (median 5.0, 2.5–97.5 percentile 2.0–10.5), which might not be sufficient for adequate assessment of TTR and INR-variability. Simultaneous correction for both INR-variability and TTR did not result in a further decrease towards unity for any of the endpoints comparing severe and moderate CKD to non-CKD patients, indicating no additive effect of TTR over INR-variability, and vice versa. This indicates that the increased risks in patients with severe CKD for stroke or TIA, major bleeds and MACE were mediated via suboptimal anticoagulation control.

Discussion

Our study has three important findings. First, risks of stroke or TIA, MACE and major bleeding complications during VKA therapy were high in AF patients with severe non-dialysis dependent CKD, when compared to those without renal impairment, or with moderate CKD. Second, stroke or TIA, MACE and major bleeding risks were similar for patients with moderate CKD and those with normal renal function. Third, patients with CKD spent more time above INR target range and

Table 2. Risk of stroke, TIA, MACE and major bleeding events during vitamin K-antagonist treatment stratified by renal function within the entire population.

Endpoint	No. of events	N/100 py‡ (95% CI)	Crude HR (95% CI)	Adjusted HR (95% CI)
Stroke or TIA				
No CKD	19	1.62(1.03–2.54)	ref	ref
Moderate CKD	15	1.20(0.71–1.99)	0.72(0.36–1.41)	0.70(0.35–1.41)
Severe CKD	11	4.24(2.30–7.53)	2.40(1.13–5.07)	2.75(1.25–6.05)
Overall MACE*				
No CKD	36	3.48(2.51–4.80)	ref	ref
Moderate CKD	41	3.79(2.80–5.12)	1.06(0.68–1.67)	1.05(0.66–1.67)
Severe CKD	30	15.4(10.95–21.16)	3.78(2.31–6.19)	3.57(2.10–6.06)
Fatal MACE†				
No CKD	7	0.64(0.28–1.35)	ref	ref
Moderate CKD	12	1.05(0.58–1.85)	1.68(0.66–4.27)	1.64(0.64–4.17)
Severe CKD	4	1.67(0.50–4.38)	2.09(0.60–7.23)	1.92(0.55–6.67)
Overall major bleeding*				
No CKD	46	4.45(3.34–5.89)	ref	ref
Moderate CKD	45	4.11(3.07–5.46)	0.91(0.60–1.37)	0.90(0.59–1.37)
Severe CKD	22	8.84(5.85–13.07)	1.88(1.13–3.14)	1.66(0.97–2.86)
Fatal bleeding†				
No CKD	9	0.83(0.41–1.59)	ref	ref
Moderate CKD	8	0.70(0.33–1.40)	0.85(0.33–2.21)	0.82(0.32–2.13)
Severe CKD	4	1.67(0.50–4.38)	1.62(0.49–5.33)	1.52(0.46–5.02)

Definitions: no-CKD = estimated glomerular filtration rate (eGFR) >60 ml/min, moderate CKD = eGFR 30–60 ml/min, severe CKD = eGFR <30 ml/min.
Abbreviations: CKD = chronic kidney disease, PY = patient years, CI = confidence interval, HR = hazard ratio, MACE = major adverse cardiovascular event, TIA = transient ischemic attack.
‡Reported incidences for patients with an eGFR 30–60 or eGFR >60 ml/min are influenced by sampling of patients matched for age and gender to those with an eGFR <30 ml/min.
* HR adjusted for age, gender, hypertension, the use of platelet-inhibitors, diabetes mellitus and congestive heart failure.
†HR adjusted for age and gender. Further correcting resulted in non-converging coefficients.

had a higher INR-variability. Consequently, in a nested case-control study we have shown additionally that poor anticoagulation control was associated with increased risks of stroke or TIA, MACE and major bleeds in severe CKD patients. Our study therefore provides important insights into the efficacy and safety of VKA treatment in patients with CKD and AF.

CKD is a common comorbid condition in AF patients and increases a patient's risk for both stroke and major bleeds. Suggested mechanisms for this higher stroke and bleeding risk are endothelial dysfunction, hypercoagulability, and chronic inflammation [8,11,12]. We demonstrated in a nested case-control study that impaired anticoagulation control might be an important additional determinant. Interestingly, within the total study population of 724 patients, CKD patients were spending more time above INR target range and had a higher INR variability compared with non-CKD patients, despite frequent INR monitoring. We hypothesize several explanations for this observation. CKD by itself may affect the quality of anticoagulant treatment. First, renal impairment might influence hepatic VKA metabolism, as has been shown in animal models for hepatic cytochrome P-450 metabolism [26,27]. Second, CKD influences the pharmacokinetic characteristics of VKA, as warfarin half-life was reported to be shorter in CKD compared with non-CKD patients with a greater unbound warfarin fraction [28,29]. Third, we cannot exclude that anticoagulant control is impaired in patients with CKD by poor patient compliance. Regardless of the mechanism by which CKD

influences the quality of VKA therapy, our nested case-control study indicates that the increased risks of stroke or TIA, MACE and major bleeding complications in severe CKD patients are mediated through suboptimal anticoagulation control. This suggests that although warfarin has been shown to be effective in preventing stroke in CKD patients with AF in two observational and one randomized study [7,8,12], there is a great need for better tailored anticoagulant treatment approaches for this specific population, involving either better INR control, or the use of anticoagulants other than VKAs.

The use of computer-assisted dosage programs surveying both INR-variability and TTR during VKA treatment may help to identify patients with poor anticoagulant control in order to prevent them from developing stroke, TIA or major bleeding events [30]. Further, patient education and self-monitoring of INRs might improve patient compliance [31].

The novel oral anticoagulants have demonstrated less inter- and intra-individual variability in their pharmacokinetic properties compared with VKA. Within the Phase-3 trials, subgroup analyses have been performed for the efficacy and safety of these new agents compared with standard warfarin or aspirin treatment in AF patients with moderate CKD (i.e. eGFR >25 or >30 ml/min) [32]. These analyses demonstrated either a reduced risk of stroke and systemic thromboembolism compared with warfarin (Dabigatran 150 mg twice daily) or aspirin (Apixaban 5 mg twice daily), or a similar efficacy compared with warfarin treatment for AF

Table 3. Time within therapeutic range and INR variability within the entire population of 724 patients with atrial fibrillation.

	No CKD	Moderate CKD	P-value comparison	Severe CKD	P-value comparison	P-value comparison with
	eGFR>60 ml/min	eGFR 30-60 ml/min	with no CKD patients	eGFR<30 ml/min	with no CKD patients	moderate CKD patients
Time spend within therapeutic range, %						
First six weeks of VKA therapy	39.4(13.2-73.5)	49.7(24.1-81.3)	0.01	44.1(26.4-77.9)	0.10	0.60
First eighteen weeks of VKA therapy	57.9(29.8-79.3)	65.5(42.1-83.9)	0.01	60.7(39.4-80.6)	0.37	0.19
First twenty-six weeks of VKA therapy	61.5(38.7-79.8)	67.1(46.7-82.4)	0.02	64.7(41.5-75.6)	0.92	0.07
Entire treatment period	67.0(43.1-81.1)	75.1(57.8-82.9)	<0.01	70.3(49.2-81.1)	0.41	0.10
Time under target range (entire treatment), %	8.7(2.6-35.5)	6.2(2.1-13.0)	<0.001	5.5(2.3-12.9)	0.001	0.77
Time above target range (entire treatment), %	11.7(3.9-21.2)	15.2(9.8-24.0)	<0.001	20.8(11.7-32.7)	<0.001	<0.01
INR variability (2.5-97.5 percentiles)						
First six weeks of VKA therapy	0.5(0.1-1.6)	0.6(0.2-1.6)	0.10	0.7(0.4-2.3)	0.001	0.03
First eighteen weeks of VKA therapy	0.4(0.2-1.3)	0.6(0.2-1.5)	0.08	0.8(0.4-1.8)	<0.001	0.01
First twenty-six weeks of VKA therapy	0.5(0.3-1.2)	0.7(0.4-1.2)	0.24	0.8(0.4-1.8)	<0.001	<0.01
Entire treatment period	0.5(0.3-1.2)	0.7(0.4-1.2)	0.03	0.9(0.5-1.8)	<0.001	<0.01

Data are presented as median, (Interquartile range), P-values were computed using Mann-Whitney test, after proof of significant differences between groups using a Kruskal-Wallis test. CKD = chronic kidney disease, VKA = vitamin K-antagonists, eGFR = estimated glomerular filtration rate, INR = international normalized ratio.

Table 4. Mediation analysis on effect of INR-variability on the increased risks of major adverse cardiovascular events and major bleeding complications in patients with chronic kidney disease in a nested case-control study.

Outcome	Crude OR (95% CI)	Adjusted OR 1 (95% CI)	Adjusted OR 2 (95% CI)	Adjusted OR 3 (95% CI)	Adjusted OR 4 (95% CI)
Stroke or TIA					
No CKD (N=91, of whom 67 unique)	ref	ref	ref	ref	ref
Moderate CKD (N=90, of whom 70 unique)	0.76(0.36–1.61)	0.76(0.35–1.67)	0.79(0.36–1.76)	1.06(0.41–2.75)	1.02(0.40–2.56)
Severe CKD (N=25, of whom 22 unique)	2.98(1.17–7.60)	2.56(0.92–7.10)	2.23(0.73–6.84)	1.96(0.50–7.74)	2.50(0.69–9.07)
MACE					
No CKD (N=210, of whom 125 unique)	ref	ref	ref	ref	ref
Moderate CKD (N=205, of whom 134 unique)	1.21(0.74–1.98)	1.14(0.68–1.93)	1.15(0.66–1.99)	1.05(0.58–1.91)	1.10(0.62–1.96)
Severe CKD (N=58, of whom 49 unique)	5.18(2.76–9.70)	5.07(2.57–10.02)	5.37(2.58–11.19)	3.58(1.59–8.03)	3.77(1.71–8.32)
Major bleeding					
No CKD (N=211, of whom 128 unique)	ref	ref	ref	ref	ref
Moderate CKD (N=245, of whom 137 unique)	0.81(0.51–1.28)	0.76(0.47–1.23)	0.74(0.45–1.22)	0.88(0.52–1.52)	0.83(0.49–1.40)
Severe CKD (N=60, of whom 42 unique)	2.08(1.12–3.85)	1.77(0.91–3.43)	1.82(0.93–3.56)	1.55(0.70–3.44)	1.57(0.72–3.40)
Major bleeding or MACE					
No CKD (N=361, of whom 179 unique)	ref	ref	ref	ref	ref
Moderate CKD (N=419, of whom 192 unique)	0.87(0.62–1.25)	0.85(0.59–1.24)	0.87(0.59–1.27)	0.93(0.61–1.41)	0.88(0.59–1.34)
Severe CKD (N=122, of whom 80 unique)	2.92(1.88–4.54)	2.61(1.64–4.16)	2.67(1.64–4.34)	2.49(1.40–4.41)	2.31(1.33–4.03)

Model 1 includes age, gender, hypertension, the use of platelet-inhibitors, diabetes mellitus and congestive heart failure.
Model 2 includes model 1 + INR VAR entire treatment period, Model 3 includes model 1 + INR variability over six months prior to event.
Model 4 includes model 1 + INR variability over three months prior to event.
Abbreviations: CKD = chronic kidney disease, MACE = major adverse cardiovascular event, OR = odds ratio, TIA = transient ischemic attack.

Table 5. Mediation analysis on effect of time within therapeutic range on the increased risks of major adverse cardiovascular events and major bleeding complications in patients with chronic kidney disease in a nested case-control study.

Outcome	Crude OR (95% CI)	Adjusted OR 1 (95% CI)	Adjusted OR 2 (95% CI)	Adjusted OR 3 (95% CI)	Adjusted OR 4 (95% CI)
Stroke or TIA					
No CKD (N=91, of whom 67 unique)	ref	ref	ref	ref	ref
Moderate CKD (N=90, of whom 70 unique)	0.76(0.36–1.61)	0.76(0.35–1.67)	0.94(0.41–2.13)	1.31(0.52–3.37)	1.01(0.40–2.56)
Severe CKD (N=25, of whom 22 unique)	2.98(1.17–7.60)	2.56(0.92–7.10)	1.95(0.64–5.88)	2.49(0.65–9.55)	2.46(0.68–8.88)
MACE					
No CKD (N=210, of whom 125 unique)	ref	ref	ref	ref	ref
Moderate CKD (N=205, of whom 134 unique)	1.21(0.74–1.98)	1.14(0.68–1.93)	1.16(0.67–2.01)	1.06(0.58–1.93)	1.11(0.62–1.98)
Severe CKD (N=58, of whom 49 unique)	5.18(2.76–9.70)	5.07(2.57–10.02)	4.98(2.42–10.23)	3.26(1.45–7.34)	3.42(1.55–7.55)
Major bleeding					
No CKD (N=211, of whom 128 unique)	ref	ref	ref	ref	ref
Moderate CKD (N=245, of whom 137 unique)	0.81(0.51–1.28)	0.76(0.47–1.23)	0.73(0.44–1.21)	0.87(0.51–1.50)	0.83(0.49–1.41)
Severe CKD (N=60, of whom 42 unique)	2.08(1.12–3.85)	1.77(0.91–3.43)	1.55(0.79–3.07)	1.48(0.67–3.29)	1.50(0.68–3.28)
Major bleeding or MACE					
No CKD (N=361, of whom 179 unique)	ref	ref	ref	ref	ref
Moderate CKD (N=419, of whom 192 unique)	0.87(0.62–1.25)	0.85(0.59–1.24)	0.93(0.62–1.40)	0.96(0.63–1.46)	0.93(0.62–1.40)
Severe CKD (N=122, of whom 80 unique)	2.92(1.88–4.54)	2.61(1.64–4.16)	2.22(1.27–3.88)	2.37(1.33–4.21)	2.22(1.27–3.88)

Model 1 includes age, gender, hypertension, the use of platelet-inhibitors, diabetes mellitus and congestive heart failure.
Model 2 includes model 1 + time within therapeutic range over entire treatment period, Model 3 includes model 1 + time within therapeutic range over six months prior to event, Model 4 includes model 1 + time within therapeutic range over three months prior to event.
Abbreviations: CKD = chronic kidney disease, MACE = major adverse cardiovascular event, OR = odds ratio, TIA = transient ischemic attack.

(rivaroxaban 20 mg per day, or apixaban 5 mg twice daily). In terms of safety, the Aristotle trial demonstrated a lower risk of major bleeds in the apixaban compared with the warfarin group, whereas for all other novel oral anticoagulants, bleeding risks were comparable with the risks on warfarin or aspirin treatment [32]. Though, it is unknown whether these new agents would provide a better tailored anticoagulant treatment strategy compared with warfarin in severe CKD patients as they have been excluded systematically from the Phase-3 trials [33–35]. In terms of renal clearance, apixaban (25%) and betrixaban (17%) might be most suitable for use in patients with CKD. Although betrixaban has not been studied yet in a Phase-3 trial for stroke prevention in AF, the results of the Phase-2 trial, in which only CKD patients on dialysis were excluded, were promising in terms of a lower risk of bleeding compared with standard warfarin treatment in the group receiving the lowest betrixaban dose (i.e. 40 mg daily) [36]. However, the use of novel oral anticoagulants may not be advisable when the insufficient anticoagulant control in the CKD population is caused by poor patient compliance, which might even more be difficult to manage when laboratory monitoring of anticoagulant therapy is no longer required.

Our study has limitations. First, we had no information on alterations in renal function during follow-up, which might have led to misclassification of patients and consequently a misestimation of the reported hazard ratios. Second, events were recorded from chart review given the design of the study and we cannot fully exclude that some events were missed. However, our endpoints of stroke or TIA, MACE and major bleeding were clearly defined and are both serious medical events, requiring evaluation in a hospital setting and are thus likely to be reported in medical charts. Third, our primary and secondary outcomes were not adjudicated by an independent committee. Fourth, our sample size was too small to make further subdivisions in the stages of CKD other than moderate and severe CKD, or to demonstrate statistical differences in fatal MACE and bleeding rates. Fifth, we did not investigate the influence of co-medication interacting with VKAs

on study outcomes. However, the majority of medication used by severe CKD patients is not known for interactions with VKAs. Sixth, we missed serum creatinine values at time of VKA initiation in 1894 of 9633 patients (19.6%) but we selected all patients with severe CKD (for whom serum creatinine values are highly unlikely to be lacking) and sampled controls matched for age and gender with moderate or without CKD. As patients without serum creatinine values are unlikely to have severe CKD it is implausible that lacking creatinine values in 1894 patients influenced the reported HRs on study outcomes.

In conclusion, patients with severe non-dialysis dependent CKD (i.e. eGFR <30 ml/min) are at higher risk for stroke or TIA, MACE and major bleeding complications during VKA treatment for AF, compared with those with moderate CKD (i.e. eGFR 30–60), or without renal impairment. Our study suggests that suboptimal anticoagulation control is a determinant in their poor cardiovascular prognosis. These study findings stress the need for more advanced tailored anticoagulant treatment approaches for AF patients with severe CKD. Whether the use of computer-assisted VKA dosage programs monitoring both INR-variability and TTR, or the use of novel oral anticoagulants are the answer to this issue remains to be studied.

Acknowledgments

The authors thank Dr. T.J. Römer (Department of Cardiology, Diaconessenhuis, Leiden, the Netherlands) for his help with data collection.

Author Contributions

Conceived and designed the experiments: JK NVR SCC TJR GYHL MVH. Performed the experiments: JK BS KAJVB JRB WRVDP AIDS SCC. Analyzed the data: JK NVR BS KAJVB JRB WRVDP AIDS SCC TJR GYHL MVH. Contributed reagents/materials/analysis tools: JK BS KAJVB JRB WRVDP AIDS. Wrote the paper: JK NVR SCC TJR GYHL MVH FAK. Interpretation of study results: FAK.

References

1. Koren-Morag N, Goldbourt U, Tanne D (2006) Renal dysfunction and risk of ischemic stroke or TIA in patients with cardiovascular disease. Neurology 67: 224–228. 67/2/224 [pii];10.1212/01.wnl.0000229099.62706.a3 [doi].

2. Tsukamoto Y, Takahashi W, Takizawa S, Kawada S, Takagi S (2012) Chronic kidney disease in patients with ischemic stroke. J Stroke Cerebrovasc Dis 21: 547–550. S1052-3057(10)00277-6 [pii];10.1016/j.jstrokecerebrovasdis.2010.12.005 [doi].

3. Kooiman J, van de Peppel WR, van der Meer FJ, Huisman MV (2011) Incidence of chronic kidney disease in patients with atrial fibrillation and its relevance for prescribing new oral antithrombotic drugs. J Thromb Haemost 9: 1652–1653. 10.1111/j.1538-7836.2011.04347.x [doi].

4. McManus DD, Rienstra M, Benjamin EJ (2012) An update on the prognosis of patients with atrial fibrillation. Circulation 126: e143–e146. 126/10/e143 [pii];10.1161/CIRCULATIONAHA.112.129759 [doi].

5. Herzog CA, Asinger RW, Berger AK, Charytan DM, Diez J, et al. (2011) Cardiovascular disease in chronic kidney disease. A clinical update from Kidney Disease: Improving Global Outcomes (KDIGO). Kidney Int 80: 572–586. ki2011223 [pii];10.1038/ki.2011.223 [doi].

6. Winkelmayer WC (2013) More evidence on an abominable pairing: atrial fibrillation and kidney disease. Circulation 127: 560–562. 127/5/560 [pii];10.1161/CIRCULATIONAHA.112.000640 [doi].

7. Hart RG, Pearce LA, Asinger RW, Herzog CA (2011) Warfarin in atrial fibrillation patients with moderate chronic kidney disease. Clin J Am Soc Nephrol 6: 2599–2604. CJN.02400311 [pii];10.2215/CJN.02400311 [doi].

8. Olesen JB, Lip GY, Kamper AL, Hommel K, Kober L, et al. (2012) Stroke and bleeding in atrial fibrillation with chronic kidney disease. N Engl J Med 367: 625–635. 10.1056/NEJMoa1105594 [doi].

9. Camm AJ, Lip GY, De CR, Savelieva I, Atar D, et al. (2012) 2012 focused update of the ESC Guidelines for the management of atrial fibrillation: an update of the 2010 ESC Guidelines for the management of atrial fibrillation—developed with the special contribution of the European Heart Rhythm Association. Europace 14: 1385–1413. eus305 [pii];10.1093/europace/eus305 [doi].

10. Abdelhafiz AH, Myint MP, Tayek JA, Wheeldon NM (2009) Anemia, hypoalbuminemia, and renal impairment as predictors of bleeding complications in patients receiving anticoagulation therapy for nonvalvular atrial fibrillation: a secondary analysis. Clin Ther 31: 1534–1539. S0149-2918(09)00228-8 [pii];10.1016/j.clinthera.2009.07.015 [doi].

11. Ng KP, Edwards NC, Lip GY, Townend JN, Ferro CJ (2013) Atrial Fibrillation in CKD: Balancing the Risks and Benefits of Anticoagulation. Am J Kidney Dis. S0272-6386(13)00784-1 [pii];10.1053/j.ajkd.2013.02.381 [doi].

12. Lai HM, Aronow WS, Kalen P, Adapa S, Patel K, et al. (2009) Incidence of thromboembolic stroke and of major bleeding in patients with atrial fibrillation and chronic kidney disease treated with and without warfarin. Int J Nephrol Renovasc Dis 2: 33–37.

13. Roldan V, Marin F, Fernandez H, Manzano-Fernandez S, Gallego P, et al. (2013) Renal impairment in a "real-life" cohort of anticoagulated patients with atrial fibrillation (implications for thromboembolism and bleeding). Am J Cardiol 111: 1159–1164. S0002-9149(12)02648-3 [pii];10.1016/j.amjcard.2012.12.045 [doi].

14. Wieloch M, Jonsson KM, Sjalander A, Lip GY, Eriksson N, et al. (2013) Estimated glomerular filtration rate is associated with major bleeding complications but not thromboembolic events, in anticoagulated patients taking warfarin. Thromb Res 131: 481–486. S0049-3848(13)00008-X [pii];10.1016/j.thromres.2013.01.006 [doi].

15. Levey AS, Coresh J, Greene T, Stevens LA, Zhang YL, et al. (2006) Using standardized serum creatinine values in the modification of diet in renal disease study equation for estimating glomerular filtration rate. .Ann Intern Med 145: 247–254. 145/4/247 [pii].

16. Pottelbergh van G, Van HL, Mathei C, Degryse J (2010) Methods to evaluate renal function in elderly patients: a systematic literature review. Age Ageing 39: 542–548. afq091 [pii];10.1093/ageing/afq091 [doi].

17. Schulman S, Kearon C (2005) Definition of major bleeding in clinical investigations of antihemostatic medicinal products in non-surgical patients. J Thromb Haemost 3: 692–694. JTH1204 [pii];10.1111/j.1538-7836.2005.01204.x [doi].

18. Klok FA, Zondag W, van Kralingen KW, van Dijk AP, Tamsma JT, et al. (2010) Patient outcomes after acute pulmonary embolism. A pooled survival analysis of different adverse events. Am J Respir Crit Care Med 181: 501–506. 200907-1141OC [pii];10.1164/rccm.200907-1141OC [doi].

19. Amouyel P, Mismetti P, Langkilde LK, Jasso-Mosqueda G, Nelander K, et al. (2009) INR variability in atrial fibrillation: a risk model for cerebrovascular events. Eur J Intern Med 20: 63–69. S0953-6205(08)00136-2 [pii];10.1016/j.ejim.2008.04.005 [doi].

20. Cannegieter SC, Rosendaal FR, Wintzen AR, van der Meer FJ, Vandenbroucke JP, et al. (1995) Optimal oral anticoagulant therapy in patients with mechanical heart valves. N Engl J Med 333: 11–17. 10.1056/NEJM199507063330103 [doi].

21. Hylek EM, Go AS, Chang Y, Jensvold NG, Henault LE, et al. (2003) Effect of intensity of oral anticoagulation on stroke severity and mortality in atrial fibrillation. N Engl J Med 349: 1019–1026. 10.1056/NEJMoa022913 [doi];349/11/1019 [pii].

22. Reynolds MW, Fahrbach K, Hauch O, Wygant G, Estok R, et al. (2004) Warfarin anticoagulation and outcomes in patients with atrial fibrillation: a systematic review and metaanalysis. Chest 126: 1938–1945. 126/6/1938 [pii];10.1378/chest.126.6.1938 [doi].

23. Rosendaal FR, Cannegieter SC, van der Meer FJ, Briet E (1993) A method to determine the optimal intensity of oral anticoagulant therapy. Thromb Haemost 69: 236–239.

24. Leeuwen van Y, Rosendaal FR, Cannegieter SC (2008) Prediction of hemorrhagic and thrombotic events in patients with mechanical heart valve prostheses treated with oral anticoagulants. J Thromb Haemost 6: 451–456. JTH2874 [pii];10.1111/j.1538-7836.2007.02874.x [doi].

25. Ibrahim S, Jespersen J, Poller L (2013) The clinical evaluation of International Normalized Ratio variability and control in conventional oral anticoagulant administration by use of the variance growth rate. J Thromb Haemost 11: 1540–1546. 10.1111/jth.12322 [doi].

26. Dreisbach AW, Lertora JJ (2003) The effect of chronic renal failure on hepatic drug metabolism and drug disposition. Semin Dial 16: 45–50. 3011 [pii].

27. Leblond F, Guevin C, Demers C, Pellerin I, Gascon-Barre M, et al. (2001) Downregulation of hepatic cytochrome P450 in chronic renal failure. J Am Soc Nephrol 12: 326–332.

28. Bachmann K, Shapiro R, Mackiewicz J (1976) Influence of renal dysfunction on warfarin plasma protein binding. J Clin Pharmacol 16: 468–472.

29. Bachmann K, Shapiro R, Mackiewicz J (1977) Warfarin elimination and responsiveness in patients with renal dysfunction. J Clin Pharmacol 17: 292–299.

30. Ibrahim S, Jespersen J, Poller L (2013) The clinical evaluation of International Normalized Ratio variability and control in conventional oral anticoagulant administration by use of the variance growth rate. J Thromb Haemost 11: 1540–1546. 10.1111/jth.12322 [doi].

31. Beyth RJ, Quinn L, Landefeld CS (2000) A multicomponent intervention to prevent major bleeding complications in older patients receiving warfarin. A randomized, controlled trial. Ann Intern Med 133: 687–695. 200011070-00010 [pii].

32. Hart RG, Eikelboom JW, Brimble KS, McMurtry MS, Ingram AJ (2013) Stroke prevention in atrial fibrillation patients with chronic kidney disease. Can J Cardiol 29: S71–S78. S0828-282X(13)00222-5 [pii];10.1016/j.cjca.2013.04.005 [doi].

33. Connolly SJ, Ezekowitz MD, Yusuf S, Eikelboom J, Oldgren J, et al. (2009) Dabigatran versus warfarin in patients with atrial fibrillation. N Engl J Med 361: 1139–1151. NEJMoa0905561 [pii];10.1056/NEJMoa0905561 [doi].

34. Patel MR, Mahaffey KW, Garg J, Pan G, Singer DE, et al. (2011) Rivaroxaban versus warfarin in nonvalvular atrial fibrillation. N Engl J Med 365: 883–891. 10.1056/NEJMoa1009638 [doi].

35. Granger CB, Alexander JH, McMurray JJ, Lopes RD, Hylek EM, et al. (2011) Apixaban versus warfarin in patients with atrial fibrillation. N Engl J Med 365: 981–992. 10.1056/NEJMoa1107039 [doi].

36. Connolly SJ, Eikelboom J, Dorian P, Hohnloser SH, Gretler DD, et al. (2013) Betrixaban compared with warfarin in patients with atrial fibrillation: results of a phase 2, randomized, dose-ranging study (Explore-Xa). Eur Heart J 34: 1498–1505. eht039 [pii];10.1093/eurheartj/eht039 [doi].

8

Induction of Atrial Fibrillation by Neutrophils Critically Depends on CD11b/CD18 Integrins

Kai Friedrichs[1,2,9], Matti Adam[3,9], Lisa Remane[1,2], Martin Mollenhauer[1,2], Volker Rudolph[1,2], Tanja K. Rudolph[1,2], René P. Andrié[4], Florian Stöckigt[4], Jan W. Schrickel[4], Thorben Ravekes[1,2], Florian Deuschl[3], Georg Nickenig[4], Stephan Willems[5], Stephan Baldus[1,2], Anna Klinke[1,2*]

1 Heart Center, University of Cologne, Cologne, Germany, 2 Cologne Cardiovascular Research Center, University of Cologne, Cologne, Germany, 3 Department of General and Interventional Cardiology, University Heart Center Hamburg, Hamburg, Germany, 4 Department of Medicine-Cardiology, University Hospital of Bonn, Bonn, Germany, 5 Department of Electrophysiology, University Heart Center Hamburg, Hamburg, Germany

Abstract

Background: Recent observational clinical and *ex-vivo* studies suggest that inflammation and in particular leukocyte activation predisposes to atrial fibrillation (AF). However, whether local binding and extravasation of leukocytes into atrial myocardium is an essential prerequisite for the initiation and propagation of AF remains elusive. Here we investigated the role of atrial CD11b/CD18 mediated infiltration of polymorphonuclear neutrophils (PMN) for the susceptibility to AF.

Methods and Results: C57bl/6J wildtype (WT) and CD11b/CD18 knock-out (CD11b$^{-/-}$) mice were treated for 14 days with subcutaneous infusion of angiotensin II (Ang II), a known stimulus for PMN activation. Atria of Ang II-treated WT mice were characterized by increased PMN infiltration assessed in immunohistochemically stained sections. In contrast, atrial sections of CD11b$^{-/-}$ mice lacked a significant increase in PMN infiltration upon Ang II infusion. PMN infiltration was accompanied by profoundly enhanced atrial fibrosis in Ang II treated WT as compared to CD11b$^{-/-}$ mice. Upon *in-vivo* electrophysiological investigation, Ang II treatment significantly elevated the susceptibility for AF in WT mice if compared to vehicle treated animals given an increased number and increased duration of AF episodes. In contrast, animals deficient of CD11b/CD18 were entirely protected from AF induction. Likewise, epicardial activation mapping revealed decreased electrical conduction velocity in atria of Ang II treated WT mice, which was preserved in CD11b$^{-/-}$ mice. In addition, atrial PMN infiltration was enhanced in atrial appendage sections of patients with persistent AF as compared to patients without AF.

Conclusions: The current data critically link CD11b-integrin mediated atrial PMN infiltration to the formation of fibrosis, which promotes the initiation and propagation of AF. These findings not only reveal a mechanistic role of leukocytes in AF but also point towards a potential novel avenue of treatment in AF.

Editor: Ali A. Sovari, University of Illinois at Chicago, United States of America

Funding: This work was supported by the Deutsche Forschungsgemeinschaft, http://www.dfg.de/index.jsp (DFG BA 1870/7-1, BA 1870/9-1 and BA 1870/10-1 And DFG KL 2516/1-1 And DFG RU 1876/1-1) and the Deutsches Zentrum für Herz-Kreislaufforschung, http://dzhk.de/(DZHK). The funders had no role in study design, data collection and analysis, decision to publish, or preparation of the manuscript.

Competing Interests: The authors have declared that no competing interests exist.

* E-mail: anna.klinke@uk-koeln.de

⑨ These authors contributed equally to this work.

Introduction

Atrial fibrillation (AF) stands out as the most prevalent human rhythm disorder. Atrial fibrillation is associated with an increased long-term risk of heart failure, remains a principal and common cause of stroke and doubles mortality [1–4]. Despite its prevalence and its contribution to morbidity and mortality, treatment strategies still remain scarce. Ion channel directed therapies as well as interventional strategies are most effective only in a subset of patients: whereas patients with non permanent, paroxysmal AF can be treated in the majority of cases, individuals with permanent AF in large part do not derive benefit from anti-arrhythmic and interventional therapy, respectively, calling for adjunct therapies [5,6].

Therefore, a better understanding of the underlying pathophysiology is of foremost importance. An accumulating body of evidence suggests that atrial fibrosis plays a major role in the pathogenesis of atrial fibrillation: Increased deposition of interstitial matrix such as collagen I and III and fibronectin impedes atrial conduction, allowing for an increased electrical ectopy and reentry. Moreover, matrix turnover - by exposing cytokines, adhesion molecules and growth factors – propagates a proinflammatory milieu [7–9]. In fact, inflammation appears to be a critical confounder for structural remodeling of the atria and thus for the genesis of atrial fibrillation [10,11]. Clinical studies support this view by revealing a predictive role of biomarkers such as C-reactive protein (CRP), interleukin (IL)-6 and tumor necrosis factor (TNF)-α with respect to AF occurrence, persistence, recurrence and left atrial dimensions. [12–22]. More so, clinical observations revealed leukocytes to be of critical significance for this disease in humans: Leukocytes were identified in atrial tissue of AF patients even without an underlying structural heart disease [11], and postoperative atrial leukocyte infiltration independently predicted postsurgery AF [23,24]. Of note, enzyme systems stored in leukocytes such as myeloperoxidase (MPO) and matrix metalloproteinase (MMP)-2, enzymes known to accelerate tissue remodeling, were also predictive of AF burden and recurrence of this disease following interventional ablation [25,26].

Activation and extravasation of leukocytes and in particular of polymorphonuclear neutrophils (PMN), the most abundant subset of leukocytes and the major constituents of the innate immune system, depend on the activation state of the local endothelium – which releases local cytokines and expresses adhesion molecules. As of at least similar importance, PMN adhesion critically relies on the expression of integrins on the leukocytes outer membrane: PMN express CD11b/CD18 integrins (Mac1), which allow binding to adhesion molecules like intercellular adhesion molecule-1 (ICAM-1) on the endothelial cell surface – the principal prerequisite for the leukocytes subsequent extravasation [27–29]. Notably, CD11b/CD18 integrins not only interact with cellular proteins, they also bind with high affinity to components of the extracellular matrix like fibrinogen/fibrin and collagen and to polysaccharides like heparan sulfates [30–32]. Furthermore, CD11b/CD18 takes central stage in PMN activation: Effector pathways downstream of CD11b/CD18 include NADPH-oxidase activation with concomitant formation of superoxide and release of granular proteins [33,34]. Interestingly, it has been shown lately, that PMN release MPO to endothelial cells via a direct CD11b/CD18-integrin mediated intercellular link [35].

We observed recently, that MPO promotes fibrosis and thereby increases AF susceptibility [25]. However, to date a direct mechanistic link between AF and PMN localization within the atrial tissue has not been established. Here we tested the impact of CD11b/CD18 integrins on AF susceptibility in a murine model of AF.

Methods

Ethics Statement

All animal studies were approved by the local authorities: (Behörde für Soziales, Familie, Gesundheit und Verbraucherschutz, Fachabteilung Veterinärwesen und Lebensmittelsicherheit, Hamburg, G09/064 and Landesamt für Natur, Umwelt und Verbraucherschutz Nordrhein-Westfalen, 84-02.04.2012.A307) and the Universities of Hamburg and Cologne Animal Care and Use Committees. All surgical interventions were performed under isoflurane anaesthesia and buprenorphine analgesia to minimize suffering of animals.

Patient studies were approved by the local Ethics Committee (Hamburg) and were performed in accordance with the Declaration of Helsinki and with written informed consent.

Animals and experimental design

Male C57bl/6J WT and CD11b/CD18-deficient (Itgam_tm1-Myd/J, CD11b$^{-/-}$) mice (8–10 weeks of age, Jackson Laboratory) were treated with either angiotensin II (Ang II, 1.3 ng/g/min) or vehicle via subcutaneously implanted osmotic minipumps (Alzet, model 1002) for 2 weeks. We did not observe any differences in mortality, wound infection or wound healing after minipump implantation in CD11b$^{-/-}$ compared to WT mice. These findings were consistent with previous work that reported similar observations [36].

Electrophysiological investigation

Mice were anaesthetized with isoflurane and placed in supine position on a heating pad. An octapolar electrophysiological catheter (1.1 F, Scisense) was inserted via the right jugular vein to the right atrium and ventricle. Surface ECG was analyzed under stable baseline conditions for at least 3 min. Heart rate, P wave duration, QRS duration and QTc interval were measured by successive evaluation of 10 RR complexes in the most distinguishable tracings. Electrophysiological investigation with induction of arrhythmias was performed as described previously [37]. Intracardiac atrial and ventricular recording and atrial stimulation maneuvers were performed using a CardioTek EPTracer (Biotronik). Bipolar electrograms were obtained from each electrode pair during the whole procedure. Programmed atrial stimulation was performed at pacing stimulus amplitudes of 1.0 and 2.0 mA with 7 stimuli fixed rate at S1S1 cycle length of 120 ms, 110 ms and 100 ms, respectively, with one short coupled extra stimulus with a 10 ms-stepwise S1S2 reduction starting at cycle length of 80 ms down to 10 ms. Atrial refractory period (ARP) was determined, which was defined as longest S1S2 with absent atrial response in the most representative intracardiac tracing. Atrial burst stimulation was performed for 1 sec (three times consecutively) at S1S1 stimulation cycle lengths starting at 50 ms with 10-ms stepwise reduction down to 10 ms at pacing stimulus amplitudes of 1.0 and 2.0 mA. Between these stimulation procedures, a 10-sec recovery period was maintained. Atrial fibrillation was defined by presence of rapid and fragmented atrial electrograms in combination with irregular AV-nodal conduction and ventricular rhythm with a duration of these atrial electrograms of more than one second [38]. Number of AF episodes and AF duration (last stimulus-spike to the first sinus-rhythm P wave) were analyzed.

Thereafter, blood was drawn from the caval vein into heparinized syringes, hearts were flushed with saline via left ventricular puncture and hearts were excised. Hearts were either fixed in 3.7% paraformaldehyde solution and embedded in paraffin, embedded in optimal cutting temperature compound (OCT) and frozen to −80°C or atria and ventricles were dissected and snap frozen in liquid nitrogen.

Langendorff-perfused hearts and epicardial mapping

For investigation of myocardial conduction velocities and homogeneity of conduction, hearts were Langendorff-perfused and epicardial activation mapping (EAM) using a 36-electrode array (FlexMEA36, Multi Channel Systems, interelectrode distance: 300 μm) was performed [37]. For this, hearts were excorporated and dissected from surrounding tissue in ice-cold Krebs-Henseleit buffer. Following cannulation of the aorta, the heart was immersed in a water-jacketed chamber and further fixed on a moisturized support. Hearts were then retrogradely perfused in a Langendorff-apparatus (Radnoti Technologies Inc.) at constant pressure perfusion (80 mmHg, resulting in coronary flow between 2–2.5 ml/min). The perfusate composition was (in mM): NaCl 110, KCl 4.6, MgSO$_4$ 1.2, CaCl 2, NaH$_2$PO$_4$ 2, NaHCO$_3$ 25, glucose 8.3, Na-pyruvate 2 and gassed with carbogen (O$_2$ 95%, CO$_2$ 5%), pH, 7.35–7.45 at constantly 37°C. 36 unipolar electrograms were recorded from the epicardial surface of both atria with regard to a reference electrode in the water-bath. Electrograms were recorded using a computer assisted recording system (Multi Channel Systems) with a sampling rate of up to 25 kHz. Data were band-pass filtered (50 Hz), digitized with 12 bit and a range of 20 mV.

Activation maps were calculated from these data using Cardio 2D Software (version 2.0.3, Multi Channel Systems). The first derivative of each unipolar electrogram was evaluated and maximal negative dV/dt activation was defined as the time-point of maximum local activation. With regard to myocardial fiber orientation, longitudinal and transversal conduction velocities (CV) were evaluated by calculating latencies between two electrodes, divided by the interelectrode distance.

Immunofluorescence analysis

OCT embedded samples were cut to 3 μm sections and fixed with 3.7% formaldehyde. Tissue was permeabilized with 0.1% Triton-X 100 and treated with primary antibodies to murine Ly6G (Hycult Biotechnology, 1:40) and MPO (Thermo Scientific, 1:100) or for human sections to MPO (Calbiochem, 1:200) and Alexa-Fluor-conjugated secondary antibodies (Invitrogen, 1:200). Nuclei were stained with DAPI. Images of MPO and PMN in atrial tissue were captured with a CCD camera mounted on a Leica DMLB microscope with IVision software. Number of PMN was counted in 4–5 fields of view (magnification ×40) per atrium.

Determination of MPO levels in heart perfusates

To release MPO from its binding to the vascular endothelium of the coronary circulation, hearts of anaesthetized mice were explanted and immediately cannulated via the aorta. Hearts were rinsed retrogradely with 200 μl of PBS followed by perfusion with 2 ml of heparin solution (5 I.U./ml). The perfusate was concentrated by vacuum centrifugation to 40 μl and the MPO concentration was determined by ELISA following manufacturer's instructions (Hycult Biotechnology).

Determination of MPO levels in atrial homogenates

Samples were homogenized in lysis buffer (20 mM Tris-HCl pH 7.5, 250 mM succrose, 20 mM ETDA, 3 mM EGTA, 0.1% Triton X-100, supplemented with 10× ETDA-free Protease Inhibitor Tablets and 10× PhoSTOP; Roche Diagnostics) using the Tissue Lyzer (Qiagen). Homogenates were centrifuged at 14,000 g (4°C, 10 min) and the supernatant was recovered. MPO was quantified using an ELISA (Hycult Biotechnology) according to the manufacture's instruction. Total protein amount in samples was assessed with BCA-protein assay (Pierce). MPO levels were related to total protein.

Immunoblot

Hearts were explanted from anaesthetized mice, rinsed in ice cold PBS and atria were dissected from ventricles. The tissue was snap frozen in liquid nitrogen and stored at −80°C. Samples were homogenated in lysis buffer as described above. Homogenates were centrifuged at 14,000 g (4°C, 10 min) and the supernatant was recovered. Proteins were separated by SDS-PAGE and transferred to nitrocellulose membranes. After blocking with 5% nonfat milk in TBST (20 mM Tris-HCl pH 7.5, 137 mM NaCl, 0.1% (v/v) Tween 20), membranes were incubated with primary antibodies to ICAM-1 (1:200, Santa Cruz Biotechnology), VCAM-1 (1:200, Santa Cruz Biotechnology) or GAPDH (1:2,500, Cell Signaling Technology), followed by horseradish peroxidase-conjugated secondary antibodies (1:10,000, Vector Laboratories) and chemiluminescence signals were detected with a Fusion FX Advance (Vilber Lourmat) and analyzed densitometrically with Fusion-CAPT software (Vilber Lourmat).

Determination of atrial fibrosis

Longitudinal sections (4 μm) of paraffin embedded hearts were prepared and stained with Trichrome stain following a standard protocol. The area in atrial sections, which was stained in light blue (excluding pericardium), was quantified using color threshold and planimetry with Keyence BZII Analyzer (Keyence) software.

Patients with AF

Right atrial appendages were obtained from patients undergoing elective coronary artery bypass surgery, either from patients with persistent AF or without AF.

Statistical analysis

Continuous variables were tested for normal distribution by using the Kolmogorov-Smirnoff test. Data are presented as mean ± SEM or as median (line) and interquartile range (box); whiskers indicate 5% and 95% percentiles. Statistical analysis was performed by one-way ANOVA followed by Bonferroni or LSD post hoc test for normally distributed data, or Kruskal-Wallis test with Mann-Whitney-U post hoc test, as appropriate. For comparison of two groups of non-normally distributed data, Mann-Whitney U test was used. A value of $P < 0.05$ was considered statistically significant. All calculations were carried out by using SPSS Statistics 20 for Mac.

Results

To induce leukocyte activation in wild type (WT) and CD11b/CD18 integrin-deficient (CD11b$^{-/-}$) mice, Ang II was infused subcutaneously for 14 days by osmotic minipumps. Immunohistochemical analysis of atrial sections revealed increased atrial infiltration of PMN in WT mice (n = 13) as compared to vehicle treated animals (n = 6; p<0.05). This Ang II-dependent increase in PMN extravasation proved to be CD11b-dependent, since mice devoid of the integrin did not demonstrate any significant increase in extravascular deposition of PMN in the atria (Ang II: n = 15, vehicle: n = 7; p = 0.09) (**Fig. 1A, B**). Immunoblot analyses of the amount of endothelial CD11b/CD18 binding partners revealed that the protein amounts of ICAM-1 (WT ctrl, Ang II: n = 6, 9; CD11b$^{-/-}$ ctrl, Ang II: 6, 6) and vascular cell adhesion molecule-1 (VCAM-1) (WT ctrl, Ang II: n = 5, 10; CD11b$^{-/-}$ ctrl, Ang II: n = 5, 5) were slightly enhanced following Ang II application as compared to untreated animals, but were not different between Ang II treated WT and Ang II treated CD11b$^{-/-}$ mice (ICAM-1 p = 0.12; VCAM-1 p = 0.98) (**Fig. 1C, D**). Analysis of cardiac MPO deposition in the different treatment groups revealed significantly lower MPO concentrations in atrial homogenates of CD11b$^{-/-}$ mice upon Ang II treatment (n = 5) as compared to Ang II treated WT mice (n = 11, p<0.05) (**Fig. 1E**). Likewise, the amount of endothelial bound MPO within the coronary vasculature was markedly lower in Ang II treated CD11b$^{-/-}$ (n = 4) as compared to Ang II treated WT mice (n = 7; p<0.01), thereby also indicating a decrease in cardiac MPO accumulation due to CD11b/CD18 deficiency (**Fig. 1F**).

To investigate whether increased atrial PMN infiltration and enhanced cardiac MPO deposition translates into aggravated atrial remodeling, we analyzed atrial fibrosis in WT and CD11b$^{-/-}$ mice. Evidenced by increased deposition of matrix proteins, Ang II treatment resulted in profoundly augmented atrial fibrosis compared to vehicle treated WT mice (n = 13, 12; p<0.001). Remarkably, the genesis of atrial fibrosis in Ang II treated CD11b$^{-/-}$ mice was blunted (WT Ang II vs. CD11b$^{-/-}$ Ang II p<0.05) and not different if compared to vehicle-treated CD11b$^{-/-}$ mice (n = 6; p = 0.24; **Fig. 2A–C**).

Next, we tested whether increased presence of PMN and aggravated atrial fibrosis translate into a lower threshold for initiation of atrial fibrillation. Therefore, we performed in-vivo electrophysiological investigations as described previously [37].

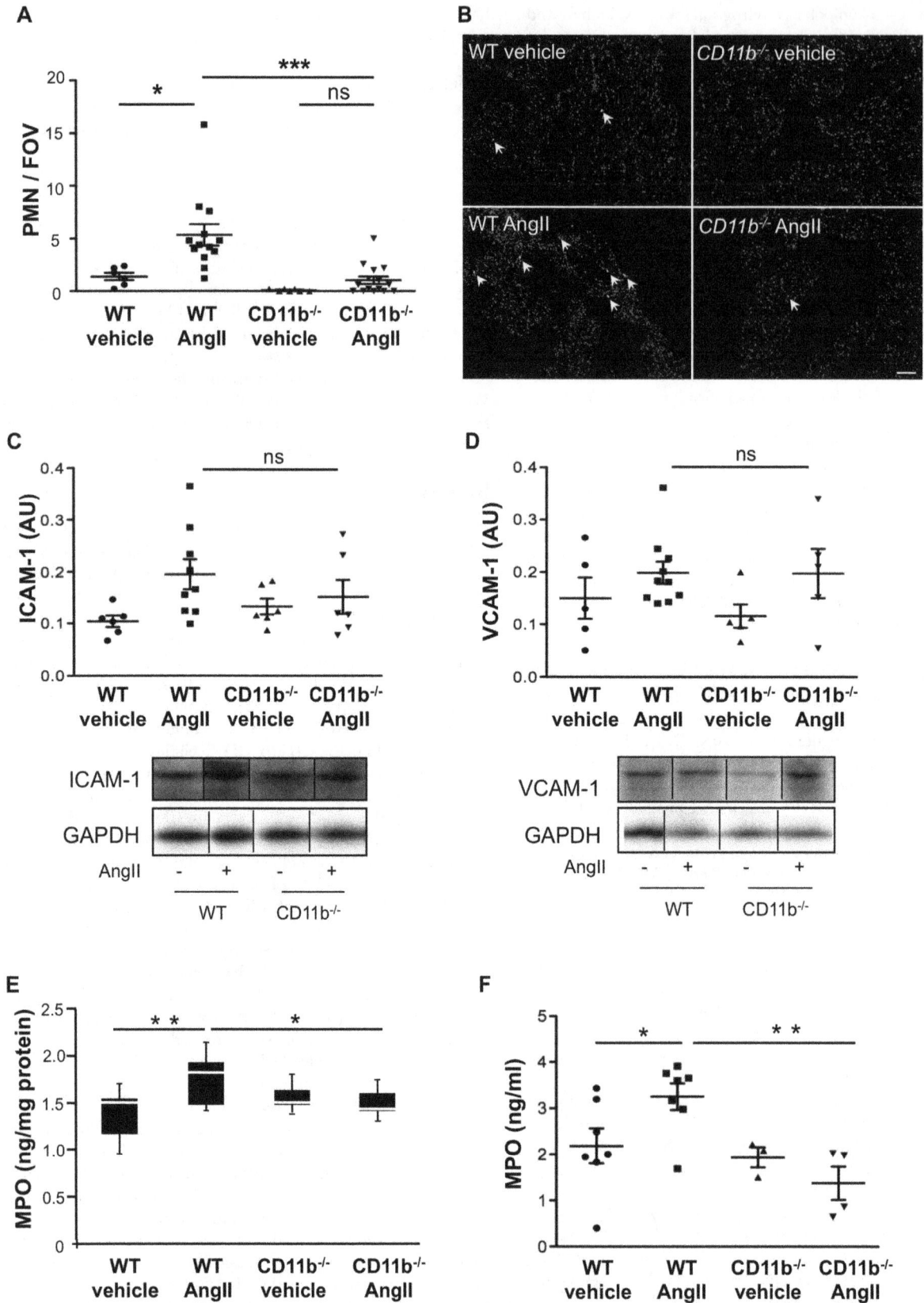

Figure 1. Atrial PMN infiltration and MPO accumulation was attenuated by CD11b-deficiency. (A) Number of MPO- and Ly6G-positive leukocytes in atrial sections of WT and CD11b$^{-/-}$ mice upon vehicle or Ang II treatment was quantified in 4–5 FOVs per atrium (FOV = field of view, ×40). * = p<0.05, *** = p<0.001. (B) Representative images of immunofluorescence staining of PMN in mouse atrial tissue: blue = DAPI, red = Ly6G, green = MPO. Arrowheads indicate leukocytes. Scale bar = 50 μm. (C, D) Protein expression of ICAM-1 and VCAM-1 in atrial tissue of WT and

CD11b$^{-/-}$ mice upon vehicle or Ang II infusion. Representative immunoblots are shown, where bands are spliced together as they were noncontinuous but were run on the same gel. **(E)** MPO in atrial tissue of WT and CD11b$^{-/-}$ mice. * = p<0.05, ** = p<0.01. **(F)** Amount of MPO deposition in the coronary circulation of WT and CD11b$^{-/-}$ mice. * = p<0.05, ** = p<0.01.

Upon controlled local right atrial burst stimulation, inducibility and length of atrial fibrillation was captured. As shown in Fig. 3 WT mice exposed to Ang II (n = 18) revealed markedly increased vulnerability to AF: Number of AF episodes as well as the length of AF episodes were significantly increased as compared to vehicle treated animals (n = 10; p<0.05). In contrast, CD11b$^{-/-}$ mice were protected from the AF-provoking effect of Ang II (n = 8, 12; WT Ang II vs. CD11b$^{-/-}$ Ang II p<0.05) **(Fig. 3 A–C)**. In line with this, P-wave duration was prolonged in Ang II treated WT mice in contrast to CD11b$^{-/-}$ mice (p<0.01) **(Table 1)**. In support of these results from electrophysiological investigations, epicardial mapping analyses revealed, that electrical conduction velocity was decreased following chronic Ang II infusion in WT mice (n = 7, 6; Ang II vs. vehicle p<0.001). This deceleration was blunted in CD11b$^{-/-}$ mice (p = 0.6; n = 7; Ang II WT vs. CD11b$^{-/-}$ p<0.001) **(Fig. 3D, E)**.

Finally, we determined the amount of MPO-positive leukocytes in right atrial appendage tissue of patients with persistent AF (n = 5) or without AF (n = 4), which revealed a significantly increased number of leukocytes with enhanced MPO-deposition in sections of patients with AF as compared to control subjects (p<0.05) **(Fig. 4A, B)**.

Discussion

In the current study we revisited the biological significance of CD11b/CD18 integrin-dependent cardiac recruitment of PMN for atrial fibrosis and AF.

We have reported recently that MPO, stored in primary granules of PMN and released by the cells upon activation, links atrial fibrosis and the susceptibility for atrial fibrillation [25]. However, whether leukocytes are critical for the local distribution of MPO into the tissue has not been answered so far. The current data now show that reduced PMN infiltration in CD11b$^{-/-}$ mice

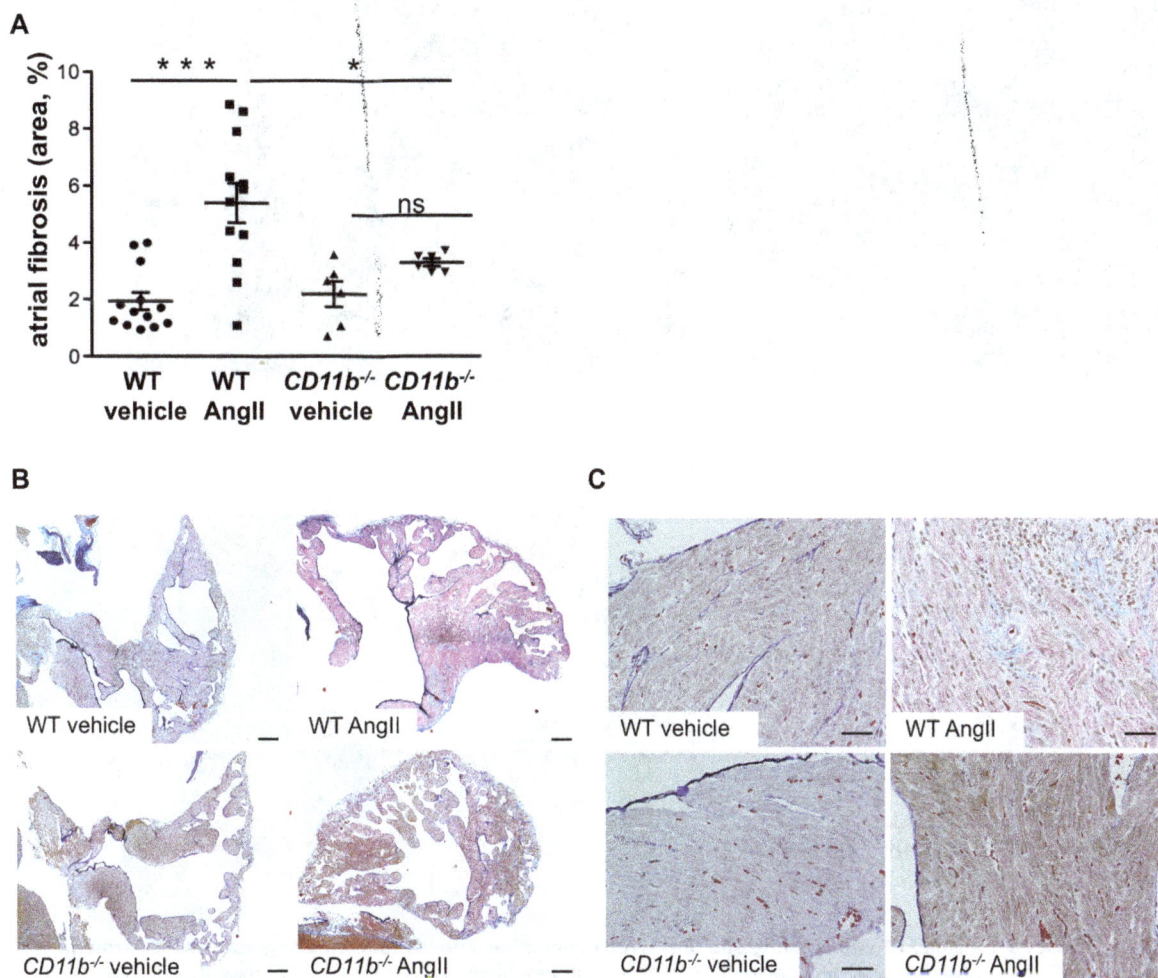

Figure 2. Angiotensin II-induced atrial fibrosis was reduced in CD11b$^{-/-}$ mice. (A) Percentage of fibrotic area in atrial sections of WT and CD11b$^{-/-}$ mice upon vehicle or Ang II treatment. * = p<0.05, *** = p<0.001. **(B, C)** Representative images of Trichrome stained atrial sections with fibrotic tissue stained in light blue merged from 6 individual images with 10× magnification **(B)**, scale bar = 200 μm and with 40× magnification **(C)**, scale bar = 40 μm.

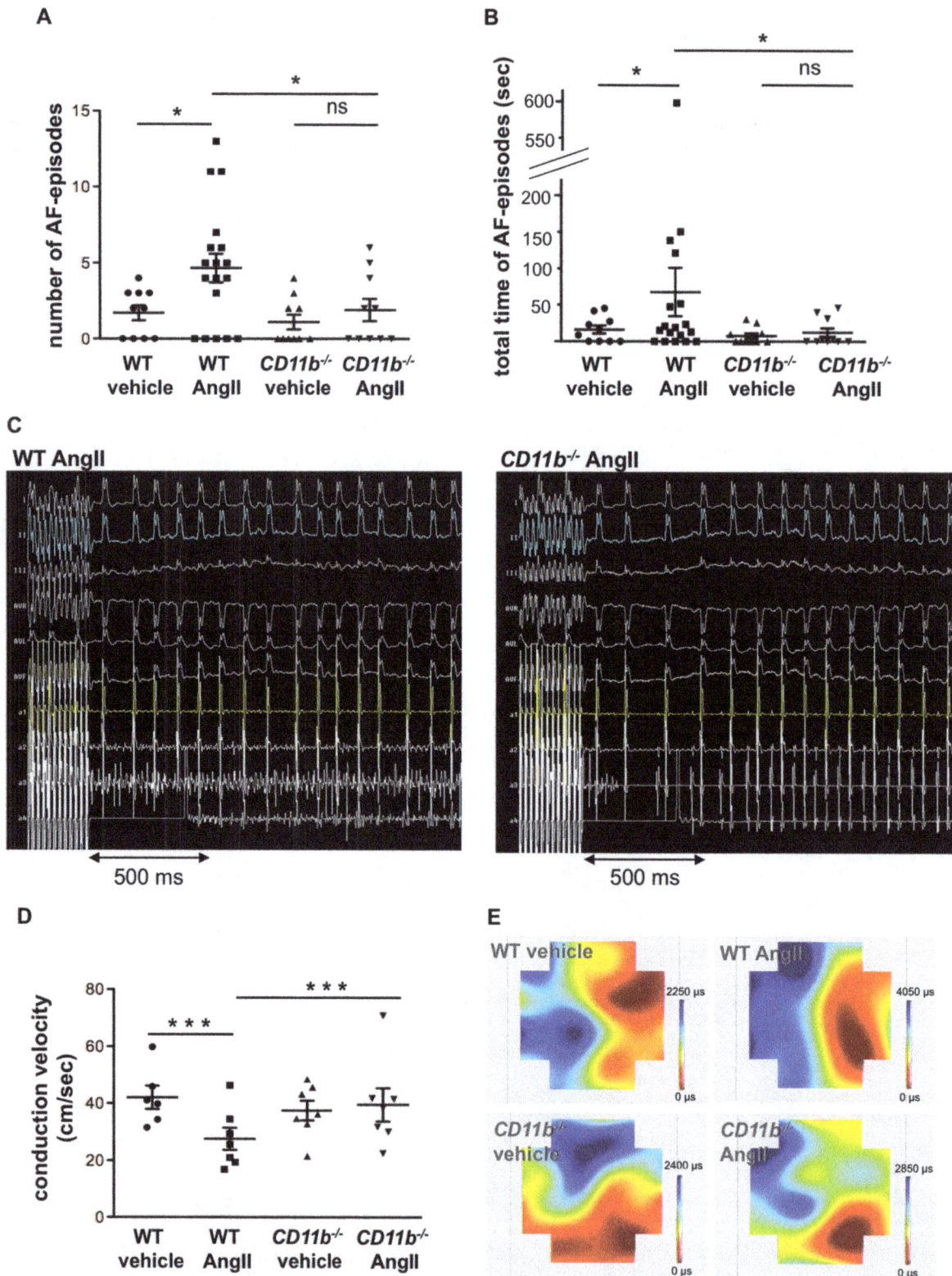

Figure 3. CD11b-deficiency diminished AF vulnerability and preserved conduction velocity following angiotensin II treatment. (A, B) Number and total time of AF-episodes during an electrophysiological stimulation procedure in WT and CD11b$^{-/-}$ mice upon vehicle or Ang II application. * = p<0.05. (C) Example electrical tracings of surface and intracardiac leads from Ang II treated WT and CD11b$^{-/-}$ mice during electrophysiological burst stimulation with cycle length of 20 ms. (D) Electrical conduction velocity in propagation direction as assessed by epicardial mapping of Langendorff-perfused hearts of WT and CD11b$^{-/-}$ mice. *** = p<0.001. (E) Representative examples of conduction properties of epicardial activation mapping.

Table 1. Electrophysiological parameters derived from surface ECGs.

	WT vehicle	WT Ang II	$CD11b^{-/-}$ vehicle	$CD11b^{-/-}$ Ang II	P-value
P (ms)	12.6±0.4*	14.1±0.3	12.3±0.3#	12.8±0.5‡	*0.003; #<0.001; ‡0.009 vs. WT Ang II
ARP (ms)	37±5.4	38.8±2.3	37.8±3.2	43.7±3.2	n.s.
QRS (ms)	12.6±0.5	13.2±0.4	12.4±0.3	12.5±0.4	n.s.
QTc (ms)	153.8±8.1	156.2±5.5	158.3±3.0	143.3±5.9	n.s.
HR (bpm)	334±14	345±11	330±12	327±14	n.s.

P, P-wave duration; ARP, atrial refractory period; QRS, QRS duration; QTc, QT interval corrected for heart rate; HR, heart rate; bpm, beats per minute; n.s., not significant.

indeed is firmly connected to atrial remodeling and inducibility of AF. Whereas WT mice exposed to 14 days of Ang II infusion exhibited increased atrial fibrosis and concomitantly were noted for decreased threshold for atrial fibrillation, $CD11b^{-/-}$ mice not only displayed attenuated atrial PMN accumulation after Ang II treatment, but also less fibrosis, which translated into reduced susceptibility to atrial fibrillation. Mechanistically, CD11b/CD18 integrin knockout has repeatedly been shown to prevent local PMN extravasation [36,39,40], implying a direct negative effect of attenuated atrial PMN infiltration on atrial remodeling. Other potential mechanisms include impaired leukocyte - extracellular matrix interactions [41] and diminished responses of other CD11b expressing cells like macrophages and natural killer cells. Interestingly, a more recent study also supports CD11b-dependent internalization of MPO by endothelial cells [35], thereby providing an additional pathobiological mechanism for a decreased inflammatory atrial milieu in $CD11b^{-/-}$ mice, independently of PMN infiltration itself.

The current study now expands our understanding on the basic mechanisms linking inflammation, atrial remodeling and the development of atrial fibrillation in an important way: The current data reveal that leukocytes, in particular PMN are not only bystanders of AF but at best function as circulating carriers of effector proteins, which then propagate atrial remodeling. Moreover, our results reveal that intimate contact of PMN with the atrial vasculature and PMN recruitment into atrial tissue represent relevant components of atrial fibrosis. Whereas this is accompanied with release of MPO, the enzyme is most probably not the exclusive effector, by which PMN increase the burden of

fibrosis in the atria. Superoxide, generated by the cells NADPH oxidase, by uncoupled NO-synthases or released by mitochondria is closely linked to the initiation of fibrosis and AF [42,43]. However the contribution of leukocytes as critical effectors in the pathophysiology of AF has probably been underestimated so far.

Angiotensin II is appreciated as a central effector peptide allowing for atrial remodeling and ultimately the induction of AF [44]. However, these proarrhythmic effects were mainly attributed to the local, myocyte-directed effects of Ang II yielding increased superoxide generation, matrix production and cellular hypertrophy. Interestingly, acute Ang II-mediated proarrhythmic effects in a rat model of ventricular arrhythmia were shown to be dependent on the presence of an aged and more fibrotic myocardium rather than on the occurrence of Ang II induced early afterdepolarisations alone [45]. Given that Ang II-mediated leukocyte activation in the absence of CD11b/CD18-integrins exerted only a slight proarrhythmic effect suggests, that the cytokine-like, leukocyte-activating properties of this peptide contribute to its arrhythmogenicity. Certainly, this does not necessarily imply that inhibition of Ang II-signaling is beneficial in the prevention or therapy of AF, as PMN can be activated by various other stimuli. In fact, inflammatory markers like high-sensitive CRP (hsCRP) and IL-6 are elevated in patients with recurrent AF in an early non-permanent stage of AF [46], but these particular patients did not benefit from Ang II receptor inhibition [47]. However, meta-analyses show an overall beneficial effect for Angiotensin-converting enzyme (ACE) inhibitors and angiotensin receptor blockers (ARBs) in primary and secondary prevention of AF [48,49], especially in patients already suffering from recurrent AF

A

B

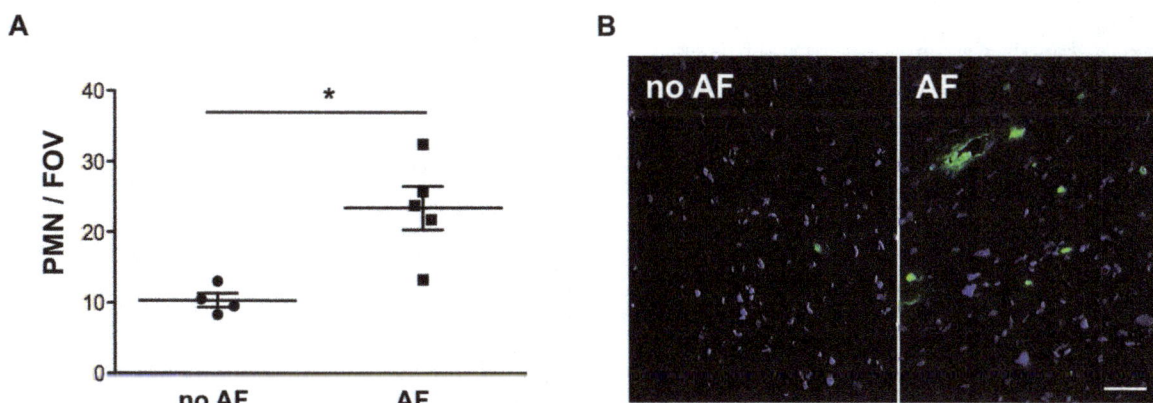

Figure 4. Atrial PMN-infiltration was enhanced in patients with AF. (A) Number of MPO-positive leukocytes in sections of atrial appendages of control subjects and patients with persistent AF (FOV = field of view, ×40). **(B)** Representative images of immunoreactivity for MPO (green) in human atrial appendage sections. Scale bar = 15 μm.

or with concomitant diseases like hypertension or heart failure. Given the increasing effects of ACE inhibitors and ARBs in patients with exaggerated disease in humans, augmented atrial fibrosis is most likely the result of a variety of pathways, with one of them being mediated by PMN.

Limitations of the current study arise from the fact that we only studied rodents and do not provide data helping to translate the current results into a clinical setting. Furthermore, we investigated AF, which was induced by electrical stimulation instead of detecting spontaneous occurrence of the arrhythmia, e.g. in an ageing cohort of animals.

However, the data clearly reveal the significance of CD11b/CD18 integrins for the initiation and perpetuation of AF, furthermore underscore the role of fibrosis for this disease and call for a more in-depth evaluation of inflammatory mechanisms underlying AF in human pathophysiology.

Acknowledgments

The authors want to thank Hartwig Wieboldt and Gülsah Duman for expert technical assistance.

Author Contributions

Conceived and designed the experiments: KF MA SB AK. Performed the experiments: KF MA AK MM LR VR TKR TR FS FD. Analyzed the data: KF MA AK MM RPA JWS GN SW. Wrote the paper: KF MA AK SB.

References

1. Kannel WB, Abbott RD, Savage DD, McNamara PM (1982) Epidemiologic features of chronic atrial fibrillation: the Framingham study. N Engl J Med 306: 1018–1022.

2. Stewart S, Hart CL, Hole DJ, McMurray JJ (2002) A population-based study of the long-term risks associated with atrial fibrillation: 20-year follow-up of the Renfrew/Paisley study. Am J Med 113: 359–364.

3. Kirchhof P, Auricchio A, Bax J, Crijns H, Camm J, et al (2007) Outcome parameters for trials in atrial fibrillation: executive summary. Eur Heart J 28: 2803–2817.

4. Camm AJ, Kirchhof P, Lip GY, Schotten U, Savelieva I, et al (2010) Guidelines for the management of atrial fibrillation: the Task Force for the Management of Atrial Fibrillation of the European Society of Cardiology (ESC). Europace 12: 1360–1420.

5. Weerasooriya R, Khairy P, Litalien J, Macle L, Hocini M, et al (2011) Catheter ablation for atrial fibrillation: are results maintained at 5 years of follow-up? J Am Coll Cardiol 57: 160–166.

6. Ouyang F, Tilz R, Chun J, Schmidt B, Wissner E, et al (2010) Long-term results of catheter ablation in paroxysmal atrial fibrillation: lessons from a 5-year follow-up. Circulation 122: 2368–2377.

7. Goudis CA, Kallergis EM, Vardas PE (2012) Extracellular matrix alterations in the atria: insights into the mechanisms and perpetuation of atrial fibrillation. Europace 14: 623–630.

8. Friedrichs K, Klinke A, Baldus S (2011) Inflammatory pathways underlying atrial fibrillation. Trends Mol Med 17: 556–563.

9. Friedrichs K, Baldus S, Klinke A (2012) Fibrosis in Atrial Fibrillation - Role of Reactive Species and MPO. Front Physiol 3: 214.

10. Spodick DH (1976) Arrhythmias during acute pericarditis. A prospective study of 100 consecutive cases. JAMA 235: 39–41.

11. Frustaci A, Chimenti C, Bellocci F, Morgante E, Russo MA, et al (1997) Histological substrate of atrial biopsies in patients with lone atrial fibrillation. Circulation 96: 1180–1184.

12. Aviles RJ, Martin DO, Apperson-Hansen C, Houghtaling PL, Rautaharju P, et al (2003) Inflammation as a risk factor for atrial fibrillation. Circulation 108: 3006–3010.

13. Conway DS, Buggins P, Hughes E, Lip GY (2004) Prognostic significance of raised plasma levels of interleukin-6 and C-reactive protein in atrial fibrillation. Am Heart J 148: 462–466.

14. Dernellis J, Panaretou M (2004) Relationship between C-reactive protein concentrations during glucocorticoid therapy and recurrent atrial fibrillation. Eur Heart J 25: 1100–1107.

15. Henningsen KM, Therkelsen SK, Bruunsgaard H, Krabbe KS, Pedersen BK, et al (2009) Prognostic impact of hs-CRP and IL-6 in patients with persistent atrial fibrillation treated with electrical cardioversion. Scand J Clin Lab Invest 69: 425–432.

16. Leftheriotis DI, Fountoulaki KT, Flevari PG, Parissis JT, Panou FK, et al (2009) The predictive value of inflammatory and oxidative markers following the successful cardioversion of persistent lone atrial fibrillation. Int J Cardiol 135: 361–369.

17. Letsas KP, Weber R, Bürkle G, Mihas CC, Minners J, et al (2009) Pre-ablative predictors of atrial fibrillation recurrence following pulmonary vein isolation: the potential role of inflammation. Europace 11: 158–163.

18. Marcus GM, Smith LM, Ordovas K, Scheinman MM, Kim AM, et al (2010) Intracardiac and extracardiac markers of inflammation during atrial fibrillation. Heart Rhythm 7: 149–154.

19. Psychari SN, Apostolou TS, Sinos L, Hamodraka E, Liakos G, et al (2005) Relation of elevated C-reactive protein and interleukin-6 levels to left atrial size and duration of episodes in patients with atrial fibrillation. Am J Cardiol 95: 764–767.

20. Schnabel RB, Larson MG, Yamamoto JF, Sullivan LM, Pencina MJ, et al (2010) Relations of biomarkers of distinct pathophysiological pathways and atrial fibrillation incidence in the community. Circulation 121: 200–207.

21. Smith JG, Newton-Cheh C, Almgren P, Struck J, Morgenthaler NG, et al (2010) Assessment of conventional cardiovascular risk factors and multiple biomarkers for the prediction of incident heart failure and atrial fibrillation. J Am Coll Cardiol 56: 1712–1719.

22. Bruins P, te Velthuis H, Yazdanbakhsh AP, Jansen PG, van Hardevelt FW, et al (1997) Activation of the complement system during and after cardiopulmonary bypass surgery: postsurgery activation involves C-reactive protein and is associated with postoperative arrhythmia. Circulation 96: 3542–3548.

23. Ramlawi B, Otu H, Mieno S, Boodhwani M, Sodha NR, et al (2007) Oxidative stress and atrial fibrillation after cardiac surgery: a case-control study. Ann Thorac Surg 84: 1166–72; discussion 1172–3.

24. Lamm G, Auer J, Weber T, Berent R, Ng C, et al (2006) Postoperative white blood cell count predicts atrial fibrillation after cardiac surgery. J Cardiothorac Vasc Anesth 20: 51–56.

25. Rudolph V, Andrié RP, Rudolph TK, Friedrichs K, Klinke A, et al (2010) Myeloperoxidase acts as a profibrotic mediator of atrial fibrillation. Nat Med 16: 470–474.

26. Okumura Y, Watanabe I, Nakai T, Ohkubo K, Kofune T, et al (2011) Impact of biomarkers of inflammation and extracellular matrix turnover on the outcome of atrial fibrillation ablation: importance of matrix metalloproteinase-2 as a predictor of atrial fibrillation recurrence. J Cardiovasc Electrophysiol 22: 987–993.

27. Ding ZM, Babensee JE, Simon SI, Lu H, Perrard JL, et al (1999) Relative contribution of LFA-1 and Mac-1 to neutrophil adhesion and migration. J Immunol 163: 5029–5038.

28. Harris ES, McIntyre TM, Prescott SM, Zimmerman GA (2000) The leukocyte integrins. J Biol Chem 275: 23409–23412.

29. Mocsai A, Ligeti E, Lowell CA, Berton G (1999) Adhesion-dependent degranulation of neutrophils requires the Src family kinases Fgr and Hck. J Immunol 162: 1120–1126.

30. Murdoch C, Finn A (2000) Chemokine receptors and their role in inflammation and infectious diseases. Blood 95: 3032–3043.

31. Hughes BJ, Hollers JC, Crockett-Torabi E, Smith CW (1992) Recruitment of CD11b/CD18 to the neutrophil surface and adherence-dependent cell locomotion. J Clin Invest 90: 1687–1696.

32. Ross GD (2002) Role of the lectin domain of Mac-1/CR3 (CD11b/CD18) in regulating intercellular adhesion. Immunol Res 25: 219–227.

33. Zhou MJ, Brown EJ (1994) CR3 (Mac-1, alpha M beta 2, CD11b/CD18) and Fc gamma RIII cooperate in generation of a neutrophil respiratory burst: requirement for Fc gamma RIII and tyrosine phosphorylation. J Cell Biol 125: 1407–1416.

34. Lau D, Mollnau H, Eiserich JP, Freeman BA, Daiber A, et al (2005) Myeloperoxidase mediates neutrophil activation by association with CD11b/CD18 integrins. Proc Natl Acad Sci U S A 102: 431–436.

35. Jerke U, Rolle S, Purfürst B, Luft FC, Nauseef WM, et al (2013) β2 integrin-mediated cell-cell contact transfers active myeloperoxidase from neutrophils to endothelial cells. J Biol Chem 288: 12910–12919.

36. Coxon A, Rieu P, Barkalow FJ, Askari S, Sharpe AH, et al (1996) A novel role for the beta 2 integrin CD11b/CD18 in neutrophil apoptosis: a homeostatic mechanism in inflammation. Immunity 5: 653–666.

37. Schrickel JW, Brixius K, Herr C, Clemen CS, Sasse P, et al (2007) Enhanced heterogeneity of myocardial conduction and severe cardiac electrical instability in annexin A7-deficient mice. Cardiovasc Res 76: 257–268.

38. Sah VP, Minamisawa S, Tam SP, Wu TH, Dorn GW, et al (1999) Cardiac-specific overexpression of RhoA results in sinus and atrioventricular nodal dysfunction and contractile failure. J Clin Invest 103: 1627–1634.

39. Soriano SG, Coxon A, Wang YF, Frosch MP, Lipton SA, et al (1999) Mice deficient in Mac-1 (CD11b/CD18) are less susceptible to cerebral ischemia/reperfusion injury. Stroke 30: 134–139.

40. Gao XP, Liu Q, Broman M, Predescu D, Frey RS, et al (2005) Inactivation of CD11b in a mouse transgenic model protects against sepsis-induced lung PMN infiltration and vascular injury. Physiol Genomics 21: 230–242.

41. Walzog B, Schuppan D, Heimpel C, Hafezi-Moghadam A, Gaehtgens P, et al (1995) The leukocyte integrin Mac-1 (CD11b/CD18) contributes to binding of human granulocytes to collagen. Exp Cell Res 218: 28–38.

42. Reil JC, Hohl M, Oberhofer M, Kazakov A, Kaestner L, et al (2010) Cardiac Rac1 overexpression in mice creates a substrate for atrial arrhythmias characterized by structural remodelling. Cardiovasc Res 87: 485–493.

43. Sovari AA, Morita N, Karagueuzian HS (2008) Apocynin: a potent NADPH oxidase inhibitor for the management of atrial fibrillation. Redox Rep 13: 242–245.

44. Novo G, Guttilla D, Fazio G, Cooper D, Novo S (2008) The role of the renin-angiotensin system in atrial fibrillation and the therapeutic effects of ACE-Is and ARBS. Br J Clin Pharmacol 66: 345–351.

45. Bapat A, Nguyen TP, Lee JH, Sovari AA, Fishbein MC, et al (2012) Enhanced sensitivity of aged fibrotic hearts to angiotensin II- and hypokalemia-induced early afterdepolarization-mediated ventricular arrhythmias. Am J Physiol Heart Circ Physiol 302: H2331–H2340.

46. Masson S, Aleksova A, Favero C, Staszewsky L, Bernardinangeli M, et al (2010) Predicting atrial fibrillation recurrence with circulating inflammatory markers in patients in sinus rhythm at high risk for atrial fibrillation: data from the GISSI atrial fibrillation trial. Heart 96: 1909–1914.

47. Disertori M, Latini R, Barlera S, Franzosi MG, Staszewsky L, et al (2009) Valsartan for prevention of recurrent atrial fibrillation. N Engl J Med 360: 1606–1617.

48. Khatib R, Joseph P, Briel M, Yusuf S, Healey J (2013) Blockade of the renin-angiotensin-aldosterone system (RAAS) for primary prevention of non-valvular atrial fibrillation: a systematic review and meta analysis of randomized controlled trials. Int J Cardiol 165: 17–24.

49. Huang G, Xu JB, Liu JX, He Y, Nie XL, et al (2011) Angiotensin-converting enzyme inhibitors and angiotensin receptor blockers decrease the incidence of atrial fibrillation: a meta-analysis. Eur J Clin Invest 41: 719–733.

9

Atrial Fibrillation-Linked Germline *GJA5*/Connexin40 Mutants Showed an Increased Hemichannel Function

Yiguo Sun[9]**, Matthew D. Hills**[9]**, Willy G. Ye, Xiaoling Tong, Donglin Bai***

Department of Physiology and Pharmacology, The University of Western Ontario, London, Ontario, Canada

Abstract

Mutations in *GJA5* encoding the gap junction protein connexin40 (Cx40) have been linked to lone atrial fibrillation. Some of these mutants result in impaired gap junction function due to either abnormal connexin localization or impaired gap junction channels, which may play a role in promoting atrial fibrillation. However, the effects of the atrial fibrillation-linked Cx40 mutants on hemichannel function have not been studied. Here we investigated two atrial fibrillation-linked germline Cx40 mutants, V85I and L221I. These two mutants formed putative gap junction plaques at cell-cell interfaces, with similar gap junction coupling conductance as that of wild-type Cx40. Connexin deficient HeLa cells expressing either one of these two mutants displayed prominent propidium iodide-uptake distinct from cells expressing wild-type Cx40 or other atrial fibrillation-linked Cx40 mutants, I75F, L229M, and Q49X. Propidium iodide-uptake was sensitive to $[Ca^{2+}]_o$ and the hemichannel blockers, carbenoxolone, flufenamic acid and mefloquine, but was not affected by the pannexin 1 channel blocking agent, probenecid, indicating that uptake is most likely mediated via connexin hemichannels. A gain-of-hemichannel function in these two atrial fibrillation-linked Cx40 mutants may provide a novel mechanism underlying the etiology of atrial fibrillation.

Editor: Alexander V. Panfilov, Gent University, Belgium

Funding: This work was supported by the Canadian Institutes of Health Research (MOP86649 to D.B.); Heart and Stroke Foundation of Canada (G-13-0003066 to D.B.); and an Early Researcher Award from Ontario government (to D.B.). The funders had no role in study design, data collection and analysis, decision to publish, or preparation of the manuscript.

Competing Interests: The authors have declared that no competing interests exist.

* E-mail: donglin.bai@schulich.uwo.ca

[9] These authors contributed equally to this work.

Introduction

Gap junctions are intercellular channels formed by dodecamers of integral membrane protein subunits known as connexins (Cxs). Gap junctions allow direct exchange of ions and small molecules between apposing cells [1]. The Cx family of proteins all share a common structural topology, which consists of an intracellular amino-terminus, four transmembrane domains, two extracellular loops, a cytoplasmic loop and an intracellular carboxyl-terminus [2]. The oligomerization of six Cxs forms a hemichannel (also known as connexon) and two hemichannels on the plasma membrane of neighbouring cells can dock end-to-end to form a gap junction channel.

In addition to forming gap junction channels, Cxs are able to form undocked hemichannels on the plasma membrane. These hemichannels can provide a direct passage between the intracellular environment and the extracellular space, which allows for the release of small intracellular molecules such as ATP [3], glutamate [4], NAD^+ [5] and prostaglandin E2 [6]. These signaling molecules can then act on their respective receptors located on the same cell (autocrine) or its neighbouring cells (paracrine). A common feature of all hemichannels is that under physiological conditions they have a low open probability, but can be opened by a number of different stimuli including reduced concentrations of extracellular divalent cations, such as Ca^{2+} and Mg^{2+}, large and prolonged membrane depolarization, mechanical membrane stress and/or metabolic inhibition [7,8].

In the heart, gap junctions mediate direct electrical coupling between cardiomyocytes, allowing for rapid propagation of action potentials in the atria and ventricles, which is essential for synchronous contractions [9]. The human heart expresses three main Cx isoforms: Cx40, Cx43 and Cx45. Both Cx40 and Cx43 are expressed in the atria and Cx43 is the major connexin in the ventricles. In contrast, Cx45 is mainly found in the sinoatrial and atrioventricular nodes [10]. In addition to its extensive expression in the atria, Cx40 is also found in parts of the ventricular conduction system, such as the His-bundle, the upper and lower bundle branches and the Purkinje fibres. Several recent studies indicate somatic and germline mutations in the Cx40 gene (*GJA5*) are associated with lone atrial fibrillation (AF) [11,12,13,14,15]. Studies by us and others on these AF-linked Cx40 mutants revealed various changes in cellular distribution and gap junction function [11,12,15,16]. However, it is not known if there are any changes in the hemichannel function for any of the AF-linked Cx40 mutants. Here we investigated two novel germline Cx40 mutations, V85I and L221I, identified by Yang et al. (2010b) from two Chinese families with inherited lone AF. These mutations were autosomal dominantly inherited and mutant carriers in the family showed early onset of AF. These mutations were not found in other members in the family or in 200 unrelated, healthy, ethnic- and age-matched control subjects [13]. We observed little change in the gap junction distribution and function of these two Cx40 mutants in HeLa and N2A cells. However, these two

AF-linked Cx40 mutants showed an increase in propidium iodide (PI) uptake under conditions favoring hemichannel opening. Interestingly, we did not observe any PI-uptake in wild-type Cx40 expressing cells, indicating that the mutants showed a gain-of-hemichannel function, which may play a role in the pathogenesis of AF.

Methods

Plasmid Construction

The human Cx40-YFP, Cx40-IRES-GFP, Cx43-IRES-GFP and Cx26-GFP constructs were created as previously described [12,17]. The C-terminal fusion YFP-tagged (V85I-YFP and L221I-YFP) and the non-fusion GFP-tagged (V85I-IRES-GFP and L221I-IRES-GFP) constructs were generated by the Quick-Change site directed mutagenesis kit (Stratagene, La Jolla, CA) on the respective template with the following primers: the forward 5'-CAGATCATCTTCATCTCCACGCCCT-3' and the reverse 5'-AGGGCGTGGAGATGAAGATGATCTG-3' for V85I and the forward 5'-CTGTCCCTCCTCATTAGCCTGGCTG-3' and the reverse 5'-CAGCCAGGCTAATGAGGAGGGACAG-3' for L221I. All connexin clones were sequenced to confirm the accuracy of the nucleotide sequence and no additional variations were introduced.

Cell Culture and Transfection

HeLa (human cervical carcinoma, American Type Culture Collection, Manassas, VA) cells were grown in Dulbecco's modified Eagle's medium (DMEM, Invitrogen, Burlington, ON) containing 4.5 g/L D-glucose, 584 mg/L L-glutamine, 110 mg/L sodium pyruvate, 10% fetal bovine serum and 1% penicillin and streptomycin, in an incubator with 5% CO_2 at 37°C. HeLa cells were plated at 60–80% confluence on 35 mm Petri dishes 12–24 hours before transfection. For each transfection, HeLa cells were incubated with 1.5 μg of a cDNA construct and 3 μl of X-tremeGENE HP DNA transfection reagent (Roche, Mississauga, ON) in Opti-MEM I+GlutaMAX-I medium supplemented with HEPES and 2.4 g/L sodium bicarbonate (Invitrogen) for 4 hours. Medium was then changed back to the modified DMEM and cells were used for either localization studies or dye uptake assays approximately 18–24 hours after transfection.

Localization Study

To observe the localization of Cx40-YFP, V85I-YFP and L221I-YFP, HeLa cells were cultured on glass bottom dishes and were transfected individually with the respective cDNA constructs. After culturing for 24 hours, the cells were fixed with a solution of 80% methanol and 20% acetone for 20 minutes at −20°C. Wild-type Cx40-YFP and YFP-tagged mutants were imaged using a Zeiss LSM 510-META confocal microscope as described earlier [12]. To quantify the percentage of gap junction plaque-like structures at the cell-to-cell interfaces of successfully transfected cells, approximately 20–30 cells were counted for each transfection.

To observe the localization of untagged Cx40 and mutants, HeLa and N2A cells (American Type Culture Collection) were transfected with Cx40-IRES-GFP, V85I-IRES-GFP or L221I-IRES-GFP. After culturing for 24 h, cells were rinsed with PBS and fixed for 10 minutes in a 1:1 solution of acetone and methanol at −20°C. Cells were then blocked for 1 hour with 5% BSA in PBS. Anti-Cx40 antibody (Millipore, Billerica, MA) was incubated for 1 h at room temperature. The cells were washed and subsequently stained for 30 min with the secondary Alexa 594–conjugated antibody (Invitrogen) prior to confocal microscopy.

Dye Uptake Assay

Propidium iodide (PI)-uptake assay was used to assess the hemichannel function of YFP-tagged Cx40 and mutants. HeLa cells were plated at a low density to allow for isolated, single cells to be transiently transfected as described above. The cells were washed with regular extracellular solution (ECS) (also known as divalent cation-containing ECS, DCC-ECS) containing 142 mM NaCl, 5.4 mM KCl, 1.4 mM $MgCl_2$, 2 mM $CaCl_2$, 10 mM HEPES and 25 mM D-Glucose. The pH of ECS was adjusted to 7.35 and the osmolarity was adjusted to 298 mOsm. The cells were then washed with divalent cation free-ECS (DCF-ECS), which contains no Ca^{2+} or Mg^{2+} and 2 mM EGTA to chelate the remaining ambient divalent cations. The cells were incubated in DCF-ECS-containing PI (150 μM) at 37°C for 15 minutes to assess PI-uptake. After incubation, the cells were washed three times with regular ECS and the percentage of transfected cells (green with either GFP or YFP) showing PI-uptake was measured under a fluorescent microscope (DMIRE2, Leica). Cells in pairs and clusters were excluded from measurement to avoid errors produced by gap junctions. Negative controls (untransfected cells and YFP-transfected cells) and positive control (Cx26-GFP transfected cells) and the various incubation conditions (e.g. with hemichannel blockers carbenoxolone, flufenamic acid, mefluquine or different $[Ca^{2+}]_o$) were indicated in each experiment. For each experiment approximately 30–50 cells were counted to obtain a percentage of PI-uptake. The bar graphs were generated with 5–15 transfections. Similar PI-uptake experiments were performed on HeLa cells transfected with the mutant-IRES-GFP constructs with a slightly longer PI-incubation time (20 minutes).

For the experiment with continuous measurement of PI-uptake, HeLa cells were cultured in glass bottom dishes. Fluorescence measurements of PI were performed with a confocal microscope (LSM 510 Meta, Zeiss, Germany). Baseline fluorescence (F0) in regular ECS and the increase of PI-uptake during the incubation of DCF-ECS (F) were collected at 1 minute intervals for 20 minutes. The obtained images were quantitatively analyzed using ZEN software for changes in fluorescence intensities within regions of interest (ROIs) of isolated GFP-positive cells, which expressed mutant-IRES-GFP. The intracellular fluorescence changes during PI incubation are expressed as the ratio of current fluorescence intensity over that of the baseline (F/F_0).

Electrophysiological Studies

Electrophysiological recordings for measuring gap junction coupling were carried out in connexin-deficient neuroblastoma (N2A) cells. N2A cells were grown at 37°C in 35-mm culture dishes to 70% confluence in Dulbecco's modified Eagle's medium containing 10% FBS. Cells were transiently transfected with mutant or wild-type connexin DNA by X-tremeGENE HP reagent. The dual whole-cell patch clamp technique was performed at room temperature to assess the gap junctional conductance (G_j) between cell pairs 24 hours after transfection [12,18]. For co-transfection experiments, cell pairs showing successful co-expression with V85I-IRES-GFP (or L221I-GFP) and Cx43mRFP were selected for recording as described earlier [12]. The junctional current (I_j) was amplified via a MultiClamp 700A amplifier (Molecular Devices, Sunnyvale, CA) and was digitized at a sampling rate of 10 kHz with a Digidata 1322A (Molecular Devices, Sunnyvale, CA). Data were analyzed with pClamp9 software. Each cell of a pair was initially held at a common holding potential of 0 mV. To evaluate junctional coupling, 20 mV pulses for 7 seconds were applied to one cell to establish a transjunctional voltage (V_j), while the junctional currents (I_j) were measured in the other cell. Macroscopic junctional conductance (G_j) was calculated as follows: $G_j = I_j/V_j$. In all cases, cells were studied after multiple independent transfections and only cell pairs with fluorescent protein signals were selected for double patch clamp recording.

Hemichannel currents were studied in the mutant and control connexins (all with untagged GFP in pIRES2-GFP vector) transfected HeLa cells using a voltage ramp protocol (from −110 to +110 mV in 6 seconds, 36.7 mV/s) similar to that previously reported [19]. DCF-ECS was used to facilitate the hemichannel opening. Pipette solution and extracellular saline were the same as those described earlier [12]. Carbenoxolone (CBX 100 μM) was used to block the hemichannel current.

Statistical Analysis

One-way ANOVA followed by Newman-Keuls test was used to compare the multiple groups of data on G_j and PI-uptake percentage. Statistical significance is denoted with asterisks (*, $P < 0.05$ or ***, $P < 0.001$) on the graphs. The data presented on the graphs are expressed as mean ± standard error of the mean (SEM). Unless specified, all experiments were performed at least three times.

Results

Localization of YFP-tagged Cx40 Mutants

The localization of wild-type Cx40-YFP and the AF-linked Cx40 mutants, V85I-YFP or L221I-YFP, were examined in connexin-deficient HeLa cells. As shown in Fig. 1A, Cx40-YFP, V85I-YFP and L221I-YFP were all able to traffic to the plasma membrane and form gap junction plaque-like structures at cell-cell interfaces. Free YFP did not form gap junction plaque-like structures at cell-cell interfaces (data not shown). To further quantify the probability of gap junction plaque formation, we calculated the percentage of the cell pairs/clusters displaying putative gap junction plaques at cell-cell interfaces. The percentage of successful formation of gap junction plaques of V85I-YFP- and L221I-YFP-expressing cells were 65±2% (n = 7) and 46±2% (n = 7), respectively and were found to be statistically lower than that of the cells expressing Cx40-YFP (89±2%, n = 7; $P < 0.001$ for both mutants), indicating that these two AF-linked mutants showed a modest but statistically significant decrease in the formation of gap junction plaque-like structures at cell-cell interfaces.

G_js of the V85I- and L221I-expressing Cell Pairs Were the Same as that of Cell Pairs Expressing Wild-type Cx40

Dual patch clamp technique was used to measure the coupling conductance (G_j) of N2A cell pairs expressing Cx40-YFP, V85I-YFP or L221I-YFP. Transjunctional currents (I_js) in response to a 20 mV transjunctional voltage pulse (V_j) are shown in Fig. 1B. Our results indicate that the averaged coupling conductance (G_js) for each mutant was not statistically different from the control (Cx40), demonstrating that the gap junction function of these two mutants was not impaired in the N2A cells.

V85I- and L221I-expressing Cells Showed Increased Propidium Iodide-uptake

Since we observed no apparent gap junction function defects of these two Cx40 mutants in our model cells, this prompted us to look into possible changes in non-gap junction linked functions, including hemichannel function. To facilitate the opening of undocked Cx40 gap junction hemichannels in HeLa cells, we removed both Ca^{2+} and Mg^{2+} and added EGTA (2 mM) to chelate the ambient low level of divalent cations. This solution was defined as divalent cation free-extracellular solution (DCF-ECS or DCF). HeLa cells expressing Cx26-GFP, incubated in DCF-ECS and PI, showed a prominent PI-uptake in 86% of cells (Fig. 2A, B), while the majority of untransfected HeLa cells or YFP-expressing HeLa cells failed to show PI-uptake (Fig. 2A, B), suggesting that undocked Cx26 hemichannels may be responsible for the PI-uptake. Interestingly, positive PI-uptake was identified in the majority of HeLa cells expressing YFP-tagged Cx40 mutants, V85I (67.6±6.6%, n = 10) and L221I (83.2±2.8%, n = 10). In contrast to these findings, Cx40-YFP-expressing cells failed to show a significant PI-uptake under the same conditions (4.6±1.2%, n = 14). This was significantly different from the PI-uptake observed for the two mutants ($P < 0.001$), but was similar to that of the negative control, YFP-expressing cells (4.0±1.6%, $P > 0.05$).

Our previous studies showed that AF-linked Cx40 mutants, I75F and Q49X, impaired homotypic gap junction function, while L229M did not impair homotypic gap junction function, but specifically impaired the gap junction function when co-expressed with Cx43 [12,15]. Here we tested PI-uptake of HeLa cells expressing these Cx40 mutants individually. As shown in Fig. 2B, these mutants all failed to show any substantial PI-uptake, indicating that either their undocked hemichannels were unlikely to be in the open state during the incubation with DCF-ECS or in the case of Q49X, it is probably unable to oligomerize to form hemichannels, and even if it could form hemichannels, they would be unlikely to reach the plasma membrane.

The Role of Extracellular Divalent Cations and Carbenoxolone on PI-uptake

Previous studies indicated that several gap junction hemichannel-mediated dye-uptake could be blocked by the elevation of extracellular calcium concentration or addition of the hemichannel blocker, carbenoxolone (CBX) [8]. We hypothesized that PI-uptake was due to the undocked connexin hemichannels on the plasma membrane. To test this, transfected HeLa cells were incubated with PI in the presence of divalent cation containing solution (DCC-ECS or DCC) or CBX (100 μM). Both DCC-ECS and CBX effectively eliminated PI-uptake in cells expressing Cx26-GFP and the Cx40 mutants, V85I and L221I (Fig. 3A).

To quantitatively assess $[Ca^{2+}]_o$ dependence of the PI-uptake, several $[Ca^{2+}]_o$ concentrations from nominal Ca^{2+}-free to 2 mM were tested. Our data indicated that cells expressing Cx26 or the Cx40 mutants, V85I and L221I, displayed $[Ca^{2+}]_o$ concentration-dependent PI-uptake (Fig. 3B). In the range of 0.2 and 0.02 mM $[Ca^{2+}]_o$, Cx26-expressing cells showed a higher level, L221I-expressing cells showed an intermediate level and V85I-expressing cells showed a lower level of PI-uptake (Fig. 3B), suggesting that these hemichannels may have different sensitivities to $[Ca^{2+}]_o$. For Cx40-expressing cells, no PI-uptake was observed for any of the calcium concentrations tested (Fig. 3B).

Hemichannel Characterizations Using Untagged Cx40 Mutants

Fusion of fluorescent proteins at the carboxyl terminus of connexins is very useful in determining the distribution and function of connexins in live cells. However, to verify our results obtained by using YFP-tagged Cx40, we also studied untagged Cx40 mutants using mutant-IRES-GFP constructs. We expressed V85I-IRES-GFP and L221I-IRES-GFP in HeLa and N2A cells. Anti-Cx40 antibody was used to reveal the localization of expressed Cx40 mutants. As shown in Fig. 4A, V85I and L221I

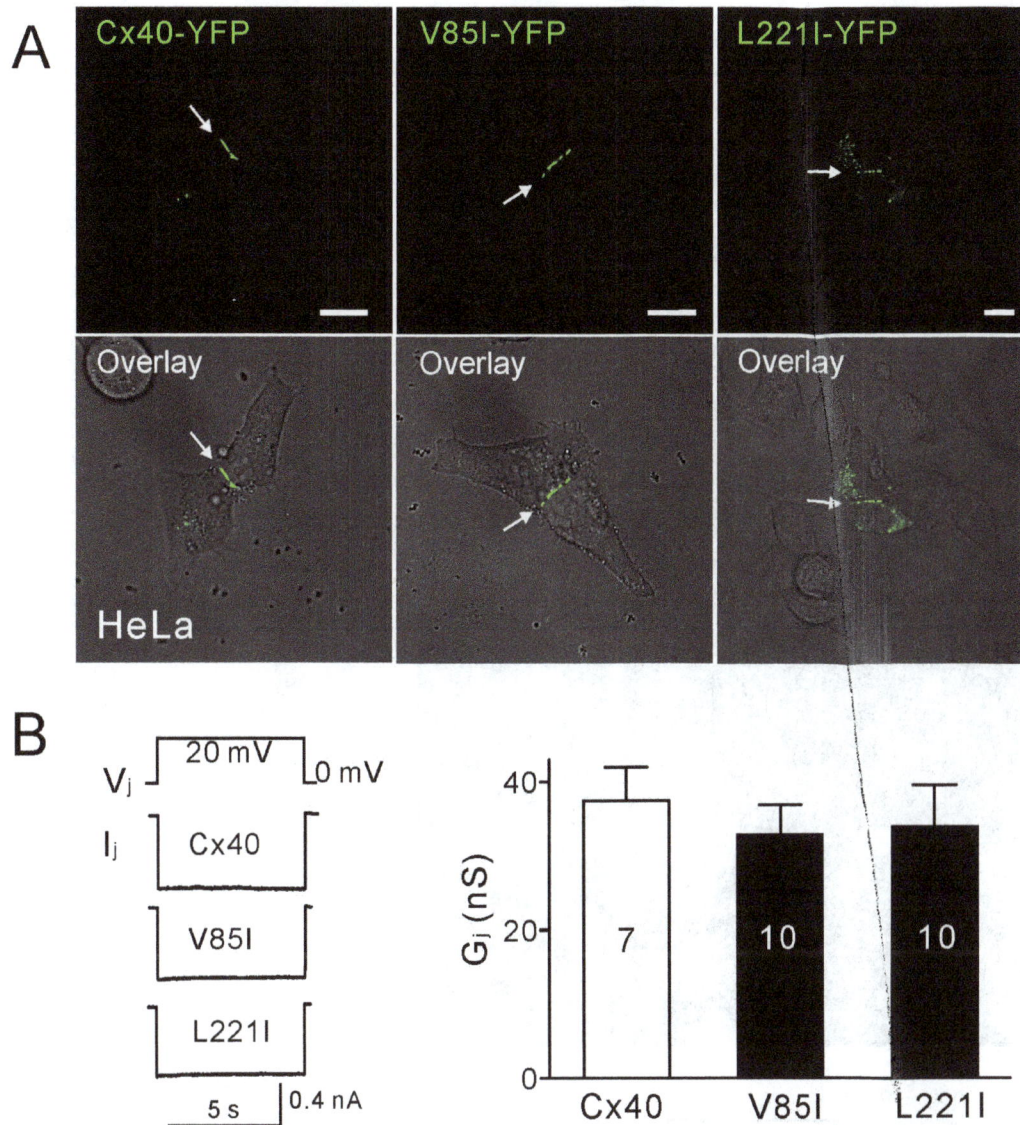

Figure 1. The localization and macroscopic dual whole-cell patch clamp recordings of YFP-tagged homotypic Cx40 and Cx40-mutant gap junctions. (A) Representative fluorescent confocal images of Cx40-YFP, V85I-YFP and L221I-YFP (top panels). The overlaid fluorescent images on top of phase contrast images are also shown (bottom panels). All three constructs were able to form gap junction plaque-like structures at the cell-cell junction. Scale bar = 10 μm. (B) Voltage steps of 20 mV were applied to one cell of a transfected N2A cell pair and the junctional current (I_j) was recorded in the second cell. There was no significant difference between the I_j in cell pairs expressing Cx40-YFP, V85I-YFP or L221I-YFP. The junctional conductance (G_j) was calculated and there was no significant difference between the G_j of cell pairs expressing Cx40-YFP, V85I-YFP or L221I-YFP.

showed a similar intracellular distribution pattern and both of them were able to reach cell-cell interfaces to form gap junction plaque-like structures, similar to that observed for wild-type Cx40, in both HeLa and N2A cells.

The coupling conductance (G_j) of N2A cell pairs expressing either one of these mutants showed a similar level as that of Cx40-expressing cells (Fig. 4B). In contrast, GFP-expressing cells failed to display any gap junction coupling (Fig. 4B). Co-expression of either one of these mutants with Cx43 in N2A cell pairs did not show any change in the coupling conductance compared to that of cell pairs expressing Cx43 (Fig. 4C).

PI-uptake was assessed the same way as described earlier by incubating HeLa cells in DCF-ECS. Both V85I and L221I showed a significantly higher level of PI-uptake than that of Cx40 (Fig. 5A).

We also found that cells expressing these two mutants displayed higher levels of PI-uptake than that of wild-type Cx43 (Fig. 5A). Adding divalent cations (DCC) or CBX (100 μM) virtually eliminated PI-uptake, while the pannexin 1 channel blocker, probenecid (200 μM), failed to decrease PI-uptake (Fig. 5B). In addition, flufenamic acid (FFA, 50 μM) or mefloquine (MFQ, 25 μM) blocked the majority of PI-uptake in either V85I or L221I-expressing cells (Fig. 5C). These results confirmed that PI-uptake was due to undocked hemichannels and unlikely to be pannexin 1 channels.

To evaluate the time course of PI-uptake during the incubation with DCF medium, we monitored the cellular PI-fluorescent level changes. L221I- and V85I-expressing cells showed a time-dependent increase in PI-uptake and saturated near the end of

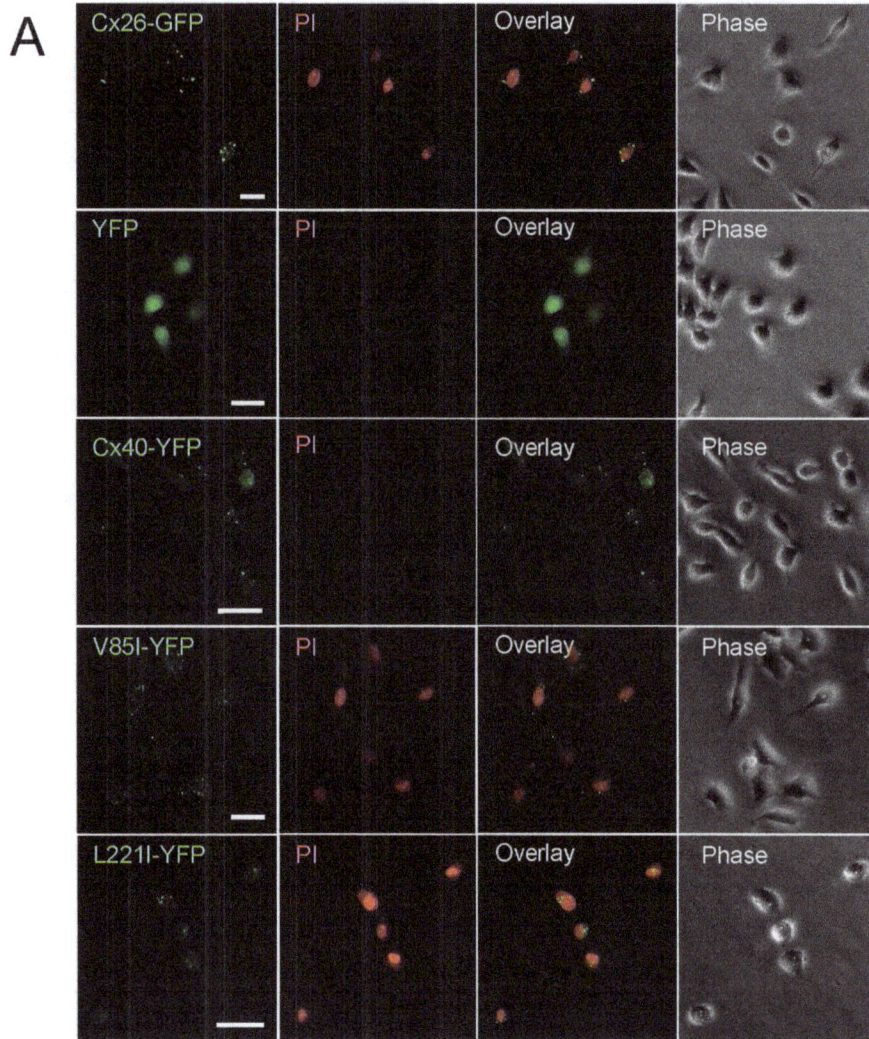

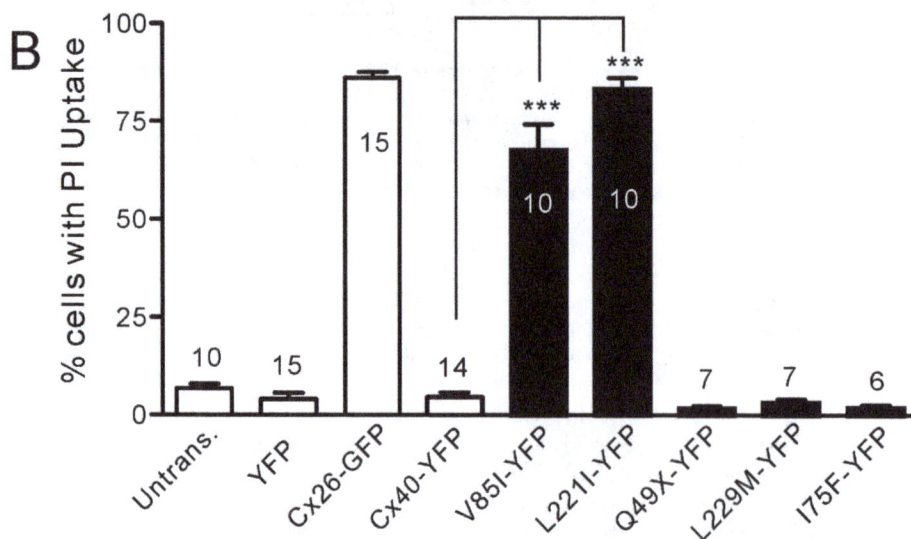

Figure 2. Propidium iodide-uptake under divalent cation-free conditions. (A) Representative images of propidium iodide (PI)-uptake under divalent cation-free (DCF) conditions for isolated, individual, transfected HeLa cells. Successful transfection can be identified by their tagged green/yellow fluorescent proteins (green colour in the first column images). PI-uptake (red colour in the second column images) can be seen in cells expressing Cx26-GFP, V85I-YFP and L221I-YFP, but no uptake was seen in cells expressing YFP alone or Cx40-YFP. Scale bar = 20 μm. **(B)** Quantification of PI-uptake under DCF conditions. V85I-YFP (67.6%, n = 10) and L221I-YFP (83.2%, n = 10) showed a significant increase in PI-uptake

compared to Cx40-YFP (4.6%, n = 14, ***indicates P<0.001). Other AF-linked Cx40 mutants, Q49X, L229M and I75F, were also studied and did not show any PI-uptake.

the 20 minute incubation (Fig. 6). V85I-expressing cells showed a slightly slower rate of PI-uptake within the first 10 minutes than that of L221I-expressing cells. However, they both reach a similar level of PI-uptake near the end of 20 minute-incubation. Addition of CBX (100 μM) virtually abolished the PI-uptake of mutant-expressing cells.

Patch Clamp Recording of Putative Hemichannel Current in Mutant-expressing HeLa Cells

Voltage-clamp recording was used to study hemichannel current on HeLa cells expressing the Cx40 mutants and Cx40. A voltage ramp protocol induced an extra outward current in positive voltages (+20 mV or higher) after exchanging the saline

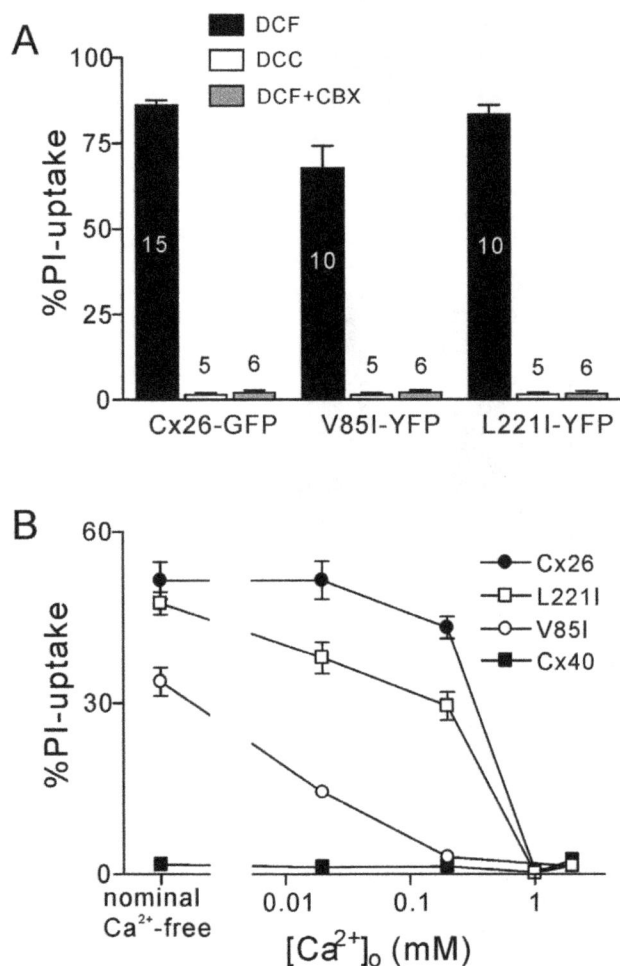

Figure 3. The effect of external Ca²⁺ concentration on PI-uptake. (**A**) Comparison of PI-uptake for divalent cation containing (DCC) and divalent cation-free (DCF) conditions. The PI-uptake for cells expressing Cx26-GFP, V85I-YFP and L221I-YFP was significantly increased under DCF conditions compared to DCC conditions. Also the addition of the hemichannel blocker carbenoxolone (CBX, 100 μM) under DCF conditions significantly decreased PI-uptake. (**B**) [Ca²⁺]$_o$ dose-dependent PI-uptake. Cx26-GFP, V85I-YFP and L221I-YFP all showed [Ca²⁺]$_o$ dependent PI-uptake. Cx40-YFP did not show PI-uptake for any concentrations tested.

(DCC) with DCF saline in the majority of mutant-expressing cells (Fig. 7A, B). The DCF-dependent currents in these V85I- or L221I-expressing cells were largely blocked by CBX (100 μM). Although the DCF-dependent currents were also observed in Cx43 or Cx40-expressing cells, the incidence was lower, especially in Cx40-expressing cells, where most of cells displayed no change in the voltage ramp-induced current in DCF (Fig. 7C, D). None of the GFP-expressing cells showed DCF-dependent current (Fig. 7D). These results support a model where the DCF-dependent and CBX-sensitive current are mediated, at least in part, by the mutant (or wild-type connexin) hemichannels. Both V85I and L221I increased the incidences of observing the hemichannel current compared to that of Cx40.

Discussion

Here we studied two AF-linked germline mutations in the Cx40 gene. Our data indicated that V85I and L221I showed a statistically significant reduction in gap junction plaque formation at cell-cell interfaces. However, the functional inspection of the coupling conductance in N2A cell pairs expressing any of the mutants did not show a change from that of the wild-type Cx40, indicating that these mutants are unlikely to impair gap junction function. To further evaluate if there were any changes in the hemichannel function, we performed PI-uptake assays in the divalent cation-free medium. Cells expressing wild-type Cx40 did not show any PI-uptake, but V85I- and L221I-expressing cells showed pronounced PI-uptake. PI-uptake was eliminated or significantly reduced by the elevation of [Ca²⁺]$_o$ or hemichannel blocking agents, carbenoxolone, FFA and MFQ, but was not blocked by probenecid, indicating that the PI-uptake is likely due to the opening of connexin hemichannels. Patch clamp recording also showed an increased incidence of the putative hemichannel current in the mutant-expressing cells during large membrane depolarizations. Lack of expression of pannexin 2 and 3 and no change in pannexin 1 expression with the expression of either Cx40 or L221I, indicating that pannexins are unlikely to play a major role in the observed hemichannel functions. The gain-of-function on hemichannels for these two AF-linked Cx40 mutants provided a completely novel mechanism for possible AF-pathogenesis. Our tests on several previously studied AF-linked germline Cx40 mutants suggested that a number of different mechanisms could link these mutants to AF, including impaired steady-state localization to the gap junction site, reduced/eliminated gap junction channel function or increased hemichannel function (Fig. 8). A detailed understanding of the AF-linked Cx40 mutants will be crucial in developing proper, effective strategies to treat AF.

Atrial fibrillation is the most common sustained cardiac arrhythmia and the prevalence is predicted to increase due to the aging of our population [20]. AF is characterized by rapid and irregular atrial activations, which are followed by uncoordinated and ineffective atrial contractions. This can lead to stagnant blood pooling in the atria and lead to thrombosis formation and is therefore a leading cause of embolic stroke [21]. Approximately 30% of AF patients have a form of AF that is not secondary to other cardiovascular problems, such as hypertension, heart failure or myocardial infarction, and this is known as lone or idiopathic AF [20,22]. Although most of the Cx40 mutants show some sort of impairment in terms of forming functional gap junction channels, V85I and L221I show normal channel function when expressed

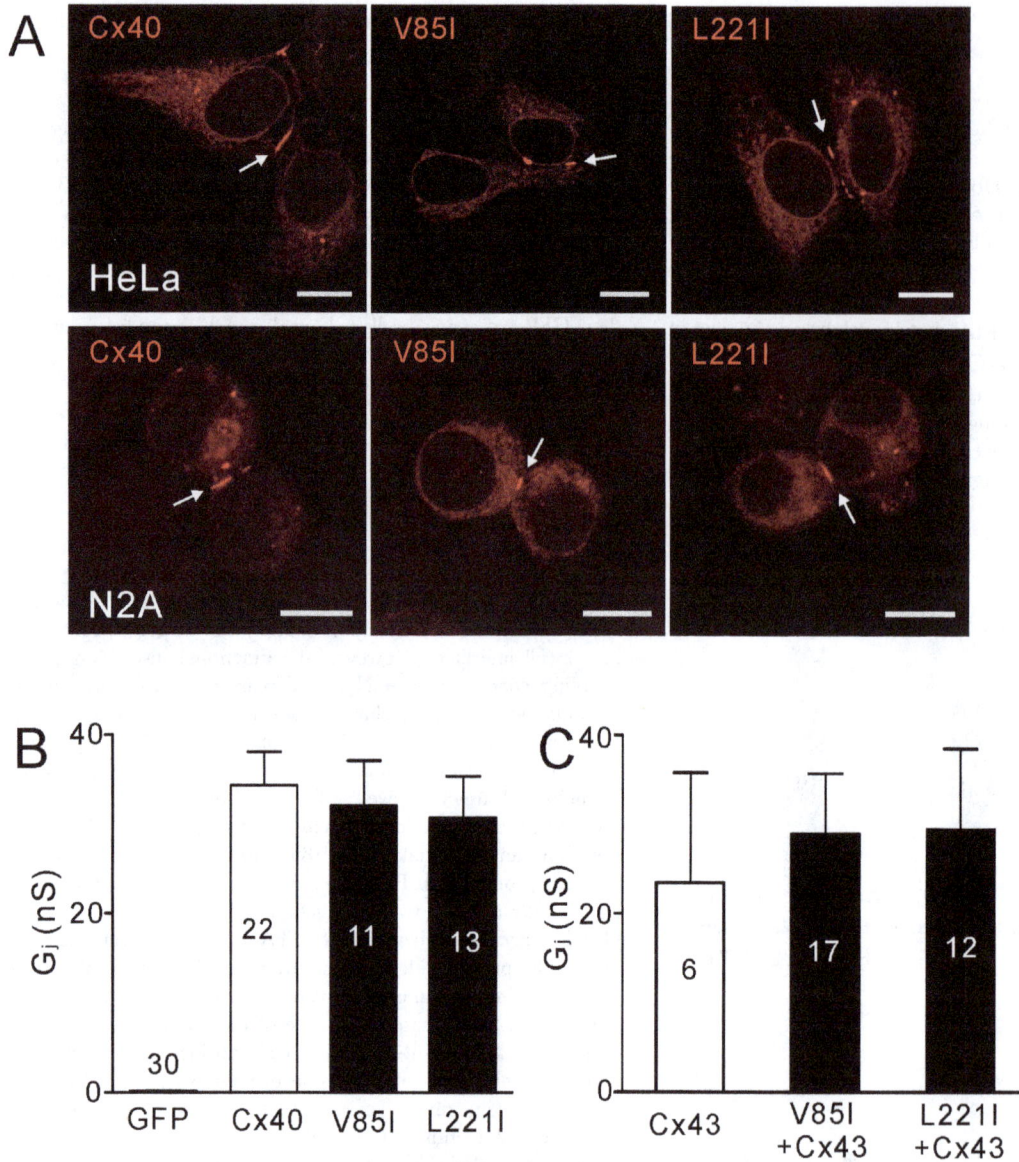

Figure 4. The localization and function of untagged homotypic Cx40 and Cx40-mutant gap junctions. (**A**) Representative confocal images showing the anti-Cx40 antibody localizations of untagged Cx40, V85I and L221I expressed in HeLa (top panels) and N2A (bottom panels) cells. In both cell lines, Cx40, V85I and L221I were all able to traffic to the cell-cell interface and form gap junction plaque-like structures. Scale bar = 10 µm. (**B**) There was no significant difference between the G_j of cell pairs expressing Cx40, V85I or L221I. (**C**) Co-expression of Cx40V85I-IRES-GFP or L221I-IRES-GFP with Cx43-mRFP (V85I+Cx43 or L221I+Cx43) in N2A cell pairs showed a similar G_j with cell pairs expressing Cx43-mRFP. The number of cell pairs are indicated on the bars.

alone or together with Cx43, but are gain of hemichannel function mutants. With this result comes the question of how this gain of hemichannel function can contribute to AF. Several possibilities associated with the opening of hemichannels may directly or indirectly change electrical properties of the cardiomyocytes, which could promote atrial arrhythmias. 1) Open hemichannels would allow for the inward and outward fluxes of Na^+ and K^+ ions according to their electrochemical gradient, respectively, the result of which is membrane depolarization. Transient membrane depolarization brings the cell closer to/over the threshold of firing an action potential, while sustained depolarization may lead to substantial Na^+ channel inactivation, which can reduce the excitability of cardiomyocytes and lead to a slower conduction velocity. Both actions could increase the heterogeneity of

cardiomyocyte excitability, increasing the susceptibility to arrhythmias [23]. 2) Open hemichannels may lead to the release of ATP to the extracellular space. The released ATP could act in an autocrine and paracrine manner to cause intracellular Ca^{2+} wave propagation via purinergic receptors [3]. 3) It is well-documented that most of the characterized gap junction hemichannels are large enough to allow leakage of small signaling and nutrient/metabolic molecules. The mutant Cx40 hemichannels may provide a passage to lose some of these important molecules, which may be critical for normal cardiomyocyte function. All of the above possibilities have the potential to lead to abnormal activities of the cardiomyocytes and may play a role in generating arrhythmias in patients carrying these mutations. It is noted that in normal physiological conditions these mutant hemichannels are unlikely to

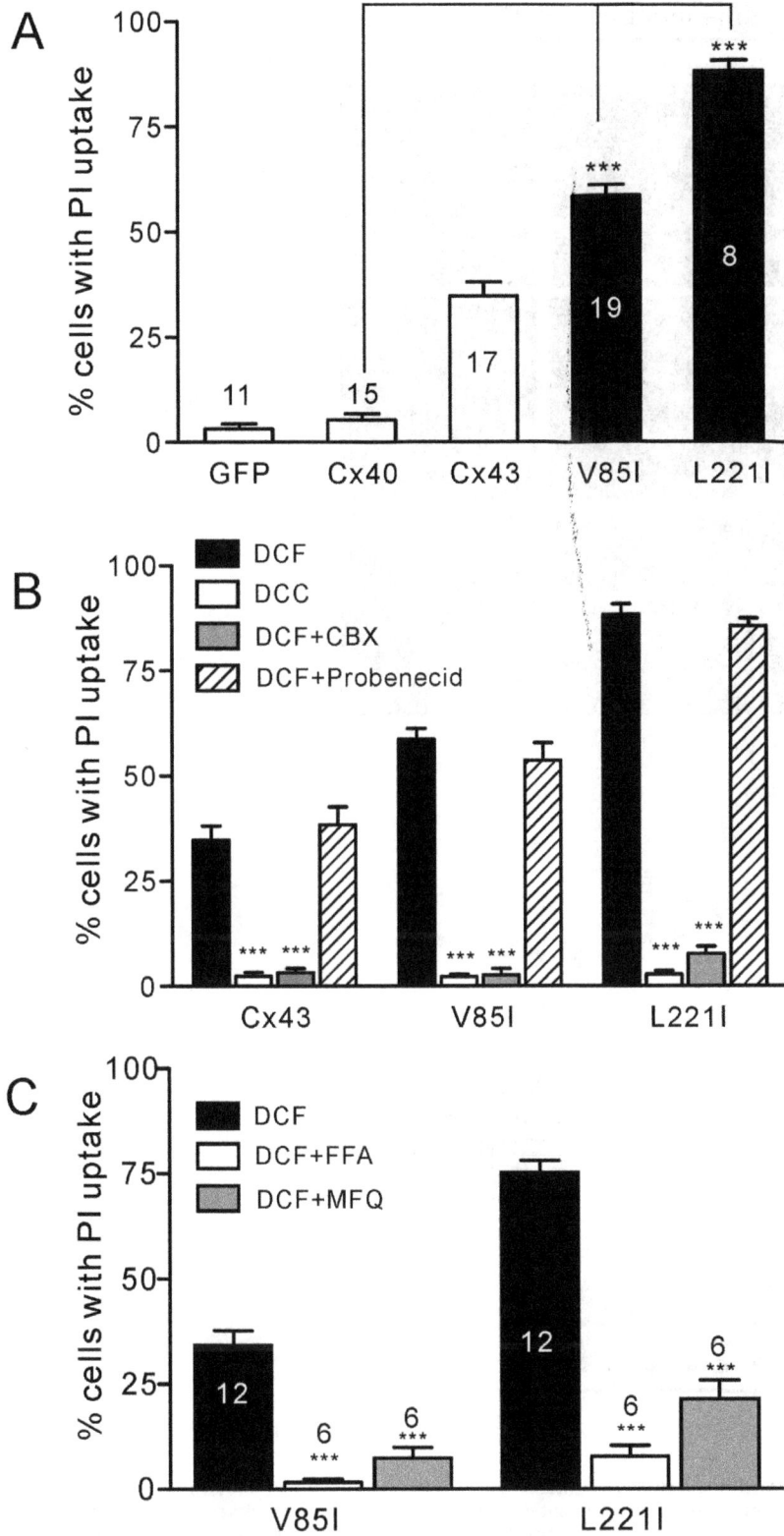

Figure 5. PI-uptake of untagged Cx40 and Cx40 mutants. (**A**) Untagged V85I and L221I showed a significant increase in PI-uptake compared to both wild-type Cx40 and Cx43 under the divalent cation-free (DCF) conditions. (**B**) The addition of divalent cations (DCC, open bars) or CBX (100 µM, gray bars) blocked the PI-uptake from cells expressing Cx43, V85I and L221I. However, the addition of the pannexin 1 channel blocker probenecid (200 µM, hatched bars) did not affect PI-uptake. (**C**) PI-uptake in cells expressing untagged V85I or L221I under DCF were significantly (P<0.001 in both cases) reduced by the addition of flufenamic acid (FFA, 50 µM) or mefloquine (MFQ, 25 µM). The total number of experiments are indicated on the bar.

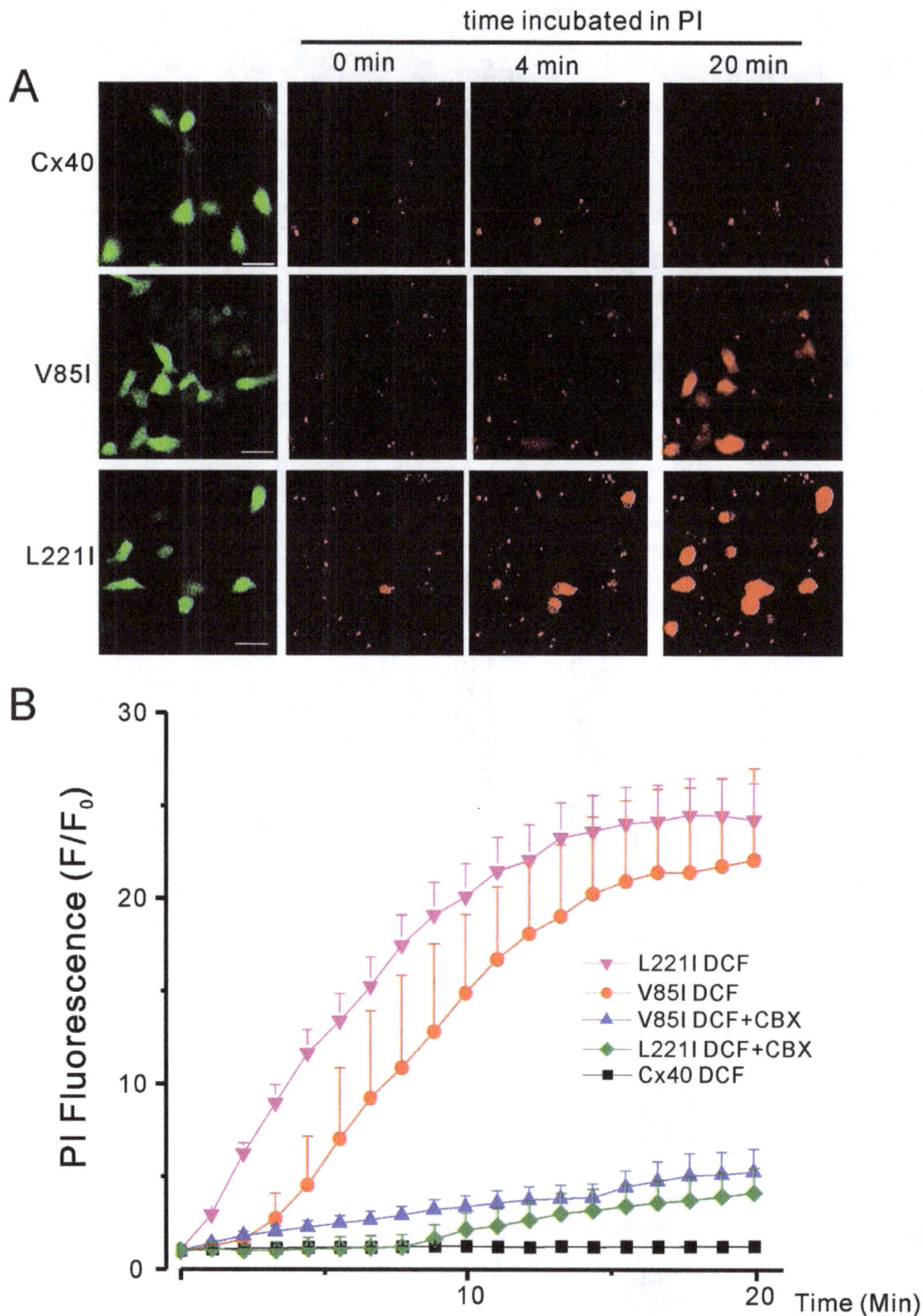

Figure 6. Time course of PI-uptake under the DCF conditions. (**A**) Representative confocal images of PI-uptake for HeLa cells transfected with wild-type Cx40 or Cx40 mutants (V85I or L221I). Time points of 0, 4 and 20 minutes of incubation with PI are displayed. During 20 minutes of incubation with PI, only cells expressing the V85I and L221I mutants showed PI uptake. Scale bar = 50 μm. (**B**) Ratio of current PI fluorescence intensity over the initial baseline fluorescence over a 20 minute incubation. L221I showed the fastest rate of PI-uptake, with V85I having a slightly slower rate of uptake, however, both L221I and V85I had similar levels of PI-uptake near the end of 20 minute incubation. The addition of 100 μM CBX blocked PI-uptake. Cx40 expressing cells failed to show any PI-uptake.

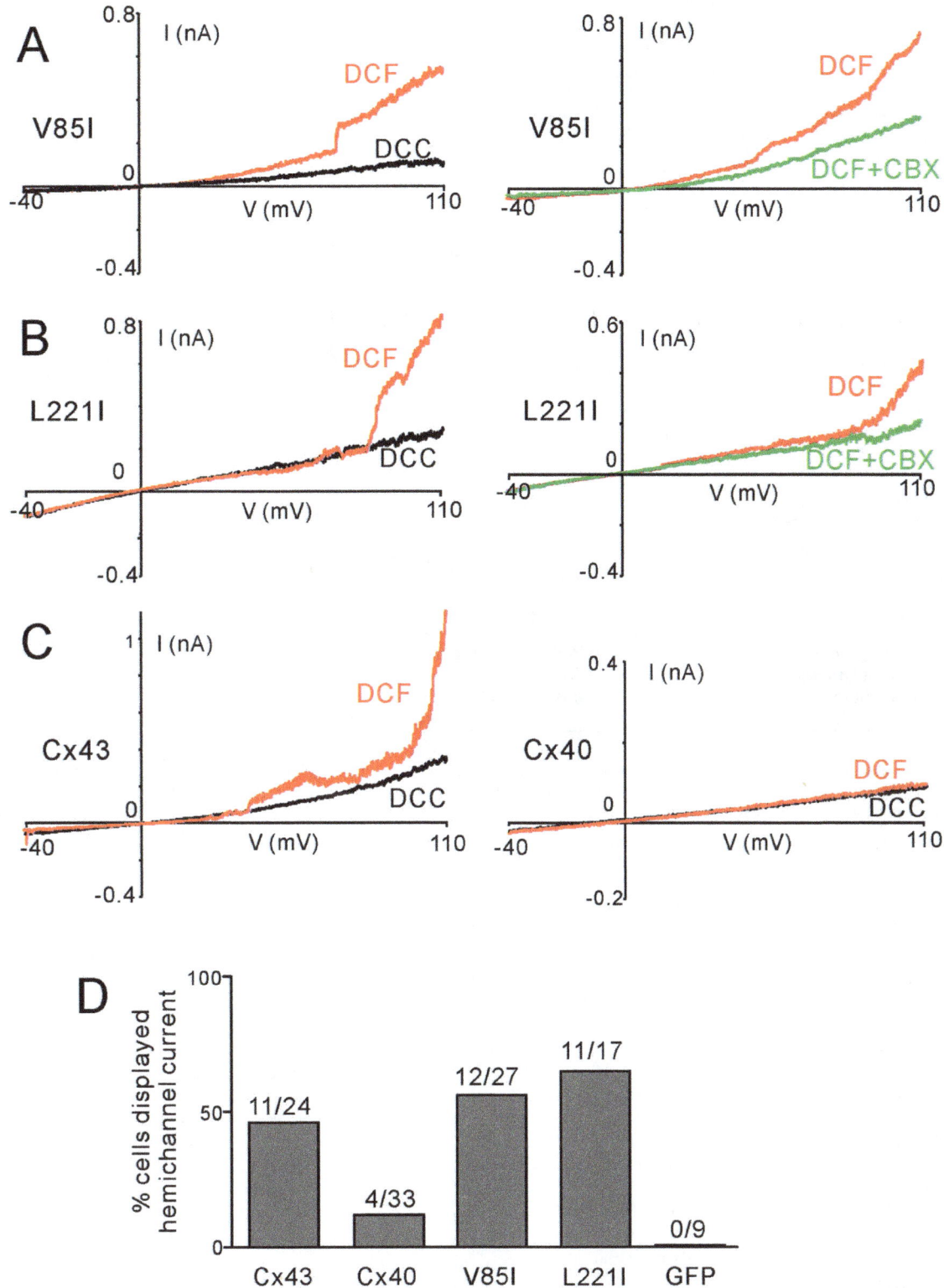

Figure 7. Putative hemichannel currents were increased in the HeLa cells-expressing AF-linked Cx40 mutants. Voltage clamp ramp protocol (−40 to 110 mV) was used to study currents under divalent cation containing saline (DCC, black traces) and the divalent-cation free saline (DCF, red traces). Putative hemichannel currents (the current amplitude differences between red and black traces) were observed in cells expressing AF-linked Cx40 mutants, V85I (A), L221I (B) and wild-type Cx43 (C, left panel). Most of Cx40-expressing cells failed to show the current (C, right panel). The DCF-dependent currents in the mutant-expressing cells were largely blocked by carbenoxolone (CBX, 100 μM, green traces). Bar graph summarized the percentages of cells displayed hemichannel current during the voltage ramp under DCF conditions (D). The connexin constructs expressed and the numbers of cells recorded are indicated. Note only 4/33 cells expressing Cx40 displayed putative hemichannel current (data not shown).

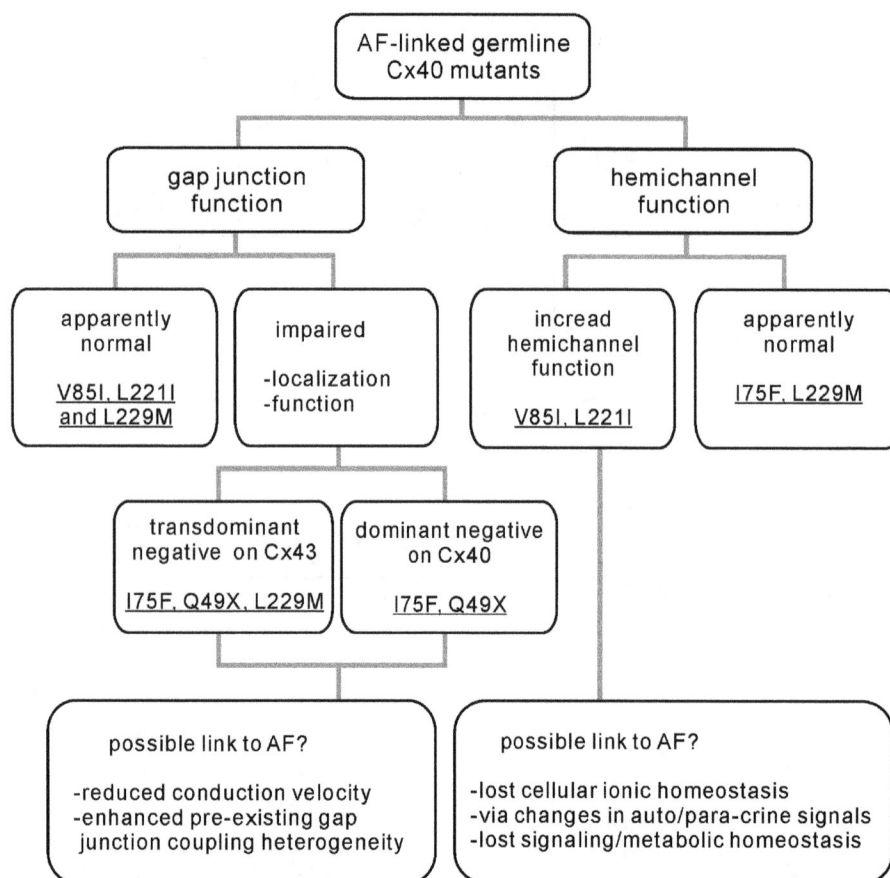

Figure 8. Overall summary of AF-linked germline Cx40 mutants. AF-linked germline Cx40 mutants have been shown to impair gap junction function via impaired localization (Q49X) or channel function (I75F). Dominant negative on Cx40 (Q49X and I75F) and/or transdominant negative actions on Cx43 were also observed (Q49X, I75F and L229M) [12,15]. Present study showed that AF-linked Cx40 mutants, V85I and L221I, increased hemichannel function.

be opened, however, our data indicate that both reduction of $[Ca^{2+}]_o$ and large membrane depolarization (e.g. during the peak of action potentials) can promote the mutant hemichannel opening.

Previous studies on AF-linked gap junction mutants are focused on the localization and function of gap junction channels. Cx40 mutants, P88S and Q49X, as well as the Cx43 mutant, G60S, showed impaired trafficking to the cell surface [11,15,24], while Cx40 mutants, I75F, A96S, L229M and G38D did not show any alterations in their localization, but displayed various degrees of reduction of the GJ coupling conductance [11,12]. In any case, the GJ function is impaired via different underlying mechanisms. It is predicted that the connexin mutants with impaired localization would also likely eliminate/reduce their hemichannel function. However, it is not known whether hemichannel function is reduced, increased or unchanged in those mutants with impaired gap junction function because other disease-linked Cx43 and Cx30 mutants with GJ impairment can increase [25] or decrease hemichannel function [26]. Here we tested AF-linked Cx40 mutants, Q49X, I75F and L229M, PI-uptake in DCF conditions and found no measurable increase in PI-uptake in our experimental conditions. At this time we are unable to identify if there is a decrease in the hemichannel function for these mutants due to the fact that we did not observe any substantial PI-uptake in wild-type Cx40 hemichannels. This is in contrast to the results seen with V85I or L221I, which show no obvious defect in gap junctional conductance when expressed alone or co-expressed with wild-type Cx43; however they showed prominent PI-uptake under DCF conditions, indicating a gain-of-hemichannel function.

Although many Cxs have been investigated for their hemichannel function, a number of them have not yet been properly characterized to our knowledge, including Cx40. Our current study is the first functional study of wild-type Cx40 and its mutant hemichannels. One study by Allen et al. (2011), used atomic force microscopy to evaluate the three-dimensional molecular topology and calcium-dependent conformational changes of Cx40 hemichannels [27]. They demonstrated that at low $[Ca^{2+}]_o$ (<10 μM), Cx40 hemichannels showed surface openings. The increase of external Ca^{2+} concentration closed most of the Cx40 hemichannels, suggesting that Ca^{2+} ions cause conformational rotation of Cx40 subunits, which act to close the pore. They also noted that the addition of EDTA, which acts as a Ca^{2+} chelator in a similar way to EGTA, led to Cx40 hemichannel opening [27]. Although this study reported the structural hemichannel opening of Cx40, they did not study if the morphological changes observed can translate into functional changes of Cx40 hemichannels. Here we provide experimental evidence that eliminating extracellular Ca^{2+}, Mg^{2+} and a large membrane depolarization may lead to the opening of Cx40 hemichannels in a small fraction of cells (4/33, Fig. 7D), however, this open state may be too small to allow the large fluorescent dye, PI, to pass through.

There is an apparent contradiction in our electrophysiological data (both DCF and substantial membrane depolarization are required to activate the hemichannel current) and the PI-uptake data (DCF at resting membrane potential is sufficient to show PI-uptake via hemichannels). However, it is important to note that there is a key difference in temporal domain between these two hemichannel-mediated processes: hemichannel current is rapid and observable in milliseconds time scale, while the PI-uptake is much slower to develop, requires 15 minutes to reach a saturation level. It is possible that each hemichannel may have two gates (could be those described slow 'loop'-gate on the extracellular end and the fast V_j-gate on the cytosol end of a hemichannel) [28], hemichannel currents could only be recorded when both gates are open, e.g. during depolarized membrane potentials in DCF. While these two gates could be opened sequentially to transfer PI dye at resting membrane potential, but they might rarely open both gates simultaneously to produce hemichannel current. An alternative possibility could be that the hemichannel could be opened at resting membrane potential, but the probability of opening is too low to be recorded during the short ramp protocols. Future systematic studies may help to understand the molecular mechanisms of hemichannel gating of these AF-linked Cx40 mutants.

Specific increases in connexin hemichannel function have been associated with human disease-linked mutations in several connexin genes. For example, two Clouston syndrome-linked Cx30 mutants, G11R and A88V, have been previously reported to increase hemichannel function while maintaining normal gap junction function. Under physiological conditions, both G11R and A88V show increased ATP release via hemichannels compared to wild-type Cx30 [29]. The Cx32 mutation S85C, which is associated with X-linked Charcot-Marie-Tooth (CMTX) disease, has shown large hemichannel-mediated voltage-dependent currents that are not seen with wild-type Cx32 [30]. Another CMTX Cx32 mutation, F235C, also forms leaky hemichannels that contribute to a very severe neuropathy [31]. Leaky hemichannels have also been reported in Cx26 mutations linked to keratitis-ichthyosis-deafness syndrome, G45E [32] and A40V [33]. Both

mutants exhibit normal gap junction function, but A40V has altered extracellular Ca^{2+} regulation leading to a higher hemichannel open probability and G45E shows increased permeability to Ca^{2+} [34]. Finally, three oculodentodigital dysplasia-linked Cx43 mutants, I31M, G138R and G143S, all showed greater than a 2-fold increase in hemichannel activity compared to wild-type Cx43 as demonstrated by an increase in ATP release [35]. It should be noted that the G138R mutant also impaired GJ function in addition to increasing hemichannel activity. Our current study provides the first demonstration of Cx40 mutant hemichannel function, giving us new insights into the etiology of lone AF.

Conclusion

Two germline Cx40 mutations, V85I and L221I, were identified and each was linked to a Chinese family suffering from lone AF. These mutations showed impaired trafficking to the cell surface, but did not significantly impair gap junction function. Wild-type Cx40 did not show any PI-uptake, signifying a likely closed hemichannel under our experimental conditions. Both the Cx40 mutants showed significantly increased PI-uptake and hemichannel current compared to wild-type Cx40, suggesting a gain of hemichannel function. These findings demonstrate the first functional study of Cx40 hemichannels and also describe a novel mechanism by which Cx40 mutants may contribute to the pathogenesis of lone AF.

Acknowledgments

We thank Drs. Weixiong Huang, Xiang-Qun Gong and Silvia Penuela, as well as Ms. Honghong Chen for technical help on some experiments.

Author Contributions

Conceived and designed the experiments: YS MDH DB. Performed the experiments: YS MDH WGY XT. Analyzed the data: YS MDH WGY XT DB. Contributed reagents/materials/analysis tools: YS DB. Wrote the paper: YS MDH DB. Principal investigator for this project: DB.

References

1. Goodenough DA, Goliger JA, Paul DL (1996) Connexins, connexons, and intercellular communication. Annual review of biochemistry 65: 475–502.
2. Kumar NM, Gilula NB (1996) The gap junction communication channel. Cell 84: 381–388.
3. Dale N (2008) Dynamic ATP signalling and neural development. The Journal of physiology 586: 2429–2436.
4. Parpura V, Scemes E, Spray DC (2004) Mechanisms of glutamate release from astrocytes: gap junction "hemichannels", purinergic receptors and exocytotic release. Neurochemistry international 45: 259–264.
5. Bruzzone S, Guida L, Zocchi E, Franco L, De Flora A (2001) Connexin 43 hemi channels mediate Ca2+-regulated transmembrane NAD+ fluxes in intact cells. FASEB journal : official publication of the Federation of American Societies for Experimental Biology 15: 10–12.
6. Cherian PP, Siller-Jackson AJ, Gu S, Wang X, Bonewald LF, et al. (2005) Mechanical strain opens connexin 43 hemichannels in osteocytes: a novel mechanism for the release of prostaglandin. Molecular biology of the cell 16: 3100–3106.
7. Evans WH, De Vuyst E, Leybaert L (2006) The gap junction cellular internet: connexin hemichannels enter the signalling limelight. The Biochemical journal 397: 1–14.
8. Wang N, De Bock M, Decrock E, Bol M, Gadicherla A, et al. (2013) Paracrine signaling through plasma membrane hemichannels. Biochimica et biophysica acta 1828: 35–50.
9. Davis LM, Rodefeld ME, Green K, Beyer EC, Saffitz JE (1995) Gap junction protein phenotypes of the human heart and conduction system. Journal of cardiovascular electrophysiology 6: 813–822.
10. Jansen JA, van Veen TA, de Bakker JM, van Rijen HV (2010) Cardiac connexins and impulse propagation. Journal of molecular and cellular cardiology 48: 76–82.

11. Gollob MH, Jones DL, Krahn AD, Danis L, Gong XQ, et al. (2006) Somatic mutations in the connexin 40 gene (GJA5) in atrial fibrillation. The New England journal of medicine 354: 2677–2688.
12. Sun Y, Yang YQ, Gong XQ, Wang XH, Li RG, et al. (2013) Novel germline GJA5/connexin40 mutations associated with lone atrial fibrillation impair gap junctional intercellular communication. Human mutation 34: 603–609.
13. Yang YQ, Liu X, Zhang XL, Wang XH, Tan HW, et al. (2010) Novel connexin40 missense mutations in patients with familial atrial fibrillation. Europace : European pacing, arrhythmias, and cardiac electrophysiology : journal of the working groups on cardiac pacing, arrhythmias, and cardiac cellular electrophysiology of the European Society of Cardiology 12: 1421–1427.
14. Yang YQ, Zhang XL, Wang XH, Tan HW, Shi HF, et al. (2010) Connexin40 nonsense mutation in familial atrial fibrillation. International journal of molecular medicine 26: 605–610.
15. Sun Y, Tong X, Huang T, Shao Q, Huang W, et al. (2014) An endoplasmic reticulum-retained atrial fibrillation-linked connexin40 mutant impairs atrial gap junction channel function. (online published).
16. Thibodeau IL, Xu J, Li Q, Liu G, Lam K, et al. (2010) Paradigm of genetic mosaicism and lone atrial fibrillation: physiological characterization of a connexin 43-deletion mutant identified from atrial tissue. Circulation 122: 236–244.
17. Thomas T, Telford D, Laird DW (2004) Functional domain mapping and selective trans-dominant effects exhibited by Cx26 disease-causing mutations. The Journal of biological chemistry 279: 19157–19168.
18. Roscoe W, Veitch GI, Gong XQ, Pellegrino E, Bai D, et al. (2005) Oculodentodigital dysplasia-causing connexin43 mutants are non-functional and exhibit dominant effects on wild-type connexin43. J Biol Chem 280: 11458–11466.
19. Contreras JE, Saez JC, Bukauskas FF, Bennett MV (2003) Gating and regulation of connexin 43 (Cx43) hemichannels. Proc Natl Acad Sci U S A 100: 11388–11393.

20. Chaldoupi SM, Loh P, Hauer RN, de Bakker JM, van Rijen HV (2009) The role of connexin40 in atrial fibrillation. Cardiovascular research 84: 15–23.

21. Wakili R, Voigt N, Kaab S, Dobrev D, Nattel S (2011) Recent advances in the molecular pathophysiology of atrial fibrillation. The Journal of clinical investigation 121: 2955–2968.

22. Saffitz JE (2006) Connexins, conduction, and atrial fibrillation. The New England journal of medicine 354: 2712–2714.

23. Rudy Y (2008) Molecular basis of cardiac action potential repolarization. Annals of the New York Academy of Sciences 1123: 113–118.

24. Manias JL, Plante I, Gong XQ, Shao Q, Churko J, et al. (2008) Fate of connexin43 in cardiac tissue harbouring a disease-linked connexin43 mutant. Cardiovascular research 80: 385–395.

25. Dobrowolski R, Sasse P, Schrickel JW, Watkins M, Kim JS, et al. (2008) The conditional connexin43G138R mouse mutant represents a new model of hereditary oculodentodigital dysplasia in humans. Human molecular genetics 17: 539–554.

26. Lai A, Le DN, Paznekas WA, Gifford WD, Jabs EW, et al. (2006) Oculodentodigital dysplasia connexin43 mutations result in non-functional connexin hemichannels and gap junctions in C6 glioma cells. Journal of cell science 119: 532–541.

27. Allen MJ, Gemel J, Beyer EC, Lal R (2011) Atomic force microscopy of Connexin40 gap junction hemichannels reveals calcium-dependent three-dimensional molecular topography and open-closed conformations of both the extracellular and cytoplasmic faces. J Biol Chem 286: 22139–22146.

28. Bukauskas FF, Verselis VK (2004) Gap junction channel gating. Biochim Biophys Acta 1662: 42–60.

29. Essenfelder GM, Bruzzone R, Lamartine J, Charollais A, Blanchet-Bardon C, et al. (2004) Connexin30 mutations responsible for hidrotic ectodermal dysplasia cause abnormal hemichannel activity. Human molecular genetics 13: 1703–1714.

30. Abrams CK, Bennett MV, Verselis VK, Bargiello TA (2002) Voltage opens unopposed gap junction hemichannels formed by a connexin 32 mutant associated with X-linked Charcot-Marie-Tooth disease. Proceedings of the National Academy of Sciences of the United States of America 99: 3980–3984.

31. Liang GS, de Miguel M, Gomez-Hernandez JM, Glass JD, Scherer SS, et al. (2005) Severe neuropathy with leaky connexin32 hemichannels. Annals of neurology 57: 749–754.

32. Stong BC, Chang Q, Ahmad S, Lin X (2006) A novel mechanism for connexin 26 mutation linked deafness: cell death caused by leaky gap junction hemichannels. The Laryngoscope 116: 2205–2210.

33. Gerido DA, DeRosa AM, Richard G, White TW (2007) Aberrant hemichannel properties of Cx26 mutations causing skin disease and deafness. Am J Physiol Cell Physiol 293: C337–345.

34. Sanchez HA, Mese G, Srinivas M, White TW, Verselis VK (2010) Differentially altered Ca2+ regulation and Ca2+ permeability in Cx26 hemichannels formed by the A40V and G45E mutations that cause keratitis ichthyosis deafness syndrome. The Journal of general physiology 136: 47–62.

35. Dobrowolski R, Sommershof A, Willecke K (2007) Some oculodentodigital dysplasia-associated Cx43 mutations cause increased hemichannel activity in addition to deficient gap junction channels. The Journal of membrane biology 219: 9–17.

10

Non-Alcoholic Fatty Liver Disease Is Associated with an Increased Incidence of Atrial Fibrillation in Patients with Type 2 Diabetes

Giovanni Targher[1]*, Filippo Valbusa[2], Stefano Bonapace[3], Lorenzo Bertolini[4], Luciano Zenari[4], Stefano Rodella[5], Giacomo Zoppini[1], William Mantovani[6,7], Enrico Barbieri[3], Christopher D. Byrne[8,9]

1 Division of Endocrinology, Diabetes and Metabolism, Department of Medicine, University and Azienda Ospedaliera Universitaria Integrata of Verona, Verona, Italy, 2 Division of General Medicine, "Sacro Cuore" Hospital of Negrar, Verona, Italy, 3 Division of Cardiology, "Sacro Cuore" Hospital of Negrar, Verona, Italy, 4 Diabetes Unit, "Sacro Cuore" Hospital of Negrar, Verona, Italy, 5 Division of Radiology, "Sacro Cuore" Hospital of Negrar, Verona, Italy, 6 Section of Hygiene and Preventive, Environmental and Occupational Medicine, Department of Public Health and Community Medicine, University of Verona, Verona, Italy, 7 Department of Prevention, Public Health Trust, Trento, Italy, 8 Nutrition and Metabolism, Faculty of Medicine, University of Southampton, Southampton, United Kingdom, 9 Southampton National Institute for Health Research Biomedical Research Centre, University Hospital Southampton, Southampton, United Kingdom

Abstract

Background: The relationship between non-alcoholic fatty liver disease (NAFLD) and atrial fibrillation (AF) in type 2 diabetes is currently unknown. We examined the relationship between NAFLD and risk of incident AF in people with type 2 diabetes.

Methods and Results: We prospectively followed for 10 years a random sample of 400 patients with type 2 diabetes, who were free from AF at baseline. A standard 12-lead electrocardiogram was undertaken annually and a diagnosis of incident AF was confirmed in affected participants by a single cardiologist. At baseline, NAFLD was defined by ultrasonographic detection of hepatic steatosis in the absence of other liver diseases. During the 10 years of follow-up, there were 42 (10.5%) incident AF cases. NAFLD was associated with an increased risk of incident AF (odds ratio [OR] 4.49, 95% CI 1.6–12.9, $p < 0.005$). Adjustments for age, sex, hypertension and electrocardiographic features (left ventricular hypertrophy and PR interval) did not attenuate the association between NAFLD and incident AF (adjusted-OR 6.38, 95% CI 1.7–24.2, $p = 0.005$). Further adjustment for variables that were included in the 10-year Framingham Heart Study-derived AF risk score did not appreciably weaken this association. Other independent predictors of AF were older age, longer PR interval and left ventricular hypertrophy.

Conclusions: Our results indicate that ultrasound-diagnosed NAFLD is strongly associated with an increased incidence of AF in patients with type 2 diabetes even after adjustment for important clinical risk factors for AF.

Editor: Melania Manco, Scientific Directorate, Bambino Hospital, Italy

Funding: The authors have no support or funding to report.

Competing Interests: The authors have declared that no competing interests exist.

* E-mail: giovanni.targher@univr.it

Introduction

Non-alcoholic fatty liver disease (NAFLD) has reached epidemic proportions and is the most common cause of chronic liver disease in clinical practice [1,2]. The prevalence of NAFLD has been estimated to be in the 20 to 35% range in the general adult population in Western countries and is almost certainly increasing [1,2]. Compared with nondiabetic subjects, patients with type 2 diabetes seem to be at increased risk for developing NAFLD and certainly have a higher risk for developing advanced fibrosis and cirrhosis. It has been estimated that approximately 60 to 70% of persons with type 2 diabetes have some form of NAFLD [1–3].

To date, growing clinical evidence indicates that NAFLD is linked to an increased risk of cardiovascular disease (CVD) both in patients without diabetes and in those with type 2 diabetes [3,4]. Recent studies also suggest that NAFLD is associated with early left ventricular (LV) diastolic dysfunction, independently of

hypertension and other cardiometabolic risk factors [5–7]. More recently, two large community-based cohort studies that used serum levels of gamma-glutamyltransferase (GGT) to diagnose NAFLD have shown that this disease is associated with an increased incidence of heart failure, independently of several established risk factors [8,9].

In parallel, it is well recognized that atrial fibrillation (AF) is the most common sustained arrhythmia and its prevalence is expected to rise substantially over the next few decades because of ageing population and improvements in cardiovascular treatments [10,11]. The prevalence of AF increases from about 1% in individuals less than 55 years of age to about 10–12% in those older than 80 years of age [10]. Along with older age, many pathologic conditions such as obesity, hypertension, coronary heart disease, heart failure and valvular heart disease have been reported to be among the strongest risk factors for new-onset AF

[12–14], which is a disease associated with high rates of hospitalisation and death [10,15].

Thus, although NAFLD correlates with abnormalities in cardiac structure and function and shares with AF multiple cardiometabolic risk factors, there is currently a lack of available information on the relationship between NAFLD and AF in people with type 2 diabetes, a group of individuals in which these two diseases are highly prevalent. Very recently, the Framingham Heart Study investigators have reported an independent association between mildly elevated serum transaminase concentrations, a surrogate marker of NAFLD, and increased risk of new-onset AF in the community [16].

The aim of this study was to test the hypothesis that NAFLD as diagnosed by ultrasonography (the most widely used imaging test for diagnosing hepatic steatosis) predicts subsequent development of incident AF in people with type 2 diabetes.

Materials and Methods

Participants

In this exploratory analysis, we followed for 10 years a sample of 400 patients with type 2 diabetes, who were clinically free from AF at baseline. As detailed in Figure 1, these participants were selected by a simple random sampling technique (using a random number generator) from the whole cohort ($n = 1,718$) of outpatients with type 2 diabetes attending the diabetes clinic at the 'Sacro Cuore' Hospital of Negrar (Verona) during 2000–2001, after excluding subjects who did not meet the inclusion criteria for the study. In particular, we excluded (1) patients who had a history of AF or atrial flutter, (2) those who were taking any anti-arrhythmic drugs, (3) those who had a history of previous moderate-to-severe aortic and mitral valvular disease, hyperthyroidism, malignancy and end-stage renal disease, (4) those who had known causes of chronic liver disease (i.e., alcohol-induced or drug-induced liver disease, viral hepatitis, hemochromatosis or other known causes of liver diseases), and (5) those with missing liver ultrasound or laboratory data.

The sample size of this study was calculated with the specific aim of constructing a confidence interval around the incidence proportion of AF in patients with analogous characteristics. In a similar patient cohort the proportion with AF has been estimated to be approximately 7% [14]. Therefore, with a precision of 2.5% and a confidence interval of 95%, we calculated that a sample size of 400 patients would be needed, taking also into account a cumulative proportion of losses to follow-up of 20%. Thus, a sample size of 400 patients from a population of 1,718 patients produces a 95% confidence interval equal to the population proportion, plus or minus 2.5%, when the estimated proportion of patients with AF is 7% and the expected cumulative proportion of losses to follow-up is 20%. As specified in the Results section (1st paragraph), the random sampling procedure allowed us to select a sample of 400 patients that was well representative of the 1,718 type 2 diabetic patients initially eligible.

All participants were periodically seen at the diabetes clinic (every 6–12 months) for medical examinations of glycemic control, chronic diabetic complications and routine 12-lead electrocardiograms (ECG). The ascertainment at the end of the follow-up period (January 2011) for the whole sample was 100%.

The local ethics committee of the 'Sacro Cuore' Hospital of Negrar approved the study and all participants gave their written informed consent for participation in this medical research.

Clinical and Laboratory Data

BMI was calculated by dividing weight in kilograms by the square of height in meters. Blood pressure was measured in duplicate by a physician with a mercury sphygmomanometer (at the right upper arm using an appropriate cuff size) after patient had been seated quietly for at least 5 minutes. Subjects were considered to have hypertension if their blood pressure was ≥140/90 mmHg or if they were taking any anti-hypertensive drugs. Information on medical history, alcohol consumption, smoking and use of medications was obtained from all patients by interviews during medical examinations.

Venous blood was drawn in the morning after an overnight fast. Serum liver enzymes, lipids and other biochemical blood measurements were determined by standard laboratory procedures (DAX 96; Bayer Diagnostics, Milan, Italy). Most participants (92% of total) had serum liver enzyme levels within the reference ranges in our laboratory. No participants had seropositivity for viral hepatitis B and C. LDL-cholesterol was calculated by the Friedewald's equation. HbA1c was measured by an automated high-performance liquid chromatography analyzer (HA-8140; Menarini Diagnostics, Florence, Italy); the upper limit of normal for our laboratory was 5.8%. Albuminuria was measured by an immuno-nephelometric method on a morning spot urine sample and expressed as the albumin-to-creatinine ratio.

At baseline, the diagnosis of left ventricular hypertrophy (LVH) was made by a single cardiologist on the basis of a resting 12-lead ECG according to Sokolow-Lyon's voltage criteria (SV1+RV5 or RV6≥3.5 mV) and/or Cornell's voltage criteria (SV3+RaVL >2.0 mV in women and >2.8 mV in men, respectively) [17]. In all participants the electrocardiographic PR interval was also recorded. Coronary heart disease (CHD) was defined as a documented history of myocardial infarction, angina, coronary artery bypass grafts, percutaneous trans-luminal coronary angioplasty or typical ECG abnormalities (according to the Minnesota code). The history of previous congestive heart failure and mild valvular heart disease were confirmed by reviewing medical records of the hospital, including diagnostic symptoms patterns, echocardiograms and results of other laboratory exams. Chronic kidney disease (CKD) was defined as the presence of abnormal albuminuria (urine albumin-to-creatinine ratio ≥30 mg/g) and/or glomerular filtration rate <60 ml/min/1.73 m^2 as estimated by the four-variable Modification of Diet in Renal Disease (MDRD) study equation [18].

Liver and Carotid Ultrasonography

At baseline, hepatic ultrasonography was performed in all patients by a single experienced radiologist, who was blinded to the participants' details. Hepatic steatosis was diagnosed on the basis of characteristic sonographic features, i.e., evidence of diffuse hyper-echogenicity of the liver relative to the kidneys, ultrasound beam attenuation and poor visualization of intra-hepatic vessel borders and diaphragm [19]. It is known that ultrasonography has good sensitivity and specificity for detecting moderate and severe hepatic steatosis (~90–95%), but its sensitivity is reduced when the hepatic fat infiltration upon liver biopsy is <33% [19]. Semi-quantitative sonographic scoring for the degree of hepatic steatosis (mild, moderate or severe) was not available in this study. Grading of hepatic fat content using ultrasonography has been used in previous studies but remains somewhat subjective [19].

The presence of atherosclerotic plaques (i.e., stenosis of 30% or more) at the level of either internal or common carotid arteries was diagnosed by echo-Doppler scanning, which was

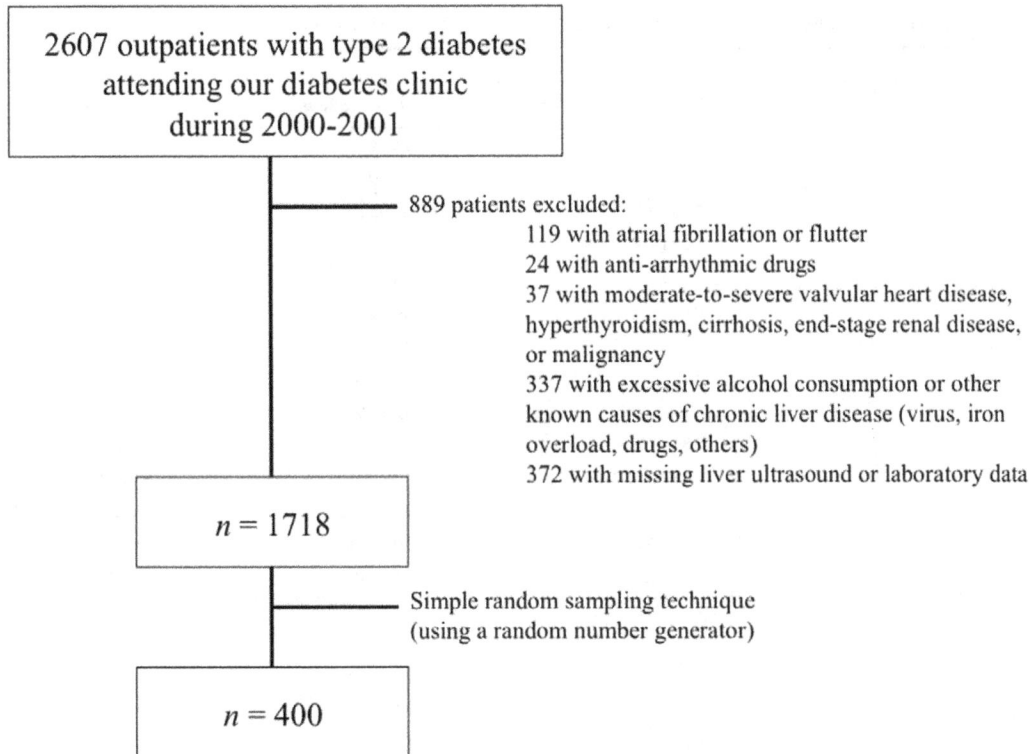

Figure 1. Details of the study design.

performed by a single specialist physician, who was blind to subjects' characteristics.

Diagnosis of Incident Atrial Fibrillation

At baseline, all participants were free from AF as documented by a standard 12-lead ECG. A 24-hour Holter monitor examination was not routinely performed either at baseline or during the follow-up period. During the follow-up, participants were diagnosed with AF if AF or atrial flutter was present on a standard ECG that was obtained either from a routine clinic examination in our diabetes clinic (i.e., a 12-lead resting ECG was performed annually in all participants) or from reviewing hospital and physician charts from all participants. The diagnosis of AF was confirmed in affected participants by an experienced cardiologist, who was blinded to clinical characteristics of participants, including NAFLD status.

Statistical Analysis

Data are expressed as means ± SD, medians (interquartile range) or percentages. Skewed variables (serum liver enzymes, triglycerides and diabetes duration) were transformed using natural logarithmic transformation to improve normality prior to analysis. The unpaired-t test (for continuous variables) and the chi-squared test or the Fisher's exact test when appropriate (for categorical variables) were used to analyze the differences among the characteristics of the participants at the time of enrollment in relation to their status of either future development of AF (Table 1) or presence of NAFLD at baseline (Table 2). Binary logistic regression analysis was used to study the association between NAFLD and incident AF (Table 3). We preferred to perform a logistic regression analysis instead of a time-dependent Cox regression analysis since in presence of a small number of events

a time-to-event type of analysis, such as Cox regression, is more susceptible to bias than binary logistic regression analysis when adjusted for predictor variables since there is the potential for a marked difference in time to event in the exposed versus the unexposed group. In addition, since the precise time to event (AF) may not be known in some people with asymptomatic AF (e.g. in those with slow AF), we undertook logistic regression analysis. Nevertheless, our results remained essentially unchanged when we used either Cox regression analysis or robust Poisson regression analysis. Compared with logistic regression analysis, both of these time-dependent regression analyses yielded similar estimates of regression coefficients for the association between NAFLD and risk of AF (data not shown). For prediction of incident AF, men and women were combined and first-order interaction terms for sex-by-NAFLD interactions on risk for AF were examined. Because the interactions were not statistically significant ($p = 0.38$), a sex-pooled multivariable logistic regression analysis was used. Four forced-entry regression models were performed: an unadjusted model; a model adjusted for age and sex (model 1); a model further adjusted for hypertension (blood pressure $\geq 140/90$ mmHg or treatment), and electrocardiographic LVH and PR interval (model 2); and, finally, a regression model (model 3) adjusted for variables included in the 10-year Framingham Heart Study-derived AF risk score (i.e. age, sex, BMI, systolic BP, hypertension treatment, electrocardiographic PR interval and history of heart failure) [20]. As sensitivity analyses, we restricted our association analysis between NAFLD and incident AF to patients at the baseline examination who did not have a documented history of ischemic heart disease and heart failure ($n = 353$). A Kaplan-Meier analysis of incidence curves for AF during 10 years of follow-up was undertaken; in patients with, and without NAFLD at baseline. Differences between groups was tested by the log-rank test.

Table 1. Baseline clinical characteristics of participants stratified by atrial fibrillation (AF) status at follow-up.

	No AF at follow-up	AF at follow-up	p value
Sex (male/female, n)	211/147	24/18	0.85
Age (years)	63±9	69±9	<0.001
BMI (kg/m²)	29.6±4.7	30.0±5.1	0.54
Diabetes duration (years)	5.0 (1–17)	9.0 (1–24)	<0.01
Systolic BP (mmHg)	139±15	147±15	<0.001
Diastolic BP (mmHg)	81±7	80±8	0.81
Pulse pressure (mmHg)	58±12	67±13	<0.001
Hemoglobin A1c (%)	7.7±1.6	7.7±1.7	0.92
HDL-cholesterol (mmol/L)	1.24±0.3	1.32±0.3	0.16
LDL-cholesterol (mmol/L)	2.84±1.3	2.81±1.3	0.82
Triglycerides (mmol/L)	1.45 (0.41–2.49)	1.41 (0.52–2.42)	0.20
ALT (U/L)	24 (5–39)	27 (8–44)	0.56
GGT (U/L)	29 (6–53)	39 (7–90)	<0.05
PR interval (msec)	166±23	210±36	<0.001
Current smokers (%)	21	17	0.45
History of coronary heart disease (%)	9	10	0.98
History of mild valvular disease (%)	1	2	0.38
History of congestive heart failure (%)	1	10	<0.001
Hypertension (%)	68	90	<0.01
Electrocardiographic LVH (%)	21	52	<0.001
Carotid artery stenoses ≥30% (%)	50	81	<0.005
Chronic kidney disease (%)	24	36	0.10
ACE-inhibitors or sartans (%)	61	71	0.18
Calcium channel blockers (%)	22	31	0.20
Alpha blockers (%)	5	12	0.08
Beta blockers (%)	12	14	0.70
Diuretics (%)	26	41	<0.05
Anti-platelet drugs (%)	62	76	0.28
Lipid-lowering drugs (%)	27	19	0.23
Oral hypoglycemic drugs (%)	71	69	0.67
Insulin therapy (%)	20	26	0.33
NAFLD (%)	68	90	<0.001

Sample size, n = 400. Data are means ± SD, medians (interquartile range) or percentages. Differences between the groups were tested by the unpaired-t test (for continuous variables), the chi-squared or the Fisher's exact test (for categorical variables) when appropriate.
ALT, alanine aminotransferase; GGT, gamma-glutamyl-transferase; LVH, left ventricular hypertrophy; NAFLD, non-alcoholic fatty liver disease.
Hypertension was defined as blood pressure ≥140/90 mmHg and/or treatment. Electrocardiographic LVH was diagnosed according to Sokolow-Lyon and/or Cornell's voltage criteria.

All analyses were performed using statistical package SPSS 19.0 and statistical significance was assessed at the two-tailed 0.05 threshold.

Results

Overall, the 400 randomly selected participants did not significantly differ from the initially eligible sample of 1,718 type 2 diabetic patients in terms of baseline demographics (age: 64±10 vs. 66±4 years; male sex: 58.7 vs. 60.5%; duration of diabetes: 6±7 vs. 8±4 years), HbA1c (7.6±1.6 vs. 7.4±1.0%), documented history of CHD (9.3 vs. 10.6%) and heart failure (2 vs. 3.5%), proportion of obesity (43.9 vs. 46.7%), hypertension (70 vs. 73.6%) and NAFLD on ultrasound (70.2 vs. 72.4%).

Of the 400 participants included in the study, 281 (70.2%) patients met the clinical criteria for diagnosis of NAFLD (i.e., hepatic steatosis on ultrasound among persons who drank less than 20 g/day of alcohol, and who did not have viral hepatitis, drug-induced liver disease, iron overload or other secondary causes of liver disease) and 119 (29.8%) patients did not.

During the 10 years of follow-up, 42 patients developed incident AF (i.e., cumulative incidence of 10.5%). The baseline characteristics of participants stratified by AF status at follow-up are displayed in Table 1. At baseline, patients who developed AF at follow-up were older, had longer duration of diabetes, longer electrocardiographic PR interval, and greater frequencies of hypertension, electrocardiographic LVH and carotid artery stenoses ≥30% than those who did not. Patients who developed

Table 2. Baseline clinical characteristics of participants stratified by NAFLD status at baseline.

	Without NAFLD	With NAFLD	p value
Sex (male/female, n)	68/51	167/114	0.73
Age (years)	64±9	63±9	0.28
BMI (kg/m²)	27.1±4.4	30.7±4.5	<0.001
Diabetes duration (years)	7.0 (1–10)	5.0 (1–13)	0.68
Systolic BP (mmHg)	138±14	141±15	<0.05
Diastolic BP (mmHg)	80±7	81±7	0.28
Pulse pressure (mmHg)	57±12	60±13	<0.05
Hemoglobin A1c (%)	7.6±1.6	7.8±1.6	0.42
HDL-cholesterol (mmol/L)	1.30±0.3	1.24±0.3	<0.05
LDL-cholesterol (mmol/L)	2.88±1.3	3.02±1.3	0.43
Triglycerides (mmol/L)	1.26 (0.96–1.81)	1.56 (1.14–2.22)	<0.001
ALT (U/L)	22 (16–31)	30 (24–41)	<0.05
GGT (U/L)	28 (20–43)	33 (25–50)	<0.05
PR interval (msec)	161±25	173±29	<0.01
Current smokers (%)	17	22	0.07
History of coronary heart disease (%)	9	9	0.95
History of mild valvular disease (%)	1	1	0.95
History of congestive heart failure (%)	1	3	0.50
Hypertension (%)	65	73	<0.05
Electrocardiographic LVH (%)	23	25	0.86
Carotid artery stenoses ≥30% (%)	54	55	0.93
Chronic kidney disease (%)	19	23	0.06
ACE-inhibitors or sartans (%)	54	66	<0.05
Calcium channel blockers (%)	27	27	0.98
Alpha blockers (%)	5	7	0.91
Beta blockers (%)	19	12	0.12
Diuretics (%)	33	31	0.79
Anti-platelet drugs (%)	66	61	0.27
Lipid-lowering drugs (%)	27	27	0.97
Oral hypoglycemic drugs (%)	63	74	<0.05
Insulin therapy (%)	22	20	0.48

Sample size, n = 400. Data are means ± SD, medians (interquartile range) or percentages.

AF at follow-up were also more likely to have a documented history of heart failure and had higher values of systolic BP and pulse pressure. Notably, 90% of patients who developed AF at follow-up had NAFLD on ultrasound at baseline. Patients who developed AF also had higher serum GGT levels, although the vast majority of patients (~90%) had baseline serum ALT and GGT levels within the laboratory reference ranges. Sex, BMI, smoking, serum lipids, HbA1c, CKD, history of previous CHD and mild valvular heart disease, and use of ACE-inhibitors, angiotensin receptor antagonists, beta blockers, lipid-lowering, anti-platelet and hypoglycemic drugs did not significantly differ between the groups.

As expected, when the study participants were grouped according to their NAFLD status at baseline (Table 2), patients with NAFLD were more likely to be obese, to be hypertensive, and had higher systolic BP, higher pulse pressure, higher plasma triglycerides and lower HDL-cholesterol than those without NAFLD. They also were more frequently treated with oral hypoglycemic drugs and ACE-inhibitors or angiotensin receptor antagonists and had higher serum liver enzyme levels, although the vast majority of patients with NAFLD had normal serum ALT and GGT levels.

Notably, as shown in Figure 2, there was also a marked difference in the overall cumulative incidence of AF in patients with NAFLD compared with those without NAFLD ($p<0.001$).

Figure 3 shows a Kaplan-Meier analysis of incidence curves for AF during 10 years of follow-up in patients with and without NAFLD at baseline. The difference between the two groups was statistically significant and the incidence of AF increased markedly after 6 years of follow-up ($p<0.005$ by the log-rank test).

Table 3 shows the effect of the adjustment for known risk factors on the relationship between NAFLD and risk of incident AF. In univariate analysis (unadjusted model), NAFLD was significantly associated with an increased risk of incident AF. After adjustment for age and sex (model 1), NAFLD maintained a significant association with risk of incident AF. Importantly, the strength of the association between NAFLD and incident AF was not attenuated after additional adjustment for hypertension and electrocardiographic features, i.e. LVH and PR interval (model 2). Notably, in this regression model, other independent predictors of incident AF were older age, LVH and longer PR interval (Table 3). As also shown in Table 3, in a less parsimonious regression model (model 3), the adjustment for variables that were included in the 10-year Framingham Heart Study-derived AF risk score did not appreciably weaken the association between NAFLD and incident AF. However, given the relatively small number of events, the results of this latter regression model should be interpreted with some caution.

Notably, the significant association between NAFLD and increased risk of incident AF remained essentially unchanged even after excluding those ($n=47$) with documented history of CHD and heart failure: unadjusted model (OR 4.03, 95% CI 1.4–11.6, $p<0.01$), adjusted model 1 (adjusted-OR 4.83, 95% CI 1.6–14.5, $p<0.01$), model 2 (adjusted-OR 4.05, 95% CI 1.1–15.3, $p<0.05$) and model 3 (adjusted-OR 3.78, 95% CI 1.1–13.2, $p<0.05$), respectively.

We also conducted other sensitivity analyses to evaluate the robustness of our findings (p values for interaction >0.15 in all subgroups analyses). Almost identical results were found when the results were stratified by sex (OR 2.98, 95% CI 1.1–12.2, for women, and OR 10.4, 95% CI 1.4–80 for men, respectively); by age (OR 8.62, 95% CI 1.1–65 for those aged ≤70 years, and OR 3.94, 95% CI 1.1–14.5 for those older than 70 years of age); by status of electrocardiographic PR interval (OR 3.43, 95% CI 1.1–14.6 for those with PR interval <200 msec, and OR 6.01, 95% CI 1.2–29.7 for those with PR interval ≥200 msec); and by electrocardiographic LVH status (OR 5.31, 95% CI 1.2–25.0 for those without LVH, and OR 4.23, 95% CI 1.02–18.2 for those with LVH, respectively).

Discussion

NAFLD and AF are two pathologic conditions that are highly prevalent in Western countries and that share multiple cardiometabolic risk factors. Presently, the published research on the association between AF and NAFLD (or liver function tests) is

Table 3. Logistic regression models for NAFLD as a predictor for development of AF in patients with type 2 diabetes.

Logistic Regression Models	Odds Ratios (95% CI)	p value
NAFLD (yes *vs.* no)		
unadjusted model	4.49 (1.6–12.9)	<0.005
adjusted model 1	5.40 (1.8–15.9)	<0.005
adjusted model 2	6.38 (1.7–24.2)	=0.005
adjusted model 3	4.96 (1.4–17.0)	=0.01
Other independent predictors of incident AF in regression model 2		
Age (years)	1.06 (1.01–1.12)	<0.01
Electrocardiographic PR interval (msec)	1.05 (1.03–1.06)	<0.001
Electrocardiographic LVH (yes *vs.* no)	4.29 (1.8–10.4)	<0.001

Sample size, n = 400. Data are expressed as odds ratios ±95% confidence intervals as assessed by univariable (unadjusted) or multivariable logistic regression analyses. Other covariates included in multivariable logistic regression models were as follows: **model 1:** age and sex; **model 2:** age, sex, hypertension (blood pressure ≥140/90 mmHg or treatment), electrocardiographic PR interval and LVH; **model 3:** adjustment for variables included in the 10-year Framingham Heart Study-derived AF risk score (i.e. age, sex, BMI, systolic BP, hypertension treatment, electrocardiographic PR interval and history of heart failure).

sparse. In a large retrospective cohort study, it has been reported that the prevalence of ALT elevations (i.e. defined as serum ALT >40 U/L), as surrogate markers of NAFLD, among a routine clinical care population with AF was high (i.e. 27.6%), although the incidence of new persistent and significant ALT elevations was uncommon [21]. More interestingly, the Framingham Heart Study investigators have recently shown that moderately elevated serum ALT or AST levels (>40 U/L for either marker) were independently associated with an increased incidence of AF over a 8-year follow-up period in a community-based cohort of 3,744 adults, who were free of clinical heart failure at baseline [16].

To our knowledge, this is the first prospective study to examine the role of NAFLD as detected by ultrasonography (which is a more accurate measure of liver fat than serum transaminase levels) in predicting development of incident AF in patients with type 2 diabetes, who were clinically free from AF at baseline. The major finding of our study was that NAFLD was significantly associated with an increased risk of incident AF during a follow-up period of 10 years. Notably, and more importantly, this association was independent of numerous clinical risk factors for AF.

In accordance with previously published reports, we found that older age, LVH and longer PR interval on ECG (i.e. a measure of left atrial size) were strong predictors of incident AF [12–14,22,23]. It is well known that LVH causes LV dysfunction and left atrial enlargement, which may lead to fibrosis and electrical remodelling of the atrium, providing a pathophysiological substrate for subsequent development of AF [10,24]. Recently, the Framingham Heart Study investigators published a clinical risk score for development of AF in 10 years that incorporated the presence of age, sex, BMI, systolic BP, hypertension treatment, longer PR interval and history of heart failure [20]. Similarly, the Atherosclerosis Risk in Communities study showed that a 10-year clinical risk score incorporating age, race, smoking, systolic BP, hypertension treatment, electrocardiographic LVH, electrocardiographic left atrial enlargement, diabetes, CHD and heart failure was predictive for development of AF in a multi-ethnic, community-based cohort of individuals [25].

Although there are few data on cardiac function among patients with NAFLD, preliminary evidence indicates that there is a strong relationship between NAFLD and early LV diastolic dysfunction in both non-diabetic and type 2 diabetic individuals [5–7]. It is likely that LV diastolic dysfunction plays a role in AF pathogenesis either by increasing pressure that can affect stretch receptors in pulmonary veins triggers and other areas of the atria or by inducing direct structural changes in atrial myocardium [10,24]. Interestingly, two large population-based studies have also shown that moderately elevated serum GGT levels, as surrogate markers of NAFLD, are independently associated with an increased risk of incident heart failure [8,9]. Collectively, as reported above, our findings confirm and extend to patients with type 2 diabetes, using

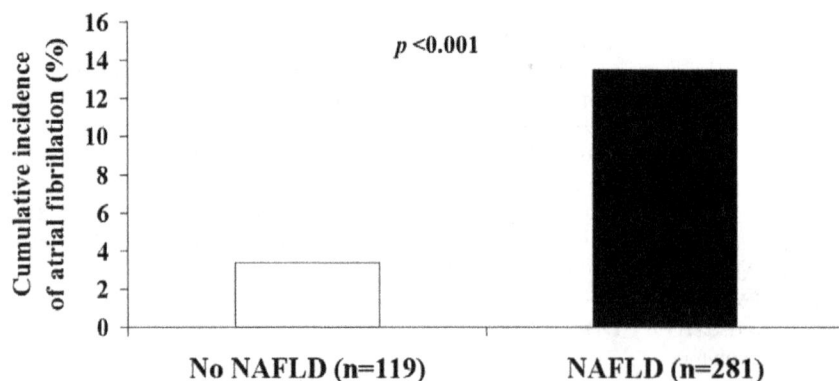

Figure 2. Cumulative incidence rates of atrial fibrillation by NAFLD status.

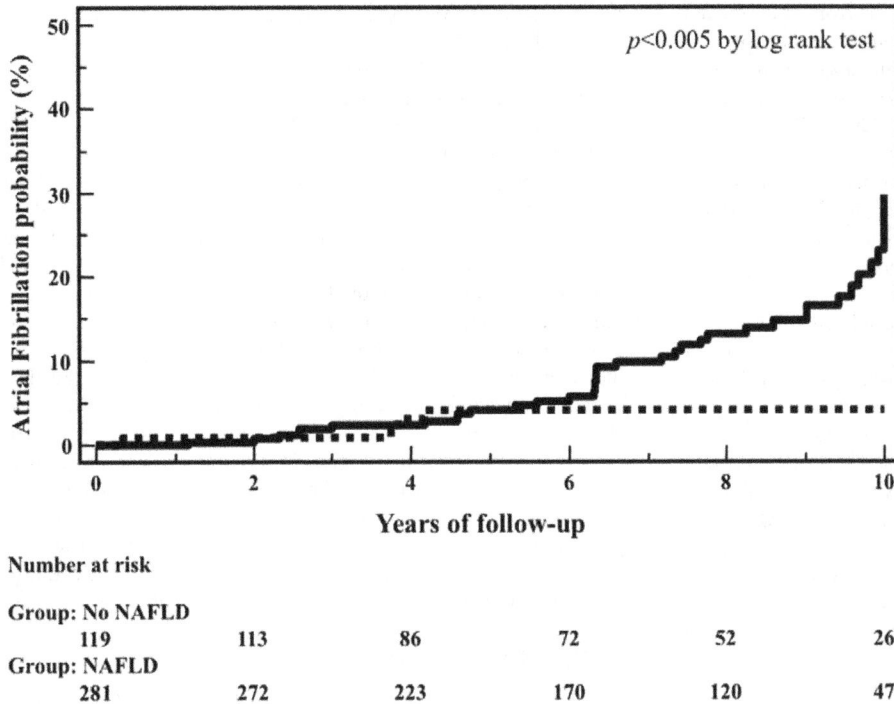

Figure 3. Incidence curves for atrial fibrillation during follow-up, in patients with (solid line) and without (dotted line) NAFLD at baseline.

liver ultrasound for diagnosing NAFLD, the recent results reported by Sinner *et al.* [16] demonstrating that NAFLD (as detected by serum transaminase levels) is an independent predictor of new-onset AF in the adult general population.

The underlying mechanisms responsible for the association between NAFLD and increased risk of incident AF require further study. Speculatively, they could include some of the following. Firstly, the association between NAFLD and incident AF is simply a consequence of the shared risk factors and comorbid conditions. However, it is important to underline that in our study NAFLD was associated with an increased risk of incident AF, independently of age, sex, hypertension, electrocardiographic LVH and other clinical risk factors included in the 10-year Framingham Heart Study-derived AF risk score. The odds ratio was not attenuated after adjustment for these potential confounders, thus suggesting that the increased risk of incident AF associated with NAFLD, cannot be fully explained by these shared AF risk factors. Again, the increased risk of AF associated with NAFLD also remained, even after excluding participants with a documented history of previous CHD and heart failure. Secondly, it could be postulated that NAFLD is a marker of ectopic fat accumulation in other tissues, including both the myocardium and pericardium. Rijzewijk *et al.* [26] and Ng *et al.* [27] showed that the intra-myocardial fat content, as detected by proton magnetic resonance spectroscopy, was greater in patients with type 2 diabetes than in nondiabetic controls, and was associated with LV diastolic dysfunction. Interestingly, in the study by Rijzewijk *et al.* [26] there was also a significant, positive association between intra-myocardial and intra-hepatic fat content. Recently, it has been also reported that increased pericardial fat volume was associated with both increased left atrial dimensions [28] and increased prevalence of AF [29], independently of multiple established risk factors. Moreover, Shin *et al.* reported that total and inter-atrial epicardial adipose tissues were larger in AF patients than in

matched controls and were independently associated with left atrial remodeling among patients with AF [30]. Preliminary experimental evidence suggests that adipocytes from epicardial or retro-sternal adipose tissues could directly modulate the electro-physiological properties and ion currents, causing higher arrhyth-mogenesis, in isolated rabbit left atrial myocytes [31]. Thirdly, because in our study NAFLD was associated with increased AF incidence, independently of multiple potential confounders, it is also possible to speculate that NAFLD is not only associated with the risk of AF as the consequence of the shared risk factors but that NAFLD *per se* might partly contribute to the development and persistence of AF. This process might occur through the systemic release of pathogenic mediators from the steatotic and inflamed liver, including C-reactive protein, interleukin-6, tumor necrosis factor-alpha, plasminogen activator inhibitor-1 and other inflam-matory cytokines. Importantly, several studies have shown that these pathogenic mediators are remarkably higher in patients with NAFLD than in those without [6,7,32], and may play a role in the development and persistence of AF, possibly by inducing structural and/or electrical remodeling of the atria [33–36]. These pathways may represent a novel pathogenic mechanism by which structural changes resulting from chronic inflammation can perpetuate AF. These findings require further testing and confirmation in larger clinical trials. Nevertheless, these pathways might provide a potential target for pharmacological interruption or reversal of atrial structural remodeling [33–36].

Our study has some important limitations. First, our cohort comprised of type 2 diabetic patients of European extraction, so that the results cannot be generalized directly to other ethnic groups. Second, there were a relatively small number of clinical events during the follow-up and, therefore, the results should be interpreted with some caution. Third, the diagnosis of NAFLD was based on ultrasonography that is relatively insensitive to the presence of smaller amounts of hepatic steatosis (<33% liver fat infiltration) and that cannot distinguish NASH from other forms of NAFLD (although, that said, the overall sensitivity and specificity of ultrasonography for detecting moderate and severe hepatic steatosis are ~85% and ~95% respectively, when compared to liver biopsy as a gold-standard) [19]. Although some non-differential misclassification of NAFLD on the basis of ultrasonography is likely (i.e., some of the control patients with diabetes could have mild hepatic steatosis and undetected NAFLD, despite normal serum liver enzymes and a negative ultrasonography examination); this limitation would serve to attenuate the magnitude of our effect measures towards the null. Thus, we reason that our results can probably be considered a conservative estimate of the relationship between NAFLD and increased AF incidence. Since hepatic ultrasonography was assessed at baseline only, we could not investigate the relationship of changes (development or resolution) in hepatic steatosis over time to incident AF risk. Fourth, the diagnosis of LVH was based on widely accepted ECG criteria (that have a very high specificity but a relatively low sensitivity when compared with echocardiographic findings) [17]. Unfortunately, no echocardiographic measurements were available in this study. However, our data have been also adjusted for systolic BP and hypertension treatment, which are likely to capture almost all patients with LVH not detected by classical ECG voltage criteria. In addition, it is important to recognise that the additional incorporation of echocardiographic measurements only slightly improved the predictive ability of the 10-year Framingham Heart Study-derived risk score for the development of AF [20]. Finally, we cannot exclude residual confounding.

Notwithstanding these limitations, our study has important strengths, including its prospective design, the long duration of follow-up (10 years), the relatively large number of participants of both sexes, the diagnosis of hepatic steatosis by ultrasonography (which was performed in all patients by a single experienced radiologist), the complete nature of the dataset, and the ability to adjust for baseline AF risk factors included in the 10-year Framingham risk prediction model [20].

In conclusion, our study is the first to demonstrate that ultrasound-diagnosed NAFLD is closely associated with an increased incidence of AF in patients with type 2 diabetes, independently of important clinical risk factors for AF. Further studies are needed to confirm this finding in other populations, to elucidate the responsible mechanisms for this association, and to explore whether pharmacological interventions aimed at improving NAFLD effectively reduce the incidence of AF in patients with type 2 diabetes. In the interim, from the perspective of clinical practice, it is important that specialists and practicing clinicians be aware of the link between NAFLD and AF, especially because of the high and growing prevalence of these two pathologies.

Author Contributions

Conceived and designed the experiments: GT FV SB GZ CDB. Performed the experiments: GT FV SB LB LZ SR WM EB. Analyzed the data: GT WM GZ CDB. Wrote the paper: GT GZ CDB.

References

1. Ratziu V, Bellentani S, Cortez-Pinto H, Day C, Marchesini G (2010) A position statement on NAFLD/NASH based on the EASL 2009 special conference. J Hepatol 53: 372–384.

2. Chalasani N, Younossi Z, Lavine JE, Diehl AM, Brunt EM, et al. (2012) The diagnosis and management of non-alcoholic fatty liver disease: practice Guideline by the American Association for the Study of Liver Diseases, American College of Gastroenterology, and the American Gastroenterological Association. Hepatology 55: 2005–2023.

3. Targher G, Day CP, Bonora E (2010) Risk of cardiovascular disease in patients with nonalcoholic fatty liver disease. N Engl J Med 363: 1341–1350.

4. Bhatia LS, Curzen NP, Calder PC, Byrne CD (2012) Non-alcoholic fatty liver disease: a new and important cardiovascular risk factor? Eur Heart J 33: 1190–1200.

5. Goland S, Shimoni S, Zornitzki T, Knobler H, Azoulai O, et al. (2006) Cardiac abnormalities as a new manifestation of nonalcoholic fatty liver disease: echocardiographic and tissue Doppler imaging assessment. J Clin Gastroenterol 40: 949–955.

6. Bonapace S, Perseghin G, Molon G, Canali G, Bertolini L, et al. (2012) Nonalcoholic fatty liver disease is associated with left ventricular diastolic dysfunction in patients with type 2 diabetes. Diabetes Care 35: 389–395.

7. Hallsworth K, Hollingsworth KG, Thoma C, Jakovljevic D, Macgowan GA, et al. (2012) Cardiac structure and function are altered in adults with non-alcoholic fatty liver disease. J Hepatol doi: 10.1016/j.jhep.2012.11.015 [Epub ahead of print].

8. Dhingra R, Gona P, Wang TJ, Fox CS, D'Agostino RB, et al. (2010) Serum gamma-glutamyl-transferase and risk of heart failure in the community. Arterioscler Thromb Vasc Biol 30: 1855–1860.

9. Wannamethee SG, Whincup PH, Shaper AG, Lennon L, Sattar N (2012) Gamma-glutamyltransferase, hepatic enzymes and risk of incident heart failure in older men. Arterioscler Thromb Vasc Biol 32: 830–835.

10. Lip GY, Tse HF, Lane DA (2012) Atrial fibrillation. Lancet 379: 648–661.

11. Miyasaka Y, Barnes ME, Gersh BJ, Cha SS, Bailey KR, et al. (2006) Secular trends in incidence of atrial fibrillation in Olmsted Country, Minnesota, 1980 to 2000, and implications on the projections for future prevalence. Circulation 114: 119–125.

12. Benjamin EJ, Levy D, Vaziri SM, D'Agostino RB, Belanger AJ, et al. (1994) Independent risk factors for atrial fibrillation in a population-based cohort: the Framingham Heart Study. JAMA 271: 840–844.

13. Psaty BM, Manolio TA, Kuller LH, Kronmal LA, Cushman M, et al. (1997) Incidence of and risk factors for atrial fibrillation in older adults. Circulation 96: 2455–2461.

14. Nichols GA, Reinier K, Chugh SS (2009) Independent contribution of diabetes to increased prevalence and incidence of atrial fibrillation. Diabetes Care 32: 1851–1856.

15. Jabre P, Roger VL, Murad MH, Chamberlain AM, Prokop L, et al. (2011) Mortality associated with atrial fibrillation in patients with myocardial infarction: a systematic review and meta-analysis. Circulation 123: 1587–1593.

16. Sinner MF, Wang N, Fox CS, Fontes JD, Rienstra M, et al. (2013) Relation of circulating liver transaminase concentrations to risk of new-onset atrial fibrillation. Am J Cardiol 111: 219–224.

17. Vanezis AP, Bhopal R (2008) Validity of electrocardiographic classification of left ventricular hypertrophy across adult ethnic groups with echocardiography as a standard. J Electrocardiol 41: 404–412.

18. American Diabetes Association (2012) Standards of medical care in diabetes - 2012. Diabetes Care 35 (suppl 1): S11–S63.

19. Mehta SR, Thomas EL, Bell JD, Johnston DG, Taylor-Robinson SD (2008) Non-invasive means of measuring hepatic fat content. World J Gastroenterol 14: 3476–3483.

20. Schnabel RB, Sullivan LM, Levy D, Pencina MJ, Massaro JM, et al. (2009) Development of a risk score for atrial fibrillation (Framingham Heart Study): a community-based cohort study. Lancet 373: 739–745.

21. Makar GA, Weiner MG, Kimmel SE, Bennet D, Burke A, et al. (2008) Incidence and prevalence of abnormal liver associated enzymes in patients with atrial fibrillation in a routine clinical care population. Pharmacoepidemiol Drug Saf 17: 43–51.

22. Tsang TS, Gersh BJ, Appleton CP, Tajik AJ, Barnes ME, et al. (2002) Left ventricular diastolic dysfunction as a predictor of the first diagnosed non-valvular atrial fibrillation in 840 elderly men and women. J Am Coll Cardiol 40: 1636–1644.

23. Darbar D, Jahangir A, Hammill SC, Gersh BJ (2002) P wave signal-averaged electrocardiography to identify risk for atrial fibrillation. Pacing Clin Electrophysiol 25: 1447–1453.

24. Rosenberg MA, Gottdiener JS, Heckbert SR, Mukamal KJ (2012) Echocardiographic diastolic parameters and risk of atrial fibrillation: the Cardiovascular Health Study. Eur Heart J 33: 904–912.

25. Chamberlain AM, Agarwal SK, Folsom AR, Soliman EZ, Chambless LE, et al. (2011) A clinical risk score for atrial fibrillation in a biracial prospective cohort (from the Atherosclerosis Risk in Communities [ARIC] study). Am J Cardiol 107: 85–91.

26. Rijzewijk LJ, van der Meer RW, Smit JW, Diamant M, Bax JJ, et al. (2008) Myocardial steatosis is an independent predictor of diastolic dysfunction in type 2 diabetes mellitus. J Am Coll Cardiol 52: 1793–1799.

27. Ng AC, Delgado V, Bertini M, van der Meer RW, Rijzewijk LJ, et al. (2010) Myocardial steatosis and biventricular strain and strain rate imaging in patients with type 2 diabetes mellitus. Circulation 122: 2538–2544.

28. Fox CS, Gona P, Hoffmann U, Porter SA, Salton CJ, et al. (2009) Pericardial fat, intrathoracic fat, and measures of left ventricular structure and function: the Framingham Heart Study. Circulation 119: 1586–1591.

29. Thanassoulis G, Massaro JM, O'Donnell CJ, Hoffmann U, Levy D, et al. (2010) Pericardial fat is associated with prevalent atrial fibrillation: the Framingham Heart Study. Circ Arrhythm Electrophysiol 3: 345–350.

30. Shin SY, Yong HS, Lim HE, Na JO, Choi CU, et al. (2011) Total and interatrial epicardial adipose tissues are independently associated with left atrial remodeling in patients with atrial fibrillation. J Cardiovasc Electrophysiol 22: 647–655.

31. Lin YK, Chen YC, Chen JH, Chen SA, Chen YJ (2012) Adipocytes modulate the electrophysiology of atrial myocytes: implications in obesity-induced atrial fibrillation. Basic Res Cardiol 107: 293.

32. Targher G, Chonchol M, Miele L, Zoppini G, Pichiri I, et al. (2009) Non-alcoholic fatty liver disease as a contributor to hypercoagulation and thrombophilia in the metabolic syndrome. Semin Thromb Hemost 35: 277–287.

33. Chung MK, Martin DO, Sprecher D, Wazni O, Kanderian A, et al. (2001) C-reactive protein elevation in patients with atrial arrhythmias. Inflammatory mechanisms and persistence of atrial fibrillation. Circulation 104: 2886–2891.

34. Liu T, Li G, Li L, Korantzopoulos P (2007) Association between C-reactive protein and recurrence of atrial fibrillation after successful electrical cardioversion: a meta-analysis. J Am Coll Cardiol 49: 1642–1648.

35. Schnabel RB, Larson MG, Yamamoto JF, Sullivan LM, Pencina MJ, et al. (2010) Relations of biomarkers of distinct pathophysiological pathways and atrial fibrillation incidence in the community. Circulation 121: 200–207.

36. Conen D, Ridker PM, Everett BM, Tedrow UB, Rose L, et al. (2010) A multimarker approach to assess the influence of inflammation on the incidence of atrial fibrillation in women. Eur Heart J 31: 1730–1736.

11

Computational Model of Erratic Arrhythmias in a Cardiac Cell Network: The Role of Gap Junctions

Aldo Casaleggio[1]*, Michael L. Hines[2], Michele Migliore[3]

1 Institute of Biophysics, National Research Council, Genova, Italy, **2** Dept. of Neurobiology, Yale University School of Medicine, New Haven, Connecticut, United States of America, **3** Institute of Biophysics, National Research Council, Palermo, Italy

Abstract

Cardiac morbidity and mortality increases with the population age. To investigate the underlying pathological mechanisms, and suggest new ways to reduce clinical risks, computational approaches complementing experimental and clinical investigations are becoming more and more important. Here we explore the possible processes leading to the occasional onset and termination of the (usually) non-fatal arrhythmias widely observed in the heart. Using a computational model of a two-dimensional network of cardiac cells, we tested the hypothesis that an ischemia alters the properties of the gap junctions inside the ischemic area. In particular, in agreement with experimental findings, we assumed that an ischemic episode can alter the gap junctions of the affected cells by reducing their average conductance. We extended these changes to include random fluctuations with time, and modifications in the gap junction rectifying conductive properties of cells along the edges of the ischemic area. The results demonstrate how these alterations can qualitatively give an account of all the main types of non-fatal arrhythmia observed experimentally, and suggest how premature beats can be eliminated in three different ways: *a)* with a relatively small surgical procedure, *b)* with a pharmacological reduction of the rectifying conductive properties of the gap-junctions, and *c)* by pharmacologically decreasing the gap junction conductance. In conclusion, our model strongly supports the hypothesis that non-fatal arrhythmias can develop from post-ischemic alteration of the electrical connectivity in a relatively small area of the cardiac cell network, and suggests experimentally testable predictions on their possible treatments.

Editor: Maxim Bazhenov, University of California, Riverside, United States of America

Funding: This work has been supported by the Institute of Biophysics of the National Research Council (Italy) and by NINDS grant R01-NS11613 to MLH. The funders had no role in study design, data collection and analysis, decision to publish, or preparation of the manuscript.

Competing Interests: The authors have declared that no competing interests exist.

* Email: casaleggio@ge.ibf.cnr.it

Introduction

Understanding the basic cellular mechanisms underlying cardiac pathophysiology is of increasing importance, as the aging of the population predicts an increasing prevalence of cardiac morbidity and mortality. For this purpose, an important complement to experimental and clinical investigations is the mathematical modeling and simulation of the mechanisms responsible for cardiac electrophysiology [1], especially those that can underlie alterations in the propagation of electrical activity leading to arrhythmias. Although there are many types of arrhythmic cardiac behavior, most of the current models give emphasis to those with severe or fatal complications, such as atrial fibrillation [2] or ventricular fibrillation [3], and are based on the so-called reentry model. Reentry was first defined by Mines [4] as a persisting electrical impulse that reactivates an area of previously activated myocardial tissue that is no longer refractory, resulting in a circular movement of activation. The length of the circle depends on the impulse wavelength, defined as the product of the refractory period and conduction velocity (plus an excitable gap when present) [5]. The requirements for reentrant activation in the intact heart are a region of unidirectional block and a (regionally) slow-enough conduction velocity allowing an impulse to travel around or inside the affected region. The ultimate proof of reentry is its termination by interruption of the circle [4]. Our

understanding of reentry has been extended by the introduction of different initiation mechanisms such as single rotor reentry [6], fibrillatory conduction [7–8], and the leading circle concept [9]. These mechanisms have been recently explored [3], cardiac tissue simulators have been presented [10], and the use of modeling in helping clinical practice has been suggested [11–13].

To explain the mechanisms underlying the initiation of a reentrant arrhythmic behavior, most models assume permanent changes in the intrinsic electrophysiological parameters of cardiac cells, such as altered intracellular Calcium dynamics [14] or ion channel modifications [15]. Other models consider alternative mechanisms, such as mitochondrial membrane potential oscillations and waves [16], or the roles played by individual sarcolemmal ion channels in atrial and ventricular fibrillation [17]. The major problem with these approaches is that the arrhythmic behavior is reproduced in an all-or-none fashion. In these models, the arrhythmia (usually a tachyarrhythmia) is often systematic, triggered by a single stimulus and, once initiated, does not stop spontaneously. This contrasts with what is observed in clinical practice, where thousands of relatively brief non-fatal episodes of arrhythmias occur during the life of a subject. Isolated premature ventricular beats (iPVB), bi- or tri-geminy sequences, couplets, triplets, and ventricular tachyarrhythmias (see the MIT-BIH Arrhythmia data base [18]), are commonly observed during the life of a subject without immediate life threatening conditions, although an increased rate of premature ventricular beats have been associated with an increased risk of sudden death in patients with heart failure [19]. Since these conditions are widespread in the population, it is important to investigate the malfunctioning mechanisms and how they can be treated.

In this paper, we explore with a computational model the possibility that non-fatal arrhythmias can originate from post-ischemic dynamic alteration of the electrical connectivity in a relatively small area of the cardiac cell network. The simulation findings show that random fluctuations of the intercellular gap junction conductance inside an ischemic area are sufficient to generate practically all of the observed types of transient arrhythmia. The model suggests possible treatments to reduce or eliminate these conditions.

Methods

All simulations were carried out with the NEURON simulation environment (v7.3) [20] on a parallel BlueGene/Q IBM super-computer (CINECA, Bologna, Italy). A typical 130 sec simulation required about 3 hours using 1024 processors. Model and simulation files will be available for public download on the ModelDB section of the Senselab suite (http://senselab.med.yale.edu/ModelDB/, acc.n.150691).

We modeled a relatively small two-dimensional cardiac tissue of 12.8×4.1 mm, composed of 128×256 cardiac cells implemented as a single-compartment of 100×16 μm, corresponding to the real size of canine ventricular myocardial cells [21]. Electrophysiological passive and active properties were identical to those used in the Beeler-Reuter model [21], with model files downloaded from the public ModelDB database (http://senselab.med.yale.edu/modeldb, acc.n. 97863). This is one of the simplest realistic electrophysiology models for a single ventricular canine myocyte. It describes the cell activity on the basis of 4 trans-membrane currents: a sodium current, two potassium currents, and a calcium current which is responsible for the plateau potential occurring during a cell's depolarization. A typical action potential generated in this cardiac cell model by a short (4 nA, 5 ms) current injection is shown in Fig. 1A. Each cell was connected via gap junctions with its 4 neighbors, as schematically represented in Fig. 1B. A gap junction between any two given cells under control conditions was modeled as a bidirectional, time-independent, ohmic conductance of 30 nS under control conditions, in agreement with experimental data [22] and within the wide range experimentally measured in mammals, which ranges from the 500 nS measured in ventricular pairs to the 8 nS in SA nodal pairs [23–24].

To model the abnormal conditions underlying different types of arrhythmias, we first implemented an ischemic area by altering the gap junction rectifying conductive properties (Fig. 1C) of the cells along the edges of the ischemic area (as illustrated in Fig. 1D). The gap junction conductance of the cells inside the area was reduced to a lower average value, which randomly fluctuated with time during a simulation (see Results). The complex behavior of gap junction conductance involved in cardiac function has been reviewed in Moreno [25]. Rectification of the gap junction conductance has been experimentally observed in HeLa cells [26–27], whereas fluctuations in the conductance during ischemia have been observed in dogs [28], rabbits [29] and humans [30]. This is the first time that the effects of time dependent fluctuations is investigated in the context of erratic cardiac arrhythmias.

The properties of an ischemic area were constrained by experimental observations. In particular, Peters et al. [31] found altered gap junctions as part of the early remodeling of myocardium after inducing infarction and ischemia in 6 dogs.

Another study [32] proposed the existence of an entry and an exit door somewhere along the border of an ischemic region. We thus implemented a generic ischemic area as a region with propagation properties slower than normal tissue [33] (represented in yellow in Fig. 1D). The affected area was delimited by an almost completely closed contour which blocks signal propagation (black cells in Fig. 1D). Entry and exit doors were implemented along the contour with two small sections (grey cells in Fig. 1D) having strong rectification properties which allow only mono-directional communication between the normal external tissue and the ischemic inner region. Two different ischemic areas, of the same width (3.9 mm, corresponding to 39 cells) but different height (0.5–0.75 mm, corresponding to 30–45 cells) have been simulated.

During a typical 130 sec simulation, a pacemaker signal was generated by a periodic (every 800 ms) short current injection (4 nA, 5 ms) to cell (1,1) (indicated with a red marker in Fig. 1D). Gap junctions of cells belonging to the normal region were fixed to their control value of 30 nS, whereas the values of each gap junction inside the ischemic region were randomly chosen, every 500+/−50 ms, from a normal distribution with a given average and variance. Change the gap junction conductance to an average interval shorter than the normal periodic signal simplifies the analysis of the results. However, different intervals and mechanisms were also tested (see Results). Several combinations of gap conductance average value (range 4.5–5 nS) and variance (range 0.3–0.8 nS^2) were tested. The membrane potential of cell(25,100) (indicated with a blue marker in Fig. 1D) under control conditions (i.e. no ischemic area) is shown in Fig. 1E. A movie illustrating the propagation of the activity following an external stimulation of cell(1,1) is reported in Movie S1.

It is important to stress that a number of additional mechanisms can be affected by an ischemic episode. Virtually all of them, from increased intracellular acidity [34] to changes in channel functioning [35], may independently contribute to the emergence of a PVB, and can lead to the generation of life-threatening arrhythmias. This is precisely why we did not include them in the model, at this stage. Rather, we were interested in studying the role, and isolating the effect, of random gap junction fluctuations. This is a process that is quite difficult to study experimentally. In this paper we have chosen to investigate only the functional consequences of an ischemic episode on gap junctions. It would be interesting to include the modulation of other mechanisms in a future study, to study how and to what extent they affect the basic findings shown in this paper.

Comparison with Experimental Findings on Non-fatal Arrhythmias

For a qualitative comparison of our model with experimental data we selected several representative electrocardiographic signals (ECG) from the Physionet Data Base [36] and shown in Fig. 2. In particular, we considered several 10 sec recordings from different patients with non-fatal arrhythmias commonly related to increasing cardiac electrical activity deterioration. These include: single premature ventricular beat (PVB), trigeminy sequences (a sequence of normal and premature beats with the ratio of 2:1), bigeminy sequences (a sequence of normal and premature beats with the ratio of 1:1), couplets (two consecutive premature beats), triplets (three consecutive premature beats) and, finally, a short run of non-sustained Ventricular Tachycardia (VT, a sequence of more than 3 premature beats that spontaneously recover to the normal condition).

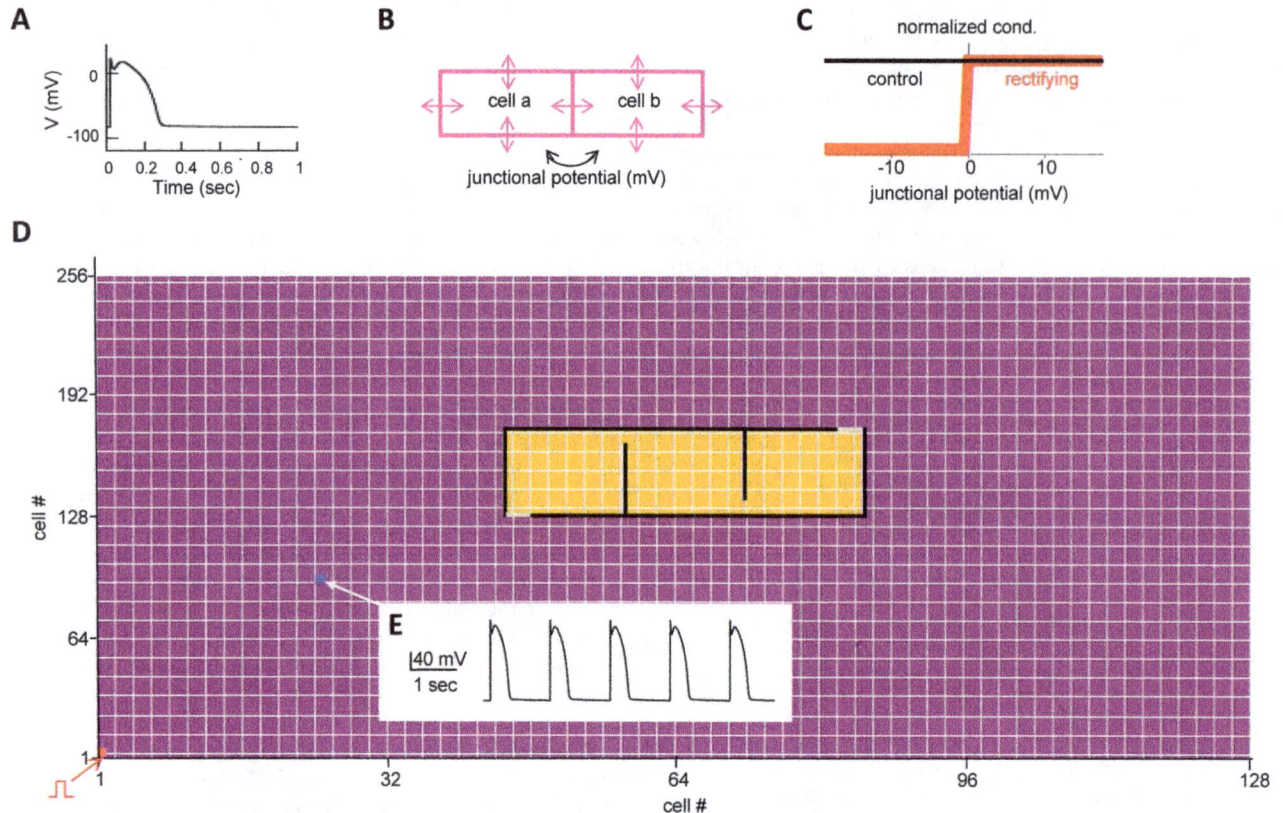

Figure 1. Model implementation. A) the action potential of an isolated cell in response to a short current pulse injection (4 nA, 5 ms); **B)** schematic representation of the gap junctions connecting neighbor cells, represented by arrows; **C)** the gap junction conductance as a function of the junctional potential under control conditions (black line) and for cells forming the edges of the fibrotic area (red line); **D)** Schematic representation of the full 128×256 cell network; individual cells are represented with small purple (normal) or yellow (ischemic) rectangles; the black lines identify the contour of the lesion, composed by non-conducting cells (i.e. g = 0). Cells with rectifying gap junctions, implementing entry and exit doors are shown in gray. Physiological input signals from Purkinje cells were modeled by periodically stimulating with a short current pulse cell(1,1) (bottom left of the network, shown in red); **E)** typical membrane potential of cell(25,100) under physiological conditions (i.e. no ischemic area).

Results

The main mechanism underlying the generation of premature beats suggested by our model is a direct consequence of the differential signal propagation inside an ischemic area. This process is illustrated in Fig. 3, where we show a few snapshots from Movie S2 and the membrane potential of cell(25,100) (indicated with a yellow mark in Fig. 3), outside the ischemic area. Under control conditions (i.e. without an ischemic area) each wave of activity generated by pacemaker cells will freely flow without interference (as shown in Movie S1). In the presence of a lesion (delimited by the yellow lines in Fig. 3), the signal propagation around the scar (see snapshots A-C and the corresponding time points in the bottom plot of Fig. 3) generates a secondary wave of activity inside the ischemic area (Fig. 3, snapshots D-E). Once it reaches the normal region (Fig. 3, snapshot F), it causes the generation of a premature beat. The activity spreads backward (Fig. 3, snapshots G-H) and negatively interferes with the generation of the expected beat in cell(1,1) (green arrow at t = 1800 ms in the bottom plot of Fig. 3), which is still within the refractory period. Activity returns to normal afterwards (Fig. 3, snapshot I). The arrhythmia does not occur every heart cycle because the gap junction random fluctuations do not allow reliable propagation of the signal inside the ischemic area (see Movie S2). These results show that an alteration in the gap junction conductance, caused for example by an ischemic episode in a

relatively small area of cardiac tissue, can generate premature beats leading to arrhythmias.

To investigate this mechanism in greater detail, we carried out a systematic set of simulations using different values for the average and variance of the gap junction conductance inside the ischemic area. It should be stressed that, in all cases, the normal electrophysiological properties of all cells were not changed. Typical simulation findings exhibiting different kinds of arrhythmia are shown in Fig. 4A, where we plot selected excerpts of single cell recordings (cell 25,100) from simulations using different values for the average and variance of the gap junctions conductance in the ischemic area. The different types of arrhythmias where classified as shown in Table 1, by considering the sequence of interspike intervals having an abnormal duration with respect to that expected for normal cells. As can be seen, the model was able to qualitatively reproduce all types of experimentally observed arrhythmias (see Fig. 2). During each simulation we observed that, just as it occurs in the real system, different types of arrhythmias can appear at different times, and that their relative proportion depended on the average and variance of the gap conductance. A typical example is shown in Fig. 4B, where we show the membrane potential of cell(25,100) during a 25 sec time window of a simulation with a gap conductance of g = 4.7±0.7 nS. More or less organized premature beats appear throughout the simulation (labels above the trace in Fig. 4B). Taken together these results demonstrate that a single mechanism, namely the dynamical

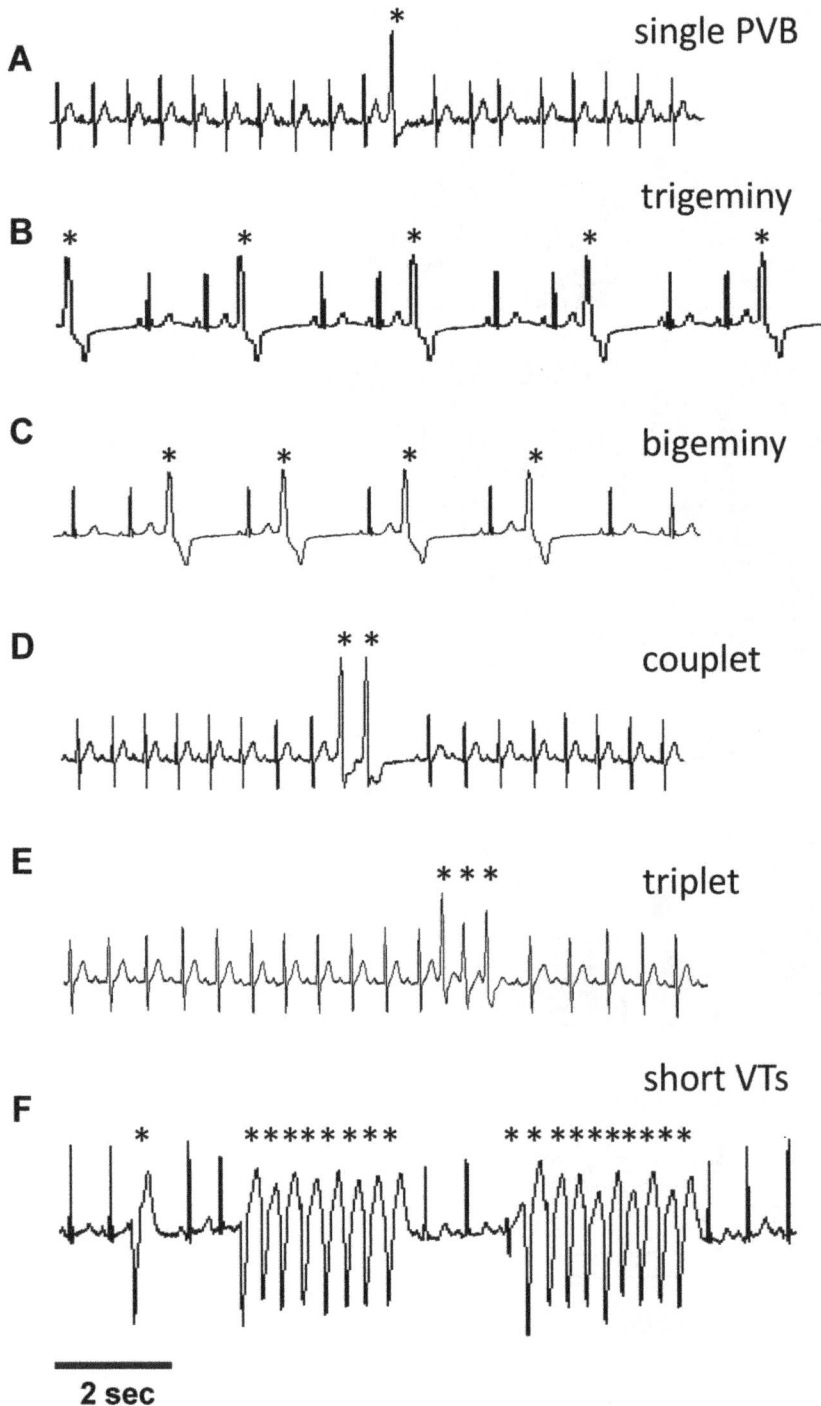

Figure 2. Typical experimental ECG recordings showing the different arrhythmias taken into account by our model. A) single premature ventricular beat; **B)** trigeminy complexes; **C)** bigeminy complexes; **D)** couplet episode; **E)** triplet episode; **F)** two short runs of tachyarrhythmias. In all cases, markers highlight arrhythmic complexes.

fluctuation of the gap junction conductance inside an ischemic area, is able to explain practically all kinds of non-fatal arrhythmias experimentally observed in cardiac cells.

A more systematic exploration of the gap conductance parameter space is presented in Fig. 5A, where we report the proportion of PVB as a function of the average and variance of the fluctuations inside the ischemic area. The range of values for the gap conductance reproducing the arrhythmias is drastically lower

than the value for normal cells. To the best of our knowledge, there are no direct measurements of the gap conductance within a cardiac ischemic area, except for the obvious case of dead cells (scars), which can safely be assumed to have a 0 conductance. Since one of the conditions that may affect this value is an anisotropic distribution of gap junctions on individual cells [37], we tested different anisotropy ratios (calculated as the ratio between the longitudinal and transversal gap conductance in a

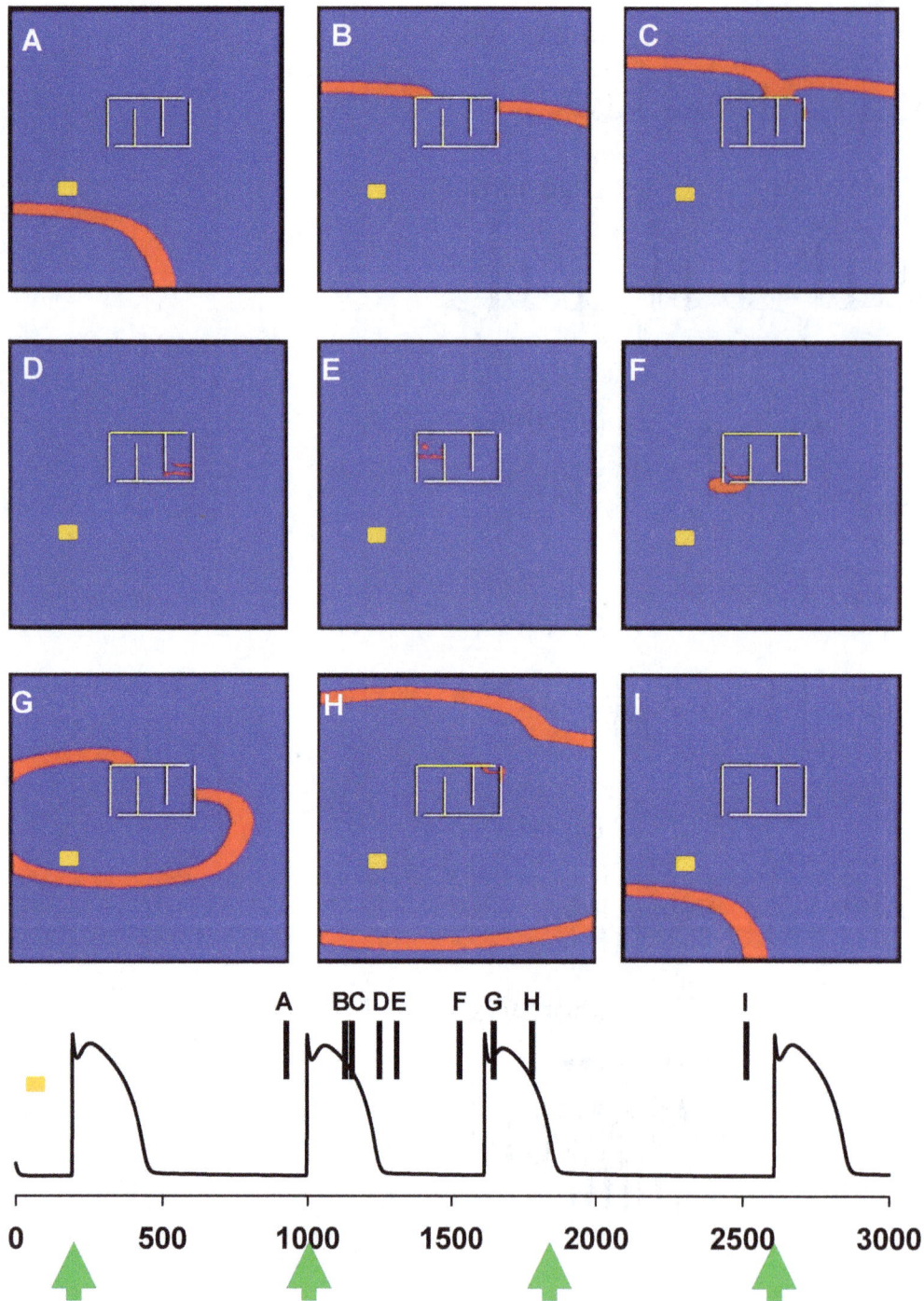

Figure 3. Typical onset of a premature beat. A–I) snapshots from Movie S2, illustrating the propagation of two normal beats (panels A-B-C and I) and a premature beat (panels D through H); *(bottom plot):* membrane potential of cell(25,100), marked in yellow in the snapshots, during the simulation shown in Movie S2. Vertical markers show the time points at which the snapshots in panels A-I were taken.

given cell). For this purpose, we started from a configuration with an average total gap conductance in each cell of $4 \times 4.5 = 18$ nS. An isotropic distribution resulted in 5% of PVB (Fig. 5A, left). As shown in Fig. 5A (right), a similar proportion of PVB (red labels in Fig. 5A, right) was obtained for increasing values of anisotropy with a corresponding increase in the average gap conductance. Interestingly, we found that the relative distribution of premature beats corresponding to the different kind of arrhythmias can be

directly related to the variance of the gap conductance fluctuations. This is illustrated in the top plot of Fig. 5B, where we show that (for an average gap conductance of 4.7 nS) a progressively higher variance in the fluctuation results in a decrease of isolated premature beats (Fig. 5B, iPVB, white bars), and an increase of those involved with episodes of bigeminy, couplet, triplet, and tachycardia. The same effect, although less pronounced, was observed as a function of the average value (with a fixed variance

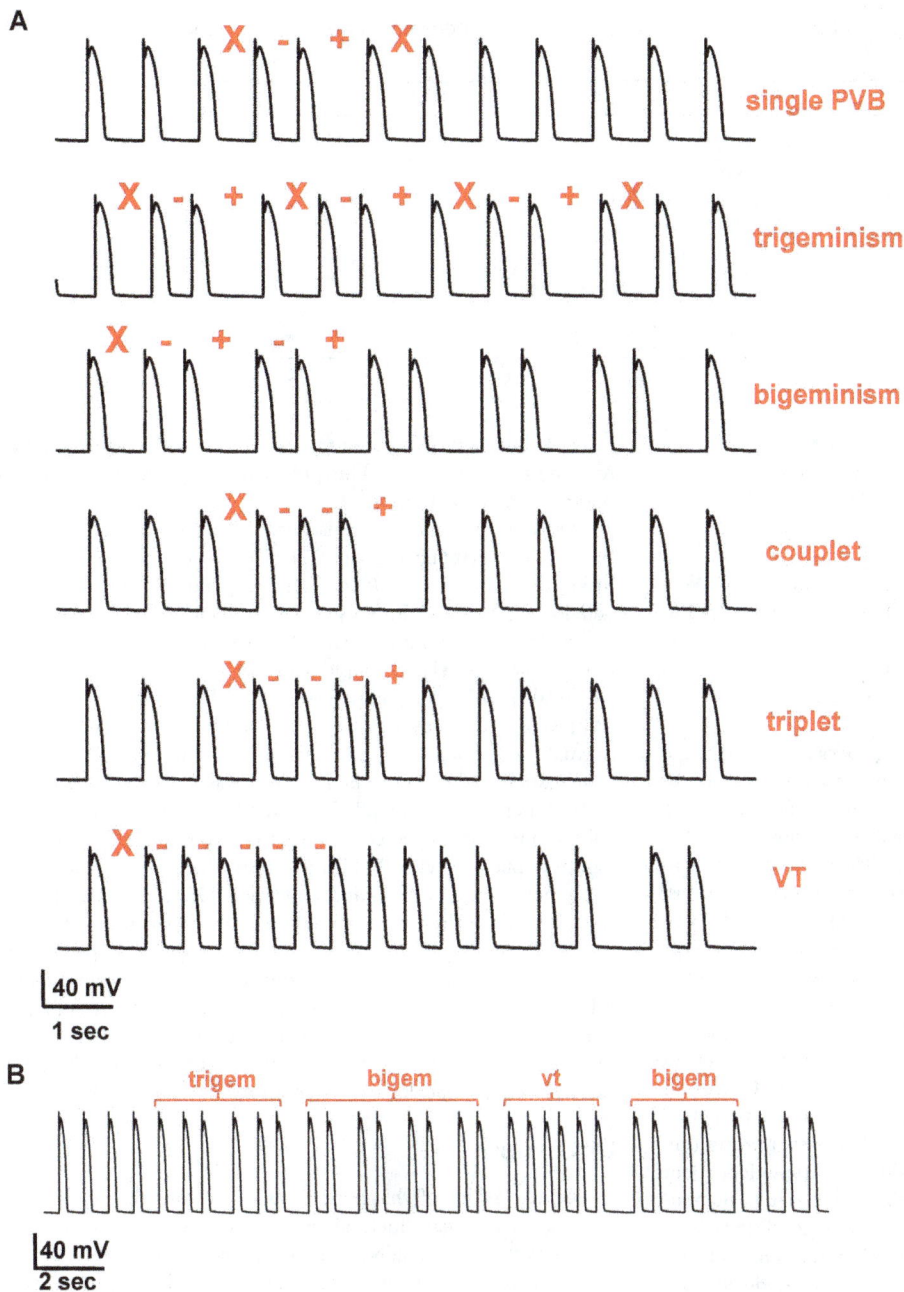

Figure 4. Our model suggests that all kinds of arrhythmia can be explained by dynamical fluctuations of the gap junctions. A) (top to bottom) isolated arrhythmia, trigeminy complex, bigeminy complex, couplet, triplet, short runs of tachyarrhythmias followed by a bigeminism; compare all panels with those in Fig. 2; **B)** 25 sec simulation exhibiting different types of arrhythmic behavior. In all cases, red markers highlight abnormal sequences (see Table 1); traces represent the membrane potential of cell(25,100), from simulations with the following average gap junction conductance and variance: (4.7, 0.3) iPVB, (4.9, 0.3) trigeminy, bigeminy, and triplet, (4.7, 0.6) couplet, (4.7, 0.8) VT.

of 0.3 nS^2, bottom plot in Fig. 5B). These results suggest that random fluctuations in the gap conductance inside an ischemic area can promote and modulate the development of specific types of arrhythmic behavior.

To investigate the possible effects of ischemic areas of different sizes and positions with respect to the propagation of the normal electrical activity, we carried out a set of simulations using a different cell (O2 instead of O1, Fig. 6A) for the pacemaker stimulation. Simulations were also carried out using a 30% smaller area (Fig. 6A, Is_S), involving 1200 instead of 1800 cells. In these

cases, the average value for the gap conductance was fixed at 4.7 nS. The results are shown in Figure 6B, where the fraction of premature beats is plotted as function of conductance variance. They suggest that when an ischemic episode creates a sufficiently large area of altered gap junctions (Fig. 6B, Is_B plots), the occurrence of premature beats does not depend on the direction of propagation of the physiological electrical activity. In contrast, a relatively smaller area (Fig. 6A, Is_S), may be much more sensitive to the propagation direction (Fig. 6B, Is_S). This occurs because the signal propagation delay inside a larger damaged area is

Table 1. Specific sequences of interspike interval (ISI) define normal or abnormal behavior; X normal ISI; −, shorter than normal; +, longer than normal.

normal	X X X X X
single PVB	X −+X
trigeminism	X −+X −+X
bigeminism	X −+−+X
couplet	X − − X
triplet	X − − − X
vt	X − − − −

sufficiently long to reach the normal region after the end of the refractory period of the normal tissue, independently from the origin of the external stimulation; for a smaller area (such as Is_S) this occurs when the signal arrives from O1 but not from O2. The phenomenon is illustrated in Movie S3 and Movie S4, respectively. Furthermore, consistent with the experimental findings of Woie et al. [38] showing that larger myocardial infarction areas lead to slower ventricular tachyarrhythmias, in our simulations the average interval during tachycardia events increased from 362±13 ms for the smaller Is_S case, to 545±21 ms for the larger Is_B.

To show the robustness of the results we carried out additional simulations. Starting from the typical configuration discussed in Fig. 3 we applied different variations, one at a time. We tested anisotropic gap junctions [37] concentrated at the ends (Movie S5) or at the sides (Movie S6) of the cells, 10% fluctuation of gap junctions in the entire tissue (Movie S7), and shorter (250 ms, Movie S8) or longer (1000 ms, Movie S9) average intervals for gap conductance fluctuations. One particularly intriguing possibility is for gap junction fluctuations to be an activity-dependent process. The implementation of a long- or short-term plasticity mechanism (analogous to what occurs in chemical synapses) was outside the scope of this work. However, as proof of principle, we ran an additional simulation in which gap fluctuations (4.7±0.5 nS) in each cell occurred on the rising phase of the action potential, corresponding to the heart contraction. We obtained a proportion of PVB similar to that obtained with the time-dependent fluctuations (19% vs 25%). Taken together these results demonstrate the robustness of our model under different conditions, with the emergence of a number of PVBs at random times in all cases.

Finally, assuming that ischemic areas can be modeled with regions of cells with malfunctioning gap junctions, we considered ways to reduce or eliminate premature beats and, thus, arrhythmias. Clinically, severe cases of ventricular arrhythmias are treated by the relatively minor surgical procedure of radiofrequency ablation [39], whereas quite extensive and invasive maze cuts are used for cases of atrial fibrillation [40].

Our model suggests that premature beats can be eliminated in three different ways: a) by closing the exit door from the ischemic region, as it is usually done at the hospital with the radio-frequency ablation procedure, b) by pharmacologically opening the entry/exit doors to the ischemic area, and c) by pharmacologically decreasing the gap junction conductance. To implement the surgical procedure (case a), we created additional lesions by setting to 0 the gap junction conductance of the cells surrounding the exit door of the ischemia. This precluded the propagation of an ischemic beat outside the ischemic area and prevented the generation of premature beats (see Movie S10). Case b) was implemented by strongly reducing the gap rectification property of

the cells involved with the entry/exit doors, making them similar to those of normal cells. This practically removed the entry/exit doors, and had the effect of stopping the generation and propagation of abnormal beats outside the ischemic area (Movie S11). The remaining propagation of abnormal electrical activity inside the ischemic area (and the corresponding heart contractile activity) might explain why the infarction zone may appear relatively small during myocardial ischemia/reperfusion injury in open-chest dogs [41]. To implement case c), we ran a simulation in which all gap junction conductances (including those of normal cells) were reduced by 10%. The results (Movie S12) show that the normal propagation of the signal was unaffected, but its propagation inside the ischemic area was severely hindered. A 10% change may seem relatively small to result in macroscopic effects, but it should be considered that the suggested pharmacological application would affect (by 10%) the entire population of gap junctions (i.e. normal and ischemic). This is sufficient (in our model) to affect the behavior of the signal propagation within the ischemic region (which is already barely able to propagate the signal) without interfering with the propagation in normal tissue. Of course this change may not be enough in the presence of larger ischemic regions. Taken together these results show that it could be possible to treat non-fatal arrhythmias using relatively minor surgical or pharmacological procedures.

Discussion

The main aim of this paper was to explore the role of gap junction dynamical fluctuations in the occasional onset and termination of the (usually) non-fatal arrhythmias widely observed in the heart. In patients with ischemic cardiomyopathy, these events arise from an abnormal generation and propagation of electrical activity caused by more or less important ischemic episodes [42]. Because signal propagation in the heart occurs via gap-junctions mediating the interaction among neighbor cardiac cells, a deeper understanding of the functional consequences of gap-junction malfunctioning can be an important step to understand cardiac arrhythmias. In general, the dynamic reconfiguration of gap junction conductance can have non-trivial consequences in defining normal and pathological activity of a network of connected cells in the heart and also in the central nervous system [43].

With our model, we have demonstrated how the degradation of gap junctions inside an ischemic area is able to explain practically all kinds of non-fatal arrhythmias experimentally observed in cardiac cells. The average value and variability of the gap junction conductance can be directly related to the type and seriousness of the arrhythmic behavior, whereas their fluctuation with time determines the length of the episode. There is considerable

A

B

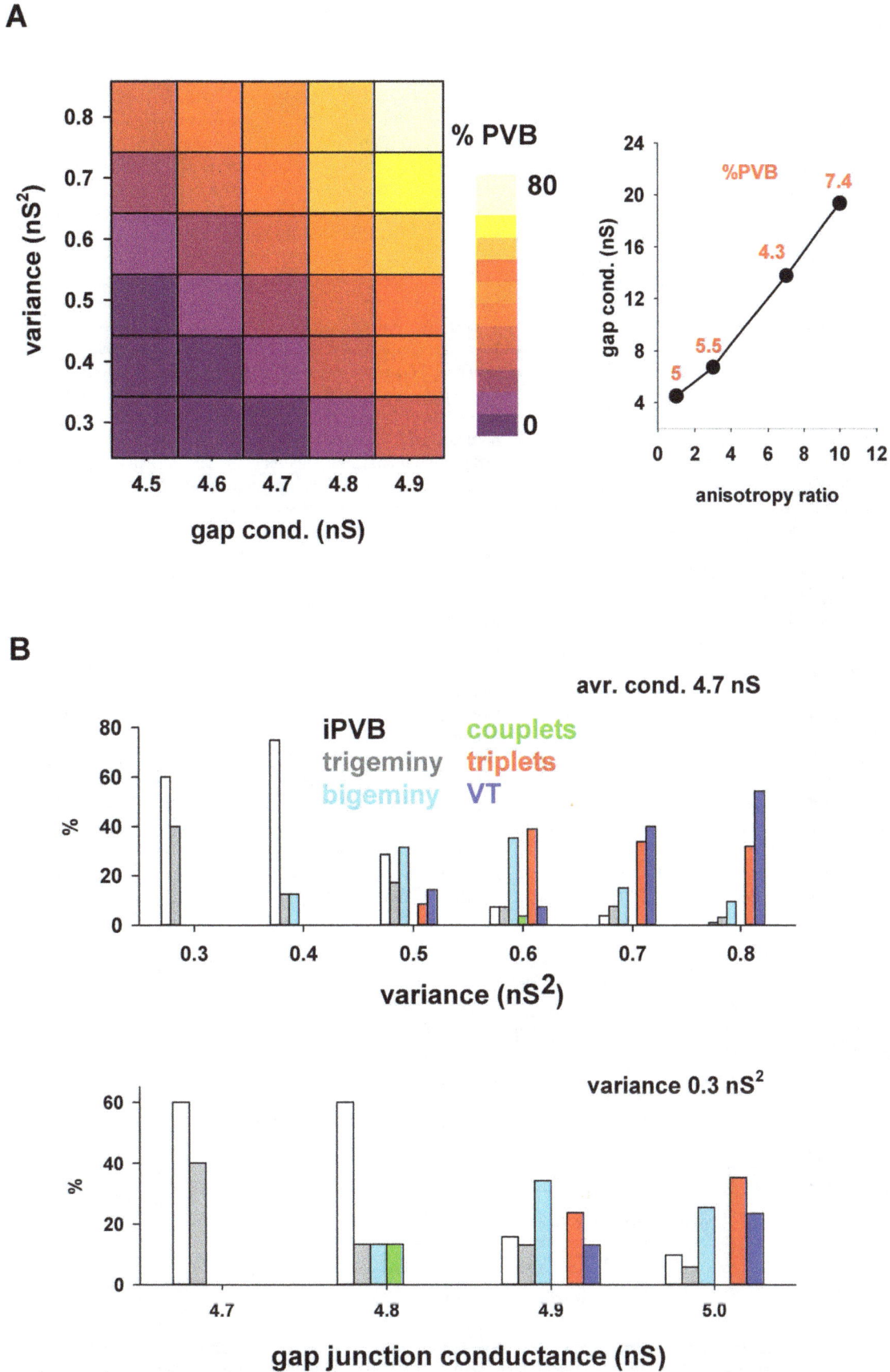

Figure 5. Gap junction modulations and fluctuations inside an ischemic area determine the relative proportion of premature beats.
A) Percent of premature beats, with respect to the total number of beats, generated by different average and variance values of the gap junction

conductance inside the ischemic area; **B)** Distribution of abnormal events as a function of the variance (top graph) or the average value (bottom graph) of the gap junctions conductance inside the ischemic area. White bars represent iPVB.

experimental evidence for the role of gap junction conductance changes in cardiac arrhythmias. From a general point of view, gap junctions consist of transmembrane proteins called connexins, which assemble to form homomeric or heteromeric hemichannels (connexons) with an aqueous pore. In mammals, there are many types of connexins, and several of them (e.g. Connexin 40, Connexin 43, Connexin 45) are present in the cardiac tissue [25], [44]. The docking of two connexons leads to the establishment of a homotypic or heterotypic gap junction channel, according to the different possible combinations of connexins that can form a channel [25], [27]. For example, it has been shown that various pathological disorders can be associated with alterations in expression and modulation of connexin proteins [45–47]. In particular, in end-stage failing human hearts, Connexin43 expression is decreased, with respect to normal conditions, at both the mRNA and protein levels, due to both ischemic and dilated cardiomyopathy [48], and Connexin 40 plays a role in atrial fibrillation [49–50]. Furthermore, arrhythmogenic remodelling of activation and repolarization in the failing human heart has been associated with changes in the expression of connexins [51]. Finally, the atrial myocardium susceptible to atrial fibrillation can be distinguished from its non-susceptible counterpart by a reduced Connexin 40 expression [47].

A critical property suggested by our model, for the generation of premature beats, is the anisotropy of conductance in the cells forming the entry and exit doors to the ischemic area. Experimental evidence for this rectifying effect has been reported in studying the electrical properties of cells coupled by Connexin 40, Connexin 43 and Connexin 45 [25–27]. The post-ischemia formation of entry and exit doors, from an area with slower signal propagation properties, has been suggested by experimental findings [31–32]. The alteration of gap junction properties is also supported by a number of experimental findings and observations. For example, heterotypic gap-junction channels may exhibit rectification with respect to the junction potential [26], especially when the Connexons include Connexin 45 together with

Connexin 40 or Connexin 43 [25], [27]. Also, ischemia has been associated with a reduced amount of active Connexin 43 [45], [52–53] and Connexin 40 [47]. Furthermore, the novel drug Rotigaptide has been shown to increase gap junction conductance [54] by increasing Connexin 43 activity [55]. Our model suggests that this drug is effective because, by increasing the fraction of phosphorylated Connexin 43, it contributes to the formation of homotypic gap junctions with symmetrical properties, rather than heterotypic gap junction. This mechanism can thus inhibit the formation of entry/exit doors.

Both gap junction alterations and the mechanism of re-entry have been previously explored with computational models to explain cardiac arrhythmic behavior [2–3], [14]. However, to take into account the initiation of arrhythmias, all these models assume a number of modifications to different model mechanisms. None of them take into account the spontaneous termination of the arrhythmic behavior. Different models for the human atrial fibrillation were reviewed and compared [2] and, in agreement with our study, the results suggest that a reduced conductance of the gap-junctions inside a damaged area may promote non-fatal arrhythmias. Another review [56] also focused on the atrial fibrillation and the role of re-entry, originating from the presence of an obstacle and correlated with the presence of a fibrotic area within the myocardium. In this case, two types of re-entry mechanisms were considered [32]: an inner loop, in which the ischemic region acts as a delay line of the front-wave, and an outer loop where the reentry originates around an obstacle. The outer loop [2], [56] has been shown to be a useful way to explain the initiation (but not the termination) of atrial and ventricular tachycardia or fibrillation. With our model we have shown that all types of non fatal arrhythmias and slow tachycardia can also initiate and terminate by assuming an inner loop as their origin.

The treatment of at least the most severe forms of arrhythmia is usually carried out with surgical procedures that can be quite invasive [39–40]. It is thus important to develop alternatives to reduce or eliminate the occurrence of more or less organized

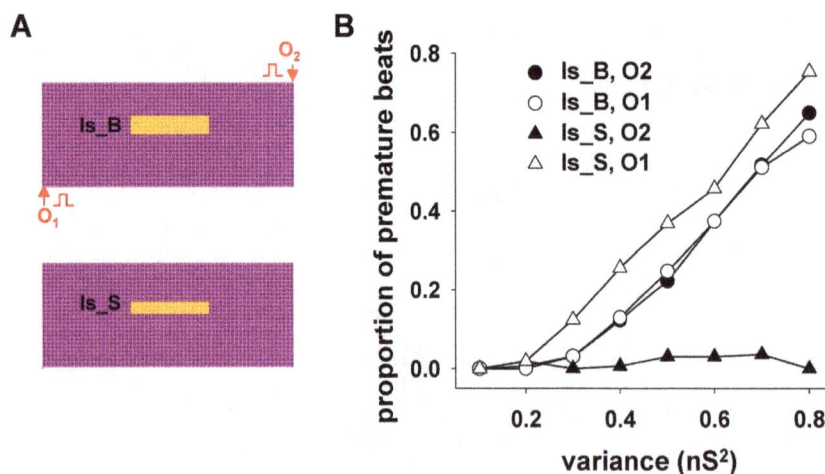

Figure 6. The generation of premature beats may depend on the direction of signal propagation. A) schematic representation of the two ischemic areas investigated, and the two stimulation points (O1 and O2) used to model different directions for the propagation of a physiological signal; **B)** Proportion of premature beats as function of the variance of the gap junction conductance inside the ischemic area for different stimulation points. The average value of the gap junction conductance of the cells inside the ischemic area was 4.7 nS in all cases.

premature beats. Our model suggests a few experimentally testable predictions on the possible actions that, in principle, can be used: *a)* relatively minor surgery to close the exit door to the ischemic area (Movie S10), *b)* pharmacological actions to reduce or eliminate the rectification properties of the gap junctions (Movie S11) and, *c)* a relatively small (10%) pharmacological reduction of the gap junctions conductance (Movie S12). In all cases, the propagation of the activity inside the ischemic area would be hindered while propagation in the normal tissue remains essentially unaffected.

Supporting Information

Movie S1 Simulation under control conditions.

Movie S2 Simulation in the presence of an ischemic area (Is_B).

Movie S3 Simulation in the presence of an ischemic area of smaller size (Is_S) with origin in O1.

Movie S4 Simulation in the presence of an ischemic area of smaller size (Is_S) with origin in O2.

Movie S5 Simulation in the presence of an ischemic area and the total gap junction's conductance for each cell distributed with 3:1 ratio, between the ends and the sides of a cell, to represent a higher concentration of gap junctions at the ends of a cell.

Movie S6 Simulation in the presence of an ischemic area and the total gap junction's conductance for each cell distributed with 1:3 ratio, between the ends and the sides of a cell, to represent a higher concentration of gap junctions at the sides of a cell.

Movie S7 Simulation in the presence of an ischemic area, with all gap junction conductances independently

undergoing an average 10% random fluctuation every 500±50 ms.

Movie S8 Simulation in the presence of an ischemic area, with all gap junction conductances independently undergoing an average 10% random fluctuation every 250±25 ms.

Movie S9 Simulation in the presence of an ischemic area, with all gap junction conductances independently undergoing an average 10% random fluctuation every 1000±100 ms.

Movie S10 Simulation in the presence of an ischemic area with ablation of the exit door.

Movie S11 Simulation in the presence of an ischemic area (Is_B) but without anisotropy of the gap junction's conductance of the cells forming the entry/exit doors.

Movie S12 Simulation in the presence of an ischemic area (Is_B), but with all gap junctions conductance reduced by 10%.

Acknowledgments

AC and MM thank Franco Gambale for useful and productive discussions during the early stages of this work. We thank the CINECA consortium (Bologna, Italy) for access to their Fermi IBM BG/Q supercomputer system (Bologna, Italy).

Author Contributions

Conceived and designed the experiments: AC MM. Performed the experiments: AC. Analyzed the data: AC MM. Contributed reagents/materials/analysis tools: MLH. Wrote the paper: AC MM MLH.

References

1. Clayton RH, Bernus O, Cherry EM, Dierckx H, Fenton FH, et al. (2011) Models of cardiac tissue electrophysiology: progress, challenges and open questions. Prog Biophys Mol Biol 104: 22–48.
2. Wilhelms M, Hettmann H, Maleckar MM, Koivumäki JT, Dössel O, et al. (2013) Benchmarking electrophysiological models of human atrial myocytes. Frontiers in Computational Physiology and Medicine 3: 487. doi: 10.3389/fphys.2012.00487.
3. Pandit SV, Jalife J (2013) Rotors and the dynamics of cardiac fibrillation. Circ Res 112: 849–862.
4. Mines GR (1914) On circulating excitations in heart muscle and their possible relation to tachycardia and fibrillation. Trans R Soc Can IV:43–52.
5. Han J, Moe GK (1964) Nonuniform recovery of excitability in ventricular muscle. Circ Res 14: 44–60.
6. Winfree AT (1994) Electrical turbulence in three-dimensional heart muscle. Science 266: 1003–1006.
7. Chen J, Mandapati R, Berenfeld O, Skanes AC, Gray RA, et al (2000) Dynamics of wavelets and their role in atrial fibrillation in the isolated sheep heart. Cardiovasc Res 48: 220–232.
8. Jalife J (2000) Ventricular fibrillation: mechanisms of initiation and maintenance. Annu Rev Physiol 62: 25–50.
9. Allessie MA, Bonke FIM, Schopman FJG (1977) Circus movement in rabbit atrial muscle as a mechanism of tachycardia: III. The "Leading Circle" concept: a new model of circus movement in cardiac tissue without the involvement of an anatomical obstacle. Circ Res 41: 9–18.
10. Cooper J, Corrias A, Gavaghan D, Noble D (2011) Considerations for the use of cellular electrophysiology models within cardiac tissue simulations. Prog Biophys Mol Biol 107: 74–80.
11. Keldermann RH, Ten Tusscher KHWJ, Nash MP, Bradley CP, Hren R, et al. (2009) A computational study of mother rotor VF in the human ventricles. Am J Physiol Heart Circ Physiol 296: H370–H379.
12. Mirams GR, Davies MR, Cui Y, Kohl P, Noble D (2012) Application of cardiac electrophysiology simulations to pro-arrhythmic safety testing. Br J Pharmacol 167: 932–945.
13. Winslow RL, Trayanova N, Geman D, Miller MI (2012) Computational medicine: translating models to clinical care. Sci Transl Med 4: 158.
14. Ten Tusscher KH, Panfilov AV (2006) Alternans and spiral breakup in a human ventricular tissue model. Am J Physiol Heart Circ Physiol 291: H1088–1100.
15. Rudy Y, Silva JR (2006) Computational biology in the study of cardiac ion channels and cell electrophysiology. Q Rev Biophys 39: 57–116.
16. Yang L, Korge P, Weiss JN, Qu ZL (2010) Mitochondrial Oscillations and Waves in Cardiac Myocytes: Insights from Computational Models. Biophys J 98: 1428–1438.
17. Vaquero M, Calvo D, Jalife J (2008) Cardiac Fibrillation: From Ion Channels to Rotors in the Human Heart. Heart Rhythm 5: 872–879.
18. Moody GB, Mark RG (2001) The impact of the MIT-BIH Arrhythmia Database. IEEE Eng in Med and Biol 20: 45–50.
19. Casaleggio A, Maestri R, La Rovere MT, Rossi P, Pinna GD (2007) Prediction of sudden death in heart failure patients: a novel perspective from the assessment of the peak ectopy rate. Europace 9: 385–390.
20. Hines M, Carnevale NT (1997) The NEURON simulation environment. Neural Comp 9: 1179–1209.
21. Beeler G, Reuter H (1977) Reconstruction of the action potential of ventricular myocardial fibres J Physiol 268, 177–210.

22. De Boer TP, van der Heyden MA, Rook MB, Wilders R, Broekstra R, et al. (2006) Pro-arrhythmogenic potential of immature cardiomyocytes is triggered by low coupling and cluster size. Cardiovasc Res 71: 704–714.

23. Spitzer KW, Pollard AE,Yang L, Zaniboni M, Cordeiro JM, et al. (2006) Cell-to-Cell Electrical Interactions During Early and Late Repolarization. J Cardiovasc Electrophysiol 17: S8–S14 (Suppl. 1).

24. Anumonwo JMB,Wang HZ, Trabka-Janik E, Dunham B, Veenstra RD, et al. (1992) Gap junctional channels in adult mammalian sinus nodal cells. Immunolocalization and electrophysiology. Circ Res 71: 229–239.

25. Moreno AP (2004) Biophysical properties of homomeric and heteromultimeric channels formed by cardiac connexins. Cardiovasc Res 62: 276–286.

26. Desplantez T, Halliday D, Dupont E, Weingart R (2004) Cardiac connexins Cx43 and Cx45: formation of diverse gap junction channels with diverse electrical properties. Pflugers Arch - Eur J Physiol 448: 363–375.

27. Rackauskas M, Kreuzberg MM, Pranevicius M, Willecke K, Verselis VK, et al. (2007) Gating properties of heterotypic gap junction channels formed of connexins 40, 43, and 45. Biophys J 92: 1952–1965.

28. Luke RA, Saffitz JE (1991) Remodeling of ventricular conduction pathways in healed canine infarct border zones. J Clin Invest 87: 1594–1602.

29. Kleber AG, Riegger CB, Janse MJ (1987) Electrical uncoupling and increase of extracellular resistance after induction of ischemia in isolated, arterially perfused rabbit papillary muscle. Circ Res 61 271–279.

30. De Groot JR, Coronel R (2004) Acute ischemia-induced gap junctional uncoupling and arrhythmogenesis. Cardiovasc Res 62: 323–334.

31. Peters NS, Coromilas J, Severs NJ, Wit AL (1997) Disturbed Connexin43 Gap Junction Distribution Correlates With the Location of Reentrant Circuits in the Epicardial Border Zone of Healing Canine Infarcts That Cause Ventricular Tachycardia. Circulation. 95: 988–996.

32. Stevenson WG, Friedman PL, Sager PT, Saxon LA, Kocoviz D, et al. (1997) Exploring Postinfarction Reentrant Ventricular Tachycardia With Entrainment Mapping. JACC 29: 1180–1189.

33. Jansen JA, van Veen TA, de Bakker JM, van Rijen HV (2010) Cardiac connexins and impulse propagation. J Mol Cell Cardiol 48: 76–82.

34. Chen FFT, Vaughan-Jones RD, Clarke K, Noble D (1998) Modelling myocardial ischaemia and reperfusion. Progress in Biophysics and Molecular Biology 69: 515–538.

35. Nerbonne JM, Kass RS (2005) Molecular physiology of cardiac repolarization. Physiol Rev 85: 1205–1253.

36. Goldberger AL, Amaral LAN, Glass L, Hausdorff JM, Ivanov PC, et al. (2000) PhysioBank, PhysioToolkit, and PhysioNet: Components of a New Research Resource for Complex Physiologic Signals. Circulation 101: e215–e220.

37. Severs NJ, Bruce AF, Dupont E, Rothery S (2008) Remodelling of gap junctions and connexin expression in diseased myocardium. Cardiovasc Res 80: 9–19.

38. Woie L, Eftestol T, Engan K, Kvaloy JT, Nilsen DWT, et al. (2011) The heart rate of ventricular tachycardia following an old myocardial infarction is inversely related to the size of scarring. Europace 13: 864–868.

39. Worley SJ (1998) Use of a real-time three-dimensional magnetic navigation system for radiofrequency ablation of accessory pathways. PACE 21: 1636–1645.

40. Prasad SM, Maniar HS, Camillo CJ, Schuessler RB, Boineau JP, et al. (2003) The Cox maze III procedure for atrial fibrillation: long-term efficacy in patients undergoing lone versus concomitant procedures. J Thorac Cardiovasc Surg 126: 1822–1828.

41. Hennan JK, Swillo RE, Morgan GA, Keith JC, Schaub RG, et al. (2006) Rotigaptide (ZP123) prevents spontaneous ventricular arrhythmias and reduces infarct size during myocardial ischemia/reperfusion injury in open-chest dogs. J Pharmacol Exp Ther 317: 236–243.

42. Eckardt L, Haverkamp W, Breithardt G (2002) Antiarrhythmic therapy in heart failure. Heart Fail Monit 2: 110–119.

43. Volman V, Perc M, Bazhenov M (2011) Gap junctions and epileptic seizures-two sides of the same coin? PLoS One. 6: e20572. doi: 10.1371/journal.pone.0020572.

44. Bruzzone R, White WT, Paul DL (1996) Connection with connexins: the molecular basis of direct intercellular signaling. Eur J Biochem 138: 1–27.

45. Fontes MS, van Veen TA, de Bakker JM, van Rijen HV (2012) Functional consequences of abnormal Cx43 expression in the heart. Biochim Biophys Acta. 1818: 2020–2029.

46. Takemoto Y, Takanari H, Honjo H, Ueda N, Harada M, et al. (2012) Inhibition of intercellular coupling stabilizes spiral-wave reentry, whereas enhancement of the coupling destabilizes the reentry in favor of early termination. Am J Physiol Heart Circ Physiol 303: H578–586. doi: 10.1152/ajpheart.00355.2012 Epub 2012 Jun 15.

47. Tchou GD, Wirka RC, Van Wagoner DR, Barnard J, Chung MK, et al. (2012) Low prevalence of connexin-40 gene variants in atrial tissues and blood from atrial fibrillation subjects. BMC Med Genet 13: 102.

48. Dupont E, Ko YS, Rothery S, Coppen SR, Baghai M, et al. (2001) The Gap-Junctional Protein Connexin40 Is Elevated in Patients Susceptible to Postoperative Atrial Fibrillation. Circulation 103: 842–849.

49. Chaldoupi SM, Loh P, Hauer RN, de Bakker JM, van Rijen HV (2009) The role of connexin40 in atrial fibrillation. Cardiovasc Res 84: 15–23.

50. Gollob MH (2006) Cardiac connexins as candidate genes for idiopathic atrial fibrillation. Curr Opin Cardiol 21: 155–158.

51. Holzem KM, Efimov IR (2012) Arrhythmogenic remodelling of activation and repolarization in the failing human heart. Europace 14: v50–v57.

52. Huang XD, Sandusky GE, Zipes DP (1999) Heterogeneous loss of connexin43 protein in ischemic dog hearts. J Cardiovasc Electrophysiol 10: 79–91.

53. Beardslee MA, Lerner DL, Tadros PN, Laing JG, Beyer EC, et al. (2000) Dephosphorylation and intracellular redistribution of ventricular connexin43 during electrical uncoupling induced by ischemia. Circ Res 87: 656–662.

54. Xing D, Kjølbye AL, Nielsen MS, Petersen JS, Harlow KW, et al. (2003) ZP123 increases gap junctional conductance and prevents Reentrant ventricular tachycardia during myocardial ischemia in open chest dogs. J Cardiovasc Electrophysiol 14: 510–552.

55. Kjølbye AL, Haugan K, Hennan JK, Petersen JS (2007) Pharmacological modulation of gap junction function with the novel compound rotigaptide: a promising new principle for prevention of arrhythmias. Basic Clin Pharmacol Toxicol 101: 215–230.

56. Schotten U, Verheule S, Kirchhof P, Goette A (2011). Pathophysiological mechanisms of atrial fibrillation: a translational appraisal. Physiol Rev 91: 265–325.

12

Bleeding Risk and Mortality of Edoxaban: A Pooled Meta-Analysis of Randomized Controlled Trials

Shuang Li[⊃], Baoxin Liu[⊃], Dachun Xu*, Yawei Xu*

Department of Cardiology, Shanghai Tenth People's Hospital, Tongji University School of Medicine, Shanghai, China

Abstract

Objective(s): Edoxaban, a factor Xa inhibitor, is a new oral anticoagulant that has been developed as an alternative to vitamin K antagonists. However, its safety remains unexplored.

Methods: Medline, Embase and Web of Science were searched to March 8, 2014 for prospective, randomized controlled trials (RCTs) that assessed the safety profile of edoxaban with warfarin. Safety outcomes examined included bleeding risk and mortality.

Results: Five trials including 31,262 patients that met the inclusion criteria were pooled. Overall, edoxaban was associated with a significant decrease in major or clinically relevant nonmajor bleeding events [risk ratio (RR) 0.78, 95% confidence interval (CI) 0.74 to 0.82, p<0.001] and any bleeding events [RR 0.82, 95% CI 0.79 to 0.85, p<0.001]. Edoxaban also showed superiority to warfarin both in all-cause mortality [RR 0.92, 95% CI0.85 to0.99, p = 0.02] and cardiovascular mortality [RR 0.87, 95% CI0.79 to 0.96, p = 0.004]. Subgroup analyses indicated that RRs of edoxaban 30, 60 or 120 mg/d were 0.67 (p<0.001), 0.87 (p<0.001) and 3.3 (p = 0.004) respectively in major or clinically relevant nonmajor bleeding; 0.71 (p<0.001), 0.89 (p< 0.001) and 2.29 (p = 0.002) respectively in any bleeding; as well as 0.86 (p = 0.01), 0.87 (p = 0.01) and 0.28 (p = 0.41) respectively in cardiovascular death... Meanwhile, paramount to note that pooled results other than the largest trial showed edoxaban was still associated with a decrease in the rate of major or clinically relevant nonmajor bleeding event (p = 0.02) and any bleeding (p = 0.002), but neither in all-cause death (p = 0.66) nor cardiovascular death (p = 0.70).

Conclusions: Edoxaban, a novel orally available direct factor Xa inhibitor, seems to have a favorable safety profiles with respect to bleeding risk and non-inferior in mortality when compared to warfarin. Further prospective RCTs are urgently needed to confirm the results of this meta-analysis.

Editor: Adrian V. Hernandez, Universidad Peruana de Ciencias Aplicadas (UPC), Peru

Funding: This work was supported partly by grants from National Natural Science Foundation of China (Grant No. 81270256 and 81070107; Grant NO. 81270194). The funders had no role in study design, data collection and analysis, decision to publish, or preparation of the manuscript.

Competing Interests: The authors have declared that no competing interests exist.

* E-mail: xdc77@aliyun.com (DX); xuyawei@tongji.edu.cn (YX)

[⊃] These author contributed equally to this work.

Introduction

For many decades, vitamin K antagonists (VKAs) were the only available therapy for long-term anticoagulation.[1,2] However, VKAs exhibit a considerable variability in dose response among patients, participate in multiple food and drug interactions, and have a narrow therapeutic window.[3,4] These limitations has prompted the development of a series of new oral anticoagulants (OACs) as alternatives to VKAs, including direct thrombin inhibitors such as dabigatran as well as direct factor Xa inhibitors including rivaroxaban, apixaban, and edoxaban. These new OACs appear to offer practical advantages over VKAs, with fewer food and drug interactions, a fixed daily or weekly dose, and no need for monitoring of the anticoagulant effect.[5] Several large randomized clinical trials (RCTs) have already been compared these new OACs with VKAs and two trials were cited by the European Society of Cardiology (ESC) to recommend a recently updated guideline for dabigatran and rivaroxaban as preferable to VKA for preventing stroke and other thromboem-bolic events in the vast majority of people with atrial fibrillation (AF) [6].

Edoxaban is a latest factor Xa inhibitor with several studies investigating the efficacy and safety for different indications. However, the risk for bleeding and mortality associated with this drug remains unexplored comprehensively. We therefore performed a systematic meta-analysis to compare the safety of rivaroxaban with standard VKAs therapy (warfarin), particularly focusing on bleeding and mortality.

Materials and Methods

Search Criteria

We performed a computerized search to identify relevant RCTs using Medline (via PubMed, from inception to March 8, 2014), Embase (via OVID, from 1966 to 2014), and Web of Science (including databases of SCI-EXPANDED, SSCI, A&HCI, CPCI-S, CCR-EXPANDED, IC, from 1984 to 2014) for comparing the safety of edoxaban with warfarin. We used the following keywords:

```
┌─────────────────────────────────────┐
│ 2,075 studies identified in database │
│   search                             │
│     412 from Medline                 │
│     601 from Embase                  │
│   1,062 from Web of Science          │
└─────────────────────────────────────┘
                │
                │              ┌────────────────────────────────┐
                │              │ 1,388 excluded as Publication  │
                │─────────────▶│ Type was not RCT based on      │
                │              │ mechanical    search    of     │
                ▼              │ individual database            │
┌─────────────────────────────┐└────────────────────────────────┘
│ 687 potential RCTs included │
└─────────────────────────────┘
                │              ┌────────────────────────────────┐
                │              │ 672 excluded based on title    │
                │─────────────▶│ and abstract                   │
                │              │     389  duplication           │
                ▼              │     167  not RCT               │
┌─────────────────────────────┐│     116  no edoxaban           │
│ 15 full-text assessed for   │└────────────────────────────────┘
│ eligibility                 │
└─────────────────────────────┘
                │              ┌────────────────────────────────┐
                │              │ 10 articles excluded:          │
                │─────────────▶│     5  no available results    │
                │              │     4  short duration          │
                ▼              │     1  secondary analysis      │
┌─────────────────────────────┐└────────────────────────────────┘
│ 5 relevant studies for      │
│ further meta-analysis       │
└─────────────────────────────┘
```

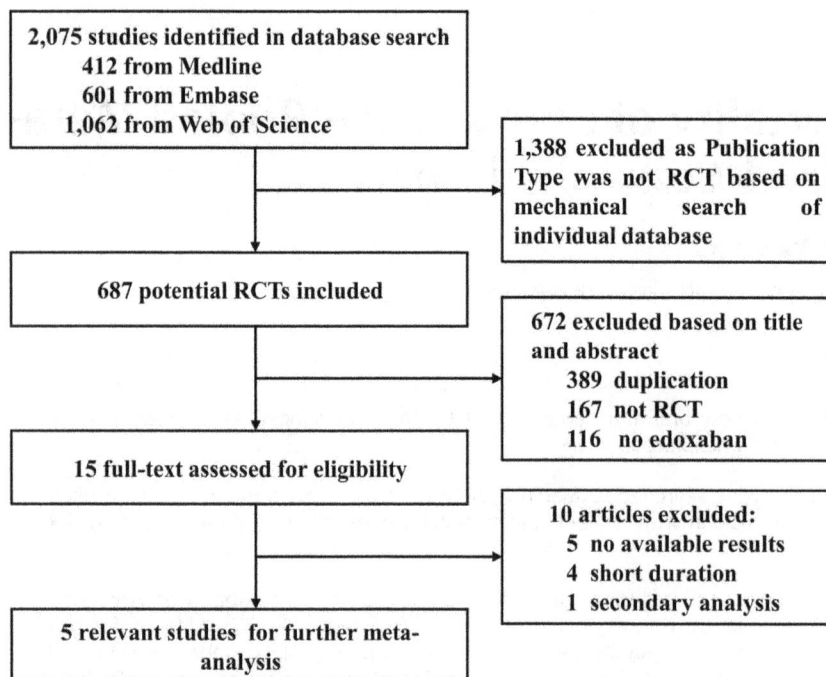

Figure 1. Flow Diagram of Selection Strategy. Flow diagram depicting the selection strategy for trials used in this meta-analysis. Please note that when we meant the phrase of 'no available data', we meant that there was no associated result that matched the end-point outcomes of our meta-analysis. **RCT** denotes randomized clinical trial, **SCIE** Science Citation Index Expanded databases.

"new oral anticoagulants", "edoxaban", "factor Xa inhibitor", and "Warfarin" No language restrictions. Publication type was limited to be RCT. We also attempted to contact authors of included study, and even asked a product manager of Daiichi Sankyo Pharma Development, the manufacturer of edoxaban for any unpublished data.

Study selection

Studies were eligible to be included in our meta-analysis if they (1) were prospectively randomized patients to receive either edoxaban or warfarin (2) had treatment duration for at least 3 months (3) had certain safety outcomes the events of bleeding risk or mortality. No restrictions were placed on population size or languages. We excluded studies that were retrospective or nonrandomized or those in which patients were not randomized to receive the edoxaban used. Letters to the editor, editorials, reviews, and abstracts from conference proceedings were also excluded from our study. All studies were reviewed independently by Dr. Yawei Xu and Dr. Dachun Xu, who have more than 30 and 20 years respectively of experience as electrophysiological cardiologists to determine whether they match the eligibility for inclusion. A kappa value was calculated to assess the degree of agreement.

Data extraction

Data were independently extracted by another two reviewers (Shuang Li, Baoxin Liu) and disagreements were resolved by consensus. Attempts were made to retrieve the data directly from the published papers or sent mails to authors for acquiring data not published. Demographic and clinical characteristics of each trial were recorded, including age, gender, numbers of subjects, information about hypertension, diabetes, congestive heart failure, previous warfarin use, prior stroke, each event of bleeding and mortality from included trials.

Risk of bias in included studies

We used the Cochrane Collaboration's recommended tool for assessing the risk of bias in included studies [7]. Trials' quality was assessed by evaluating every element of study design: blinding description, randomization process, inclusion and exclusion criteria, concealed allocation, intention-to-treat analysis, and assessment of withdrawals and dropouts. Risk for bias was assessed in duplicate, with disagreements resolved by consensus.

Assessment of Heterogeneity

We tested heterogeneity between trial results with the Cochrane Chi-square test and I^2 statistics (percentage of total variation across studies due to heterogeneity). A I^2 of 0–25% indicates no observed heterogeneity, and larger values show increasing heterogeneity, with 25–50% defined as low, 50–75% as moderate, and above 75% as high heterogeneity, respectively [8].

Data Synthesis and Analysis

All analyses were performed with review manager software (RevMan Analyses Version 5.2.4 Copenhagen; The Nordic Cochrane Center, The Cochrane Collaboration, 2013). The primary safety end-points of our meta-analysis were bleeding events (major or clinically relevant non-major bleeding event, any bleeding events) and mortality (all-cause death, cardiovascular death for patients received edoxaban or warfarin. Meanwhile, we also reported major bleeding event, clinically relevant non-major bleeding and minor bleeding.

Subgroup analyses of different fixed doses of edoxaban were performed. We calculated a weighted estimate of the typical treatment effect across trials using risk ratio (RR) by means of a

Table 1. Risk of bias in included studies.

Study	Type of Blinding	Method of Blinding Described and Appropriated	Randomization Process Described and Adequate	Adequate Concealed Allocation	Description of Withdrawals and Dropouts	Intention-to-Treat Analysis Performed	Important Baseline Differences Present	Inclusion and Exclusion Criteria Specified
ENGAGE AF-TIMI 48 [9]	Double	Yes	Yes	Yes	Yes	Yes	Yes	Yes
Hokusai-VTE [10]	Double	Yes	Yes	Yes	Yes	Yes	Yes	Yes
Yamashita, 2012 [11]	Double	Yes	NR	Yes	Yes	NR	Yes	Yes
Chung, 2011 [12]	Double	Yes	Yes	Yes	Yes	Yes	Yes	Yes
Weitz, 2010 [13]	Double	Yes	Yes	Yes	Yes	Yes	NR	NR

Risk of bias in included studies were evaluated every element of study design: blinding description, randomization process, inclusion and exclusion criteria, concealed allocation, intention-to-treat analysis, and assessment of withdrawals and dropouts. **NR** = not reported.

fixed-effect model. However, in the study with moderate to high heterogeneity ($I^2 > 50\%$), a random-effect model was performed. RRs and their two-sided 95% confidence intervals (CI) were reported. A 95% CI not including 1 and $p < 0.05$ were considered statistically significant.

Results

1. Literature searching

As shown in Figure 1, three databases were searched until March 8, 2014 (Table S1–3). A total of 2,075 articles were reviewed, of which1, 388 articles were initially rejected because they were not RCTs based on mechanical search in individual database. Then 672 potential ones were excluded based on title and abstract. Of the rest of 15 remaining studies with full-text assessment, 10 had no available data or short duration <3 months or were secondary analysis (Table S4), that might be no association with potential bias. Finally, five RCTs [9,10,11,12,13] met our inclusion criteria and were included in our study. No additional data was found either from authors' responses or the internal database of Daiichi Sankyo Pharma Development, the manufacturer of edoxaban. All included processes were performed independently by Dr. Yawei Xu and Dr. Dachun Xu. The kappa value was 0.82, reflecting excellent agreement.

2. The methodological quality of the included trials

We assessed quality of the included trials using the Cochrane Collaboration's recommended tool for assessing the risk of bias in included studies[7]. Overall, all 5 trials were designed to be randomized and double-blind with a relatively low risk for bias (Table 1).

3. Characteristics of patients and trials

A total of 31,262 subjects were included. Among the included studies, sample sizes ranged from 235[12] to 21,105[9]. Patients were predominantly men and received treatment for nonvalvular atrial fibrillation (NVAF, n = 23,022[9,11,12,13]), deep vein thrombosis (DVT, n = 4,921[10]), or pulmonary embolism (PE, n = 3,319[10]). The median treatment duration ranged from 12 weeks (3 months) [11,12,13] to 907[9] days and follow-up ranged from 2 months [11] to 1022 days[9]. Efficacy endpoints differed among those studies; however, safety outcomes (i.e., bleeding or mortality) were included. Safety analyses included all patients who received more than 30 mg/d dose of edoxaban or open-label adjusted dose of warfarin, maintaining international normalized ratio (INR) 2–3. (Table 2)

4. Outcome Measures Reporting

4.1 Definitions of Bleeding. The trials included in our study reported several bleeding and mortality outcomes (Table 3). Across all included studies, bleeding events were reported including major or clinically relevant nonmajor bleeding event, major bleeding (any, fatal, gastrointestinal and intracranial), clinically relevant nonmajor bleeding, minor bleeding, fatal bleeding, any bleeding et al. All trials stated the declaration that all suspected bleeding events were assessed by an independent blinded adjudication committee.

Definitions of bleeding event (major bleeding, clinically relevant nonmajor bleeding event and minor bleeding) among the included trials were similar. Major bleeding was defined as bleeding that was fatal or in a critical site (intracranial, intraocular, intraspinal, retroperitoneal, intra-articular, pericardial, or intramuscular with compartment syndrome) or overt and associated with a decline in haemoglobin of ≥2 g/dl or requiring transfusion of ≥2 units of

Table 2. Patient- and study-level characteristics of randomized controlled trials comparing edoxaban to warfarin.

Characteristics	ENGAGE AF-TIMI 48		Hokusai-VTE		Yamashita, 2012		Chung, 2011		Weitz, 2010	
	Edoxaban	Warfarin	Edoxaban	Warfarin	Edoxaban	Warfarin	Edoxaban	Warfarin	Edoxaban	Warfarin
Year	2013		2013		2012		2011		2010	
Country	1393 centers in 46 countries		439 centers in 37 countries		61 centers in Japan		4 Asian countries		91 centers in 12 countries	
Period	2008.11–2010.11		2010.1–2012.12		2007.4–2008.7		2007.10–2008.10		2007.7–2010.10	
Study Design	RCT, phase III		RCT, phase III		RCT, phase II		RCT, phase II		RCT, phase II	
Population	NVAF		DVT±PE		NVAF		NVAF		NVAF	
Subjects, n	21105		8240		536		235		1146	
Dose	30/60 mg/d, QD	adjusted (INR 2–3)	30/60 mg/d, QD	adjusted (INR 2–3)	30,45,60 mg/d, QD	adjusted (INR 2–3 for age <70;1.6–2.6 for age ≥70)	30,60 mg/d, QD	adjusted (INR 2–3)	30,60 mg/d, QD or BID	adjusted (INR 2–3)
Age (year)*	72(64–78)	72(64–78)	55.7±16.3	55.9±16.2	69.1	68.8	64.5±9.5	61.5±8.5	65±8.7	66±8.75
Male/Female, %	61.6/38.4	62.5/37.5	57.3/42.7	57.2/42.8	82.3/17.7	83/17	66.7/33.3	62.7/37.3	62.6/37.4	60.4/39.6
Previous warfarin use, %	59	58.8	NR	NR	84.3	86	50.3	54.7	64.3	64.8
DM, %	36.3	35.8	NR	NR	20.2	31	32.7	22.7	NR	NR
HTN, %	93.6	63.9	NR	NR	73.5	71.3	72.3	69.3	NR	NR
Prior stroke or TIA, %	28.3	28.3	NR	NR	27	30.2	25.2	22.7	NR	NR
Congestive HF, %	57.4	57.5	NR	NR	25.3	33.3	27	32	NR	NR
Treatment duration	907 days (Medium)		3–12 months		12 weeks		3 months		3 months	
Follow-up	1022 days (Medium)		12 months		8 weeks		3 months		3 months	

*measure as mean ±SD or median (interquartile range).

NVAF denotes nonvalvular atrial fibrillation; DVT deep vein thrombosis; PE pulmonary embolism; INR international normalized ratio ; QD que die; BID bis in die; NA not applicable; VKA vitamin K antagonist; TIA transient ischemic attack; HF heart failure; DM diabetes mellitus; HTN hypertension.

Table 3. Study outcomes as reported in randomized controlled trials comparing edoxaban to warfarin.

Outcome*	ENGAGE AF-TIMI 48[7]		Hokusai-VTE[8]		Yamashita, 2012[9]		Chung, 2011[10]		Weitz, 2010[11]	
	Edoxaban (n = 14014)	Warfarin (n = 7012)	Edoxaban (n = 4118)	Warfarin (n = 4112)	Edoxaban (n = 394)	Warfarin (n = 125)	Edoxaban (n = 159)	Warfarin (n = 75)	Edoxaban (n = 893)	Warfarin (n = 250)
Major or clinically relevant nonmajor bleeding event, n	2689	1761	349	423	16	4	6	5	54	8
Major bleeding, n										
Any	672	524	56	66	5	0	0	2	12	1
Fatal	52	59	2	10	NR	NR	NR	NR	NR	NR
Gastrointestinal	361	190	1	2	NR	NR	NR	NR	NR	NR
Intracranial-Fatal	36	42	NR	NR	NR	NR	NR	NR	NR	NR
Intracranial-Any	102	132	0	6	NR	NR	NR	NR	NR	NR
Clinically relevant nonmajor bleeding, n	2183	1396	298	368	NR	NR	6	3	42	7
Minor Bleeding, n	1137	714	NR	NR	76	21	48	17	NR	NR
Any bleeding, n	3564	2114	895	1056	90	25	35	22	94	20
Any-cause death, n	1612	839	132	126	NR	NR	NR	NR	NR	NR
Cardiovascular mortality, n	1057	611	15	12	NR	NR	NR	NR	6	2

*Event rates were based on the intention-to-treat population unless otherwise specified.

Study or Subgroup	Edoxaban Events	Total	Warfarin Events	Total	Weight	Risk Ratio M-H, Fixed, 95% CI	Year
2.6.1 Major or clinically relevant nonmajor bleeding event							
Weitz 2010	54	893	8	250	0.2%	1.89 [0.91, 3.92]	2010
Chung 2011	6	159	5	75	0.1%	0.57 [0.18, 1.80]	2011
Yamashita 2012	16	394	4	125	0.1%	1.27 [0.43, 3.73]	2012
ENGAGE AF-TIMI 48	2689	14014	1761	7012	34.7%	0.76 [0.72, 0.81]	2013
Hokusai-VTE	349	4118	423	4112	6.3%	0.82 [0.72, 0.94]	2013
Subtotal (95% CI)		**19578**		**11574**	**41.3%**	**0.78 [0.74, 0.82]**	
Total events	3114		2201				

Heterogeneity: Chi² = 7.93, df = 4 (P = 0.09); I² = 50%
Test for overall effect: Z = 9.98 (P < 0.00001)

2.6.2 Any bleeding events							
Weitz 2010	94	893	20	250	0.5%	1.32 [0.83, 2.09]	2010
Chung 2011	35	159	22	75	0.4%	0.75 [0.48, 1.19]	2011
Yamashita 2012	90	394	25	125	0.6%	1.14 [0.77, 1.70]	2012
ENGAGE AF-TIMI 48	3365	14014	2114	7012	41.6%	0.80 [0.76, 0.83]	2013
Hokusai-VTE	895	4118	1056	4112	15.6%	0.85 [0.78, 0.91]	2013
Subtotal (95% CI)		**19578**		**11574**	**58.7%**	**0.82 [0.79, 0.85]**	
Total events	4479		3237				

Heterogeneity: Chi² = 8.94, df = 4 (P = 0.06); I² = 55%
Test for overall effect: Z = 10.10 (P < 0.00001)

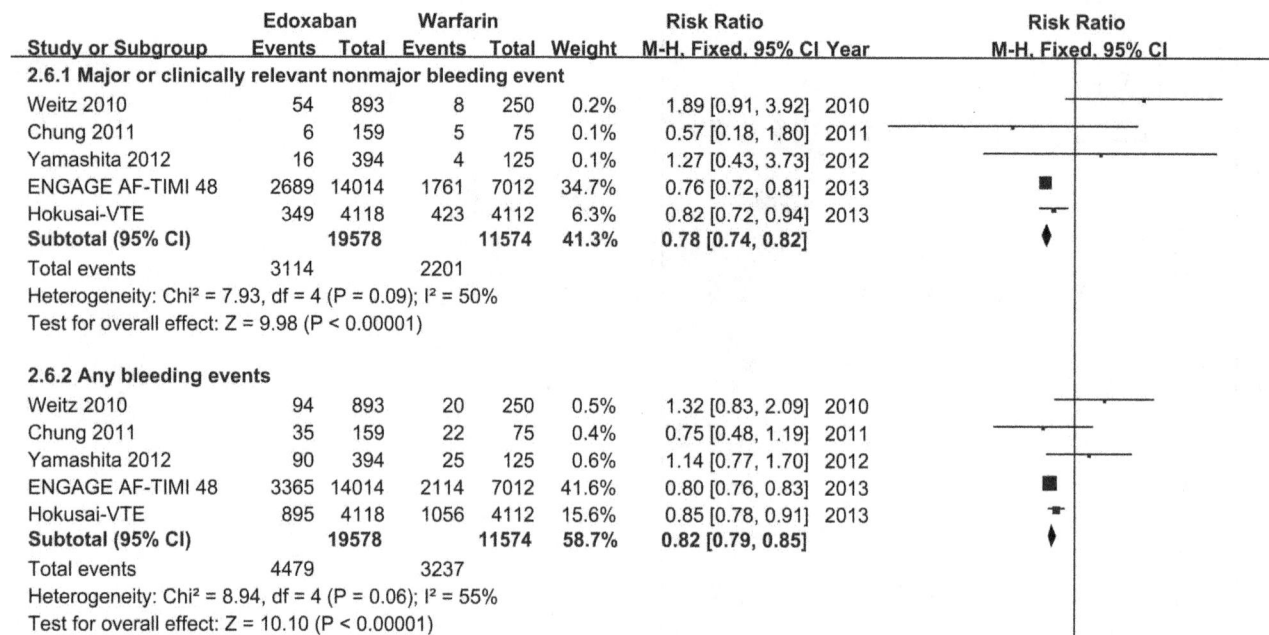

Figure 2. Forest Plot of risk ratios of bleeding events for comparison edoxaban with warfarin. A series of forest plots of risk ratios (RRs) of bleeding events for comparison of given edoxaban or warfarin according to every trial were pooled. All five trials (n = 31,262) reported events of major or clinically relevant nonmajor bleeding event and any bleeding. CI confidence interval.

blood [9,10,11,13], which consistent to the definition by the International Society on Thrombosis and Haemostasis [14] or plus transfusion≥800 ml of packed red blood cells or whole blood [12]. Clinically relevant nonmajor bleeding was defined as overt bleeding that did not meet the criteria for major bleeding but was associated with the need for medical intervention [9,10], or did not meet the criteria for major bleeding but consisting of hematoma≥5 cm in diameter/≥25 cm2; epistaxis or gingival bleeding ≥5 min in the absence of external factors[11,12,13]. Minor bleeding was defined as any bleeding that did not meet the criteria for a major or clinically relevant nonmajor bleeding event

[9,13] and included macroscopic haematuria; occult haematuria≥ 2+; occult haematuria with microscopic (RBC)≥10/high power field; ecchymosis, epistaxis and gingival bleeding occurring without any external stimuli [11,12]. Fatal bleeding was not separately defined [9,10].

4.2 The primary outcomes. All 5 trials (19,578 received edoxaban and 11,574 received warfarin) reported events of major or clinically relevant nonmajor bleeding event, and any bleeding. When data were pooled across the included studies, we found that edoxaban was associated with a decrease in major or clinically relevant nonmajor bleeding [RR 0.78, 95% CI0.74 to 0.82, p<

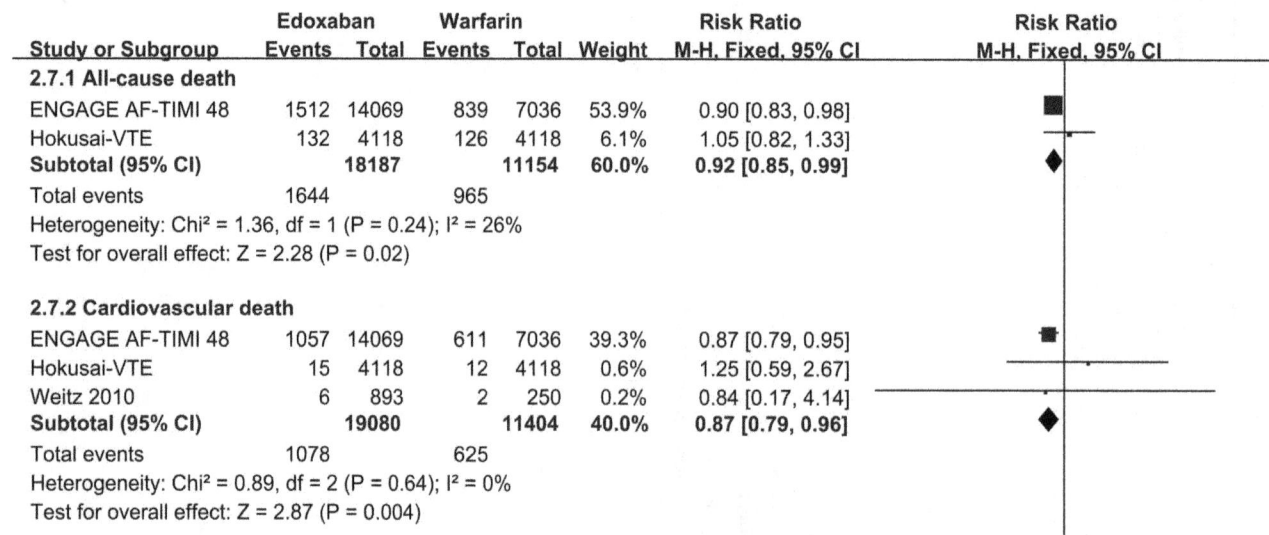

Study or Subgroup	Edoxaban Events	Total	Warfarin Events	Total	Weight	Risk Ratio M-H, Fixed, 95% CI
2.7.1 All-cause death						
ENGAGE AF-TIMI 48	1512	14069	839	7036	53.9%	0.90 [0.83, 0.98]
Hokusai-VTE	132	4118	126	4118	6.1%	1.05 [0.82, 1.33]
Subtotal (95% CI)		**18187**		**11154**	**60.0%**	**0.92 [0.85, 0.99]**
Total events	1644		965			

Heterogeneity: Chi² = 1.36, df = 1 (P = 0.24); I² = 26%
Test for overall effect: Z = 2.28 (P = 0.02)

2.7.2 Cardiovascular death						
ENGAGE AF-TIMI 48	1057	14069	611	7036	39.3%	0.87 [0.79, 0.95]
Hokusai-VTE	15	4118	12	4118	0.6%	1.25 [0.59, 2.67]
Weitz 2010	6	893	2	250	0.2%	0.84 [0.17, 4.14]
Subtotal (95% CI)		**19080**		**11404**	**40.0%**	**0.87 [0.79, 0.96]**
Total events	1078		625			

Heterogeneity: Chi² = 0.89, df = 2 (P = 0.64); I² = 0%
Test for overall effect: Z = 2.87 (P = 0.004)

Figure 3. Forest plots of studies for mortality for comparison edoxaban with warfarin. Forest plots of studies for mortality (from all causes or cardiovascular disease) for comparison edoxaban with warfarin. Two trials (n = 29,256) reported available data. CI confidence interval.

Study or Subgroup	Edoxaban Events	Total	Warfarin Events	Total	Weight	Risk Ratio M-H, Fixed, 95% CI	Risk Ratio M-H, Fixed, 95% CI
2.1.1 Edoxaban 30 mg VS.Warfarin							
Chung 2011	0	79	5	75	0.1%	0.09 [0.00, 1.54]	
ENGAGE AF-TIMI 48	1161	7002	1761	7012	43.2%	0.66 [0.62, 0.71]	
Hokusai-VTE	58	733	423	4112	3.1%	0.77 [0.59, 1.00]	
Weitz 2010	7	235	8	250	0.2%	0.93 [0.34, 2.53]	
Yamashita 2012	2	130	4	125	0.1%	0.48 [0.09, 2.58]	
Subtotal (95% CI)		8179		11574	46.8%	0.67 [0.63, 0.71]	
Total events	1228		2201				
Heterogeneity: Chi² = 3.73, df = 4 (P = 0.44); I² = 0%							
Test for overall effect: Z = 12.39 (P < 0.00001)							
2.1.2 Edoxaban 60 mg VS.Warfarin							
Chung 2011	6	80	5	75	0.1%	1.13 [0.36, 3.53]	
ENGAGE AF-TIMI 48	1528	7012	1761	7012	43.2%	0.87 [0.82, 0.92]	
Hokusai-VTE	291	3385	423	4112	9.4%	0.84 [0.72, 0.96]	
Weitz 2010	28	478	8	250	0.3%	1.83 [0.85, 3.96]	
Yamashita 2012	7	130	4	125	0.1%	1.68 [0.50, 5.61]	
Subtotal (95% CI)		11085		11574	53.1%	0.87 [0.82, 0.92]	
Total events	1860		2201				
Heterogeneity: Chi² = 5.24, df = 4 (P = 0.26); I² = 24%							
Test for overall effect: Z = 5.00 (P < 0.00001)							
2.1.3 Edoxaban 120 mg VS.Warfarin							
Weitz 2010	19	180	8	250	0.2%	3.30 [1.48, 7.37]	
Subtotal (95% CI)		180		250	0.2%	3.30 [1.48, 7.37]	
Total events	19		8				
Heterogeneity: Not applicable							
Test for overall effect: Z = 2.91 (P = 0.004)							

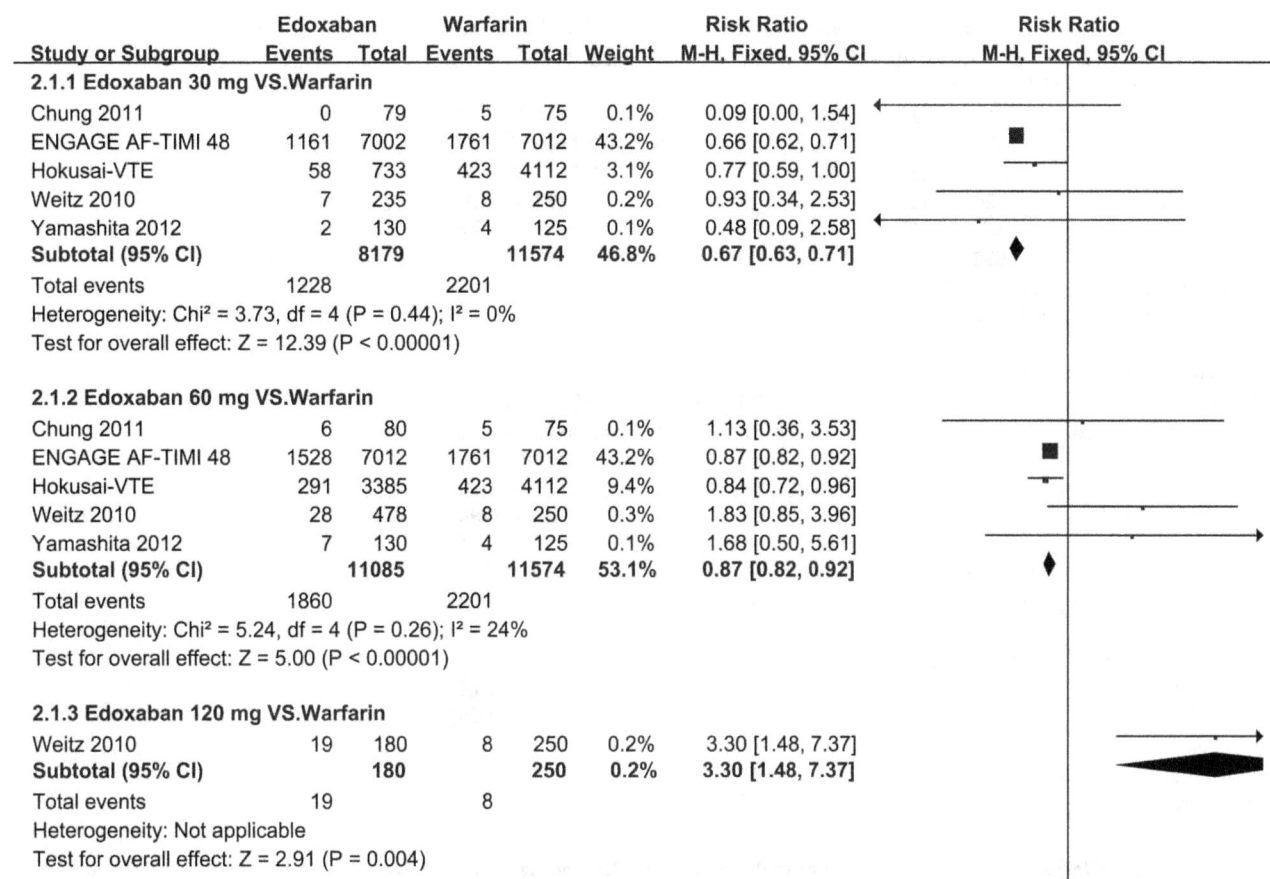

Figure 4. A series of forest plots of risk ratios of major or clinically relevant nonmajor bleeding event for comparison each fixed dose of edoxaban with warfarin. A series of forest plots of risk ratios (RRs) of major or clinically relevant nonmajor bleeding events for comparison each fixed dose of edoxaban (30, 60 or 120 mg per day) with warfarin if data were available. CI confidence interval.

0.001] and any bleeding events [RR 0.82, 95% CI 0.79 to 0.85, p<0.001]. (Figure 2)

Across all 5 studies, 2 trials[9,10] (18,132 receives edoxaban and 11,124 received warfarin) reported available events of all-cause death, and 3 trials[9,10,13] (19,025 receives edoxaban and 11,374 received warfarin) reported events of death as for cardiovascular disease (CVD). Edoxaban also showed superiority to warfarin in reduction rates of both all-cause death [RR 0.92, 95% CI 0.85 to 0.99, p = 0.02] and cardiovascular death [RR 0.87, 95% CI 0.79 to 0.96, p = 0.004]. (Figure 3)

Additionally, we also reported that edoxaban was associated with a decrease in any major bleeding [RR 67, 95% CI 0.60 to 0.74, p<0.001], clinically relevant nonmajor bleeding [RR 0.79, 95% CI 0.75 to 0.84, p<0.001], minor bleeding [RR 1.04, 95% CI 0.95 to 1.14, p = 0.35] and fatal bleeding [RR 0.42, 95% CI 0.29 to 0.60, p<0.001]. (Figure S1)

4.3 The Study of ENGAGE AF-TIMI 48. A pooled analysis of the other RCTs was also performed, other than ENGAGE AF-TIMI 48 (Figure S2 and S3), to compare with the total result. For bleeding risks, pooling results of other trials indicated consistence with the total ones. Edoxaban was still associated with a decrease in major or clinically relevant nonmajor bleeding event [RR 0.80, 95% CI 0.75 to 0.98, p = 0.02] and any bleeding [RR 0.87, 95% CI 0.80 to 0.93, P = 0.002] (Figure S2). For mortality, edoxaban showed no superiority to warfarin in reduction rate of either all-cause death [RR 1.17, 95% CI 0.59 to 2.31, p = 0.66] or

cardiovascular death [RR 1.05, 95% CI 0.82 to 1.33, p = 0.66]. (Figure S3).

4.4 Subgroup meta-analyses. Furthermore, a series of subgroup meta-analyses of different fixed doses (30, 60 or 120 mg/d) of edoxaban in comparison to warfarin were conducted (Table 4, Figure 4–6). As for Weitz 2010[13], we defined the subgroup of "edoxaban 60 mg/d" as the combination of "edoxaban 30 mg bid" and "60 mg qd" in the original protocol for medication.

Generally, relatively lower dose (30 or 60 mg/d) was associated with a decrease both in bleeding risk (Figure 4–5) and cardiovascular mortality (Figure 6) in comparison to warfarin. The RRs of bleeding risk that received edoxaban 30, 60 and 120 mg/d were 0.67 [95% CI 0.63–0.71, p<0.001], 0.87 [95% CI 0.82–0.92, p<0.001] and 3.3 [95% CI 1.48–7.37, p = 0.004] respectively in major or clinically relevant nonmajor bleeding (Figure 4); 0.71 [95% CI 0.67–0.75, p<0.001], 0.89 [95% CI 0.85–0.94, p<0.001] and 2.29 [95% CI 1.36–3.86, p = 0.002] respectively in any bleeding events (Figure 5) to that of warfarin. Meanwhile, every fixed dose was non-inferior to warfarin on reduction rate of cardiovascular mortality (Figure 6). Given 30 mg and 60 mg showed superiority to warfarin (RR 0.86 [95% CI 0.77–0.97, p = 0.01] and 0.87 95% CI 0.78–0.97, p = 0.01] respectively, Figure 6) but no significant difference between each other (p = 0.94). (Table 4)

Study or Subgroup	Edoxaban Events	Total	Warfarin Events	Total	Weight	Risk Ratio M-H, Fixed, 95% CI	Risk Ratio M-H, Fixed, 95% CI
2.3.1 Edoxaban 30 mg VS.Warfali							
Chung 2011	16	79	22	75	0.5%	0.69 [0.39, 1.21]	
ENGAGE AF-TIMI 48	1499	7002	2114	7012	48.2%	0.71 [0.67, 0.75]	
Weitz 2010	13	235	20	250	0.4%	0.69 [0.35, 1.36]	
Yamashita 2012	24	130	25	125	0.6%	0.92 [0.56, 1.53]	
Subtotal (95% CI)		**7446**		**7462**	**49.7%**	**0.71 [0.67, 0.75]**	
Total events	1552		2181				
Heterogeneity: Chi² = 1.05, df = 3 (P = 0.79); I² = 0%							
Test for overall effect: Z = 11.78 (P < 0.00001)							
2.3.2 Edoxaban 60 mg VS.Warfali							
Chung 2011	19	80	22	75	0.5%	0.81 [0.48, 1.37]	
ENGAGE AF-TIMI 48	1865	7012	2114	7012	48.2%	0.88 [0.84, 0.93]	
Weitz 2010	48	478	20	250	0.6%	1.26 [0.76, 2.07]	
Yamashita 2012	36	130	25	125	0.6%	1.38 [0.89, 2.17]	
Subtotal (95% CI)		**7700**		**7462**	**49.9%**	**0.89 [0.85, 0.94]**	
Total events	1968		2181				
Heterogeneity: Chi² = 5.81, df = 3 (P = 0.12); I² = 48%							
Test for overall effect: Z = 4.33 (P < 0.0001)							
2.3.3 Edoxaban 120 mg VS.Warfali							
Weitz 2010	33	180	20	250	0.4%	2.29 [1.36, 3.86]	
Subtotal (95% CI)		**180**		**250**	**0.4%**	**2.29 [1.36, 3.86]**	
Total events	33		20				
Heterogeneity: Not applicable							
Test for overall effect: Z = 3.12 (P = 0.002)							

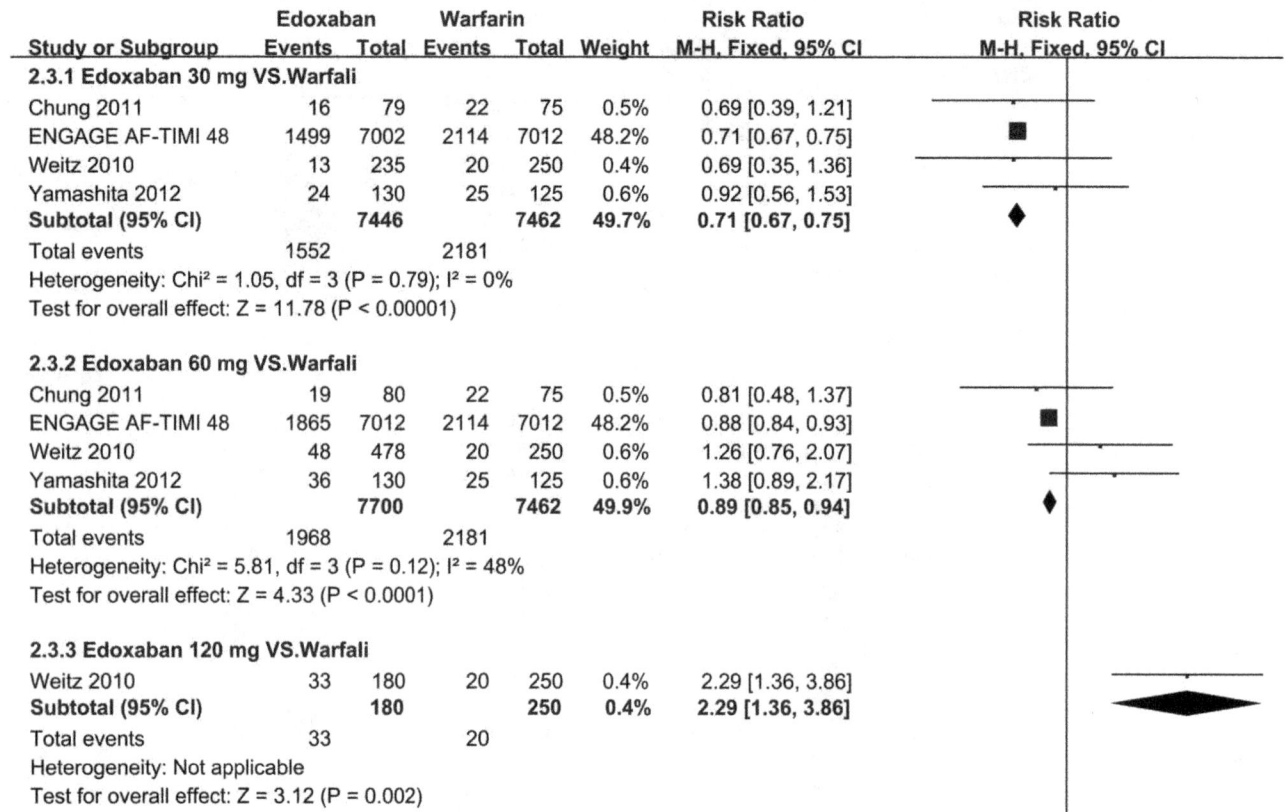

Figure 5. A series of forest plots of risk ratios of any bleeding event for comparison each fixed dose of edoxaban with warfarin. A series of forest plots of risk ratios (RRs) of any bleeding events for comparison each fixed dose of edoxaban (30, 60 or 120 mg/d) with warfarin if data were available. CI confidence interval.

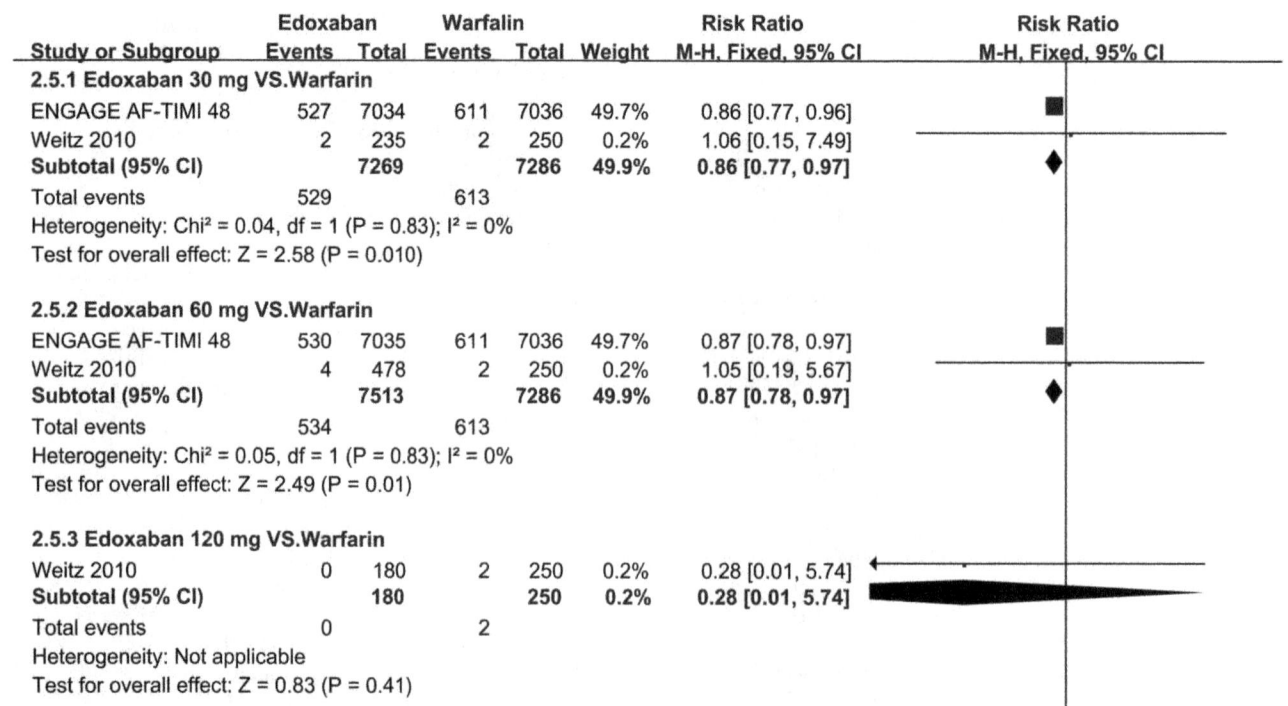

Study or Subgroup	Edoxaban Events	Total	Warfalin Events	Total	Weight	Risk Ratio M-H, Fixed, 95% CI	Risk Ratio M-H, Fixed, 95% CI
2.5.1 Edoxaban 30 mg VS.Warfarin							
ENGAGE AF-TIMI 48	527	7034	611	7036	49.7%	0.86 [0.77, 0.96]	
Weitz 2010	2	235	2	250	0.2%	1.06 [0.15, 7.49]	
Subtotal (95% CI)		**7269**		**7286**	**49.9%**	**0.86 [0.77, 0.97]**	
Total events	529		613				
Heterogeneity: Chi² = 0.04, df = 1 (P = 0.83); I² = 0%							
Test for overall effect: Z = 2.58 (P = 0.010)							
2.5.2 Edoxaban 60 mg VS.Warfarin							
ENGAGE AF-TIMI 48	530	7035	611	7036	49.7%	0.87 [0.78, 0.97]	
Weitz 2010	4	478	2	250	0.2%	1.05 [0.19, 5.67]	
Subtotal (95% CI)		**7513**		**7286**	**49.9%**	**0.87 [0.78, 0.97]**	
Total events	534		613				
Heterogeneity: Chi² = 0.05, df = 1 (P = 0.83); I² = 0%							
Test for overall effect: Z = 2.49 (P = 0.01)							
2.5.3 Edoxaban 120 mg VS.Warfarin							
Weitz 2010	0	180	2	250	0.2%	0.28 [0.01, 5.74]	
Subtotal (95% CI)		**180**		**250**	**0.2%**	**0.28 [0.01, 5.74]**	
Total events	0		2				
Heterogeneity: Not applicable							
Test for overall effect: Z = 0.83 (P = 0.41)							

Figure 6. Forest plots of risk ratios for events of cardiovascular death for comparison each fixed dose of edoxaban with warfarin. Forest plots of risk ratios (RRs) for events of cardiovascular death for comparison each fixed dose of edoxaban with warfarin. CI confidence interval.

Table 4. Subgroup analyses of safety outcomes based on different fixed doses of edoxaban.

Edoxaban*	Warfarin	Trials	Edoxaban Event,n	Edoxaban Total,n	Warfarin Event,n	Warfarin Total,n	RR	95% CI	P value	I² (%)
1. Major or clinically relevant nonmajor bleeding event										
30	Warfarin	Chung 2011	0	79	5	75	0.67	0.63–0.71	<0.001	0
		ENGAGE AF-TIMI 48	1161	7002	1761	7012				
		Hokusai-VTE	58	733	423	4112				
		Weitz 2010	7	235	8	250				
		Yamashita 2012	2	130	4	125				
60	Warfarin	Chung 2011	6	80	5	75	0.87	0.82–0.92	<0.001	24
		ENGAGE AF-TIMI 48	1528	7012	1761	7012				
		Hokusai-VTE	291	3385	423	4112				
		Weitz 2010	28	478	8	250				
		Yamashita 2012	7	130	4	125				
120	Warfarin	Weitz, 2010	19	180	8	250	3.3	1.48–7.37	0.004	NA
2. Any bleeding										
30	Warfarin	Chung 2011	16	79	22	75	0.71	0.67–0.75	<0.001	0
		ENGAGE AF-TIMI 48	1499	7002	2114	7012				
		Weitz 2010	13	235	20	250				
		Yamashita 2012	24	130	25	125				
60	Warfarin	Chung 2011	19	80	22	75	0.89	0.85–0.94	<0.001	48
		ENGAGE AF-TIMI 48	1865	7012	2114	7012				
		Weitz 2010	48	478	20	250				
		Yamashita 2012	36	130	25	125				
120	Warfarin	Weitz 2010	33	180	20	250	2.29	1.36–3.86	0.002	NA
3. Cardiovascular death										
30	Warfarin	ENGAGE AF-TIMI 48	527	7034	611	7036	0.86	0.77–0.97	0.01	0
		Weitz 2010	2	235	2	250				
60	Warfarin	ENGAGE AF-TIMI 48	530	7035	611	7036	0.87	0.78–0.97	0.01	0
		Weitz 2010	4	478	2	250				
120	Warfarin	Weitz 2010	0	180	2	250	0.28	0.01–5.74	0.41	NA

*Dose measured as mg per day.
NA not application; RR risk ratio; CI confidence interval.

Discussion

What is edoxaban?

Our systematical meta-analysis was designed to compare the safety of edoxaban with that warfarin. Edoxaban is a novel, orally available, highly specific, reversible and direct factor Xa inhibitor. It has a linear and predictable pharmacokinetic profile and 62% oral bioavailability[9,15]. It achieves maximum concentration within 1 to 2 hours, and 50% is excreted by the kidney [5,16]. Like other factor Xa inhibitors, edoxaban has a series of favorable profiles, including fewer food and drug interactions, a fixed daily dose, and no need for monitoring of the anticoagulant effect [5], which appears to offer practical advantages over vitamin K antagonists (VKAs).

Bleeding Risk

Prior RCTs have been performed to assess bleeding risk of which 4 RCTs [9,11,12,13] included patients with nonvalvular atrial fibrillation and 1trial [10] with acute venous thromboembolism. Across all studies, 2 trials [11,13] reported given 30 and 60 mg edoxaban were noninferior to warfarin on safety profiles in patients with nonvalvular atrial fibrillation, while 3 trials [9,10,12] found was associated with a significantly lower rate of bleeding. Yamashita [11] also found edoxaban 30, 45, and 60 mg/day was associated with a numerical increase in all bleeding across the dose range but not insignificantly. Hokusai-VTE [10] found similar outcomes of mortality between edoxaban and warfarin but ENGAGE AF-TIMI 48[9] pointed that edoxaban was associated with significantly lower rate of death from cardiovascular causes.

We pooled data from trials and found that (1) in comparison to traditional anticoagulation therapy with warfarin, edoxaban, a new factor Xa inhibitor, has a favorable safety profiles with respect to bleeding risk (major or clinically relevant non-major bleeding event, any bleeding event); (2) For incidence of bleeding event, it seems dose-response effect that lower dose is associated with less bleeding event significantly.

However, in spite of numerous benefits, there are concerns regarding the potential risk for bleeding with edoxaban in practice. Like other factor Xa inhibitors, rivaroxaban and apixaban, there are no standard antidotes for the reversal of edoxaban in general [17]. Some studies indicated that the availability of a reliable factor Xa assay [18] and specific reversal strategies [19] in urgent clinical situations could potentially improve the safety profile of edoxaban, but no particular strategy is well accepted in practice at this time [9]. Also, similar to edoxaban, other new OACs (i.e. dabigatran, rivaroxaban, apixaban) can also be given in fixed doses without routine laboratory monitoring and fewer drug–drug and food–drug interactions than warfarin.

Mortality profiles

Dentali [20] confirmed there were small differences among these new OACs with respect to the prevention of ischemic stroke, myocardial infarction, bleeding, or death. Some prior meta-analyses of efficacy and safety of new OACs versus warfarin have performed. Dentali [21] retrieved 12 studies (3 with dabigatran, 4 with rivaroxaban, 2 with apixaban, and 3 with edoxaban) and reported new OACs significantly reduced total mortality, cardiovascular mortality, intracranial hemorrhage but not major bleeding. Harenberg [22] made a network meta-analysis of dabigatran, rivaroxaban and apixaban from 3 trials and showed there was no difference in all-cause mortality. Miller [23] pooled 3 RCTs given dabigatran, rivaroxaban and apixaban respectively in patients of atrial fibrillation and found that new OACs were more efficacious than warfarin for the prevention of stroke and systemic embolism in patients with AF and with a decreased risk for intracranial bleeding. However, direct studies are still needed in comparison edoxaban to other new OACs to explore whether these are real differences in clinical efficacy and safety.

We found that in comparison to warfarin, edoxaban has a favorable safety profiles with respect to mortality (both all-cause death and cardiovascular death, Figure 3). Each fixed dose, even the highest dose (120 mg/d), was non-inferior to warfarin on reduction cardiovascular mortality (Figure 6). Moreover, given 30 mg and 60 mg showed superiority to warfarin (p<0.001 both, Figure 6) but no significant difference between each other (p = 0.94).

The Trial of ENGAGE AF-TIMI 48

ENGAGE AF-TIMI 48[9], as a large trial, accounted for about 67.5% of participants in the meta-analysis, and therefore its results drove much of the findings. Also, this study shows very promising results, those were almost consistent with the results of our meta-analyses. Thus, it was suspicious to wonder if it was valid of simply summing up the largest trial and smaller ones. For these considerations, a pooled sub-analysis of the other 4 trials, expect ENGAGE AF-TIMI 48[9], was conducted to compare with the total pooling. The results indicated the decrease rate of bleeding risk for edoxaban did not affect by the largest trial, while whether edoxaban could reduce mortality was largely affected. Thus, we summarized a relatively conservative conclusion that when compared with warfarin, edoxaban seems to be superior to reduce the rate of bleeding events, but non-inferior to reduce mortality, based on current evidence from RCTs.

Study strengths and limitations

The strengths of this meta-analysis are the systematic electronic search, the search criteria without language limitation and use of two review authors independently to examine and select studies.

Our meta-analysis is subject to the limitations inherent to all meta-analysis. The major limitation of our study is that the results are based on the comprehensive data of trials with heterogeneous RCTs, including patients with atrial fibrillation [9,11,12,13], deep vein thrombosis[10], and pulmonary embolism [10]. They also differed on population sizes, different protocols of medication, efficacy outcomes, treatment duration and follow-up. We have attempted to account for these differences by conducting subgroup analyses if data were available. However, some limitations still existed and cause potential bias.

Firstly, ENGAGE AF-TIMI 48, as a large trial, accounted for around 67.5% of participants in the meta-analysis, and therefore its results drove much of the findings. Secondary, we attempted to search any unpublished data through mails to authors of each included study and the manufacturer, however, found no additional data[24]. Beside, FDA was not requested for additional data. All five RCTs were funded by Daiichi Sankyo, the manuscript of edoxaban, which may also cause potential source of bias [25]. And, this meta-analysis tested heterogeneity with the Cochrane Chi-square test and I^2 statistics.

Conclusion

A pooled meta-analysis of 5 prospective RCTs and a total of 31262 patients indicated that edoxaban seems to have a favorable safety profiles with respect to bleeding risk and mortality, in comparison to warfarin. However, further prospective RCTs are urgently needed to confirm the results of this meta-analysis.

Supporting Information

Figure S1   Forest Plot of risk ratios of bleeding events for comparison edoxaban with warfarin. A series of forest plots of risk ratios (RRs) of bleeding events for comparison of given edoxaban or warfarin according to every trial were pooled. All 5 trials (n = 31152) reported events of major bleeding, clinically relevant nonmajor bleeding or minor bleeding and any bleeding, as well as 2 trials (n = 29256) reported events of fatal bleeding. CI confidence interval.

Figure S2   Forest Plot of risk ratios of bleeding events for comparison edoxaban with warfarin. A series of forest plots of risk ratios (RRs) of bleeding events for comparison of given edoxaban or warfarin according to every trial were pooled. Other than ENGAGE AF-TIMI 48, other 4 trials (n = 10,157) reported events of major bleeding, clinically relevant nonmajor bleeding, minor bleeding and any bleeding. CI confidence interval.

Figure S3   Forest plots of studies for mortality for comparison edoxaban with warfarin. Forest plots of studies for mortality of all causes or cardiovascular disease for comparison edoxaban with warfarin. Other than ENGAGE AF-TIMI 48, two trials (n = 9,386) reported available data. CVD denotes cardiovascular disease. CI confidence interval.

Table S1   Search criterion of Medline (via PubMed, from inception to March 8, 2014).

Table S2   Search criterion of Embase (via OVID, from 1966 to 2014).

Table S3   Search criterion of Web of Science (from 1984 to 2014).

Table S4   Characteristics of excluded full-text studies.

Checklist S1   PRISMA 2009 Checklist.

Acknowledgments

The authors gratefully acknowledge the assistance of Mr. Biao Zhu, a product manager of Daiichi Sankyo Pharma Development for his assistance in searching available studies, Dr. Yan Wu, MD, of department of Ophthalmology for performing statistical analyses of the data, Dr. Yi Zhang and Qing Xia, of department of Cardiology on Shanghai Tenth People's Hospital affiliated to Tongji University School of Medicine for reviewing language and writing the paper.

Author Contributions

Conceived and designed the experiments: SL DX YX. Performed the experiments: SL BL YX. Analyzed the data: SL BL DX. Contributed reagents/materials/analysis tools: SL BL YX. Wrote the paper: SL BL YX.

References

1. Buller HR, Prins MH, Lensin AW, Decousus H, Jacobson BF, et al. (2012) Oral rivaroxaban for the treatment of symptomatic pulmonary embolism. N Engl J Med 366: 1287–1297.
2. Kearon C, Akl EA, Comerota AJ, Prandoni P, Bounameaux H, et al. (2012) Antithrombotic therapy for VTE disease: Antithrombotic Therapy and Prevention of Thrombosis, 9th ed: American College of Chest Physicians Evidence-Based Clinical Practice Guidelines. Chest 141: e419S–494S.
3. Wasserlauf G, Grandi SM, Filion KB, Eisenberg MJ (2013) Meta-analysis of rivaroxaban and bleeding risk. Am J Cardiol 112: 454–460.
4. Bruins Slot KM, Berge E (2013) Factor Xa inhibitors versus vitamin K antagonists for preventing cerebral or systemic embolism in patients with atrial fibrillation. Cochrane Database Syst Rev 8: CD008980.
5. Mousa SA (2010) Oral direct factor Xa inhibitors, with special emphasis on rivaroxaban. Methods Mol Biol 663: 181–201.
6. Camm AJ, Lip GY, De Caterina R, Savelieva I, Atar D, et al. (2012) 2012 focused update of the ESC Guidelines for the management of atrial fibrillation: an update of the 2010 ESC Guidelines for the management of atrial fibrillation. Developed with the special contribution of the European Heart Rhythm Association. Eur Heart J 33: 2719–2747.
7. Higgins JPT, Green S, Cochrane Collaboration. (2008) Cochrane handbook for systematic reviews of interventions. Chichester, England ; Hoboken, NJ: Wiley-Blackwell. xxi, 649 p. p.
8. Li S, Wu Y, Yu G, Xia Q, Xu Y (2014) Angiotensin II Receptor Blockers Improve Peripheral Endothelial Function: A Meta-Analysis of Randomized Controlled Trials. PLoS One 9: e90217.
9. Giugliano RP, Ruff CT, Braunwald E, Murphy SA, Wiviott SD, et al. (2013) Edoxaban versus warfarin in patients with atrial fibrillation. N Engl J Med 369: 2093–2104.
10. Buller HR, Decousus H, Grosso MA, Mercuri M, Middeldorp S, et al. (2013) Edoxaban versus warfarin for the treatment of symptomatic venous thromboembolism. N Engl J Med 369: 1406–1415.
11. Yamashita T, Koretsune Y, Yasaka M, Inoue H, Kawai Y, et al. (2012) Randomized, multicenter, warfarin-controlled phase II study of edoxaban in Japanese patients with non-valvular atrial fibrillation. Circ J 76: 1840–1847.
12. Chung N, Jeon HK, Lien LM, Lai WT, Tse HF, et al. (2011) Safety of edoxaban, an oral factor Xa inhibitor, in Asian patients with non-valvular atrial fibrillation. Thromb Haemost 105: 535–544.
13. Weitz JI, Connolly SJ, Patel I, Salazar D, Rohatagi S, et al. (2010) Randomised, parallel-group, multicentre, multinational phase 2 study comparing edoxaban,
an oral factor Xa inhibitor, with warfarin for stroke prevention in patients with atrial fibrillation. Thromb Haemost 104: 633–641.
14. Schulman S, Kearon C (2005) Definition of major bleeding in clinical investigations of antihemostatic medicinal products in non-surgical patients. J Thromb Haemost 3: 692–694.
15. Matsushima N LF, Sat o T, Weiss D, Mendell J (2013) Bioavailability and Safety of the Factor Xa Inhibitor Edoxaban and the Effects of Quinidine in Healthy Subjects. Clin Pharm Drug 2: 358–366.
16. Ogata K, Mendell-Harary J, Tachibana M, Masumoto H, Oguma T, et al. (2010) Clinical safety, tolerability, pharmacokinetics, and pharmacodynamics of the novel factor Xa inhibitor edoxaban in healthy volunteers. J Clin Pharmacol 50: 743–753.
17. Goel R, Srivathsan K (2012) Newer oral anticoagulant agents: a new era in medicine. Curr Cardiol Rev 8: 158–165.
18. Samama MM, Mendell J, Guinet C, Le Flem L, Kunitada S (2012) In vitro study of the anticoagulant effects of edoxaban and its effect on thrombin generation in comparison to fondaparinux. Thromb Res 129: e77–82.
19. Laulicht B BS, Jiang X (2013) Antidote for new oral anticoagulants: mechanism of action and binding specif icity of PER977. Presented at the XXIV Congress of the International Society on Thrombosis and HaemostasisAmsterdam.
20. Dentali F, Riva N, Crowther M, Turpie AG, Lip GY, et al. (2012) Efficacy and safety of the novel oral anticoagulants in atrial fibrillation: a systematic review and meta-analysis of the literature. Circulation 126: 2381–2391.
21. Dogliotti A, Paolasso E, Giugliano RP (2013) Novel oral anticoagulants in atrial fibrillation: a meta-analysis of large, randomized, controlled trials vs warfarin. Clin Cardiol 36: 61–67.
22. Harenberg J, Marx S, Diener HC, Lip GYH, Marder VJ, et al. (2012) Comparison of efficacy and safety of dabigatran, rivaroxaban and apixaban in patients with atrial fibrillation using network meta-analysis. International Angiology 31: 330–339.
23. Miller CS, Grandi SM, Shimony A, Filion KB, Eisenberg MJ (2012) Meta-analysis of efficacy and safety of new oral anticoagulants (dabigatran, rivaroxaban, apixaban) versus warfarin in patients with atrial fibrillation. Am J Cardiol 110: 453–460.
24. Turner EH, Matthews AM, Linardatos E, Tell RA, Rosenthal R (2008) Selective publication of antidepressant trials and its influence on apparent efficacy. N Engl J Med 358: 252–260.
25. Lexchin J, Bero LA, Djulbegovic B, Clark O (2003) Pharmaceutical industry sponsorship and research outcome and quality: systematic review. British Medical Journal 326: 1167–1170B.

13

Systematic Review of Observational Studies Assessing Bleeding Risk in Patients with Atrial Fibrillation Not Using Anticoagulants

Luciane Cruz Lopes[1]*, **Frederick A. Spencer**[2], **Ignacio Neumann**[3,4], **Matthew Ventresca**[4], **Shanil Ebrahim**[4,5,6], **Qi Zhou**[4], **Neera Bhatnagar**[7], **Sam Schulman**[8,4], **John Eikelboom**[9], **Gordon Guyatt**[4]

1 Pharmaceutical Sciences Postgraduate Course, University of Sorocaba, Sao Paulo, Brazil, 2 Department of Medicine, Division of Cardiology, McMaster University, Hamilton, Ontario, Canada, 3 Internal Medicine Department, School of Medicine, Pontificia Universidad Catolica de Chile, Santiago, Chile, 4 Department of Clinical Epidemiology and Biostatistics, McMaster University, Hamilton, Ontario, Canada, 5 Department of Anesthesia, McMaster University, Hamilton, Ontario, Canada, 6 Stanford Prevention Research Center, Stanford University, Stanford, California, United States of America, 7 Health Sciences Library McMaster University, Hamilton, Ontario, Canada, 8 Department of Medicine, McMaster University, Hamilton, Ontario, Canada, 9 Department of Medicine, Division of Hematology and Thromboembolism, McMaster University, Hamilton, Ontario, Canada

Abstract

Background: Patients with atrial fibrillation considering use of anticoagulants must balance stroke reduction against bleeding risk. Knowledge of bleeding risk without the use of anticoagulants may help inform this decision.

Purpose: To determine the rate of major bleeding reported in observational studies of atrial fibrillation patients not receiving Vitamin K antagonists (VKA).

Data Sources: We searched MEDLINE, EMBASE and CINAHL to October 2011 and examined reference lists of eligible studies and related reviews.

Study Selection: All longitudinal cohort studies that included over 100 adult patients with atrial fibrillation not receiving VKA.

Data Extraction: Teams of two reviewers independently and in duplicate adjudicated eligibility, assessed risk of bias and abstracted study characteristics and outcomes.

Data Synthesis: Twenty-one eligible studies included 96,448 patients. Major bleeding rates varied widely, from 0 to 4.69 events per 100 patient-years. The pooled estimate in 13 studies with 78839 patients was 1.59 with a 99% confidence interval of 1.10 to 2.3 and median 1.42 (interquartile range 0.62–2.70). Pooled estimates for fatal bleeding and non-fatal bleeding from 4 studies that reported these outcomes were, respectively, 0.40 (0.34 to 0.46) and 1.18 (0.30 to 4.56) per 100 patient-years. In 9 randomized controlled trials (RCTs) the median rate of major bleeding in patients not receiving either anticoagulant or antiplatelet therapy was 0.6 (interquartile 0.2 to 0.90), and in 12 RCTs the median rate of major bleeding in patients receiving a single antiplatelet agent was 0.75 (interquartile 0.4 to 1.4).

Conclusion: Results suggest that patients with atrial fibrillation not receiving VKA enrolled in observational studies represent a population on average at higher risk of bleeding.

Editor: Dermot Cox, Royal College of Surgeons, Ireland

Funding: This study was supported by FAPESP Brazil (Process N. 2009/5308431). Shanil Ebrahim is supported by a Canadian Institutes of Health Research Fellowship Award and a MITACS Elevate Award. The funders had no role in study design, data collection and analysis, decision to publish, or preparation of the manuscript.

Competing Interests: The authors have declared that no competing interests exist.

* E-mail: luslopes@terra.com.br

Introduction

Atrial fibrillation is common, and incurs a major burden of morbidity and mortality largely as a result of associated stroke and systemic embolism. Anticoagulants reduce the risk of stroke or systemic embolism, but at a cost of inconvenience and an increased risk of serious bleeding. Choosing whether or not to use anticoagulants to reduce the risk of thromboembolism requires trading off an absolute reduction in stroke against an absolute increase in serious bleeding. Estimating the magnitude of the increased risk of bleeding using VKA is crucial in making decisions regarding anticoagulant use.

In a prior systematic review of the available observational studies, we have demonstrated that although major bleeding rates in atrial fibrillation patients receiving VKAs varied widely from study to study, the median major bleeding rate was 2.05 per 100 patient-years, interquartile range 1.57 to 3.35 [1], a value very close to that of warfarin-treated arms of randomized control trials (RCTs) (median 2.1, interquartile range 1.54 to 3.09). Applying the relative increase in bleeds with VKA from RCTs - 2.58 [2] - leads to an estimate of absolute increase in bleeding rate of 1.54 per 100 patient-years with warfarin use in atrial fibrillation.

Defining the bleeding risk in patients with atrial fibrillation not taking anticoagulants may provide further insight into the challenging decision regarding use of anticoagulants. We therefore undertook a systematic review and meta-analysis to define bleeding risk, including intracranial and extracranial, in representative patients in the community not receiving anticoagulants. Being aware that bleeding risk is likely to differ across patient and study characteristics, we, a priori, postulated explanations for possible heterogeneity in bleeding risk. We compared results to bleeding risks reported in the arms of randomized trials not receiving anticoagulants (either no antithrombotic therapy, placebo, or a single antiplatelet agent).

Methods

All methodological decisions in this review were made in advance and were recorded in a prior protocol that is available on request.

Data Sources and searches

We searched the central MEDLINE, EMBASE and CINAHL (to October 2011). We restricted the search to human subjects and adults. Medical subject headings included: hemorrhage (or bleeding$ or bleed*); atrial fibrillation (or auricular fibrillation) and risk (risk factors or risk assessment or risk*). For every eligible study, we identified, and for studies such as review articles that we identified that included citations to potentially eligible studies, one reviewer examined the reference list.

Teams of two investigators independently screened each title and abstract from this search. If either of the two screeners identified a citation as potentially relevant, we obtained the full text article for detailed review. Teams of two reviewers independently determined the eligibility of all studies that underwent full text evaluation. Disagreements were resolved through discussion between the two reviewers; when this did not resolve differences, a third reviewer made a final decision on the study's eligibility.

Study Eligibility

We included all longitudinal cohort studies or case series that included adults with atrial fibrillation. Articles met the following criteria: a) >80% of patients enrolled have atrial fibrillation and are 18 or older or b) <80% of patients included had atrial fibrillation, but results presented for the atrial fibrillation subset separately; receiving or not receiving antiplatelet agents but not receiving VKA; ≥100 patients with atrial fibrillation not using VKA; some estimate of major bleeding in an identifiable group not receiving VKA. We excluded RCTs; studies dealing only with hospitalized patients or emergency department patients; and studies with clearly unrepresentative populations with a different bleeding risk than a representative population (e.g. prior stroke, ablation).

Data abstraction and quality assessment

We abstracted the following information from each eligible study: period of data collection; country; source of funding; duration of follow-up taking or not taking antiplatelet agents; total

number of atrial fibrillation patients not taking VKA; funding of care; age. We recorded rates of major bleeding, both fatal bleeding and non-fatal which we characterized as intracranial or extra-cranial and, for extra-cranial bleeding, further characterized as gastrointestinal or other. For all major bleeding outcomes we recorded the number of patients who had a bleed, rate of bleeding (typically number of bleeds per 100 patient years) and total number of bleeds.

We assessed risk of bias using the following criteria i. patient selection random or consecutive versus other; ii. whether investigators excluded patient groups; iii. proportion lost to follow up; iv. explicitness of bleeding criteria; v. primary data collection (as opposed to administrative data base) for bleeding from patient report, physician report, or hospital records. If reported, we noted whether patients received antiplatelet agents from a prescription or over the counter.

Data synthesis and statistical analysis

We anticipated that bleeding rates would differ across studies and generated a priori hypotheses of what study features might be responsible for the differences: i. age distribution (older age, higher bleeding incidence); ii. gender distribution (women higher incidence); iii. ethnic groups (geographic area); iv. proportion nursing facility residence; v. proportion within each CHADS category (includes congestive heart failure, hypertension, age>75, diabetes = 1 point, history of stroke = 2 points); vi. proportion taking one antiplatelet agent; vii. proportion with current or remote bleeding event; alcohol/ drug abuse; viii. funding of health care (gradient of bleeding incidence if unadjusted by age Medicare, Medicaid, mixed and private payment); ix. risk of bias, in particular use of administrative data bases (claims data) versus primary data collection (primary data collection, higher bleeding incidence).

In keeping with standards for avoiding over fitting, we examined all hypotheses for which information was documented in at least 10 studies for the continuous independent (predictor) variables or at least 5 studies for each level of the independent categorical variables.

Our pooled analyses estimated the rate of bleeding per 100 patient-years of warfarin exposure for overall major bleeding and its subcategories. We used variance estimates based on confidence intervals, where provided, or the total number of patient-years of exposure. If rates, but neither confidence intervals nor total exposure, were available, we estimated total exposure from the mean years of follow-up. When total number of bleeds or total number of patients who bled, but not rates were available, we estimated rates based on the total number of bleeds or the proportion that bled and the mean follow-up. For instances in which one of a group of studies reported no events on a group, we used the 0.5 continuity correction for the calculation. We pooled estimates in log-scale units across studies using DerSimonian and Laird's random effects model weighted by the inverse of the variance and then back transformed to the rate in natural units. The pooled estimates were tested by Z-statistics and the heterogeneity, measured by Q-statistic, among the studies examined by the Chi-square test. When the heterogeneity was presented, a component of variance due to inter-study variation, D, was incorporated in the confidence interval calculation for the estimate. Studies that did not include any of the data above were not included in the pooled estimate; for such studies, we summarized bleeding rates descriptively. To examine the possibility of publication bias we constructed a funnel plot.

We made calculations for patients using or not using antiplatelet agents when studies reported these data. To explain heterogeneity, we performed univariable meta-regression analysis weighted by inverse of variance. The dependent variable was the logarithm of the bleeding rate in 100 patient-years; the independent variables are described above in our 9 a priori hypotheses regarding heterogeneity. For the purpose of interpretation, we back transformed the exponential function parameter to natural units and considered a threshold p-value of 0.01 to be significant.

Bleeding rates from randomized trials

Using the atrial fibrillation article from the 9th iteration of the American College of Chest Physicians (ACCP) antithrombotic guidelines [2], we identified randomized trials comparing anticoagulants to placebo, no antithrombotic agent, or a single antiplatelet agent for stroke prevention in atrial fibrillation and abstracted the overall rates of major bleeding among subjects not taking warfarin.

Results

Our search strategy identified 2,232 citations. Of these, 283 proved potentially eligible, and 21 fulfilled eligibility criteria and are included in this systematic review (**Figure 1**).

Study and Patient Characteristics

The 21 eligible studies, most conducted in North America and Europe, followed their patients from 1.0 to 6.0 years (mean or median), reported on between 130 and 65,477patients with a mean age varying between 63.5 and 81 years (median 67.0, interquartile range 63.5 to 76.7) of whom the majority were male, and taking at least one antiplatelet agent (Table 1, Table 2).

Risk of Bias

Most of studies enrolled consecutive or random patients, provided explicit criteria for bleeding and undertook some primary data collection. No study met all 6 risk of bias criteria; 15 studies met 3 or fewer criteria (Table 3, Table S1)

Bleeding outcomes in observational studies

Of the 21 eligible studies, 13 reported data regarding overall major bleeding that allowed pooling as bleeds per 100 patient-years [3–15]. The total bleeding rates varied widely across studies - more than an order of magnitude - from 0.0 to 4.69 per 100 patient-years (median 1.42, interquartile range 0.62–2.70). Of the 13 studies, 5 reported bleeding rates of less than 1.0 per 100 patient-year, 5 between 1.0 to 2.7, and 3 rates greater than 3 per 100 patient years (Table 2, Table S2), resulting in a pooled

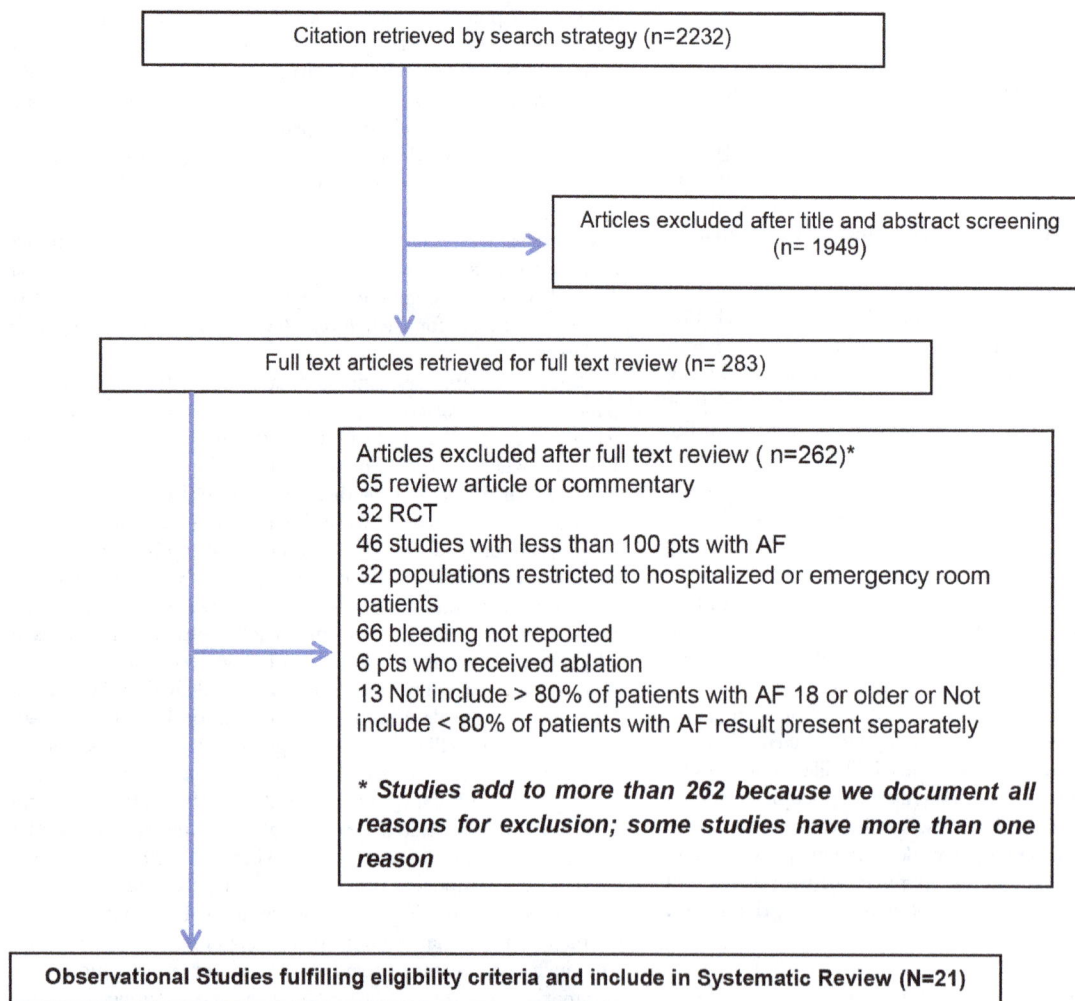

Figure 1. Literature search and study selection.

Table 1. Study characteristics of atrial fibrillation patients not taking VKA.

CHARACTERISTICS	STUDIES (N)	
SAMPLE SIZE		
Total number of AF patients	21	96,448
Total numbers of AF patients-years	9*	33,299.24
GENDER		**MEDIAN (INTERQUARTILE RANGE)**
Proportion female	11	48.6 (36.5–55.4)
AGE		**MEDIAN (INTERQUARTILE RANGE)**
	9	76.3 (69.3–79.1)
USE OF ANTIPLATELET AGENTS#		**NUMBER PTS**
Pts not taking any antiplatelet agent	9	2,602
Pts taking at least one antiplatelet agent	13	58,151
Pts taking two or more antiplatelet agent	1	2,859
Pts taking antiplatelet agents number unspecified	7	35,695
FOLLOW UP		**MEDIAN (INTERQUATILE RANGE)**
Minimum, days	3	180 (90–180)
Maximum, days	11	1,260 (720–1825)
Mean, days	6	655.5 (388.3–1095)
DEFINITION MAJOR BLEEDING		**NUMBER PTS@**
Hospitalization (initiating or prolonging)	11	75,941
Hemoglobin decrease ≥2 g/L	3	1,772
Transfusion ≥2 units blood	8	3,503
Critical area (e.g. intracranial, spinal, retroperitoneal, pericardial, hemarthrosis)	8	10,906
Surgery (requiring)	3	1,301
ICD-9 codes	10	92,230
Fatal	9	56,775
Others	5	9,313
PUBLICATIONS YEAR		**NUMBER PTS**
1998–2005	6	13,174
2006–2010	15	83,274
COUNTRY		**NUMBER PTS**
Canada	2	1,022
USA	9	34,091
Europe	7	60,616
Asia	2	422
Australia and New Zealand	1	297
SOURCE OF FUNDING		**NUMBER PTS**
For profit	5	69,600
Not for profit	10	11,268
Both	2	1,797
Not specified	4	13,783

@Some studies used more than one definition and all definitions are included.
*12 studies didn't provided the number pts-year follow up.
#some studies have more than one arm.

estimate of bleeds per 100 patient-years 1.59 with 99% confidence interval 1.10 to 2.30 (Table 4, Figure 2).

Of 21 studies, 8 reported data major bleeding in patients taking antiplatelet agents with rates from 0.0 to 3.84 per 100 patient-years (median 1.32, interquartile range 0.39 to 2.57) and pooled estimate of bleeds per 100 patient-years 1.35 with 99% confidence interval 0.55 to 3.28 (Table 2, Figure 3).

Of the 21 studies, 6 reported major bleeding in patients not taking antiplatelet agents with overall bleeding rates from 0.0 to 4.73 per 100 patient-years (median 1.54, interquartile range 1.05 to 2.10) and pooled estimate of bleeds per 100 patient-years 2.18 with 99% confidence interval 1.19 to 3.99 (Table 2, Figure 4).

Of 21 studies, 4 separately fatal (pooled estimate 0.40 per 100 patient-years) and 4 reported non-fatal (1.18 per 100 patient-years) major bleeding (Table 4, Table S2).

Table 2. Characteristics of population included in observational studies included.

AUTHOR	MEAN FOLLOW UP (year)	TOTAL NUMBER OF ATRIAL FIBRILLATION PATIENTS NOT TAKING VKA	FEMALE (%)	AGE (mean)	OUTCOME MEASURED	MAJOR BLEEDING (PER 100 PTS-YEAR)		
						All patients not taking VKA	Patients taking antiplatelet agent	Patients not taking antiplatelet
SPAFIII, 1998 [8]	2	892	22	67	Major bleeding, intracranial, extracranial gastrointestinal, extracranial others	0.44	0.44	NA
Jackson, 2001 [15]	3.14	297	39.6	77	Major bleeding	3.9	3.42	4.73
Leung, 2003 [6]	2	143	NA	NA	Major bleeding, Intracranial, extracranial, gastrointestinal	1.40	1.72	0
Sam, 2004 [19]	NA	313	50.1	NA	Major bleeding, intracranial,	NA	NA	NA
Currie, 2005 [16]	NA	3885	55.4	65.3*	Major bleeding	NA	NA	NA
Darkow, 2005 [13]	NA	7644	54.5	79.8	Major bleeding, intracraneal	3.1	NA	NA
Boulanger,2006 [10]	3.4	1787	65.1	76	Major bleeding,	0.26	NA	NA
Burton, 2006 [12]	3.1	372	NA	65*	Major bleeding, intracranial, extracranial gastrointestinal	1.67	1.66	1.31
Gage, 2006 [17]	NA	2187	NA	81	Major bleeding	NA	NA	NA
Parkash, 2007 [7]	2.1	130	40	69.2	Major bleeding	2.2	NA	NA
Shen, 2007 [20]	4.9	7851	NA	41.9*	Intracranial	NA	NA	NA
Meiltz, 2008 [3]	1.01	213	69.8	NA	Major bleeding, intracranial, extracraneal, extracraneal, others	0	0	0
Wess, 2008 [22]	NA	5622	75.1	76.7	Intracranial, extracranial, extracranial gastrointestinal	NA	NA	NA
Boccuzzi, 2009 [18]	NA	2167	NA	NA	Major Bleeding	NA	NA	NA
Lai, 2009 [9]	1.9	167	36.5	77	Major bleeding, intracranial, extracranial gastrointestinal, extracranial others	4.69	NA	NA
Singer, 2009 [21]	6	6353	48.6	48.6*	Intracranial	NA	NA	NA
Friberg, 2010 [23]	NA	617	NA	NA	Intracranial	NA	NA	NA
Hansen, 2010 [14]	NA	54,117	NA	NA	Major bleeding, intracranial, extracranial	2.7	3.84***	2.10
Lee, 2010 [4]	1.7	279	34.1	63.5	Major bleeding, intracranial, extracranial gastrointestinal, extracranial others	0.62	0.34	1.05
Ortiz, 2010 [5]	1.91	232	NA	NA	Major bleeding	0.9	NA	NA
Pisters, 2010 [11]	1	1180	NA	49.7**	Major bleeding	1.42	0.97	NA

NA – not avaliable.
*it represents proportion of pts with threshold age ≥75 yo;
**it represents proportion of pts with threshold age ≥65 yo;
***taking two antiplatelet agents.

Table 3. Risk of bias.

STUDY	CONSECUTIVE OR RANDOM	NO EXCLUSIONS	SPECIFIED LOST TO FOLLOW UP	EXPLICIT CRITERIA FOR THE BLEED	DOCUMENTATION OF ANTIPLATELET USE	PRIMARY DATA COLLECTION	CRITERIA MET
SPAFIII, 1998 [8]	✓	✗	✓	✓	✓	✓	5
Jackson, 2001 [15]	✓	✗	✗	✓	✗	✓	3
Leung, 2003 [6]	✓	✓	✗	✓	✗	✓	4
Sam, 2004 [19]	✓	✓	✗	✓	✗	✓	4
Currie, 2005 [16]	✓	✓	✗	✗	✗	✓	3
Darkow, 2005 [13]	✓	✗	✗	✓	✗	✗	2
Boulanger, 2006 [10]	✓	✗	✗	✗	✓	✗	2
Burton, 2006 [12]	✗	✗	✗	✓	✗	✓	2
Gage, 2006 [17]	✓	✗	✗	✓	✓	✗	3
Parkash, 2007 [7]	✗	✗	✗	✓	✓	✓	3
Shen, 2007 [20]	✓	✗	✗	✓	✗	✓	3
Meltz, 2008 [3]	✓	✓	✗	✗	✗	✓	3
Wess, 2008 [22]	✓	✓	✗	✗	✓	✗	3
Boccuzzi, 2009 [18]	✓	✓	✗	✓	✗	✗	3
Lai, 2009 [9]	✓	✗	✗	✓	✓	✓	4
Singer, 2009 [21]	✓	✗	✗	✓	✗	✓	3
Friberg, 2010 [23]	✓	✗	✗	✓	✗	✓	3
Hansen, 2010 [14]	✓	✓	✗	✓	✗	✗	3
Lee, 2010 [4]	✓	✗	✗	✓	✓	✗	3
Pisters, 2010 [11]	✓	✗	✓	✓	✓	✓	5

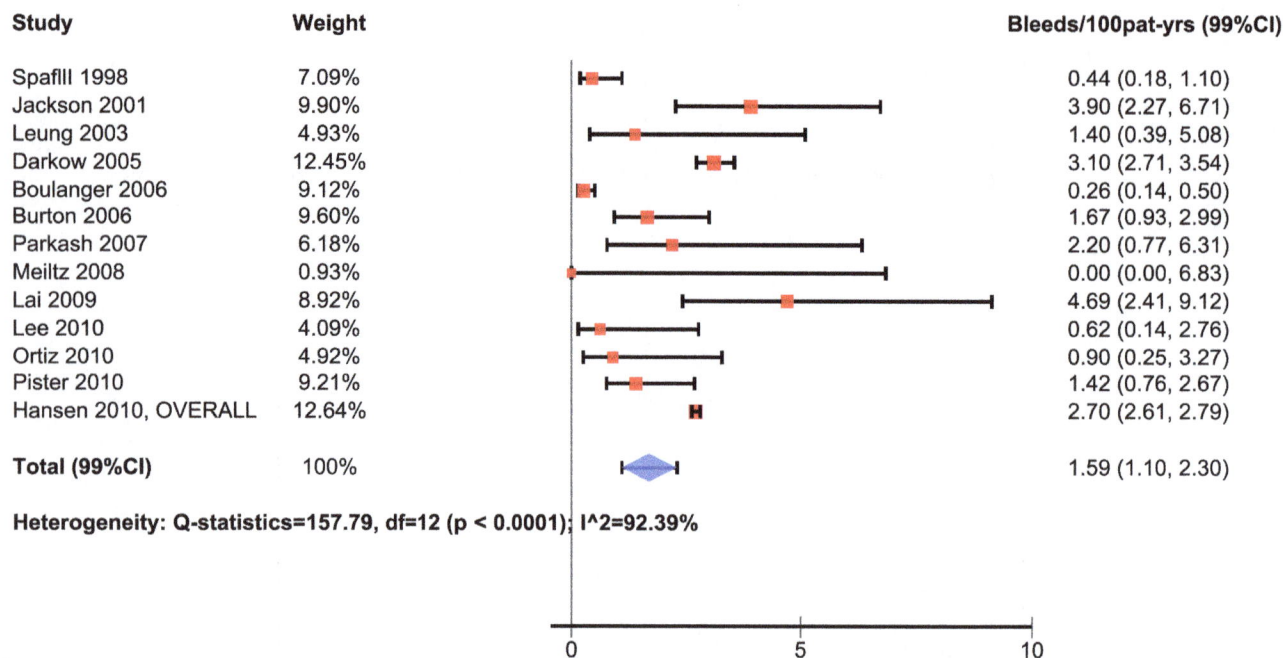

Study	Weight		Bleeds/100pat-yrs (99%CI)
Spaflll 1998	7.09%		0.44 (0.18, 1.10)
Jackson 2001	9.90%		3.90 (2.27, 6.71)
Leung 2003	4.93%		1.40 (0.39, 5.08)
Darkow 2005	12.45%		3.10 (2.71, 3.54)
Boulanger 2006	9.12%		0.26 (0.14, 0.50)
Burton 2006	9.60%		1.67 (0.93, 2.99)
Parkash 2007	6.18%		2.20 (0.77, 6.31)
Meiltz 2008	0.93%		0.00 (0.00, 6.83)
Lai 2009	8.92%		4.69 (2.41, 9.12)
Lee 2010	4.09%		0.62 (0.14, 2.76)
Ortiz 2010	4.92%		0.90 (0.25, 3.27)
Pister 2010	9.21%		1.42 (0.76, 2.67)
Hansen 2010, OVERALL	12.64%		2.70 (2.61, 2.79)
Total (99%CI)	100%		1.59 (1.10, 2.30)

Heterogeneity: Q-statistics=157.79, df=12 (p < 0.0001); I^2=92.39%

Figure 2. Major bleeding overall population not taking Vitamin K atagonist.

The 8 studies that did not report overall bleeding in a manner that allowed pooling reported overall major bleeding rates of 1.54 [16], 5.1 [17] and 6.5 [18]; the others did not report overall major bleeding rates [19–23]. Of these 8 studies, 5 reported results for intracranial bleeding [19–23] and 1 for extracranial bleeding [18] (Table S2).

Table 4. Rates of bleeding.

BLEEDING OUTCOMES	NUMBER STUDIES (PTS)	POOLED ESTIMATE BLEEDING RATES PER 100 PATIENT-YEARS (99% CI) or range
MAJOR BLEEDING (pooled)		
Total, n = 13	78839	1.59 (1.10, 2.30), 0–4.69
Fatal, n = 4	48405	0.40 (0.34, 0.46), 0.18–0.62
Non fatal, n = 4	48405	1.18 (0.30, 4.56), 0.09–3.30
MAJOR BLEEDING IN NON-POOLABLE STUDIES (RANGE)		
INTRACRANIAL BLEEDING (pooled)		
Total, n = 8	64072	0.32 (0.17, 0.59), 0.06–0.94
Fatal, n = 2	651	0.35 (0.07, 1.84), 0.17–0.62
Non fatal, n = 2	651	0.15 (0.03, 0.77), 0.09–0.17
EXTACRANIAL (pooled)		
Total, n = 3	1338	0.68 (0.05, 9.48), 0.09–3.74
Fatal, n = 2	651	0.09 (0.01, 0.72), 0.08–0.09
Non fatal, n = 1	279	0.62 (0.14, 2.76)
GATROINTESTINAL (pooled)		
Total, n = 4	48879	0.89 (0.29, 2.69), 0.09–1.87
Fatal, n = 2	651	0.09 (0.01, 0.72), 0.08–0.09
Non fatal, n = 1	279	0.62 (0.14, 2.76)
OTHERS (pooled)		
Total, n = 3	1338	0.25 (0.01, 8.34), 0.06–1.87
Fatal, n = 1	279	0.62 (0.14, 2.76)
Non fatal, n = 1	279	0.62 (0.14, 2.76)

Study	Weight		Bleeds/100pat-yrs (99%CI)
Jackson 2001	25.70%		4.73 (2.25, 9.96)
Leung 2003	2.60%		0.00 (0.02, 35.98)
Burton 2006	18.53%		1.31 (0.46, 3.76)
Meiltz 2008	2.60%		0.00 (0.05, 68.1)
Lee 2010	8.76%		1.05 (0.17, 6.53)
Hansen 2010	41.82%		2.10 (2.00, 2.20)
Total (99%CI)	100%		2.18 (1.19, 3.99)

Heterogeneity: Q-statistics=10.52, df=5 (p =0.06); I^2=52.45%

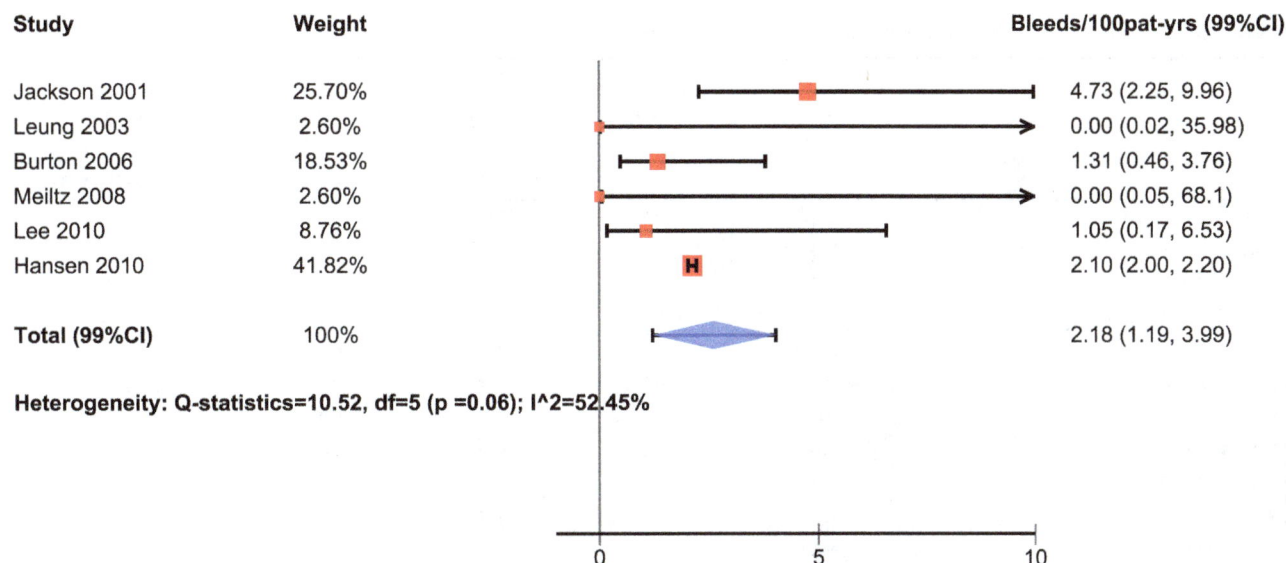

Figure 3. Subpopulation not taking antiplatelet.

Table 4 summarizes pooled results for bleeding subcategories. We observed similar large variability in bleeding rates for subcategories as we did for overall bleeding. For instance, major extracranial bleeding ranged from 0.09 to 3.74 major bleeds per 100 patient-years.

The funnel plots did not suggest publication bias (Figure S1).

Possible determinants of variability in bleeding rates

Sufficient data were available to explore only 2 categories of variables to determine whether they were predictors of major bleeding events: use of administrative data bases (claims data) versus primary data collection, and average age of patients.

With respect to data collection, studies fell into three categories: exclusively primary data collection: major bleeding rate per 100 patient-years (99%CI) 2.30 (0.27, 19.40); exclusively administrative data base data collection: 2.71 (2.20, 3.33); and both sources of data collection: 0.28 (0.04, 1.75). Bleeding rates were significantly higher with exclusively administrative data collection versus both data sources (p = 0.003) and of borderline significance in primary data collection versus both data sources (p = 0.04). There were only 2 studies with both primary and administrative data base data collection and one of these, with an extremely low bleeding rate of 0.15 per 100 patient-years, drove this result.

We were unable to demonstrate a statistical association with age and bleeding rates, estimate of relative change (relative risk for

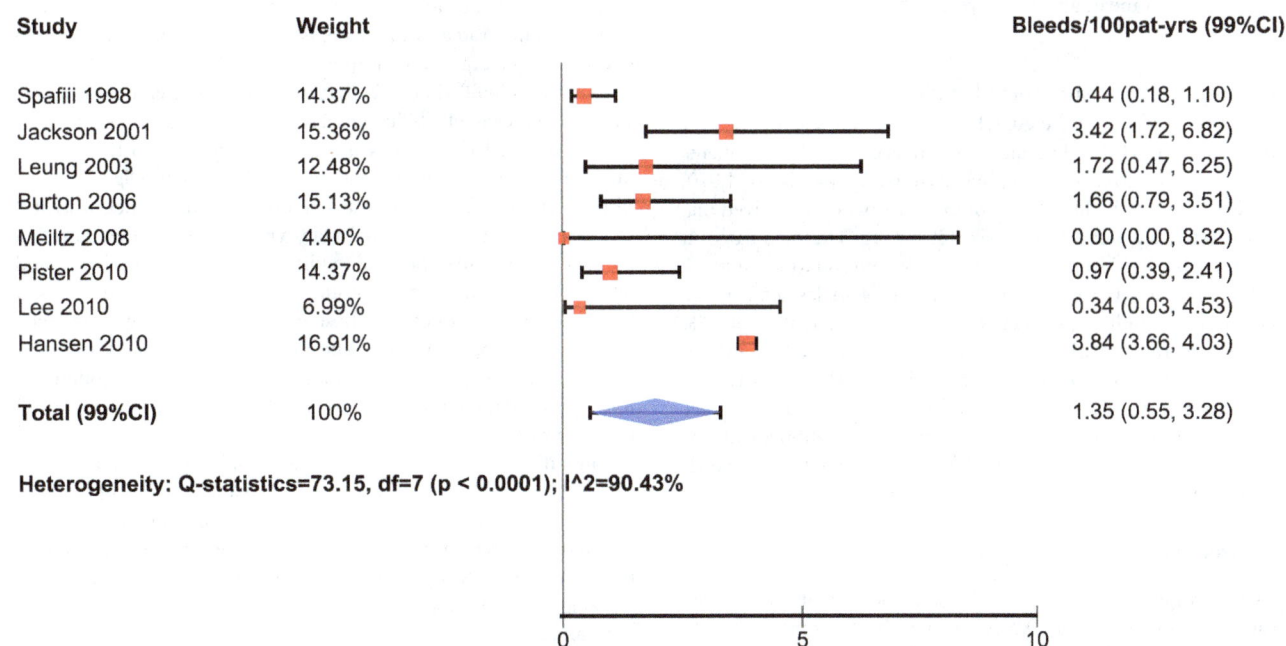

Study	Weight		Bleeds/100pat-yrs (99%CI)
Spafiii 1998	14.37%		0.44 (0.18, 1.10)
Jackson 2001	15.36%		3.42 (1.72, 6.82)
Leung 2003	12.48%		1.72 (0.47, 6.25)
Burton 2006	15.13%		1.66 (0.79, 3.51)
Meiltz 2008	4.40%		0.00 (0.00, 8.32)
Pister 2010	14.37%		0.97 (0.39, 2.41)
Lee 2010	6.99%		0.34 (0.03, 4.53)
Hansen 2010	16.91%		3.84 (3.66, 4.03)
Total (99%CI)	100%		1.35 (0.55, 3.28)

Heterogeneity: Q-statistics=73.15, df=7 (p < 0.0001); I^2=90.43%

Figure 4. Subpopulation taking at least one antiplatelet.

Table 5. Characteristics of RCTs including atrial fibrillation patients.

STUDY	PATIENTS (N)	FEMALE (%)	AGE (mean)	Major bleeding (per 100 pt year)	
				No antiplatelet	Taking at least one antiplatelet agent
AFASAK, 1989 [24]	336	53.7	72.6	0.0	
BAATAF, 1990 [25]	213	25.0	68.5	0.2	
JAST, 2006 [26]	445	30.3	64.8	0.2	
Edvardsson, 2003 [27]	334	39	73.0	0.5	
EAFT, 1993 [28],	378	47.0	73.0	0.6	
CAFA, 1991 [29]	191	26.7	67.4	0.8	
SPINAF, 1992 [30]	265	44.0	67.0	0.9	
AFI, 1994 [31]	2140	31.5	69.5	1.0	
SPAF, 1991 [32]	568	30	67.0	1.9	
Hu et al., 2006 [33]	335	40.3	63.3		0.0
SIFA, 1997 [34]	462	44.5	72.8		0.2
AFASAK, 1989 [24]	336	53.7	72.6		0.2
NASPEAF, 2004 [35]	242	43.0	69.9		0.35
EAFT, 1993 [28]*	404	42.0	71.0		0.7
EAFT, 1993 [28]*	404	42.0	71.0		0.7
JAST, 2006 [26]	426	28.9	65.5		0.8
SPAFII, 1994 [36]	357	24.0	64.0		0.9
AFI, 1994 [31]	888	35.0	70.0		1.0
AFASAK 2, 1999 [37]	336	35.0	73.1		1.4
SPAF, 1991 [32]	552	29	67.0		1.4
PATAF, 1997 [38]	319	60.0	75.6		1.4
SPAFII, 1994 [36]	188	30.3	80.0		1.6
BAFTA, 2007 [39]	485	46.0	81.1		2.0

*The EAFT study has two group of patients taking no VKA.

each increase in mean age of one year 1.02, 95% CI 0.94 to 1.11, p = 0.11).

Bleeding rates in randomized trials

The 9th iteration of the ACCP Antithrombotic guidelines [2] summarized 9 RCTs that included an arm in which patients received no antithrombotic prophylaxis (total sample size of 4,870) and 12 RCTs that included an arm in which patients received one antiplatelet agent (total sample size of 5,734). The mean age in these cohorts varied from 63.3 to 81.1 years (interquartile range 67 to 73 years) with the same preponderance of males seen in the observational studies (median proportion of females 38.2%, interquartile range 30.1 to 44.2) (Table 4). The median rate of major bleeding in patients not receiving treatment was 0.6, (interquartile range 0.20 to 0.90, total range 0.0 to 1.9 bleeds per 100 patient-years) and in the group receiving one antiplatelet was 0.75, (interquartile range 0.24 to 1.30, total range 0.0 to 2.0 bleeds per 100 patient-years).

Discussion

We identified 21 observational studies of patients with atrial fibrillation not receiving VKA of which 13 reported data contributing to pooled estimates of total major bleeding rate of 1.59 per 100 patient-years with 99% confidence interval of 1.10 to 2.3 and median 1.42 (interquartile range 0.62 to 2.70) (Table 4,

Figure 2). Patients in the NVKA arms of RCTs of alternative management strategies for patients with atrial fibrillation experienced appreciably lower bleeding rates (Table 5).

Our study fulfilled criteria for a rigorous systematic review. We specified explicit eligibility criteria; conducted a comprehensive search; assessed risk of bias using criteria specific to this review; and teams of two reviewers independently assessed eligibility, risk of bias, and checked data abstraction. Most studies met at least 3 risk of bias criteria. In particular, virtually all studies enrolled consecutive patients, specified explicit major bleeding criteria, and documented antiplatelet exposure (though most did not report bleeding rates separately for those using and not using antiplatelet agents) (Table 3, Table S1). The funnel plot for overall bleeding did not suggest publication bias (Figure S1). We conducted appropriate data analyses examining the rate of bleeding per 100 patient-years.

Limitations of our review include variability in definitions of major bleeding across studies and variability in results across studies. With only 13 studies reporting overall bleeding, some of which did not report the explanatory variables of interest, we were unable to satisfactorily explore sources of heterogeneity. The only variables we were able to formally address were the source of the data and age.

We found that studies using only administrative data and those using only primary data collection showed higher bleeding rates than studies that used both sources of information. This finding is almost certainly due to chance. The result does not conform to our a priori hypotheses, there were only two studies with both sources of data, and the result is driven almost exclusively by one of these studies. Thus, we conclude this subgroup hypothesis has low credibility.

We found no relation between mean age and bleeding risk (relative risk for each increase in mean age of one year 1.02, 95% CI 0.94 to 1.11, p = 0.11). Studies that separately reported bleeding rates in patients taking antiplately agents versus those not taking antiplatelet agents paradoxically suggested higher bleeding rates in those not taking antiplatelet agents (Figures 3 and 4).

Few studies provided information about bleeding subcategories, and those that did showed highly variable results. Once again, the paucity of studies and limited reporting precluded a systematic exploration of sources of heterogeneity.

We found no prior systematic review of bleeding rates in atrial fibrillation patients not receiving anticoagulants. Thus, our review adds original information not previously available.

Our finding that bleeding rates were appreciably higher in observational studies of atrial fibrillation patients not receiving VKAs (whether or not they received antiplatelet agents) than in the corresponding RCTs suggests that the RCTs enrolled patients at lower risk. The question then arises: which set of data is more appropriate for helping estimate bleeding risk in atrial fibrillation patients under consideration for use of anticoagulant prophylaxis?

Were we to apply the relative effect of VKAs from the RCTs (2.58) to our pooled estimate of risk of bleeding from the current observational studies (1.59) we would obtain a bleeding risk with VKAs (3.90) appreciably greater than we observed either in observational studies of patients receiving VKA or in the VKA arms of randomized trials. This strongly suggests that the cohorts enrolled in the current review included atrial fibrillation patients whose high risk of bleeding may explain their not receiving anticoagulation - that is, clinicians taking care of these patients were reluctant to prescribe anticoagulation in the face of a perceived (and it turns out accurately perceived) increased risk of bleeding.

Our results therefore highlight the limitations of observational studies in which the reasons patients did or did not receive an intervention are not completely - or not at all - transparent (sometimes referred to as confounding by indication). This lack of information is particularly limiting in the inferences that the evidence provides because of the very high variability in bleeding rates across the studies.

The bleeding incidence in patients receiving VKA from our prior review of observational studies (2.51, per 100 patient-years; median 2.05, interquartile range 1.57 to 3.35) [1] remains the best estimate of bleeding risk in patients not receiving VKA. Our prior estimate of the increase in bleeding risk with anticoagulants (1.42 per 100 patient-years) remains the best estimate of the increase in risk attendant on VKA use.

Author Contributions

Conceived and designed the experiments: LCL GG SS JE FS. Performed the experiments: LCL SE FS IN MV. Analyzed the data: LCL GG FS JE SS QZ. Wrote the paper: LCL GG SS JE FS SE IN. The strategy of the search and the search in the database: NB. The statistical analysis and all forest plot and funnel plot: QZ.

References

1. Lopes LC, Spencer FA, Neumann I, Ventresca M, Ebrahim S, et al. (2013) Bleeding risk in atrial fibrillation patients taking vitamin K antagonists: Systematic review and meta-analysis. Clin Pharmacol Ther.
2. You JJ, Singer DE, Howard PA, Lane DA, Eckman MH, et al. (2012) Antithrombotic therapy for atrial fibrillation: Antithrombotic Therapy and Prevention of Thrombosis, 9th ed: American College of Chest Physicians Evidence-Based Clinical Practice Guidelines. Chest 141: e531S–575S.
3. Meiltz A, Zimmermann M, Urban P, Bloch A, Association of Cardiologists of the Canton of G (2008) Atrial fibrillation management by practice cardiologists: a prospective survey on the adherence to guidelines in the real world. Europace 10: 674–680.
4. Lee BH, Park JS, Park JH, Park JS, Kwak JJ, et al. (2010) The effect and safety of the antithrombotic therapies in patients with atrial fibrillation and CHADS score 1. Journal of Cardiovascular Electrophysiology 21: 501–507.
5. Ruiz Ortiz M, Romo E, Mesa D, Delgado M, Anguita M, et al. (2010) Oral anticoagulation in nonvalvular atrial fibrillation in clinical practice: Impact of CHADS2 score on outcome. Cardiology 115: 200–204.
6. Leung CS, Tam KM (2003) Antithrombotic treatment of atrial fibrillation in a regional hospital in Hong Kong. Hong Kong Medical Journal 9: 179–185.
7. Parkash R, Wee V, Gardner MJ, Cox JL, Thompson K, et al. (2007) The impact of warfarin use on clinical outcomes in atrial fibrillation: a population-based study. Canadian Journal of Cardiology 23: 457–461.
8. SPAF (1998) Patients with nonvalvular atrial fibrillation at low risk of stroke during treatment with aspirin: Stroke Prevention in Atrial Fibrillation III Study. The SPAF III Writing Committee for the Stroke Prevention in Atrial Fibrillation Investigators. JAMA 279: 1273–1277.
9. Lai HM, Aronow WS, Kalen P, Adapa S, Patel K, et al. (2009) Incidence of thromboembolic stroke and of major bleeding in patients with atrial fibrillation and chronic kidney disease treated with and without warfarin. International Journal of Nephrology and Renovascular Disease 2.
10. Boulanger L, Hauch O, Friedman M, Foster T, Dixon D, et al. (2006) Warfarin exposure and the risk of thromboembolic and major bleeding events among medicaid patients with atrial fibrillation. Annals of Pharmacotherapy 40: 1024–1029.
11. Pisters R, Lane DA, Nieuwlaat R, de Vos CB, Crijns HJGM, et al. (2010) A novel user-friendly score (HAS-BLED) to assess 1-year risk of major bleeding in patients with atrial fibrillation: the Euro Heart Survey. Chest 138: 1093–1100.
12. Burton C, Isles C, Norrie J, Hanson R, Grubb E (2006) The safety and adequacy of antithrombotic therapy for atrial fibrillation: a regional cohort study. British Journal of General Practice 56: 697–702.
13. Darkow T, Vanderplas AM, Lew KH, Kim J, Hauch O (2005) Treatment patterns and real-world effectiveness of warfarin in nonvalvular atrial fibrillation within a managed care system. Current Medical Research & Opinion 21: 1583–1594.
14. Hansen ML, Sorensen R, Clausen MT, Fog-Petersen ML, Raunso J, et al. (2010) Risk of bleeding with single, dual, or triple therapy with warfarin, aspirin, and clopidogrel in patients with atrial fibrillation. Arch Intern Med 170: 1433–1441.
15. Jackson SL, Peterson GM, Vial JH, Daud R, Ang SY (2001) Outcomes in the management of atrial fibrillation: clinical trial results can apply in practice. Internal Medicine Journal 31: 329–336.
16. Currie CJ, Jones M, Goodfellow J, McEwan P, Morgan CL, et al. (2006) Evaluation of survival and ischaemic and thromboembolic event rates in patients with non-valvar atrial fibrillation in the general population when treated and untreated with warfarin. Heart 92: 196–200.
17. Gage BF, Yan Y, Milligan PE, Waterman AD, Culverhouse R, et al. (2006) Clinical classification schemes for predicting hemorrhage: results from the National Registry of Atrial Fibrillation (NRAF). American Heart Journal 151: 713–719.
18. Boccuzzi SJ, Martin J, Stephenson J, Kreilick C, Fernandes J, et al. (2009) Retrospective study of total healthcare costs associated with chronic nonvalvular atrial fibrillation and the occurrence of a first transient ischemic attack, stroke or major bleed. Current Medical Research and Opinion 25: 2853–2864.
19. Sam C, Massaro JM, D'Agostino RB Sr, Levy D, Lambert JW, et al. (2004) Warfarin and aspirin use and the predictors of major bleeding complications in

atrial fibrillation (the Framingham Heart Study). American Journal of Cardiology 94: 947–951.

20. Shen AY-J, Yao JF, Brar SS, Jorgensen MB, Chen W (2007) Racial/ethnic differences in the risk of intracranial hemorrhage among patients with atrial fibrillation. Journal of the American College of Cardiology 50: 309–315.

21. Singer DE, Chang Y, Fang MC, Borowsky LH, Pomernacki NK, et al. (2009) The net clinical benefit of warfarin anticoagulation in atrial fibrillation.[Summary for patients in Ann Intern Med. 2009 Sep 1;151(5):I36; PMID: 19721014]. Annals of Internal Medicine 151: 297–305.

22. Wess ML, Schauer DP, Johnston JA, Moomaw CJ, Brewer DE, et al. (2008) Application of a decision support tool for anticoagulation in patients with non-valvular atrial fibrillation. Journal of General Internal Medicine 23: 411–417.

23. Friberg L, Hammar N, Rosenqvist M (2010) Stroke in paroxysmal atrial fibrillation: report from the Stockholm Cohort of Atrial Fibrillation. European Heart Journal 31: 967–975.

24. AFASAK (1989) Placebo-controlled, randomized trial of warfarin and aspirin for prevention of thromboembolic complications in chronic atrial fibrillation: the Copenhagen study. Lancet 333 (8631): 175–179.

25. BAATF (1990) Boston Area Anticoagulation Trial for Atrial Fibrillation Investigators. The effect of low-dose warfarin on the risk of stroke in nonrheumatic atrial fibrillation. N Engl J Med 323: 1505–1511.

26. Sato H, Ishikawa K, Kitabatake A, Ogawa S, Maruyama Y, et al. (2006) Low-dose aspirin for prevention of stroke in low-risk patients with atrial fibrillation: Japan Atrial Fibrillation Stroke Trial. Stroke 37: 447–451.

27. Edvardsson N, Juul-Moller S, Omblus R, Pehrsson K (2003) Effects of low-dose warfarin and aspirin versus no treatment on stroke in a medium-risk patient population with atrial fibrillation. J Intern Med 254: 95–101.

28. EAFT (1993) Secundary preventionin non-rheumatic atrial fibrillation after transient ischemick attack or minor stroke. Lancet 342: 1255–1262.

29. CAFA, Connolly SJ, Laupacis A, Gent M, Roberts RS, et al. (1991) Canadian Atrial Fibrillation Anticoagulation (CAFA) Study. J Am CollCardiol 18: 349–355.

30. SPINAF, Ezekowitz MD, Bridgers SL, James KE, Carliner NH, et al. (1992) Warafarin in the preventin of stroke associated with nonrheumatic atrial fibrillation. N Engl J Med 327: 1406–1412.

31. AFI (1994) Atrial Fibrillation Investigators: Atrial Fibrillation, Aspirin, Anticoagulation Study, Boston Area Anticoagulation Trial for Atrial Fibrillation Study, Canadian Atrial Fibrillation Anticoagulation Study, Stroke Prevention in Atrial Fibrillation Study, Veterans Affairs Stroke Prevention in Nonrheumatic Atrial Fibrillation Study,Risk Factors for Stroke and Efficacy of Antithrombotic Therapy in Atrial Fibrillation: Analysis of Pooled Data From Five Randomized Controlled Trials. Arch Intern Med 154: 1449–1457.

32. SPAF (1991) Stroke Prevention in Atrial Fibrillation Study. Final results. Circulation 84: 527–539.

33. Hu DY, Zhang HP, Sun YH, Jiang LQ (2006) [The randomized study of efficiency and safety of antithrombotic therapy in nonvalvular atrial fibrillation: warfarin compared with aspirin]. Zhonghua Xin Xue Guan Bing Za Zhi 34: 295–298.

34. Morocutti C, Amabile G, Fattapposta F, Nicolosi A, Matteoli S, et al. (1997) Indobufen versus warfarin in the secondary prevention of major vascular events in nonrheumatic atrial fibrillation. SIFA (Studio Italiano Fibrillazione Atriale) Investigators. Stroke 28: 1015–1021.

35. NASPEAF (2004) Comparative Effects of Antiplatelet, Anticoagulant, or Combined Therapy in Patients With Valvular and Nonvalvular Atrial Fibrillation. J Am Coll Cardiol 44: 1557–1566.

36. SPAFII (1994) Warfarin versus aspirin for prevention of thromboembolism in atrial fibrillation: Stroke Prevention in Atrial Fibrillation II Study. Lancet 343: 687–691.

37. AFASAK 2, Gullov AL, Koefoed BG, Petersen P (1999) Bleeding During Warfarin and Aspirin Therapy in Patients With Atrial Fibrillation: The AFASAK 2 Study. Arch Intern Med 159: 1322–1328.

38. PATAF, Hellemons BSP, Langenberg M, Lodder J, Vermeer F, et al. (1997) Primary prevention of arterial thromboembolism in patients with nonrheumatic atrial fibrillation in general practice (the PATAF study). Cerebrovascular Diseases 7: 11.

39. BAFTA (2007) Warfarin versus aspirin for stroke prevention in an elderly community population with atrial fi brillation (the Birmingham Atrial Fibrillation Treatment of the Aged Study, BAFTA): a randomised controlled trial. Lancet 370: 493–503.

14

Healthcare Utilization and Clinical Outcomes after Catheter Ablation of Atrial Flutter

Thomas A. Dewland[1], David V. Glidden[2], Gregory M. Marcus[1]*

1 Department of Internal Medicine, Division of Cardiology, Electrophysiology Section, University of California San Francisco, San Francisco, California, United States of America, **2** Department of Epidemiology and Biostatistics, University of California San Francisco, San Francisco, California, United States of America

Abstract

Atrial flutter ablation is associated with a high rate of acute procedural success and symptom improvement. The relationship between ablation and other clinical outcomes has been limited to small studies primarily conducted at academic centers. We sought to determine if catheter ablation of atrial flutter is associated with reductions in healthcare utilization, atrial fibrillation, or stroke in a large, real world population. California Healthcare Cost and Utilization Project databases were used to identify patients undergoing atrial flutter ablation between 2005 and 2009. The adjusted association between atrial flutter ablation and healthcare utilization, atrial fibrillation, or stroke was investigated using Cox proportional hazards models. Among 33,004 patients with a diagnosis of atrial flutter observed for a median of 2.1 years, 2,733 (8.2%) underwent catheter ablation. Atrial flutter ablation significantly lowered the adjusted risk of inpatient hospitalization (HR 0.88, 95% CI 0.84–0.92, p<0.001), emergency department visits (HR 0.60, 95% CI 0.54–0.65, p<0.001), and overall hospital-based healthcare utilization (HR 0.94, 95% CI 0.90–0.98, p = 0.001). Atrial flutter ablation was also associated with a statistically significant 11% reduction in the adjusted hazard of atrial fibrillation (HR 0.89, 95% CI 0.81–0.97, p = 0.01). Risk of acute stroke was not significantly reduced after ablation (HR 1.09, 95% CI 0.81–1.45, p = 0.57). In a large, real world population, atrial flutter ablation was associated with significant reductions in hospital-based healthcare utilization and a reduced risk of atrial fibrillation. These findings support the early use of catheter ablation for the treatment of atrial flutter.

Editor: Ali A. Sovari, University of Illinois at Chicago, United States of America

Funding: This work was made possible by grant numbers 12POST11810036 (TAD) and 12GRNT11780061 (GMM) from the American Heart Association, and by the Joseph Drown Foundation (GMM). The funders had no role in study design, data collection and analysis, decision to publish, or preparation of the manuscript.

Competing Interests: The authors have declared that no competing interests exist.

* Email: marcusg@medicine.ucsf.edu

Introduction

The efficacy of endocardial catheter ablation for the treatment of atrial flutter (AFL) is well established. AFL ablation is associated with a high rate of acute procedural success [1] and a low incidence of AFL recurrence during follow up [2]. In addition, randomized comparisons of ablation versus medical management have shown significantly less symptoms, reduced morbidity, and enhanced quality of life with an ablation strategy [3,4].

The impact of AFL ablation on other arrhythmia related clinical outcomes, however, is less clear. Although previous investigations have found an association between AFL ablation and a reduction in subsequent healthcare visits, these small studies have been limited to single academic centers [5,6] or to carefully selected randomized trial participants [3]. Furthermore, while one randomized trial demonstrated less atrial fibrillation (AF) after AFL ablation [3], this finding was not replicated in a second study [4]. Finally, although AFL ablation could potentially reduce the risk of thromboembolic stroke through maintenance of sinus rhythm, prior investigations have not been powered to assess for differences in this endpoint.

The relationship between AFL ablation and these important clinical outcomes has not been studied in a large, real world population. We therefore used data from the Healthcare Cost and Utilization Project (HCUP) to determine if catheter ablation is associated with reductions in healthcare utilization, AF, and stroke among a contemporary population of California residents diagnosed with AFL.

Materials and Methods

Ethics Statement

Patient information was anonymized prior to analysis and certification to use this deidentified HCUP data was obtained from the University of California, San Francisco Committee on Human Research.

We identified all patients ≥18 years of age with a diagnosis of AFL who received care in a California emergency department, inpatient hospital unit, or ambulatory surgery setting between January 1, 2005 and December 31, 2009 using HCUP (Agency for Healthcare Research and Quality) California State Emergency Department Databases, State Inpatient Databases, and State Ambulatory Surgery Databases [7]. Individual databases specific to calendar year and healthcare setting were merged using an encrypted linkage variable to identify repeat visits for a given patient. Patients with missing admission date data, residence outside of the state of California, or concomitant AF (defined as an AF diagnosis either before or at the same time as an AFL diagnosis) were excluded. For the healthcare utilization outcome, individuals entered the study cohort upon their first AFL diagnosis and were censored after inpatient death or at the end of the study period (December 31, 2009). For AF and stroke analyses, patients were additionally censored at the time of the respective outcome of interest.

Age, gender, race, income level, and insurance payer were recorded at each healthcare encounter by the discharging institution. Income level was categorized by quartiles using the median household income for the patient's ZIP code. Up to 25 International Classification of Diseases-9th Edition (ICD-9) codes and 21 Current Procedural Terminology (CPT) codes were provided for each encounter. AFL and AF were defined using the ICD-9 codes 427.32 and 427.31, respectively. Because post-operative AFL and AF may have a different underlying mechanism than when observed outside of the acute surgical setting, AFL and AF were not recorded if a patient had undergone cardiothoracic surgery during the same hospitalization or within the previous 30 days [8]. Other medical comorbidities postulated to confound and/or mediate the association between AFL ablation and clinical outcomes were also recorded using ICD-9 and CPT codes (**Table S1**) [8,9]. Dichotomous medical comorbidity variables were accumulated at each healthcare encounter and carried forward over time. The Charlson Comorbidity Index was calculated at each discharge event using ICD-9 codes as previously described [10].

AFL ablation procedures were identified using the ICD-9 code for endocardial catheter ablation (37.34) in patients with a concomitant diagnosis of AFL. To maintain the specificity of AFL ablation identification, patients with a diagnosis of AF, supraventricular tachycardia, ventricular tachycardia, premature ventricular contractions, Wolf-Parkinson-White syndrome, Lown–Ganong–Levine syndrome, atrio-ventricular nodal reentrant tachycardia, or implantable pacemaker or defibrillator insertion coded at the same time of the ablation procedure were not considered to have undergone AFL ablation [9].

Healthcare utilization was defined as any inpatient hospitalization, emergency department visit without inpatient admission, or ambulatory surgery encounter. Acute ischemic stroke/transient ischemic attack and AF were identified using ICD-9 coding (**Table S1**).

Statistical Analysis

Continuous variables with a normal distribution are presented as mean ± standard deviation (SD) and were compared using t-tests. Non-normally distributed continuous variables are presented as medians with interquartile ranges (IQR) and were compared using Kruskal-Wallis tests. The association between categorical variables was determined using Chi-squared tests. Cox proportional hazards models were used to investigate the association between AFL ablation and clinical outcomes both before and after controlling for known confounders identified *a priori*. In these models, AFL ablation, insurance payer, income level, and medical comorbidities were treated as time-dependent covariates. The proportional hazards assumption was assessed using Kaplan-Meier versus predicted survival plots and log-minus-log survival plots. For the assessment of healthcare utilization, a patient who underwent AFL ablation could contribute observation time and events to both the non-ablation and ablation groups depending upon ablation status. To reduce systematic bias in favor of ablation, the AFL ablation visit was considered a post ablation healthcare encounter. AF and stroke analyses were limited to individuals with a first healthcare encounter between 2006 and 2009 to ensure adequate exclusion of patients with prevalent AF and stroke, respectively.

Several sensitivity analyses were performed to further evaluate the observed association between ablation and healthcare utilization. First, a comparison of medical visits before and after ablation was restricted to only those patients who underwent AFL ablation. Such an analysis should minimize selection bias, as healthcare utilization was compared before and after ablation within individual patients. We also recognized that non-cardiac conditions likely impact both a provider's decision to perform AFL ablation and healthcare utilization. A second analysis therefore compared healthcare utilization by AFL ablation status after adjusting for patient demographics, cardiovascular risk factors, and Charlson Comorbidity Index. The Charlson Comorbidity Index is a validated instrument that uses the presence of a wide variety of medical conditions to estimate an individual patient's relative mortality [11]. This scoring system has been adapted to administrative databases that utilize ICD-9 coding [10] and serves as an overall estimate of a patient's health status. In addition, we utilized propensity score methods to address confounding between the ablation and non-ablation groups. For these analyses, a logistic model that included age, gender, race, insurance, income, hypertension, diabetes, coronary artery disease, heart failure, valvular heart disease, pulmonary disease, chronic kidney disease, and neurologic disease was used to estimate the probability of AFL ablation for each patient at the time of index AFL diagnosis. Propensity scores were treated as either a categorical variable (expressed as quintiles) or a continuous measurement (modeled using restricted cubic splines) and included in Cox proportional hazard models to determine the adjusted association between AFL ablation and healthcare utilization. Finally, we also performed a propensity score matched analysis whereby patients undergoing ablation were matched 1:1 with non-ablated individuals using a nearest neighbor matching algorithm without replacement.

All analyses were performed using Stata 12 (StataCorp, College Station, TX, USA). A two-tailed p<0.05 was considered statistically significant.

Results

Among 33,004 patients with a diagnosis of AFL observed for a median of 2.1 (IQR 0.8 to 3.6) years, 2,733 (8.2%) underwent catheter ablation. Ablation procedures were fairly evenly distributed over the study period and were roughly equally divided between inpatient and outpatient procedural settings (**Figure 1**). The ablated group was significantly younger and had a greater proportion of men, a lower prevalence of cardiovascular comorbidities, and a lower median Charlson Comorbidity Index (**Table 1**).

AFL Ablation and Healthcare Utilization

A total of 135,614 healthcare encounters were observed among all atrial flutter patients with a median of 3 (IQR 2 to 6) visits per patient. When not ablated, there were 1.86 visits per person-year (95% CI 1.85 to 1.87). After ablation, there were 1.50 visits per person-year (95% CI 1.47 to 1.53). In multivariate analysis adjusting for patient demographics (age, gender, race, insurance, and income) and comorbidities (hypertension, diabetes, coronary artery disease, heart failure, remote history of cardiothoracic surgery, valvular heart disease, pulmonary disease, chronic kidney disease, neurologic disease, and atrial fibrillation), AFL ablation resulted in a significantly increased hazard of an ambulatory surgery encounter (HR 1.63, 95% CI 1.54 to 1.73, p<0.001). However, ablation significantly lowered the risk of inpatient hospitalization by 12% (HR 0.88, 95% CI 0.84 to 0.92, p<0.001) and cut the risk of an emergency department visit by 40% (HR

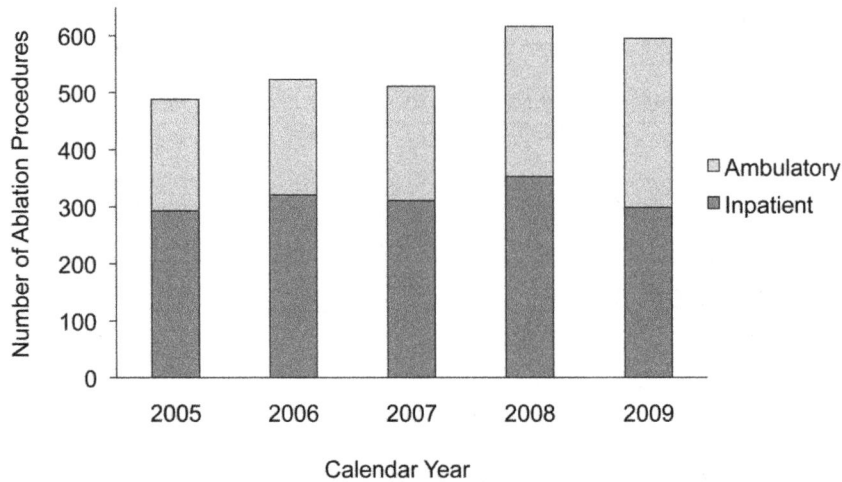

Figure 1. Atrial Flutter Ablation Procedures by Calendar Year and Healthcare Setting. The absolute number of ablation procedures performed in an ambulatory surgery (light bar) or inpatient hospitalization (dark bar) setting is shown for each calendar year included in the study.

0.60, 95% CI 0.54 to 0.65, p<0.001, **Table 2**). This resulted in a statistically significant reduction in the adjusted hazard of *overall* healthcare utilization (including ambulatory surgery encounters, inpatient hospitalizations, and emergency department visits) with AFL ablation (HR 0.94, 95% CI 0.90 to 0.98, p = 0.001, **Figure 2**).

In a sensitivity analysis controlling for the Charlson Comorbidity Index in addition to the above demographic and comorbidity variables, the hazard of healthcare utilization remained significantly reduced with ablation (HR 0.93, 95% CI 0.89 to 0.96, p< 0.001). When analysis was limited to only those patients who underwent catheter ablation (comparing visits before versus after ablation), AFL ablation was associated with a near 50% reduction

Table 1. Patient Demographics and Comorbidities at First Diagnosis of Atrial Flutter by Ablation Status.

	Ablated n = 2,733	Non-Ablated n = 30,271	P value
Age, mean (SD), years	65 (13)	70 (14)	<0.001
Female, n (%)	593 (22)	11,592 (38)	<0.001
Insurance, n (%)			<0.001
Medicare	1,614 (59)	21,670 (72)	
Medicaid	95 (3)	1,862 (6)	
Private	972 (36)	6,019 (20)	
Self-Pay	13 (1)	443 (1)	
Other	39 (1)	276 (1)	
Income Quartile, n (%)			<0.001
1 Poorest	441 (16)	5,476 (18)	
2	560 (21)	6,341 (21)	
3	749 (28)	8,665 (29)	
4 Wealthiest	951 (35)	9,476 (32)	
Hypertension, n (%)	1,211 (44)	17,292 (57)	<0.001
Diabetes, n (%)	494 (18)	8,418 (28)	<0.001
Coronary Artery Disease, n (%)	632 (23)	9,642 (32)	<0.001
Heart Failure, n (%)	465 (17)	8,861 (29)	<0.001
CTS*, n (%)	0	16 (0.1)	0.23
Valvular Disease, n (%)	363 (13)	4,265 (14)	0.24
Pulmonary Disease, n (%)	285 (10)	6,481 (21)	<0.001
Chronic Kidney Disease, n (%)	111 (4)	3,595 (12)	<0.001
Charlson Comorbidity Index, median (IQR)	0 (0 to 1)	1 (0 to 2)	<0.001

CTS, cardiothoracic surgery; IQR, interquartile range; SD, standard deviation.

Table 2. Adjusted Hazard of Healthcare Utilization by Setting.

Healthcare Setting	Adjusted HR*	95% CI	P value
Ambulatory Surgery	1.63	1.54 to 1.73	<0.001
Inpatient Hospitalization	0.88	0.84 to 0.92	<0.001
Emergency Department Visit	0.60	0.54 to 0.65	<0.001
Overall Healthcare Utilization	0.94	0.90 to 0.98	0.001

Adjusted for age, gender, race, insurance, income, hypertension, diabetes, coronary artery disease, heart failure, remote history of cardiothoracic surgery, valvular heart disease, pulmonary disease, chronic kidney disease, neurologic disease, and atrial fibrillation. Overall healthcare utilization includes ambulatory surgery, inpatient, and emergency department encounters. CI, confidence interval; HR, hazard ratio.

in the adjusted hazard of overall healthcare utilization (HR 0.51, 95% CI 0.47 to 0.55, p<0.001). In analyses treating the AFL ablation propensity score as continuous predictor, ablation was again found to be associated with a reduction in the hazard of overall healthcare utilization (HR 0.91, 0.87 to 0.95, p<0.001). This result did not substantially differ when the propensity score was modeled as a categorical variable. Similarly, in a 1:1 propensity matched analysis, AFL ablation remained associated with a significant reduction in overall healthcare utilization (HR 0.86, 0.81 to 0.90, p<0.001).

AFL Ablation and AF

From the population of AFL patients without a known diagnosis of AF, we observed 11,237 incident episodes of AF. When not ablated, the rate of incident atrial fibrillation was 23.0 per one hundred person years (95% CI 22.5 to 23.6). After flutter ablation, the rate was 16.9 per one hundred person years (95% CI 15.5 to 18.4). In multivariate analysis adjusting for age, gender, race, income, insurance status, and history of hypertension, diabetes, coronary artery disease, heart failure, cardiac surgery, valve disease, pulmonary disease, and chronic kidney disease, AFL ablation was associated with a statistically significant 11% reduction in the hazard of AF (HR 0.89, 95% CI 0.81 to 0.97, p = 0.01, **Figure 2**).

AFL Ablation and Stroke

We observed 1,203 incident acute strokes during the study period. When not ablated, the rate of incident stroke was 17.9 per thousand person years (95% CI 16.7 to 19.3). After flutter ablation, the rate was 13.1 per thousand person years (95% CI 10.0 to 17.3). In multivariate analysis adjusting for age, gender, race, insurance, income, and history of AF, hypertension, diabetes, coronary disease, heart failure, cardiac surgery, valvular heart disease, and chronic kidney disease, AFL ablation was not significantly associated with acute stroke (HR 1.09, 95% CI 0.81 to 1.45, p = 0.57, **Figure 2**).

Discussion

In a large, real world population of patients diagnosed with AFL, we found that AFL ablation significantly reduced overall healthcare utilization. The lower rate of healthcare encounters after ablation was driven by substantial reductions in all-cause inpatient hospitalization and emergency department visits. AFL ablation was also associated with a reduced incidence of post-procedural AF, although ablation did not reduce the hazard of acute stroke.

Prior observational studies and randomized trials have demonstrated decreased healthcare visits after AFL ablation [3,5,6]. Extrapolation of these previous investigations to the broad

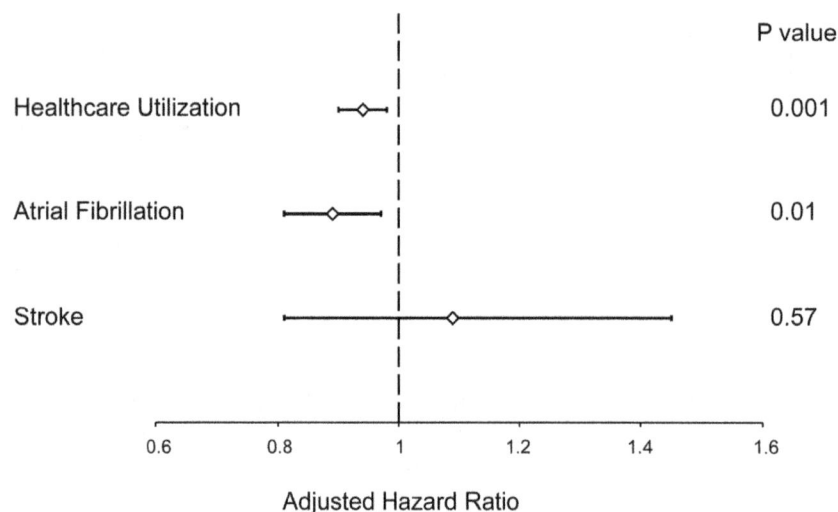

Figure 2. Adjusted Hazard of Healthcare Utilization, Atrial Fibrillation, or Stroke After Atrial Flutter Ablation. Diamonds indicate the adjusted hazard ratio point estimates and error bars denote 95% confidence intervals. The dashed vertical line represents a hazard ratio of 1 (no difference with atrial flutter ablation).

population of patients with AFL, however, is limited due to their small sample size (generally 100 or less patients), use of patient recall to identify hospitalization encounters, or selective enrollment in the context of a clinical trial. In addition, many of the studies examining this association have been performed at academic centers outside of the United States, where alternative healthcare cost and delivery forces may influence hospital utilization [5,6]. Our findings extend this prior research by demonstrating a reduction in objectively measured hospital-based encounters among real world patients treated at both community and academic hospitals across California.

We found that AFL ablation reduced the risk of overall healthcare utilization by 6%. It is important to note that our primary outcome included *all* hospital-related healthcare encounters before and after ablation. This analysis strategy was utilized to provide a conservative estimate of AFL ablation benefit, as the ablation procedure would only be expected to reduce AFL-related admissions. The ambulatory surgery encounter during which a patient underwent AFL ablation was counted as a post-ablation visit, likely accounting for the significantly increased hazard of an ambulatory surgery visit in the ablation group. Notably, AFL ablation sufficiently reduced subsequent inpatient hospitalizations and emergency department visits to offset the increased encounters incurred by the procedure itself.

Multiple sensitivity analyses were utilized to further explore the observed association between AFL ablation and healthcare outcomes. As we reasoned that a patient's overall health status would likely influence the likelihood of AFL ablation, we further adjusted our primary analysis for the Charlson Comorbidity Index. This metric was previously developed to estimate an individual patient's relative mortality using medical comorbidities identified from ICD-9 coding [10,11]. A separate analysis quantified hospital-based healthcare encounters only in patients who underwent ablation. As overall healthcare utilization was significantly decreased within individual patients after the ablation procedure, these results strongly argue against residual confounding as an explanation for our overall findings. Finally, we utilized both propensity score adjustment and matching as an additional and complementary methodology to minimize bias. Our sensitivity analyses consistently demonstrated a reduction in healthcare utilization with AFL ablation, strengthening the results of the primary analysis. The use of catheter ablation to treat a first episode of AFL is currently a Class IIa recommendation; this procedure only receives a Class I recommendation after arrhythmia recurrence [12]. Given the overall efficacy and safety of this procedure for the treatment of AFL, our findings may support the use of catheter ablation as a first-line treatment for AFL.

Although the electrophysiologic mechanisms of AFL and AF are distinct, the two arrhythmias often coexist and may share a common trigger [13–15]. Randomized trials comparing AFL ablation to medical therapy have reached divergent results, with one trial demonstrating a reduced risk of AF post-ablation [3] and a second showing no difference in AF risk [4]. Our results suggest AF risk is modestly but significantly decreased after AFL ablation, supporting the hypothesis that AFL ablation can reduce pathologic atrial changes that increase AF incidence. To our knowledge, this is the first investigation that has compared long-term stroke outcomes before and after AFL ablation. As AFL is known to increase the risk of cardiogenic thromboembolism, we hypothesized that ablation of this arrhythmia could reduce stroke incidence. The observed hazard ratio between the ablated and non-ablated groups, however, was small and did not reach statistical significance. Our findings are in agreement with a recent study from a single, experienced academic center that reported

substantial AF and stroke risk after AFL ablation [16]. This prior investigation, however, had comparatively few events and used historic controls to identify the heightened risk of these post-ablation outcomes. Our comparison of events among patients that did and did not receive an AFL ablation in a large, multicenter population extends these findings and establishes a population-based relative risk of AF and stroke outcomes after ablation.

Limitations of the present study should be recognized. Outcome and confounder variables were determined using hospital discharge coding and residual confounding cannot be excluded. Nevertheless, we believe this is less likely to explain our healthcare utilization results given that our findings persisted after sensitivity analyses. HCUP databases do not include ambulatory clinic encounters and we were therefore not able to compare such visits in our analysis. However, the most costly healthcare visits (emergency department and inpatient hospitalizations) were optimally captured by the HCUP database. We similarly did not have information regarding the use of anticoagulant or antiarrhythmic medications, which could have implications for our AF and stroke outcomes. For example, it possible that AFL ablation patients were more likely to receive care from an electrophysiologist, who may be more likely to prescribe an antiarrhythmic drug. In addition, the methodology used for AFL ablation identification in our analysis was developed to favor specificity over sensitivity. To our knowledge, there are no large, contemporary, population-based samples that define the overall proportion of AFL patients treated with catheter ablation. As such, the degree to which we have underestimated overall ablation utilization cannot be accurately quantified and the absolute rate at which this procedure is utilized in real world settings cannot be directly extrapolated from our analysis. Given the de-identified nature of the HCUP dataset, it was not possible to validate the accuracy of ICD-9 coding for AFL and AF. Notably, to bias our estimation of the association between AFL ablation and AF, the rate of misdiagnosis of these arrhythmias would need to differ by history of ablation. Because such a scenario is unlikely, we believe that widespread differential misclassification of AF and AFL by ablation status is unlikely to explain our positive results. Although we excluded arrhythmia episodes that occurred immediately after cardiac surgery, we were unable to determine which flutter diagnoses occurred in the setting of other reversible triggers (such as pneumonia or hyperthyroidism) and therefore might not be appropriately treated with an ablation procedure. Finally, because we did not have information regarding the flutter mechanism, the proportion of patients with a typical, cavotricuspid isthmus dependent arrhythmia circuit is not known (although approximately 90% of clinically observed flutter circuits are thought to involve this mechanism) [17].

In conclusion, we observed significant reductions in healthcare utilization after catheter ablation among patients with AFL. In addition, catheter ablation was associated with a reduced risk of AF. These findings support the early use of catheter ablation in the treatment of AFL.

Author Contributions

Conceived and designed the experiments: TAD DVG GMM. Performed the experiments: TAD DVG GMM. Analyzed the data: TAD DVG GMM. Contributed reagents/materials/analysis tools: TAD DVG GMM. Wrote the paper: TAD DVG GMM.

References

1. Scheinman MM, Huang S (2000) The 1998 NASPE prospective catheter ablation registry. Pacing Clin Electrophysiol 23: 1020–1028.

2. Calkins H, Canby R, Weiss R, Taylor G, Wells P, et al. (2004) Results of catheter ablation of typical atrial flutter. Am J Cardiol 94: 437–442. doi:10.1016/j.amjcard.2004.04.058.

3. Natale A, Newby KH, Pisanó E, Leonelli F, Fanelli R, et al. (2000) Prospective randomized comparison of antiarrhythmic therapy versus first-line radiofrequency ablation in patients with atrial flutter. J Am Coll Cardiol 35: 1898–1904.

4. Da Costa A, Thevenin J, Roche F, Romeyer-Bouchard C, Abdellaoui L, et al. (2006) Results from the Loire-Ardeche-Drome-Isere-Puy-de-Dome (LADIP) trial on atrial flutter, a multicentric prospective randomized study comparing amiodarone and radiofrequency ablation after the first episode of symptomatic atrial flutter. Circulation 114: 1676–1681. doi:10.1161/CIRCULATIONAHA.106.638395.

5. Lee SH, Tai CT, Yu WC, Chen YJ, Hsieh MH, et al. (1999) Effects of radiofrequency catheter ablation on quality of life in patients with atrial flutter. Am J Cardiol 84: 278–283.

6. O'Callaghan PA, Meara M, Kongsgaard E, Poloniecki J, Luddington L, et al. (2001) Symptomatic improvement after radiofrequency catheter ablation for typical atrial flutter. Heart 86: 167–171.

7. Brousseau DC, Owens PL, Mosso AL, Panepinto JA, Steiner CA (2010) Acute care utilization and rehospitalizations for sickle cell disease. JAMA 303: 1288–1294. doi:10.1001/jama.2010.378.

8. Go AS, Hylek EM, Phillips KA, Chang Y, Henault LE, et al. (2001) Prevalence of diagnosed atrial fibrillation in adults: national implications for rhythm management and stroke prevention: the AnTicoagulation and Risk Factors in Atrial Fibrillation (ATRIA) Study. JAMA 285: 2370–2375.

9. Shah RU, Freeman JV, Shilane D, Wang PJ, Go AS, et al. (2012) Procedural complications, rehospitalizations, and repeat procedures after catheter ablation for atrial fibrillation. 59: 143–149. doi:10.1016/j.jacc.2011.08.068.

10. Deyo RA, Cherkin DC, Ciol MA (1992) Adapting a clinical comorbidity index for use with ICD-9-CM administrative databases. J Clin Epidemiol 45: 613–619.

11. Charlson ME, Pompei P, Ales KL, MacKenzie CR (1987) A new method of classifying prognostic comorbidity in longitudinal studies: development and validation. J Chronic Dis 40: 373–383.

12. Blomstrom-Lundqvist C, Scheinman MM, Aliot EM, Alpert JS, Calkins H, et al. (2003) ACC/AHA/ESC guidelines for the management of patients with supraventricular arrhythmias–executive summary: a report of the American College of Cardiology/American Heart Association Task Force on Practice Guidelines and the European Society of Cardiology Committee for Practice Guidelines (Writing Committee to Develop Guidelines for the Management of Patients With Supraventricular Arrhythmias). Circulation 108: 1871–1909. doi:10.1161/01.CIR.0000091380.04100.84.

13. Morton JB, Byrne MJ, Power JM, Raman J, Kalman JM (2002) Electrical remodeling of the atrium in an anatomic model of atrial flutter: relationship between substrate and triggers for conversion to atrial fibrillation. Circulation 105: 258–264.

14. Roithinger FX, Karch MR, Steiner PR, SippensGroenewegen A, Lesh MD (1997) Relationship between atrial fibrillation and typical atrial flutter in humans: activation sequence changes during spontaneous conversion. Circulation 96: 3484–3491.

15. Waldo AL (2002) Mechanisms of atrial flutter and atrial fibrillation: distinct entities or two sides of a coin? Cardiovasc Res 54: 217–229.

16. Tomson TT, Kapa S, Bala R, Riley MP, Lin D, et al. (2012) Risk of stroke and atrial fibrillation after radiofrequency catheter ablation of typical atrial flutter. Heart Rhythm 9: 1779–1784. doi:10.1016/j.hrthm.2012.07.013.

17. Saoudi N, Cosio F, Waldo A, Chen SA, Iesaka Y, et al. (2001) Classification of atrial flutter and regular atrial tachycardia according to electrophysiologic mechanism and anatomic bases: a statement from a joint expert group from the Working Group of Arrhythmias of the European Society of Cardiology and the North American Society of Pacing and Electrophysiology. J Cardiovasc Electrophysiol 12: 852–866.

15

Isolated Insular Strokes and Plasma MR-proANP Levels Are Associated with Newly Diagnosed Atrial Fibrillation: A Pilot Study

Karl Frontzek[1,2], Felix Fluri[2,3], Jakob Siemerkus[4], Beat Müller[5], Achim Gass[6], Mirjam Christ-Crain[7], Mira Katan[3]*

1 Institute of Neuropathology, University Hospital Zurich, Zurich, Switzerland, 2 Department of Neurology, University Hospital Basel, Basel, Switzerland, 3 Department of Neurology, University Hospital Zurich, Zurich, Switzerland, 4 University Hospital of Psychiatry, Zurich, Switzerland, 5 Medical University Clinic, Cantonal Hospital Aarau, Aarau, Switzerland, 6 Department of Neurology, University Hospital Mannheim, Mannheim, Germany, 7 Department of Endocrinology, University Hospital Basel, Basel, Switzerland

Abstract

Introduction: In this study, we assessed the relationship of insular strokes and plasma MR-proANP levels with newly diagnosed atrial fibrillation (NDAF).

Methods: This study is based on a prospective acute stroke cohort (http://www.clinicaltrials.gov, NCT00390962). Patient eligibility was dependent on the diagnosis of acute ischemic stroke, absence of previous stroke based on past medical history and MRI, no history of AF and congestive heart failure (cohort A) and, additionally, no stroke lesion size $\geq$ 20 mL (sub-cohort A*). AF, the primary endpoint, was detected on 24-hour electrocardiography and/or echocardiography. Involvement of the insula was assessed by two experienced readers on MRI blinded to clinical data. MR-proANP levels were obtained through a novel sandwich immunoassay. Logistic-regression-models were fitted to estimate odds ratios for the association of insular strokes and MR-proANP with NDAF. The discriminatory accuracy of insular strokes and MR-proANP was assessed by a model-wise comparison of the area under the receiver-operating-characteristics-curve (AUC) with known predictors of AF.

Results: 104 (cohort A) and 83 (cohort A*) patients fulfilled above-mentioned criteria. Patients with isolated insular strokes had a 10.7-fold higher odds of NDAF than patients with a small ischemic stroke at any other location. The AUC of multivariate logistic regression models for the prediction of NDAF improved significantly when adding stroke location and MR-proANP levels. Moreover, MR-proANP levels remained significantly elevated throughout the acute hospitalization period in patients with NDAF compared to those without.

Conclusions: Isolated insular strokes and plasma MR-proANP levels on admission are independent predictors of NDAF and significantly improve the prediction accuracy of identifying patients with NDAF compared to known predictors including age, the NIHSS and lesion size. To accelerate accurate diagnosis and enhance secondary prevention in acute stroke, higher levels of MR-proANP and insular strokes may represent easily accessible indicators of AF if confirmed in an independent validation cohort.

Editor: Jeroen Hendrikse, University Medical Center (UMC) Utrecht, Netherlands

Funding: This work was supported by the Swiss National Science Foundation (PBZHP3-130982 [M.Katan]) as well as the Fondation Leducq (M. Katan). The funders had no role in study design, data collection and analysis, decision to publish, or preparation of the manuscript.

Competing Interests: The authors have read the journal's policy and have the following conflicts: B. Müller received financial research support as well as payments for lectures from B.R.A.H.M.S. part of Thermo Fisher Scientific. A. Gass received payments for lectures including service on speaker bureaus from Biogenldec, Novartis, Bayer and Merck. M. Katan received within the last 3 years (not related to this manuscript) an unconditional research grant form B.R.A.H.M.S. part of Thermo Fisher Scientific. K. Frontzek, F. Fluri,J. Siemerkus and M. Christ-Crain have nothing to disclose.

* E-mail: mira.katan@usz.ch

Introduction

The insular cortex plays an important role in the regulation of the autonomic nervous system. Stimulation of the right insula provokes sympathetic cardiovascular effects, whereas stimulation of the left insula leads to parasympathetic effects.[1] Insular damage has been associated with newly-detected atrial fibrillation (NDAF), atrioventricular blocks and an increased amount of ectopic beats.[2] Furthermore, insular damage is associated with adverse cardiac outcome such as sudden cardiac death and congestive heart failure.[3–5].

A-type natriuretic peptides (ANP) have been proposed as biomarkers for atrial fibrillation (AF) and midregional-proANP plasma levels correlate with the duration of AF episodes.[6,7] There are several sandwich immunoassays commercially available

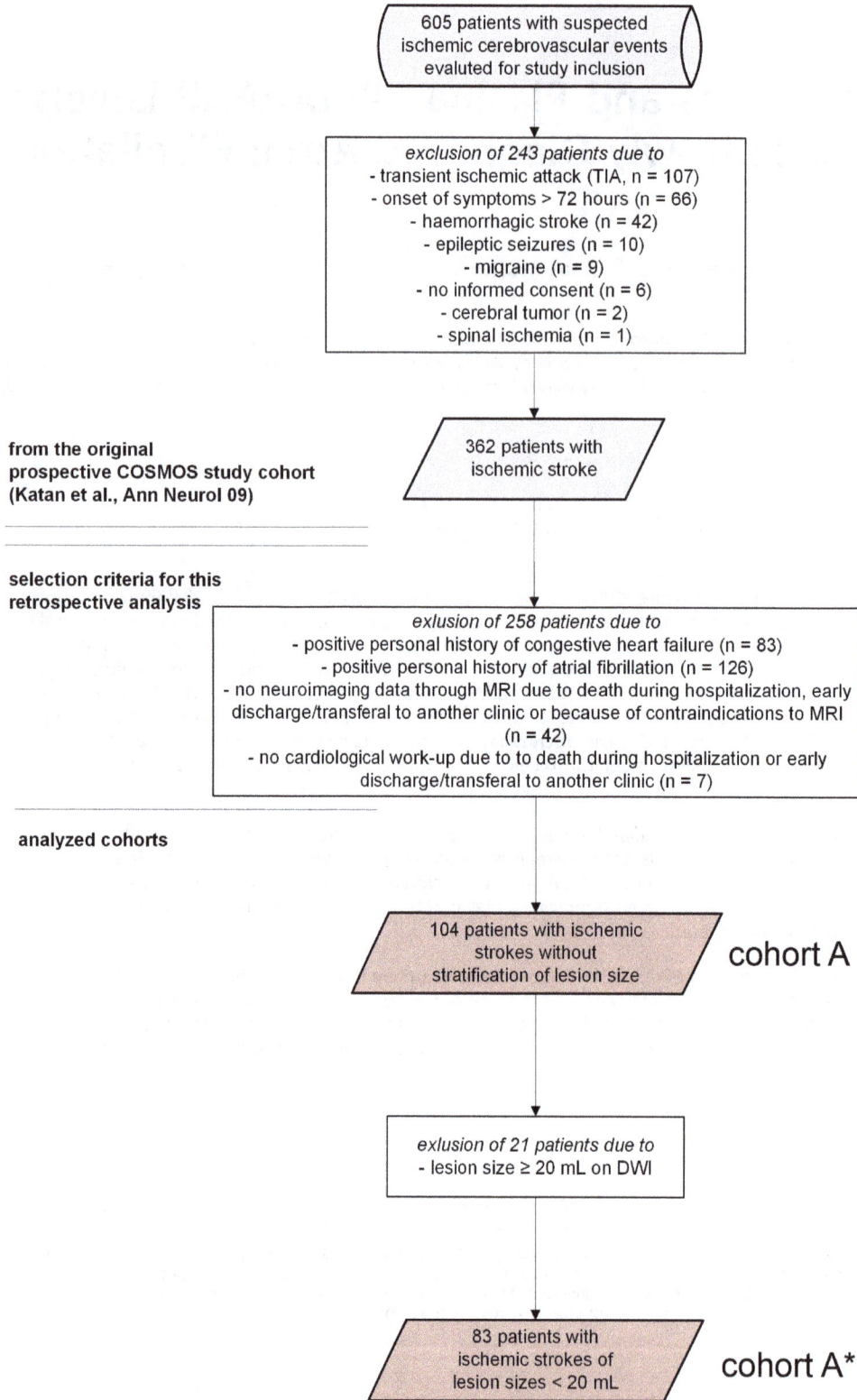

Figure 1. Patient flow chart. The upper part of the figure (as divided by 2 horizontal bars) denotes the study cohort of the original COSMOS cohort as previously described.[11] The lower part of the scheme indicates the eligibility criteria for the cohorts analyzed in this study.

that measure the concentrations of ANP and its precursor protein proANP in human plasma; however, most are prone to fragmentation and may underestimate the release of the precursor due to the early degradation of crucial epitopes at the extreme ends of the molecule. [8,9] The MR-proANP assay used in this study was designed to detect the mid-region of the prohormone, which is more stable than the N- or C-terminal part of the precursor. [10].

The aim of this study was to analyse the predictive value of isolated infarcts affecting the insular cortex in identifying patients with newly diagnosed atrial fibrillation (NDAF) during the acute hospitalization period from a large, prospectively collected stroke cohort.[11] In a second step, we aimed to investigate the putative role of plasma MR-proANP levels in predicting NDAF and its potential additive value compared to stroke location and other known predictors. Early and accurate identification of stroke patients at high risk for AF is important in selecting candidates for intensive cardiac monitoring such as implantable loop recorders. [12].

Patients and Methods

Ethics Statement

This study was based on a prospective cohort study (clinical trial registration at http://www.clinicaltrials.gov, number NCT 00390962) at the University Hospital Basel, Basel, Switzerland. The Ethics Committee of Basel, Switzerland, approved the study protocol and informed, written consent was obtained from all patients before enrollment. A complete description of the cohort has been reported previously.[11].

Description of subjects

Briefly, from 11/2006 to 11/2007, all patients with a suspected acute ischemic cerebrovascular event were consecutively screened for enrollment in the study. All patients admitted to the emergency department within 72 hours after stroke onset with an acute ischemic stroke defined according to the World Health Organization criteria were included. [13] Stroke severity on admission was assessed by stroke neurologists (MK, FF) using the National Institutes of Health Stroke Scale (NIHSS). All patients underwent a standardized diagnostic workup including brain computer tomography mainly to exclude intracranial hemorrhage, magnetic resonance imaging (MRI), standard 12-lead electrocardiography and/or 24-hour electrocardiography. Echocardiography and neurosonographic studies of the extracranial and intracranial arteries were obtained in order to classify stroke etiology according to the TOAST criteria.[14] Initially, from 605 patients with suspected cerebrovascular events admitted to the emergency department of the University Hospital of Basel, 362 patients with confirmed ischemic stroke were selected (see also *figure 1*). From this cohort, we excluded 258 patients due to positive personal history of congestive heart disease and/or atrial fibrillation (n = 209), those with no imaging data on MRI due to death

Table 1. Baseline characteristics of patient cohorts as described in figure 1.

	Cohort A					
	INS	No INS	p-value	NDAF	No NDAF	p-value
number of patients, n	18	86		13	91	
age [y], median (IQR)	72 (57 – 77)	68 (59 – 79)	0.98	71 (67 – 81)	68 (59 – 77)	0.13
NIHSS [pts], median (IQR)	11 (4 – 15)	4 (2 – 7)	0.0019*	5 (2 – 16.5)	4 (2 – 8)	0.28
female sex, % (n)	56 (10)	38 (33)	0.18	38 (5)	42 (38)	0.82
systolic blood pressure [mmHg], median (IQR)	144 (130 – 170)	168 (140 – 183)	0.10	164 (141 – 184)	166 (141 – 185)	0.88
heart rate, median [min^{-1}] (IQR)	73 (64 – 89)	68 (75 – 89)	0.66	64 (71 – 78)	76 (67 – 90)	0.31
history of coronary artery disease, % (n)	17 (3)	21 (18)	0.68	15 (2)	21 (19)	0.64
history of arterial hypertension, % (n)	78 (14)	79 (68)	0.78	77 (10)	74 (67)	0.80
lesion size on DWI [mL], median (IQR)	45.3 (9.8 – 100.5)	0.9 (0.1 – 4.1)	< 0.0001*	16.4 (2.8 – 91.1)	1.2 (0.1 – 6.6)	0.0012*
MR-proANP on admission [pM], median (IQR)	151.0 (102.1 – 255.8)	98.5 (68.7 – 169.0)	0.04*	207.0 (122.5 – 341.0)	98.1 (67.5 – 161.3)	0.0004*
Involvement of the insular cortex, % (n)	n/a	n/a		38 (5)	14 (13)	0.03*
Newly-diagnosed atrial fibrillation, % (n)	28 (5)	9 (8)	0.03*	n/a	n/a	
	Cohort A*					
	INS	**No INS**	**p-value**	**NDAF**	**No NDAF**	**p-value**
number of patients, n	7	76		8	75	
age [y], median (IQR)	65 (59 – 78)	68 (59 – 79)	0.86	70 (66 – 81)	67 (59 – 78)	0.35
NIHSS [pts], median (IQR)	4 (2 – 8)	4 (1 – 7)	0.70	4 (1 – 10)	4 (2 – 7)	0.89
female sex, % (n)	43 (3)	38 (29)	1	38 (3)	40 (30)	0.89
systolic blood pressure [mmHg], median (IQR)	162 (130 – 184)	163 (143 – 186)	0.57	162 (135 – 184)	168 (143 – 186)	0.66
heart rate, median [min^{-1}] (IQR)	87 (65 – 90)	79 (67 – 90)	0.89	74 (65 – 88)	76 (67 – 90)	0.91
history of coronary artery disease, % (n)	14 (1)	21 (16)	0.67	13 (1)	21 (16)	0.56
history of arterial hypertension, % (n)	86 (6)	70 (53)	0.47	75 (6)	71 (53)	1
MR - proANP on admission [pM], median (IQR)	122.0 (87.5 – 174.0)	98.0 (69.1 – 162.0)	0.48	195.5 (113.5 – 398.3)	93.4 (67.5 – 146.5)	0.0031*
Involvement of the insular cortex, % (n)	n/a	n/a		38 (3)	5 (4)	0.0019*
Newly-diagnosed atrial fibrillation, % (n)	43 (3)	7 (5)	0.0019*	n/a	n/a	

(INS = insular stroke, NDAF = newly diagnosed atrial fibrillation, NIHSS = National Institute of Health Stroke Scale, IQR = Interquartile Range, CAD = coronary artery disease).*p<0.05.

during hospitalization, early discharge/transferal to another hospital or due to contraindications to MR imaging (n = 42) and those without diagnostic cardiological work-up due to early death during hospitalization or early discharge or transferal to another ward (n = 7). In a second step only patients with ischemic strokes of lesion sizes under 20 mL were selected (see below) yielding a cohort of n = 83.

Neuroimaging and lesion size stratification

MRI (T1-, T2-, DWI) sequences and MR angiography was performed in all patients using a 1.5-Tesla MR Avanto system (Siemens, Erlangen, Germany). Involvement of the insular cortex was assessed on DWI and T2-weighted images by two experienced readers unaware of clinical data. Stroke lesion volumes on DWI were calculated by the commonly used semiquantitative method.[15] The insula was defined as the cortical region covered by the frontoparietal operculum and the superior temporal plane and overlying the extreme capsule and the claustrum. To obtain an estimate about the volume of the insular cortex, we performed a meta-analysis in the Internet Brain Volume Database for *in vivo* volumetric studies of non-diseased humans.[16] The query yielded 11 studies with a total of 709 investigated subjects. A cumulative meta-analysis using a random effects model for insular volume returned an estimated size of 11.38 mL (95% CI 10.12–12.64 mL). Additionally, previously conducted studies on insular strokes with published lesion sizes showed volumes of insular strokes ranging from around 30 mL [5] to 40-60 mL [4]. Taking these limits as well as our sample size into account we selected a lesion threshold of 20 mL on DWI for insular strokes.

Assays

Blood was obtained from a venous catheter and plasma was frozen at 70°C. MR-proANP was measured in a blinded batch analysis from all patients using a new sandwich immunoassay (B.R.A.H.M.S. AG), Hennigsdorf/Berlin, Germany), as described in detail elsewhere.[11] In brief, the lower detection limit of the assay is 6.0 pmol/L. The intraassay coefficient of variation was 10%. The interassay coefficient of variation was 10%. In 325 healthy individuals, the range of MR-proANP concentrations was

9.6 to 313 pmol/L. The median was 45 pmol/L (95% confidence interval [CI]: 43.0 to 49.1 pmol/L).

Statistical analysis

Baseline demographic, clinical observation, laboratory and outcome data were compared between patients with and without insular involvement as well as between those with newly-diagnosed atrial fibrillation and those without. Discrete variables are expressed as frequency (percentage) and continuous variables as medians and interquartile ranges (IQR). For two group comparison, we used Mann–Whitney U test and Chi-squared tests depending on the variable type and distribution of the variable. MR-proANP was ln-transformed to achieve a normal distribution of the variable. One-way ANOVA analysis of variance was used for multi-group comparisons of normally distributed variables with Bonferroni correction of significance for multiple testing. In order to choose the best predictive model to assess the discriminatory value of insular strokes and/or MR-proANP for newly diagnosed atrial fibrillation, we first performed univariate logistic regression analyses for already established predictors of NDAF.[17] Secondly, all variables that were significantly associated (i.e. at a p-value <0.10) with the outcome of interest (i.e. presence of new AF yes/no) in the univariate analysis were then included in a multivariate logistic regression analysis to assess their independent predictive value. The area under the receiver operating characteristic curve (AUC) was calculated to assess the discriminatory value of insular strokes and/or MR-proANP to distinguish patients with NDAF from patients without. The incremental predictive value of insular strokes and/or MR-proANP was tested by comparing the AUC between "model 1" (including all variables that have shown a significant association in the univariate logistic regression model) with the AUC of the nested models 2 and 3 (model 1 *plus* insular strokes = model 2; or model 3 = model 2 plus MR-proANP). Analogous calculations for comparison of the AUC in cohort A* are marked as model 1* (isolated insular strokes) and 2* (model 1* plus MR-proANP). For comparisons of these 3 and 2 models, respectively, we used the likelihood-ratio test as recommended [18]. Statistical analyses were undertaken using GraphPad Prism 5 (GraphPad Software, La Jolla, USA),IBM SPSS Statistics 20 (IBM, New York, USA), Comprehensive Meta-Analysis (Biostat, Englewood, USA) and custom-written scripts for MATLAB (MathWorks, Natick, USA). Testing was always two-sided and *P* values less than 0.05 were considered to indicate statistical significance.

Results

Study cohorts

We analyzed all patients from a large, prospective stroke study cohort with a known negative history of congestive heart failure and atrial fibrillation that have undergone a diagnostic cardiological work-up on admission and in whom diffusion-weighted imaging was available for volumetric analyses, yielding *cohort A*.[11] In a second step, 21 patients were excluded from cohort A due to a ischemic stroke lesion size ≥ 20 mL on diffusion-weighted imaging to be able to selectively assess the impact of isolated insular strokes, yielding cohort A*. The detailed baseline characteristics of the cohorts A and A* analyzed in this study are given in *table 1*.

Isolated insular strokes are independent predictors of newly-diagnosed atrial fibrillation

Of 104 patients taken from the original study cohort that were included for this analysis, 17% (n = 18) suffered from an ischemic stroke involving the insular cortex while it was spared in 83%

Table 2. Predictors of newly-diagnosed atrial fibrillation in cohort A.

Risk factor	OR	95% CI	p-Value
Age [y]	1.04	0.99 – 1.10	0.12
NIHSS [pts]	1.08	0.99 – 1.18	0.07[*]
Female sex (n)	0.87	0.27 – 2.87	0.82
Systolic blood pressure [mmHg]	1.00	0.98 – 1.03	0.77
Pulse [min⁻¹]	0.98	0.95 – 1.02	0.38
Coronary artery disease (n)	0.69	0.14 – 3.38	0.65
Arterial hypertension (n)	1.19	0.30 – 4.71	0.80
Lesion size [mL]	1.01	1.00 – 1.02	0.02[*]
Involvement of the insular cortex	3.75	1.06 – 13.20	0.04[*]
LnMR-proANP on admission	5.03	1.86 – 13.56	0.001[*]

Univariate logistic regression, [*]p<0.10, *p<0.05.

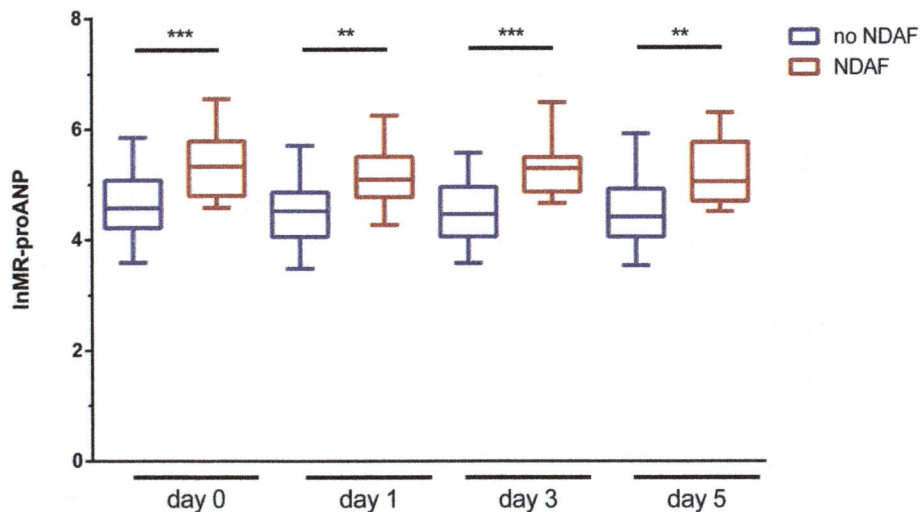

Figure 2. Timecourse of plasma MR-proANP levels. Plasma lnMR-proANP levels are plotted on the ordinate, lnMR-proANP levels were significantly different between patient groups throughout the monitored period (day 0 denotes the day of admission; ** p<0.01, *** p<0.001, one-way ANOVA with Bonferroni's multiple comparisons post-hoc test). The abscissa denotes the time points of plasma MR-proANP levels during the hospitalization period in patients with no newly-diagnosed atrial fibrillation (no NDAF, blue boxes) and those with newly-diagnosed atrial fibrillation (NDAF, red boxes). Horizontal bars indicate group means with error bars denoting 95% CI.

(n = 86) of patients (for detailed baseline characteristics see also *table 1, cohort A*). In univariate logistic regression analysis, stroke severity on admission (as determined by the NIHSS), lesion size on DWI, involvement of the insular cortex and lnMR-proANP levels on admission were significant predictors of newly diagnosed atrial fibrillation in cohort A (p<0.10 for all predictors, *table 2*). Compared to the other predictors, involvement of the insular cortex in ischemic stroke patients failed to improve the predictive value for NDAF (*tables 3, 4*). However to better investigate the association of insular involvement with NDAF we hence chose to introduce a cut-off for isolated insular strokes based on a

cumulative meta-analysis of insular cortex volumes (see also *materials and methods*, [16]) and analyzed the association of insular location with NDAF only in strokes of <20 mL including the insula (i.e. cohort A*). Herein, 8% (n = 7) of the patients suffered from an isolated insular stroke, while the insula was spared in 92% (n = 76) of patients. Of 7 patients with isolated insular strokes, 43% were diagnosed with NDAF (n = 3) while it was diagnosed in 7% of those without isolated insular strokes (n = 4). In univariate logistic regression analysis patients with isolated insular strokes were at 10-fold higher odds for NDAF than those without affection of the insula (OR 10.65, 95% CI 1.85–61.3, p<0.01, *table 5*). In subsequent multivariate logistic regression analysis of cohort A* isolated insular strokes remained an independent predictor of NDAF (OR 13.89, 95% CI 1.79–107.55, p<0.012, *table 6*) with an area under the receiver operating characteristic curve of 0.66, 95% CI 0.43–0.89 (*table 7*). Moreover, adding isolated insular strokes to the predictive model including only MRproANP-levels (in cohort A*), improved the prediction capacity (AUC 0.81 [95% CI 0.68 – 0.93] for lnMR-proANP levels on admission vs. 0.86 [95% CI 0.73 – 0.98] for lnMR-proANP levels on admission *and* isolated insular strokes, p = 0.013, likelihood-ratio test).

Table 3. Predictors of newly-diagnosed atrial fibrillation in cohort A.

Model 1			
Risk factor	**OR**	**95% CI**	**p-Value**
NIHSS	1.04	0.93 – 1.15	0.51
Lesion size [mL]	1.01	1.00 – 1.02	0.11
Model 2			
Risk factor	**OR**	**95% CI**	**p-Value**
NIHSS	1.03	0.92 – 1.15	0.60
Lesion size [mL]	1.01	1.00 – 1.02	0.19
Involvement of the insular cortex	2.28	0.57 – 9.20	0.25
Model 3			
Risk factor	**OR**	**95% CI**	**p-Value**
NIHSS	0.97	0.85 – 1.11	0.69
Lesion size [mL]	1.01	1.00 – 1.02	0.14
Involvement of the insular cortex	1.04	0.93 – 1.15	0.51
LnMR-proANP on admission	4.69	1.58 – 13.88	*0.005**

Multivariate logistic regression, *p<0.05.

Table 4. Comparison of the area under the receiver operating characteristic curve of each model in cohort A.

Model	AUC	95% CI	p-value for comparison
1	0.69	0.54 – 0.83	n/a
2	0.74	0.6 – 0.88	0.26
3	0.85	0.75 – 0.94	*0.002**

*p<0.05.

Table 5. Predictors of newly-diagnosed atrial fibrillation in cohort A*.

Risk factor	OR	95% CI	p-Value
Age [y]	1.03	0.97 – 1.09	0.34
NIHSS [pts]	1.02	0.89 – 1.17	0.74
Female sex (n)	0.90	0.20 – 4.05	0.89
Systolic blood pressure [mmHg]	1.00	0.97 – 1.03	0.79
Pulse [min^{-1}]	1.00	0.95 – 1.04	0.91
Coronary artery disease (n)	0.53	0.06 – 4.60	0.56
Arterial hypertension (n)	1.25	0.23 – 6.65	0.80
Isolated insular stroke	**10.65**	**1.85 – 61.30**	*0.008[#]*
LnMR-proANP on admission	**5.18**	**1.60 – 16.75**	*0.006[#]*

Univariate logistic regression, [#]p<0.05.

Plasma MR-proANP measured on admission is an independent predictor of newly-diagnosed atrial fibrillation

In univariate logistic regression analysis, lnMR-proANP levels on admission showed a significant association with NDAF (cohort A, OR 5.03, 95% CI 1.86–13.56, p = 0.001, table 2). In subsequent multivariate logistic regression models, lnMR-proANP levels on admission were independently associated with NDAF (OR 4.69, 95% CI 1.58–13.88, p = 0.005, table 3). LnMR-proANP levels on admission improved the predictive accuracy for NDAF in cohort A as determined by the comparison of the area under the receiver operating characteristic curve (p = 0.002, likelihood-ratio test, table 4), an effect that was also observable in cohort A* (p = 0.013, likelihood-ratio test, table 7). A cut-off value of 98.35 pM for plasma levels of MR-proANP corresponded to a detection sensitivity for NDAF of over 92.3%, thus in patients with levels below 98.4 pM atrial fibrillation is highly unlikely. A specificity of >98.9% was obtained at plasma levels over 538.5 pM, thus in these patients detection of atrial fibrillation is almost certain. LnMR-proANP levels stayed significantly different between patients with NDAF and those without throughout the monitored time course (p<0.001, day 0 [i.e. the day of admission]; p<0.01, day 1; p<0.001, day 3 and p<0.01, day 5; one-way ANOVA with Bonferroni's post-hoc adjustment of significance, figure 2).

The association of MR-proANP and insular strokes

Although patients with strokes involving the insular cortex from cohort A did have higher MR-proANP levels on admission than those without (insular strokes 151.0 pM IQR 102.1–255.8 vs. non-insular strokes 98.5 pM IQR 68.7–169.0, p = 0.04, Mann Whitney U Test, table 1), after adjusting for lesion size, MR-proANP levels were no longer associated with isolated insular strokes (in cohort A*).

Discussion

In this study, we found that patients with isolated insular strokes (i.e. ischemic strokes of the insula with a volume <20 mL on DWI) were at 10.7-fold higher odds for NDAF than those without. Insular location significantly improved the predictive model to identify NDAF when compared with other prognostic factors. Moreover we found that higher levels of lnMR-proANP were associated with 5.2-fold higher odds of newly detected AF. In

Table 6. Predictors of newly-diagnosed atrial fibrillation in cohort A*.

Model 1*			
Risk factor	**OR**	**95% CI**	**p-Value**
Isolated insular stroke	10.65	1.85 – 61.30	*0.008[#]*
Model 2*			
Risk factor	**OR**	**95% CI**	**p-Value**
Isolated insular stroke	13.89	1.79 – 107.55	*0.012[#]*
LnMR-proANP on admission	6.00	1.61 – 22.37	*0.008[#]*

Multivariate logistic regression, [#]p<0.05.

addition, the inclusion of lnMR-proANP levels in to the existing predictive model (including insular stroke) further improved differentiation between patients with NDAF and patients without NDAF.

In line with our findings, involvement of the insula in ischemic stroke patients was previously shown to be associated with severe cardiac derangement leading to complex ECG abnormalities such as premature ventricular contractions, non-sustained ventricular tachycardia and others when compared to ischemic stroke patients without insular involvement. Herein, especially right-sided insular lesions were associated with newly detected cardiac arrhythmia.[5] In another study with a smaller patient cohort, a greater increase in plasma norepinephrine concentrations was observed in patients with insular infarctions when compared to non-insular stroke patients, thus suggesting a possible direct connection of the insular lesion to activation of the sympathetic nervous system.[19] Lesion sizes of investigated subjects in the former study added up to 30 mL on average, while the latter did not adjust for lesion size at all. However, a cumulative analysis of insular volume in non-diseased patients yielded an average size of 11.38 mL (95% CI 10.12 – 12.64 mL, [16]). Above-mentioned lesions (i.e. >30 mL) are thus highly likely to affect other brain structures in the immediate anatomical neighborhood that are also described as regulators of the brain-heart-axis amongst others the caudate nucleus and the ventromedial prefrontal cortex.[20] In contrast to our study where lesion sizes was restricted to 20 mL (i.e. cohort A*) the results of these other studies might lack specificity.

Patients with AF, especially when undiagnosed and/or untreated are more prone to cardiovascular complications such as myocardial infarctions and thromboembolic events such as strokes.[21] In a prospective study with a larger cohort, patients with ischemic infarcts of the left insula were followed-up over 1 year and screened for sudden cardiac death, myocardial infarction and congestive heart failure. When compared to patients with non-insular infarcts and TIAs, left insular strokes were associated with an increased risk for adverse cardiac outcome as well as

Table 7. Comparison of the area under the receiver operating characteristic curve of each mode in cohort A*.

Model	AUC	95% CI	p-value for comparison
1*	0.66	0.43– 0.89	n/a
2*	0.86	0.73 – 0.98	0.013[#]

[#]p<0.05.

impaired cardiac wall motion. The exclusion of TIAs, however, did not yield a significant difference.[3] Increased QTc interval and the presence of left bundle branch block were also associated with higher vascular mortality rates in patients with right-sided insular infarcts.[4] These clinical implications of disturbances of the brain-heart-axis should encourage for heightened sensitivity in the acute hospitalization period in regards to selection of patients especially vulnerable towards cardiac abnormalities that may profit from a more stringent cardiological work-up and/or early detection devices amongst others implantable loop recorders. [12].

Since it is not possible to ascertain whether our patients with newly diagnosed AF had already experienced AF episodes before the stroke, we cannot make any inferences regarding causality. However, it is biologically plausible that an insular stroke in patients with paroxysmal subclinical AF or with other pre-existing but clinically unapparent cardiac dysfunction may, via activation of the sympathetic nervous system, trigger longer episodes of AF or may convert into AF, which then can be detected by monitoring. Thus, insular lesions in acute stroke patients with elevated plasma MR-proANP levels should prompt an aggressive cardiac work-up and potentially even outpatient monitoring to increase the yield for the detection of AF also in patients where the stroke etiology was not believed to be cardioembolic.

In a pilot study, mid-regional ANP precursor protein has been proven to represent a promising biomarker for determining the duration of AF episodes. More specifically, MR-proANP levels were higher in patients with AF episodes lasting longer than 48 hours compared to patients with episodes of less than 48 hours duration (321.7 IQR 236.4–425.6 versus 144.0 IQR 129.2–213.7 [pmol/L].[7] In our study, patients with elevated lnMR-proANP levels had 5.03-fold greater odds of having newly-diagnosed atrial fibrillation. Levels of brain natriuretic peptide (BNP) have been shown to be higher in patients where NDAF was documented during the hospitalization period. This association was independent of age, NIHSS and female gender.[22] In another more recently published retrospective analysis from the *Warfarin-Aspirin recurrent stroke study*, patients with plasma concentrations of amino-terminal pro-BNP (NT-proBNP) over 750 pg/mL seemed to be at lower risk for subsequent events (i.e. recurrent ischemic stroke or death over 2 years) when treated with anticoagulants other than antiplatelet agents.[23] These findings underscore the role of natriuretic peptides as serum markers of impending cardiac arrhythmias and assist in their clinical management. Although in our study, a significant difference in MR-proANP levels was

detected between patients from cohort A with ischemic strokes involving the insula and those without, insular strokes failed to be predictive for MR-proANP levels in linear regression analyses with and without lesion size stratification (*data not shown*). This suggests that the association of insular strokes with new onset of AF is not in the same causal pathway as MR-proANP and AF. Another explanation is that we were underpowered and therefore unable to find any type of mediation.

Some limitations merit attention. First, newly-diagnosed atrial fibrillation in insular stroke patients was not the primary endpoint of the original study cohort; however, all data were prospectively collected and biomarker measurements were pre-planned and assessed in a blinded manner. Second, we did not collect information on NDAF after discharge, thus we may have missed some patients with insular strokes and/or elevated MR-proANP levels that did not show signs of new-onset atrial fibrillation during their hospitalization but suffer from intermittent atrial fibrillation. [24] Hence this potential misclassification is more likely to underestimate the association of insular strokes with NDAF (i.e. bias towards the null-hypothesis) because in the group without NDAF some patients might have had atrial fibrillation thus raising the number of false negatives. Thirdly, due to sample size limitations, we did not assess insular substructures, such as anterior/posterior division or laterality, although some studies have investigated this complex and controversial topic of specifically assigned parts of the insula.[25] Finally, the results of this pilot study should be interpreted with caution due to the relatively small numbers thus an external validation in an independent larger cohort is necessary. Still, these promising results should propagate further investigation with larger patient cohorts since our findings could be of practical clinical value for the early identification of AF patients which might benefit from oral anticoagulation.

Acknowledgments

The authors wish to thank Dr. Elisabeth J. Rushing for proofreading the manuscript.

Author Contributions

Conceived and designed the experiments: MK BM MCC. Performed the experiments: MK FF KF. Analyzed the data: KF MK JS AG. Wrote the paper: KF MK.

References

1. Oppenheimer SM, Gelb A, Girvin JP, Hachinski VC (1992) Cardiovascular effects of human insular cortex stimulation. Neurology 42: 1727–1732.
2. Christensen H, Boysen G, Christensen AF, Johannesen HH (2005) Insular lesions, ECG abnormalities, and outcome in acute stroke. J Neurol Neurosurg Psychiatry 76: 269–271.
3. Laowattana S, Zeger SL, Lima JA, Goodman SN, Wittstein IS, et al. (2006) Left insular stroke is associated with adverse cardiac outcome. Neurology 66: 477–483; discussion 463.
4. Abboud H, Berroir S, Labreuche J, Orjuela K, Amarenco P (2006) Insular involvement in brain infarction increases risk for cardiac arrhythmia and death. Ann Neurol 59: 691–699.
5. Colivicchi F, Bassi A, Santini M and Caltagirone C (2004) Cardiac autonomic derangement and arrhythmias in right-sided stroke with insular involvement. Stroke 35: 2094–2098.
6. Rossi A, Enriquez-Sarano M, Burnett JC Jr, Lerman A, Abel MD, et al. (2000) Natriuretic peptide levels in atrial fibrillation: a prospective hormonal and Doppler-echocardiographic study. J Am Coll Cardiol 35: 1256–1262.
7. Meune C, Vermillet A, Wahbi K, Guerin S, Aelion H, et al. (2011) Mid-regional pro atrial natriuretic peptide allows the accurate identification of patients with atrial fibrillation of short time of onset: a pilot study. Clinical biochemistry 44: 1315–1319.
8. Katan M, Fluri F, Schuetz P, Morgenthaler NG, Zweifel C, et al. (2010) Midregional pro-atrial natriuretic peptide and outcome in patients with acute ischemic stroke. J Am Coll Cardiol 56: 1045–1053.
9. Morgenthaler NG, Struck J, Thomas B, Bergmann A (2004) Immunolumino-metric assay for the midregion of pro-atrial natriuretic peptide in human plasma. Clin Chem 50: 234–236.
10. Ala-Kopsala M, Magga J, Peuhkurinen K, Leipala J, Ruskoaho H, et al. (2004) Molecular heterogeneity has a major impact on the measurement of circulating N-terminal fragments of A- and B-type natriuretic peptides. Clin Chem 50: 1576–1588.
11. Katan M, Fluri F, Morgenthaler NG, Schuetz P, Zweifel C, et al. (2009) Copeptin: a novel, independent prognostic marker in patients with ischemic stroke. Ann Neurol 66: 799–808.
12. Cotter PE, Martin PJ, Ring L, Warburton EA, Belham M, et al. (2013) Incidence of atrial fibrillation detected by implantable loop recorders in unexplained stroke. Neurology 80: 1546–1550.
13. Hatano S (1976) Experience from a multicentre stroke register: a preliminary report. Bull World Health Organ 54: 541–553.
14. Adams HP Jr, Bendixen BH, Kappelle LJ, Biller J, Love BB, et al. (1993) Classification of subtype of acute ischemic stroke. Definitions for use in a multicenter clinical trial. TOAST. Trial of Org 10172 in Acute Stroke Treatment. Stroke 24: 35–41.

15. Broderick JP, Brott TG, Duldner JE, Tomsick T, Huster G (1993) Volume of intracerebral hemorrhage. A powerful and easy-to-use predictor of 30-day mortality. Stroke 24: 987–993.

16. Kennedy DN, Hodge SM, Gao Y, Frazier JA, Haselgrove C (2012) The internet brain volume database: a public resource for storage and retrieval of volumetric data. Neuroinformatics 10: 129–140.

17. Menezes AR, Lavie CJ, DiNicolantonio JJ, O'Keefe J, Morin DP, et al. (2013) Atrial fibrillation in the 21st century: a current understanding of risk factors and primary prevention strategies. Mayo Clin Proc 88: 394–409.

18. Vickers AJ, Cronin AM, Begg CB (2011) One statistical test is sufficient for assessing new predictive markers. BMC medical research methodology 11: 13.

19. Meyer S, Strittmatter M, Fischer C, Georg T, Schmitz B (2004) Lateralization in autonomic dysfunction in ischemic stroke involving the insular cortex. Neuroreport 15: 357–361.

20. Taggart P, Critchley H, Lambiase PD (2011) Heart-brain interactions in cardiac arrhythmia. Heart 97: 698–708.

21. Lip GY, Tse HF, Lane DA (2012) Atrial fibrillation. Lancet 379: 648–661.

22. Shibazaki K, Kimura K, Fujii S, Sakai K, Iguchi Y (2012) Brain natriuretic peptide levels as a predictor for new atrial fibrillation during hospitalization in patients with acute ischemic stroke. Am J Cardiol 109: 1303–1307.

23. Longstreth WT Jr, Kronmal RA, Thompson JL, Christenson RH, Levine SR, et al. (2013) Amino terminal pro-B-type natriuretic Peptide, secondary stroke prevention, and choice of antithrombotic therapy. Stroke 44: 714–719.

24. Nagai M, Hoshide S, Kario K The insular cortex and cardiovascular system: a new insight into the brain-heart axis. J Am Soc Hypertens 4: 174–182.

25. Butti C, Hof PR (2010) The insular cortex: a comparative perspective. Brain Struct Funct 214: 477–493.

16

Morphological and Volumetric Analysis of Left Atrial Appendage and Left Atrium: Cardiac Computed Tomography-Based Reproducibility Assessment

Mikko Taina[1,2]*, Miika Korhonen[1,2], Mika Haataja[1,2], Antti Muuronen[1,2], Otso Arponen[1,2], Marja Hedman[1,3], Pekka Jäkälä[4,5], Petri Sipola[1,2], Pirjo Mustonen[6], Ritva Vanninen[1,2]

1 Department of Clinical Radiology, Kuopio University Hospital, Kuopio, Finland, 2 Unit of Radiology, Institute of Clinical Medicine, University of Eastern Finland, Kuopio, Finland, 3 Heart Center, Kuopio University Hospital, Kuopio, Finland, 4 NeuroCenter, Kuopio University Hospital, Kuopio, Finland, 5 Unit of Neurology, Institute of Clinical Medicine, University of Eastern Finland, Kuopio, Finland, 6 Department of Cardiology, Keski-Suomi Central Hospital, Jyväskylä, Finland

Abstract

Objectives: Left atrial appendage (LAA) dilatation and morphology may influence an individual's risk for intracardiac thrombi and ischemic stroke. LAA size and morphology can be evaluated using cardiac computed tomography (cCT). The present study evaluated the reproducibility of LAA volume and morphology assessments.

Methods: A total of 149 patients (47 females; mean age 60.9 ± 10.6 years) with suspected cardioembolic stroke/transient ischemic attack underwent cCT. Image quality was rated based on four categories. Ten patients were selected from each image quality category (N = 40) for volumetric reproducibility analysis by two individual readers. LAA and left atrium (LA) volume were measured in both two-chamber (2CV) and transversal view (TV) orientation. Intertechnique reproducibility was assessed between 2CV and TV (200 measurement pairs). LAA morphology (A = Cactus, B = ChickenWing, C = WindSock, D = CauliFlower), LAA opening height, number of LAA lobes, trabeculation, and orientation of the LAA tip was analysed in all study subjects by three individual readers (447 interobserver measurement pairs). The reproducibility of volume measurements was assessed by intra-class correlation (ICC) and the reproducibility of LAA morphology assessments by Cohen's kappa.

Results: The intra-observer and interobserver reproducibility of LAA and LA volume measurements was excellent (ICCs> 0.9). The LAA (ICC = 0.954) and LA (ICC = 0.945) volume measurements were comparable between 2CV and TV. Morphological classification ($\kappa = 0.24$) and assessments of LAA opening height ($\kappa = 0.1$), number of LAA lobes ($\kappa = 0.16$), trabeculation ($\kappa = 0.15$), and orientation of the LAA tip ($\kappa = 0.37$) was only slightly to fairly reproducible.

Conclusions: LA and LAA volume measurements on cCT provide excellent reproducibility, whereas visual assessment of LAA morphological features is challenging and results in unsatisfactory agreement between readers.

Editor: Yan Li, Shanghai Institute of Hypertension, China

Funding: This study was supported by the Kuopio University Hospital (grant number 5063519). Kuopio University Hospital web site: www.psshp.fi. The funders had no role in study design, data collection and analysis, decision to publish, or preparation of the manuscript.

Competing Interests: The authors have declared that no competing interests exist.

* Email: Mikko.Taina@kuh.fi

Introduction

Stroke is the leading cause of long-term disability and the second highest cause of mortality globally [1]. The currently recognized mechanisms for ischemic stroke or transient ischemic attack (TIA) are embolism, local vascular thrombosis, and decreased brain tissue perfusion due to other reasons [2]. Cardioemboli are derived mainly from the left atrial appendage (LAA) [3]. Despite atrial fibrillation (AF) being the most common risk factor for cardioembolism, it is not always recognized during acute cardioembolic events [4]. Over one-third of ischemic strokes/TIAs remain undetermined. The role of LAA enlargement in the etiology of these strokes may be underestimated, and

cryptogenic stroke/TIA has been associated with enlarged LAA volumes [5,6]. The role of the LAA in thrombus formation and stroke risk has been studied using multiple imaging modalities [7–13]. Recent magnetic resonance imaging (MRI) studies have shown that LAA volume is strongly associated with an increased prevalence of prior stroke/TIA, and the risk differs between LAA morphologies [12,13]. Percutaneous LAA occlusion has the advantage of being a minimally invasive treatment for patients in whom long-term anticoagulation treatment is deemed unsuitable and may be equivalent to treatment with oral anticoagulant agents in those individuals considered at moderate-to-high risk of thromboembolism [14]. Increasing evidence indicates that the upper quintile of LAA volume is a powerful predictor of stroke risk

[15]. Novel low-dose computed tomography (CT) scanners may increase pressure to use cardiac CT (cCT) for both etiological assessment and risk stratification [16]. Although 2D transesophageal echocardiography (TEE) is currently the most commonly used imaging modality for preoperative assessment, the use of 3D approaches have shown to provide additive information in cases of complex morphology of the LAA [17].

The value of a measurement method is largely dependent on its ability to provide reproducible and reliable results. To the best of our knowledge, the magnitude of these errors in the assessment of LAA volume and morphology by cCT has not been fully elucidated. We analysed the intra-observer and interobserver reproducibility of LAA and left atrium (LA) volume measurements in the transversal (TV) and two-chamber view (2CV) orientations and evaluated the repeatability of visual assessments of the morphological features of the LAA.

Materials and Methods

The study was part of the EMBODETECT project [6]. The study has been approved by the Kuopio University Hospital Research Ethics Board and all clinical investigation have been conducted according to the principles expressed in the Declaration of Helsinki. Written informed consent was obtained from the participants or their legally authorized representative if a patient was unable to provide consent due to impaired mental or physical function caused by stroke.

Study Design and Population

Acute stroke/TIA patients admitted to our university hospital between March 2005 and November 2009 were evaluated as candidates for this cCT study. The neurologists involved in the study recruited 162 patients (47 females; mean age 60.9±10.6 years) with suspected cardioembolic stroke/TIA without known atrial fibrillation. Thirteen patients were excluded for the following reasons: cCT image quality was not appropriate for analysis of LAA size (n = 4), ECG synchronization was not used for cardiac imaging (n = 3), contrast media injection failed (n = 2), use of contrast media was contraindicated due to decreased renal function (n = 1), or the patients refused to participate after giving informed consent (n = 3). The remaining 149 patients were included in the present study.

CT Imaging

Contrast-enhanced cCT was performed with a 16-slice (n = 113 patients) or 64-slice (n = 36 patients) scanner (Somatom Sensation 16 and Somatom Definition AS; Siemens Medical Solutions, Forchheim, Germany). Prior to imaging, β-adrenoreceptor antagonists were not administered. The aortic arch and cervical and intracranial arteries were scanned first, immediately followed by the ascending aorta and heart. When using the 16-slice scanner, contrast agent was injected through an 18-gauge catheter into the antecubital vein at 5 mL/s, followed by a 50-mL injection at 2 mL/s and subsequent 20-mL saline chaser. With the 64-slice scanner, 100 mL of contrast agent (350 mgI/mL) was injected at 5 mL/s, followed by a 20-mL injection at 2 mL/s and subsequent 20-mL saline chaser. Cardiac imaging was performed during mid-diastole in all study subjects. In the 16-slice scanner, collimation was 16×0.75 mm, the rotation time 0.42 s, and tube potential 120 kV; the current was set to 500 mAs for the first 80 patients and reduced to 250 mAs thereafter. In the 64-slice scanner,

collimation was 64×0.6 mm, the rotation time 0.33 s, and tube potential 120 kV; the reference current was set using commercially available tube current modulation software (CAREDose4D, Siemens Medical Solutions) at 160 mAs for the first 15 patients and then reduced to 100 mAs. Mid-diastolic 0.75 to 1.0-mm-thick slices with 20–25% overlap were reconstructed.

LAA and LA Volume Measurements

Quantitative image analysis was performed on an IDS5 diagnostic workstation (version 10.2P4; Sectra Imtec, Linköping, Sweden) using magnified images on 1024×768 and 1600×1200 displays. The oblique sagittal 2CV was obtained perpendicular to the mitral valve and parallel to the cardiac septum, and set from the left ventricle (LV) apex to the centre of the mitral annulus. The TV was obtained from horizontal slices. Due to contrast agent injection, the LAA was seen as a hyperdense structure surrounded by hypodense pericardial fat with high tissue contrast between the anatomical structures. The entire LAA was fully opacified with contrast media in all study subjects. The LAA borders were traced manually on the 2CV and TV using the mitral valve annulus as a landmark to differentiate the LA from the LV. The 2CV stack and localizer tool were used to differentiate the LAA orifice from the LA in the TV. Planimetry of the entire LAA comprised a mean 10.4±2.0 slices in the 2CV and 10.8±1.9 slices in the TV, whereas planimetry of the entire LA comprised a mean 20.0±3.2 slices in the 2CV and 17.6±2.9 slices in the TV. Volumes were calculated using Simpson's method by multiplying the area of each manually traced LAA and LA by the section thickness (3 mm) and summing the volumes of the separate sections.

Intra-observer and Interobserver Reproducibility of Volume Measurements

All observers were guided by a cardioradiologist. Observer 1 performed planimetry in both the 2CV and TV. Image quality was rated as excellent, good, moderate, or poor. Forty patients were selected for reproducibility analysis based on representative image quality, resulting in 10 scans being selected from each of the four categories. To calculate intra-observer repeatability, the observer reconstructed new slices in both orientations and repeated the LAA and LA measurements one month later while blinded to the previous measurements. For interobserver reproducibility, Observer 2 reconstructed new slices and analysed the LAA and LA volumes of the same 40 patients in both orientations (Figure 1).

LAA Morphology Analysis

As originally described by Wang et al [13,18], the shape of the LAA was classified as: A) Cactus, B) ChickenWing, C) WindSock, or D) CauliFlower [19]. The Cactus is defined as a dominant central lobe, limited overall length, and one or more secondary lobes; ChickenWing as a main lobe that bends from the proximal middle part of the LAA; WindSock as one dominant lobe with several secondary, or even tertiary, lobes; and CauliFlower as limited overall length and complex internal structures. The opening height of the LAA compared to the mitral annulus, the number of LAA lobes, the amount of intra-LAA trabeculation, and the orientation of the tip of the LAA were classified into three categories.

Reproducibility of Left Atrium and Left Atrial Appendage Volume Measurements

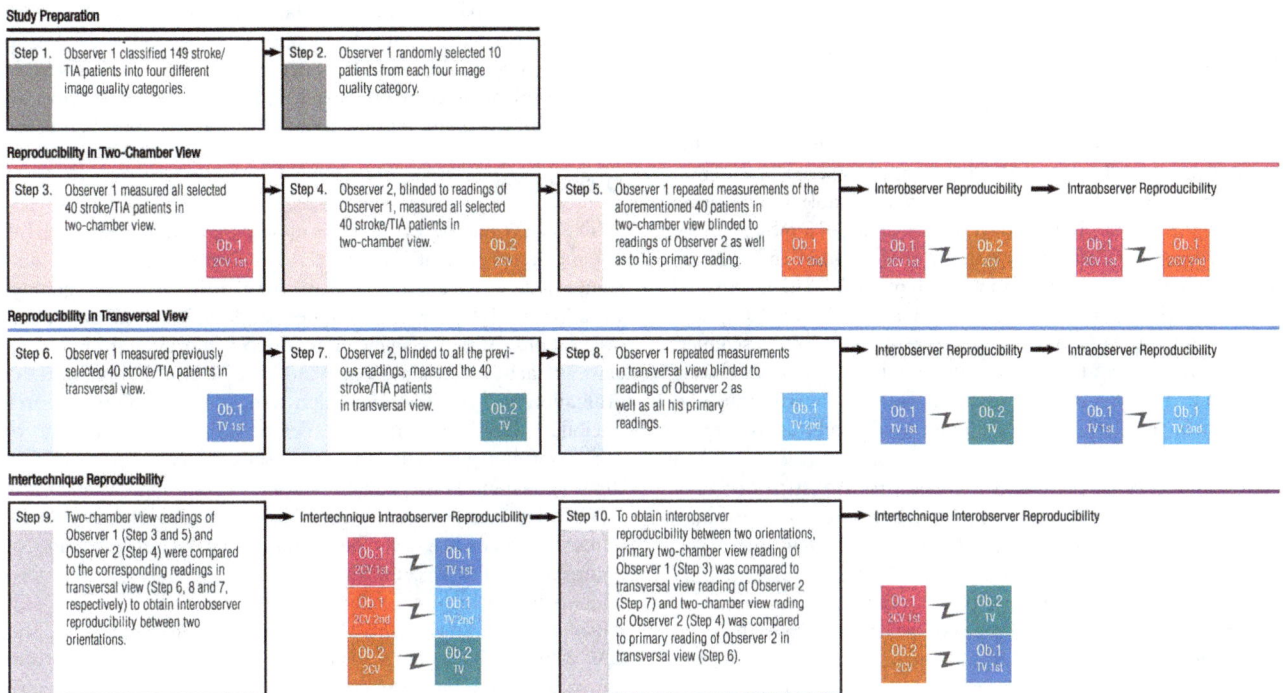

Reproducibility of Left Atrial Appendage Morphology Assessments

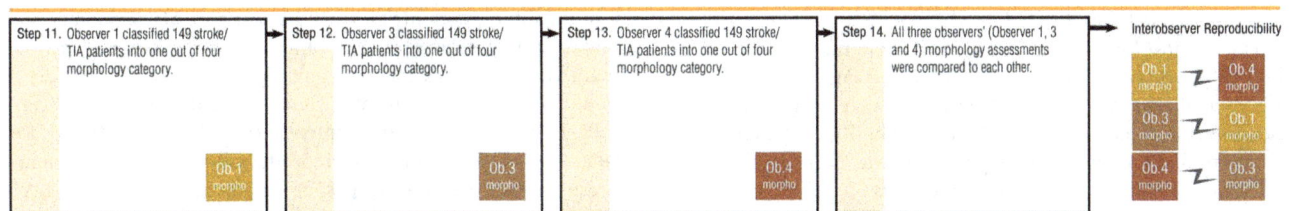

Figure 1. Study design for reproducibility analyses.

Interobserver Reproducibility of LAA Morphological Assessments

Three independent observers (Observers 1, 3, and 4) reconstructed the 2CV and visually analysed LAA morphology while blinded to collateral readings. Consequently, the reproducibility of visual classifications of LAA morphology was assessed with 447 independent classifications made by three observers (Figure 1).

Statistical Analysis

Continuous variables are presented as mean ± standard deviation (SD) and categorical variables as absolute values and percentages. Spearman's correlation coefficient was used to investigate the associations between continuous variables. Significance was set at $P<0.05$ and highly significant at $P<0.01$. In volumetric analyses, intraclass correlation coefficients (ICC) were calculated using a two-way mixed-effects model with absolute agreement to assess the interobserver and intra-observer reproducibility in both orientations and between different orientations across all four image quality categories. ICC values from 0.0 to 0.2 were considered negligible, from 0.2 to 0.4 very low, from 0.4 to

0.7 moderate, from 0.7 to 0.9 high, and from 0.9 to 1.0 very strong. Interobserver and intra-observer coefficients of variability (CV%) were assessed to evaluate the volume diversity across image quality categories for both readers in both orientations and between different orientations. CV% was calculated by dividing the SD of the differences by the mean of the parameter under consideration. In the current study, group variability with a CV% $<8\%$ was considered homogenous, from 8 to 10% average, and $>12\%$ diverse [20]. Based on a normal distribution in the Kolmogorov-Smirnov test, the Mann-Whitney U test was used to compare the ICC and CV% in dichotomous variables and the Kruskal-Wallis test in polytomous variables. The correlation between the ICC and CV% was measured to evaluate whether reproducibility is associated with volume diversity. Bland-Altman plots were created to exclude systematic bias depending on LAA and LA volume or the observers. Cohen's kappa was used to quantify the interobserver measurements for LAA morphology assessments; kappa values from 0.0 to 0.2 were considered slight, from 0.2 to 0.4 fair, from 0.4 to 0.6 moderate, from 0.6 to 0.8 substantial, and from 0.8 to 1.0 near perfect [21]. Data were analysed using SPSS for Windows (version 19, 1989–2010 SPSS Inc., Chicago, USA).

Results

Patient Characteristics and Image Quality

The characteristics of all 149 patients included in the morphological analyses and the 40 patients included in different types of reproducibility analyses are shown in Table 1. The mean radiation dose was 10.0 ± 3.5 mSv (range 2.0–16 mSv). Image quality was rated as excellent in 22 (61%), good in 8 (22%), moderate in 6 (17%), and poor in 0 (0%) of the 36 patients imaged with the 64-slice scanner, and in 8 (7%), 34 (30%), 45 (40%), and 26 (23%) of the 113 patients imaged with the 16-slice scanner, respectively. All investigated patients were in sinus rhythm during cCT scan. There was no association between hearth rate and CV% nor a correlation between image quality and heart rate.

Reproducibility of LAA and LA Volume Measurements

The results of the interobserver and intra-observer reproducibility analyses of LAA and LA volume measurements are shown in Table 2. Based on ICC values, reproducibility was very high despite variations in image quality. Volumetric measurements in 2CV and TV resulted in excellent comparability (Table 3).

Combining all reproducibility analyses, the CV% values did not indicate significant volume diversity in interobserver and intra-observer analyses, intertechnique analyses between 2CV and TV, or analyses according to image qualities (Table 2). A significant (correlation coefficient $= -0.817$; $P < 0.01$) negative correlation was observed between the ICC and CV%.

The Bland-Altman plots in Figure 2 show that the reproducibility of LAA and LA volume measurements does not depend on the volume. No systematic difference between image quality or measurement orientations was observed. The Bland-Altman plots in Figure 3 show that no systematic bias was introduced due to different readers for volume measurements in the 2CV or TV orientation.

Reproducibility of LAA Morphological Assessments

Cohen's kappa value indicated fair agreement between observers in the assessment of LAA morphology ($\kappa = 0.24$) and LAA tip orientation ($\kappa = 0.37$), and slight agreement between observers in the assessment of LAA opening height ($\kappa = 0.1$), the number of LAA lobes ($\kappa = 0.16$), and the amount of trabeculation ($\kappa = 0.15$).

Discussion

The main finding of the current study was that LAA and LA volume measurements using cCT are highly reproducible and comparable between observers, despite differing image quality, variation in LAA or LA volumes, and differing measurement orientations. Visual classification of LAA morphology into four classes (Cactus, ChickenWing, WindSock, or CauliFlower) and the evaluation of LAA tip orientation had fair interobserver reproducibility. However, the more detailed visual classifications of other morphological features were unsatisfactory, resulting in only slight agreement between the readers.

The detection of an enlarged LAA in patients with acute ischemic stroke/TIA may be useful in the risk stratification of recurrent stroke. Recent multicentre studies have shown that patients in the highest LAA volume quintile are at an increased risk of cardioembolic events [15]. In addition, increased LAA and LA volumes have been detected in patients with AF and paroxysmal AF, but also cryptogenic patients with no obvious etiology for stroke/TIA [6,12,22,23]. Some studies have also speculated whether certain LAA morphology types increase the risk for thrombus formation [13,18,24].

In the future, not only stroke/TIA, but also AF diagnostics and treatment, may take advantage of an accurate evaluation of LAA or LA volume [22–25]. To be clinically feasible, these assessments should be highly reproducible. Though considered haemodynamically more vivid, the main interest thus far has been on LA volumetry. Studies on the reproducibility of LAA volume measurements are scarce, despite increasing interest in LAA volumes [26]. Previous studies have also implied a poor correlation

Table 1. Clinical Characteristics of Patients.

Characteristic	Morphology analysis n = 149	Volumetric analysis n = 40	*Sig.*
Age, yr	60.9 ± 10.6	60.1 ± 9.7	ns.
Females, n (%)	47 (31.5)	11 (38.2)	ns.
Body mass index, kg/m^2	28.1 ± 4.4	29.2 ± 4.0	ns.
Body surface area, m^2	2.0 ± 0.2	2.0 ± 0.2	ns.
Caucasian race, n (%)	149 (100.0)	40 (100.0)	ns.
Hypertension, n (%)	88 (59.1)	21 (52.5)	ns.
Hyperlipidaemia, n (%)	61 (40.9)	18 (45.0)	ns.
Diabetes, n (%)	22 (17.8)	3 (7.5)	ns.
Smokers, n (%)	38 (25.5)	7 (17.5)	ns.
Prior stroke, n (%)	29 (19.5)	5 (12.5)	ns.
Prior myocardial infarction, n (%)	19 (12.8)	4 (10.0)	ns.
Sinus rhythm during imaging, n (%)	149 (100.0)	40 (100.0)	ns.
Heart rate, beats per minute	67.3 ± 11.2	66.7 ± 10.0	ns.
PAF in 24 hour ECG Holter, n (%)	38 (25.5)	1 (2.5)	0.033
Thrombus in LAA, n (%)	3 (2.0)	0 (0.0)	ns.

Sig = significance; ns = not significant in level P<0.05; PAF = paroxysmal atrial fibrillation.

Table 2. Interobserver and Intra-observer Reproducibility Analysis of Left Atrial Appendage (LAA) and Left Atrium (LA) Volumes.

| | Two-Chamber View | | | | | | | | Transversal View | | | | | | | |
| | LAA interobserver | | LAA intra-observer | | LA interobserver | | LA intra-observer | | LAA interobserver | | LAA intra-observer | | LA interobserver | | LA intra-observer | |
	ICC	CV%	ICC	CV%	ICC	CV%	ICC	CV%	ICC	CV%	ICC	CV%	ICC	CV%	ICC	CV%
Excellent	0.929	10.1	0.978	6.0	0.977	4.3	0.998	1.7	0.976	5.3	0.939	8.1	0.967	8.3	0.995	3.3
Good	0.970	13.3	0.988	9.1	0.987	4.6	0.988	3.6	0.943	21.0	0.988	8.2	0.948	8.9	0.979	5.8
Average	0.927	18.2	0.984	5.5	0.946	11.1	0.996	3.1	0.972	8.6	0.984	8.0	0.970	9.0	0.998	2.8
Poor	0.978	12.3	0.995	5.0	0.972	6.9	0.989	5.2	0.946	17.2	0.954	13.7	0.905	14.5	0.985	5.5
Total	0.960	13.5	0.988	6.4	0.996	6.7	0.992	3.4	0.953	13.0	0.970	9.5	0.944	10.2	0.989	4.3

Forty measurements pairs included 10 patients from each image quality category.

between LAA and LA volume, underlining the importance of separate LA and LAA evaluations [27–29]. In a previous retrospective study of 74 patients undergoing 64-slice cCT, the end-diastolic volume measurements showed significant reproducibility when evaluated with the Pearson correlation [30]. The different statistical approach makes a comparison with our results difficult. On the other hand, the Bland Altman plots did not reveal a significant bias associated with LA size [30]. In another previous study, 3D threshold-based end-diastolic volume measurements yielded ICC values of 0.961–0.997 for intra-observer and 0.867–0.926 for interobserver analyses [31], which are highly compatible with our results. Our current study was carried out with relatively old scanners. More novel 320-slice CT scanners visualize the boundaries of the LA with more advanced spatial resolution, comparable to 1.5-tesla MRI [32,33]. In a study comparing 320-slice cCT and transthoracic 2D and 3D echocardiography (TTE), the methods showed a strong positive correlation, but the absolute value of the LA volume on cCT was significantly larger than that determined by either 3D or 2D TTE, which can be due to an overestimation by cCT, underestimation by TTE, or both [34]. LAA morphology is widely used for the pre-evaluation of percutaneous LAA closure procedures [35]. The main exclusion criterion for this treatment is the presence of thrombus in the LAA [36]. TEE provides a more comprehensive tool to assess decreased blood flow velocity in LAA [14]. Nevertheless, detecting solid LAA thrombi seems feasible also with cCT [37]. According to our results, LAA volume measurements from different orientations in cCT are comparable. Although reproducible, manual LAA volume measurements are highly time-consuming, resulting in an urge to create automatized segmentation tools for clinical use. Our results indicate that an automatized segmentation tool may be based on transversal images provided automatically by the CT scan and that no specific stacks need to be formed for segmentation. LAA volumes in the 2CV seem to vary only slightly more between the different readers.

Our results yielded only slight to fair reproducibility for the visual classification of morphological features of the LAA. This result differs from the highly reproducible interobserver assessments of morphology reported by Di Biase et al [13]. They found no significant bias in classifying LAA morphology on CT ($\kappa = 0.84$). The classification method in Kimura et al [17] resulted in even higher interobserver agreement ($\kappa = 0.901$). Nevertheless, similar to our results, Khurram et al [24] reported fair interobserver reproducibility ($\kappa = 0.427$). Despite excellent tissue contrast in cCT, the more complex morphological assessments of LAA are challenging and would benefit from supporting quantitative tools or consensus readings between several specialists.

Because stroke recurrence is most probable during the first hours and days after the index stroke, it is important to determine the stroke etiology as soon as possible to prevent stroke recurrence. Compared to MRI, cCT is a faster and more widely available imaging modality with lower cost [15–16]. The radiological examination of an acute stroke patient usually includes not only CT of the brain, but also carotid artery CT angiography combined with imaging of the aortic arch [2]. Current prospective ECG-gated CT scans allow extremely low radiation doses [16]. Thus, by extending the scanned area from the carotid arteries and aortic arch down to the level of the LAA would not significantly increase the radiation dose, but may provide a valid method for evaluating the LAA in acute stroke patients [38]. While the main

Table 3. Intertechnique Reproducibility of Left Atrial Appendage and Left Atrium Volume Measurements.

	Measurement Pairs	Left Atrial Appendage		Left Atrium	
Image Quality	**N**	**ICC**	**CV%**	**ICC**	**CV%**
Excellent	50	0.917	9.8	0.965	7.3
Good	50	0.963	13.5	0.944	8.0
Average	50	0.957	12.1	0.949	9.8
Poor	50	0.953	14.1	0.930	10.6
Interobserver	80	0.949	13.0	0.931	9.4
Intra-observer	120	0.957	12.0	0.955	8.6
Total	200	0.954	12.4	0.945	8.9

Two hundred measurement pairs: 80 pairs with different observers and 120 pairs with the same observer.

indication for the cCT in these patients would be the detection or exclusion of LAA or other intracardiac thrombi, volumetric and morphological LAA assessments could provide additional information on risk stratifications of stroke recurrence [6].

Our study has several limitations. First, our imaging machinery was relatively old and represented different generations due to the long duration of patient collection. Therefore, the analysed data does not represent the cCT quality of the most modern medical care units. However, the reproducibility of volume measurements was excellent and we can assume that more modern scanners would yield even better results. Second, neither the morphological assessments nor volumetric measurements were performed by experienced cardioradiologists, but by radiology residents or research-oriented Bachelors of medicine who were guided by experts. Therefore, our study shows that LAA and LA volume measurements are robust and reproducible even in inexperienced

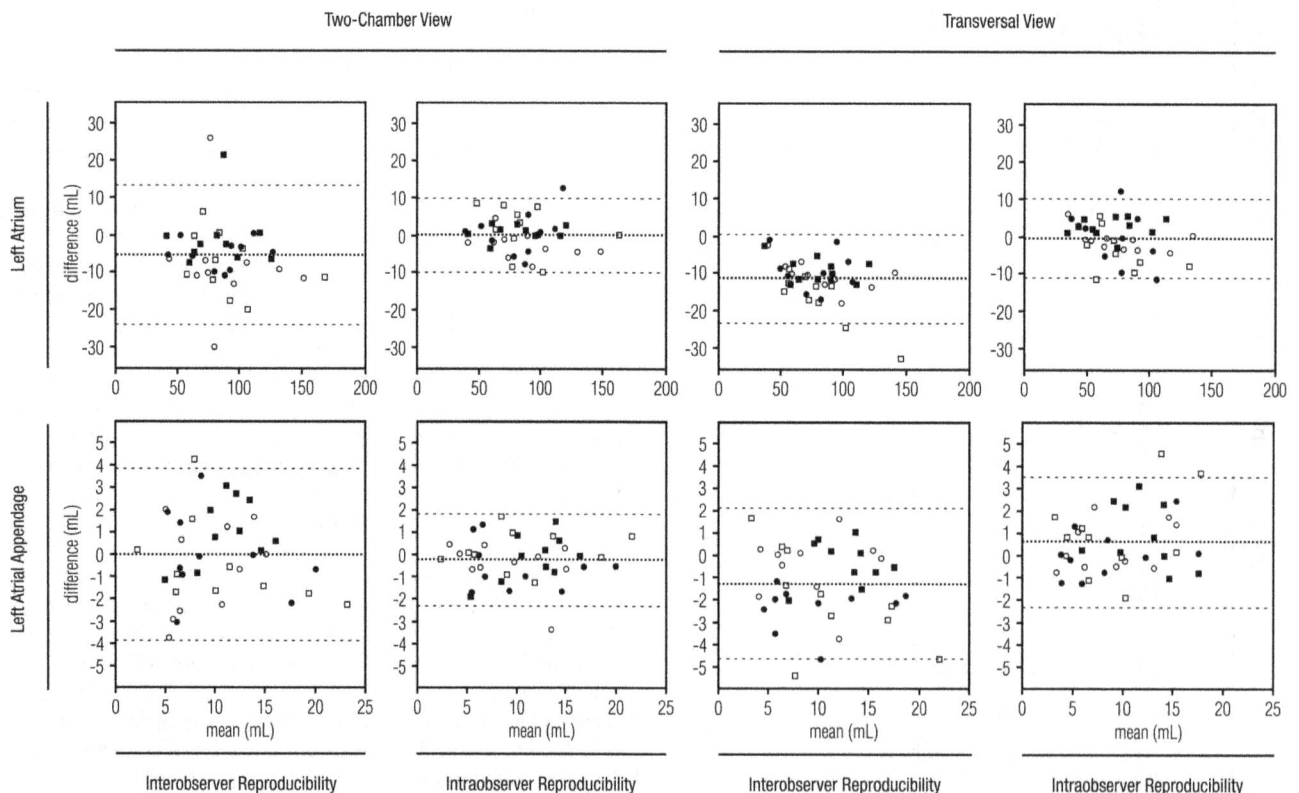

Figure 2. The reproducibility of volume measurements. Bland-Altman plots show the reproducibility of 40 left atrium and 40 left atrial appendage volume measurements for the same observer and different observers in two-chamber view and the transversal view. The X-axis shows the mean of two volume measurements and the y-axis shows a difference between respective measurements. The middle line corresponds to the mean difference and the outer lines correspond to the 95% confidence interval. Filled squares (■) indicate cardiac computed tomography images with excellent image quality; filled circles (●) indicate good image quality; empty circles (○), moderate image quality; and empty squares (□), poor image quality. Volume size and image quality had no significant influence on interobserver or intra-observer measurements in either orientation.

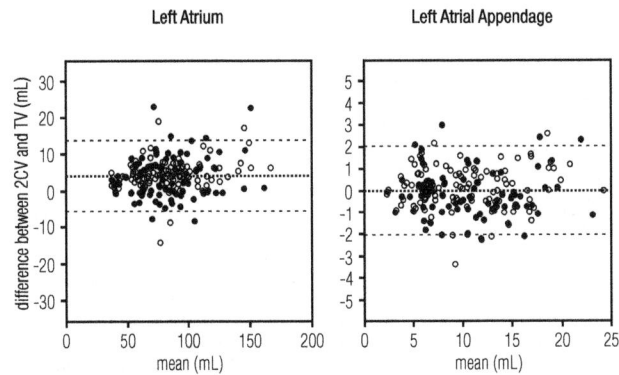

Figure 3. The intertechnique reproducibility of volume measurements. Bland-Altman plots show the intertechnique reproducibility of 200 left atrium and 200 left atrial appendage volume measurements performed in two-chamber view or transversal view. The X-axis shows the mean of two volume measurements and the y-axis shows the difference between respective measurements. The middle line corresponds to the mean difference and the outer lines correspond to the 95% confidence interval. Filled circles (●) indicate 80 interobserver measurement and empty circles (○) 120 intra-observer measurements performed in the two orientations. Volume size and observer had no significant influence on the measurements.

hands, but assessments of morphological type were more challenging and provided only fair reproducibility between clinically inexperienced observers. On the other hand, the morphological assessment of LAA is not clinically routine, and we assume that the use of more experienced readers would not have changed the results significantly. Third, intra-observer reproducibility was not analysed for LAA morphology assessments. Fourth, reproducibility analyses should be based on data both from symptomatic patients with a wide range of LAA volumes and morphological features, similar to the daily evaluation procedure in clinical practice, and a healthy normal population where the differences in assessed variable are narrower. While our study increased the radiation exposure we saw no justification to use healthy individuals.

In conclusion, LAA and LA volume measurements with cCT are robust and highly reproducible despite differing image quality, variation in LAA or LA volume, and measurements in differing orientations. The visual assessment of LAA morphology had only fair agreement between the readers and would benefit from the development of supporting quantitative tools or consensus readings between several specialists.

Author Contributions

Conceived and designed the experiments: MT MK M. Haataja AM OA M. Hedman PJ PS PM RV. Performed the experiments: MT MK M. Haataja AM OA M. Hedman PJ PS PM RV. Analyzed the data: MT MK M. Haataja AM OA M. Hedman PJ PS PM RV. Contributed reagents/materials/analysis tools: MT MK M. Haataja AM M. Hedman PS RV. Contributed to the writing of the manuscript: MT MK M. Haataja AM OA M. Hedman PJ PS PM RV.

References

1. Lloyd-Jones D, Adams RJ, Brown TM, Carnethon M, Dai S, et al. (2010) Heart disease and stroke statistics—2010 update: A report from the American Heart Association. Circulation 121: 46–215.
2. Goldstein LB, Bushnell CD, Adams RJ, Appel LJ, Braun LT, et al. (2011) Guidelines for the primary prevention of stroke: A guideline for healthcare professionals from the American Heart Association/American Stroke Association. Stroke 42: 517–584.
3. Bouzas-Mosquera A, Broullón FJ, Álvarez-García N, Méndez E, Peteiro J, et al. (2011) Left atrial size and risk for all-cause mortality and ischemic stroke. CMAJ 183: 657–664.
4. Bang OY, Lee PH, Joo SY, Lee JS, Joo IS, et al. (2003) Frequency and mechanisms of stroke recurrence after cryptogenic stroke. Ann Neurol 54: 227–234.
5. Amarenco P (2009) Underlying pathology of stroke of unknown cause (cryptogenic stroke). Cerebrovasc Dis 27: 97–103.
6. Taina M, Vanninen R, Hedman M, Jäkälä P, Kärkkäinen S, et al. (2013) Left atrial appendage volume increased in more than half of patients with cryptogenic stroke. PLoS ONE 8: e79519.
7. Al-Saady NM, Obel OA, Camm AJ (1999) Left atrial appendage: Structure, function, and role in thromboembolism. Heart 82: 547–554.
8. Kamp O, Verhorst PM, Welling RC, Visser CA (1999) Importance of left atrial appendage flow as a predictor of thromboembolic events in patients with atrial fibrillation. Eur Heart J 20: 979–985.
9. Fagan SM, Chan KL (2000) Transesophageal echocardiography risk factors for stroke in nonvalvular atrial fibrillation. Echocardiogr J Card 17: 365–372.
10. Handke M, Harloff A, Hetzel A, Olschewski M, Bode C, et al. (2005) Left atrial appendage flow velocity as a quantitative surrogate parameter for thromboembolic risk: Determinants and relationship to spontaneous echocontrast and thrombus formation—a transesophageal echocardiographic study in 500 patients with cerebral ischemia. J Am Soc Echocardiogr 18: 1366–1372.
11. Michael KA, Redfearn DP, Baranchuk A, Birnie D, Gula LJ, et al. (2009) Transesophageal echocardiography for the prevention of embolic complications after catheter ablation for atrial fibrillation. J Cardiovasc Electrophysiol 20: 1217–1222.
12. Beinart R, Heist K, Newell JB, Holmvang G, Ruskin JN, et al. (2011) Left atrial appendage dimensions predict the risk of stroke/TIA in patients with atrial fibrillation. J Cardiovasc Electrophysiol 22: 10–15.
13. Di Biase L, Santangeli P, Anselmino M, Mohanty P, Salvetti I, et al. (2012) Does left atrial appendage morphology correlate with the risk of stroke in patients with atrial fibrillation? J Am Coll Cardiol 60: 531–538.
14. Palios J, Paraskevaidis I (2014) Thromboembolism Prevention via Transcatheter Left Atrial Appendage Closure with Transeosophageal Echocardiography Guidance, Thrombosis; 832752, doi:10.1155/2014/832752.

15. Burrell LD, Horne BD, Anderson JL, Muhlestein JB, Whisenant BK (2013) Usefulness of left atrial appendage volume as a predictor of embolic stroke in patients with atrial fibrillation. Am J Cardiol 112: 1148–1152.
16. Kondratyev E, Karmazanovsky G (2013) Low radiation dose 256-MDCT angiography of the carotid arteries: Effect of hybrid iterative reconstruction technique on noise, artefacts, and image quality. Eur J Radiol 82: 2233–2239.
17. Chen OD, Wu WC, Jiang Y, Xiao MH, Wang H (2012) Assessment of the morphology and mechanical function of the left atrial appendage by real-time three-dimensional transesophageal echocardiography, Chinese Medical Journal 125: 3416–3420.
18. Wang Y, Di Biase L, Horton RP, Nguyen T, Morhanty P, et al. (2010) Left atrial appendage studied by computed tomography to help planning for appendage closure device placement. J Cardiovasc Electrophysiol 21: 973–982.
19. Kimura T, Takatsuki S, Inagawa K, Katsumata Y, Nishiyama T, et al. (2013) Anatomical characteristics of the left atrial appendage in cardiogenic stroke with low CHADS2 scores. Heart Rhythm 10: 921–925.
20. Harpreet K, Rajni A (2013) Morphological and morphometrical characterization of meloidogyne incognita from different host plants in four districts of Punjab, India. J Nematol 45: 122–127.
21. Landis JR, Koch GG (1977) The measurement of observer agreement for categorical data. Biometrics 33: 159–174.
22. Park HC, Shin J, Ban JE, Choi JI, Park SW, et al. (2013) Left atrial appendage: Morphology and function in patients with paroxysmal and persistent atrial fibrillation. Int J Cardiovasc Imaging 29: 935–944.
23. Nedios S, Tang M, Roser M, Solowjowa N, Gerds-Li JH, et al. (2011) Characteristic changes of volume and three-dimensional structure of the left atrium in different forms of atrial fibrillation: Predictive value after ablative treatment. J Interv Card Electrophysiol 32: 87–94.
24. Khurram IM, Dewire J, Mager M, Maqbool F, Zimmerman SL, et al. (2013) Relationship between left atrial appendage morphology and stroke in patients with atrial fibrillation. Heart Rhythm 10: 1843–1849.
25. Wang Y, Di Biase L, Horton RP, Nguyen T, Morhanty P, et al. (2010) Left atrial appendage studied by computed tomography to help planning for appendage closure device placement. J Cardiovasc Electrophysiol 21: 973–982.
26. Erol B, Karcaaltincaba M, Aytemir K, Cay N, Hazirolan T, et al. (2011) Analysis of left atrial appendix by dual-source CT coronary angiography: Morphologic classification and imaging by volume rendered CT images. Eur J Radiol 80: 346–350.
27. Nakajima H, Seo Y, Ishizu T, Yamamoto M, Machino T, et al. (2010) Analysis of the left atrial appendage by three-dimensional transesophageal echocardiography. Am J Cardiol 106: 885–892.
28. Nucifora G, Faletra FF, Regoli F, Pasotti E, Pedrazzini G, et al. (2011) Evaluation of the left atrial appendage with real-time 3-dimensional transesoph-

ageal echocardiography: Implications for catheter-based left atrial appendage closure. Circ Cardiovasc Imaging 4: 514–523.

29. Anwar AM, Nosir YF, Ajam A, Chamsi-Pasha H (2010) Central role of real-time three-dimensional echocardiography in the assessment of intracardiac thrombi. Int J Cardiovasc Imaging 26: 519–526.

30. Stojanovska J, Cronin P, Patel S, Gross BH, Oral H, et al. (2011) Reference normal absolute and indexed values from ECG-gated MDCT: Left atrial volume, function, and diameter. AJR Am J Roentgenol 197: 631–637.

31. Mahabadi AA, Samy B, Seneviratne SK, Toepker MH, Bamberg F, et al. (2009) Quantitative assessment of left atrial volume by electrocardiographic-gated contrast-enhanced multidetector computed tomography. J Cardiovasc Comput Tomogr 3: 80–87.

32. Artang R, Migrino RQ, Harmann L, Bowers M, Woods TD (2009) Left atrial volume measurement with automated border detection by 3-dimensional echocardiography: Comparison with magnetic resonance imaging. Cardiovasc Ultrasound 7: 16.

33. Bauer M, Bauer U, Alexi-Meskishvili V, Pasic M, Weng Y, et al. (2001) Congenital coronary fistulas: The most frequent congenital coronary anomaly. Z Kardiol 90: 535–541.

34. Kataoka A, Funabashi N, Takahashi A, Yajima R, Takahashi M, et al. (2011) Quantitative evaluation of left atrial volumes and ejection fraction by 320-slice computed-tomography in comparison with three- and two-dimensional echocardiography: A single-center retrospective-study in 22 subjects. Int J Cardiol 153: 47–54.

35. Ho IC, Neuzil P, Mraz T, Beldova Z, Gross D, et al. (2007) Use of intracardiac echocardiography to guide implantation of a left atrial appendage occlusion device (PLAATO)," Heart Rhythm 5: 567–571.

36. Landmesser U, Holmes DR (2012) Left atrial appendage closure: a percutaneous transcatheter approach for stroke prevention in atrial fibrillation. European Heart Journal 33: 698–704.

37. Hur J, Kim YJ, Lee HJ, Ha JW, Heo JH, et al. (2009) Left atrial appendage thrombi in stroke patients: detection with two-phase cardiac CT angiography versus transesophageal echocardiography. Radiology 251: 683–690.

38. Sipola P, Hedman M, Onatsu J, Turpeinen A, Halinen M, et al. (2013) Computed tomography and echocardiography together reveal more high-risk findings than echocardiography alone in the diagnostics of stroke etiology. Cerebrovasc Dis 35: 521–530.

17

Patient Self-Management of Oral Anticoagulation with Vitamin K Antagonists in Everyday Practice: Efficacy and Safety in a Nationwide Long-Term Prospective Cohort Study

Michael Nagler[1], Lucas M. Bachmann[2], Pirmin Schmid[3], Pascale Raddatz Müller[3], Walter A. Wuillemin[4]*

1 Division of Haematology and Central Haematology Laboratory, Luzerner Kantonsspital, Lucerne, and Department of Haematology and Central Haematology Laboratory, Inselspital University Hospital, Berne, Switzerland, 2 medignition Inc., Zug, Switzerland, 3 Division of Haematology and Central Haematology Laboratory, Luzerner Kantonsspital, Lucerne, Switzerland, 4 Division of Haematology and Central Haematology Laboratory, Luzemer Kantonsspital, 6000 Lucerne, and University of Berne, Berne, Switzerland

Abstract

Patient self-management (PSM) of oral anticoagulation is under discussion, because evidence from real-life settings is missing. Using data from a nationwide, prospective cohort study in Switzerland, we assessed overall long-term efficacy and safety of PSM and examined subgroups. Data of 1140 patients (5818.9 patient-years) were analysed and no patient were lost to follow-up. Median follow-up was 4.3 years (range 0.2–12.8 years). Median age at the time of training was 54.2 years (range 18.2–85.2) and 34.6% were women. All-cause mortality was 1.4 per 100 patient-years (95% CI 1.1–1.7) with a higher rate in patients with atrial fibrillation (2.5; 1.6–3.7; p<0.001), patients>50 years of age (2.0; 1.6–2.6; p<0.001), and men (1.6; 1.2–2.1; p = 0.036). The rate of thromboembolic events was 0.4 (0.2–0.6) and independent from indications, sex and age. Major bleeding were observed in 1.1 (0.9–1.5) per 100 patient-years. Efficacy was comparable to standard care and new oral anticoagulants in a network meta-analysis. PSM of properly trained patients is effective and safe in a long-term real-life setting and robust across clinical subgroups. Adoption in various clinical settings, including those with limited access to medical care or rural areas is warranted.

Editor: Terence J. Quinn, University of Glasgow, United Kingdom

Funding: The study was funded by the charitable foundation Coagulation Care, and Research Fund Haematology Luzerner Kantonsspital. The funders had no role in study design, data collection and analysis, decision to publish, or preparation of the manuscript.

Competing Interests: LMB is employed by medignition Inc., WAW has received research grants, lecture fees, and consultant fees from Roche Diagnostics, St. Jude Medical, Pfizer, Novo Nordisk, MEDA Pharma, Bayer, Boehringer Ingelheim, Bristol-Myers Squibb, GlaxoSmithKline, and sanofi-avensis.

* E-mail: walter.wuillemin@luks.ch

Introduction

Patient self-management (PSM) has become a promising concept for various chronic illnesses such as diabetes, high blood pressure or chronic obstructive pulmonary disease [1–3]. For patients with arthritis and perhaps also for patients with asthma PSM has shown to improve outcomes and also reduce cost (summarised in Bodenheimer et al. 2002 [1]). The role of PSM in long-term anticoagulation therapy to prevent thromboembolic events has been vividly discussed recently [4–10]. Proponents claim that PSM should be seen as the new benchmark for other management schemes and anticoagulation therapies. They draw on several clinical trials and meta-analyses documenting better anticoagulation control, less thromboembolic complications, increased quality of life, and, in part, a reduced mortality if compared with usual care [4–6,11–16] Some large scientific societies have adopted their view and recommend discussing PSM with eligible patients [17–20].

Opponents in return interpose that evidence on long-term safety and treatment control in clinical subgroups is sparse. Moreover, several authors recently questioned the generalizability of available trial evidence, because patients included in randomised-controlled studies are prone being heavily selected [4,5,7–10,15,18,21,22]. Discrepancies between data obtained in clinical trials and daily practice is regarded as a particular issue in anticoagulation therapy [21,22]. A recent systematic review, identifying a relevant lack of evidence thus called for population-based cohort studies to clarify the long-term efficacy and safety in a real-life setting [4].

To contribute to the discussion, we performed a nationwide, prospective cohort study determining efficacy and safety of PSM in a long-term real-life setting and with view to salient clinical subgroups such atrial fibrillation, mechanical heart valves, venous thrombosis and in elderly patients. To contextualize the results of our cohort, we additionally performed a network meta-analysis of major thromboembolism trials to compare efficacy parameters with VKA standard care, rivaroxaban, dabigatran, and apixaban.

Methods

Study Population

In this prospective cohort study, all patients trained for PSM within the initiative "coagulationcare" in Switzerland between 1998 and 2009 were included. This nationwide initiative is maintained by the charitable foundation of the same name. It trains about 90% of all Swiss patients and 95% of patients in German-speaking Switzerland. Observation period was the time span between PSM training and 31th of December 2010.

Patient Selection

All patients that were referred for PSM training have been trained without applying any type of selection. Patients were referred by the family physician, a specialist, or hospital staff. Information on PSM training was provided by presentations at scientific meetings, articles of national journals, websites, and in particular by patient organisations. Although, theses information were prepared in accordance with existing guidelines [18,19,23,24], systematic selection criteria were not provided.

Ethics Statement

The study received Ethics approval by the local review board (Kantonale Ethikkommission Luzern; #422) and all participants provided written informed consent.

PSM Training

With a view on international PSM practice and in accordance with published guidelines, a structured training programme was developed [18,19,23–25]. Details of the programme have been published previously [26]. In brief, patients had to attend a one-day training course at one of the study centres (Lucerne, Berne, Basel, Zurich, or Olten). A team of specialized physicians and paramedic staff taught all aspects of oral anticoagulation in several theoretical and practical sessions. In the theoretical part, participants learned about interactions with other drugs, interference with nutrition, the effects of concomitant illness on VKA treatment, the most common adverse events and safety measures when travelling. Moreover, instructions on the proper handling of the coagulation monitor were provided. Participants also learned how to interpret and document the results, how to use the dosing algorithm and adjustment dosages, and aspects of quality control. Practical training followed the lectures. After completion of the one-day course, participants entered the training phase for several weeks that included consultations with the family physician and parallel determinations of the international normalised ratio (INR) value.

Within this second phase, patients and family physicians were supported by online-material, e-mail contact and a 24-hour hotline. After completion of the training phase, all participants returned to the study centre for a one-hour check-up visit with a specialised physician. During the visit participants repeated the learning matters and performed an INR testing and dose

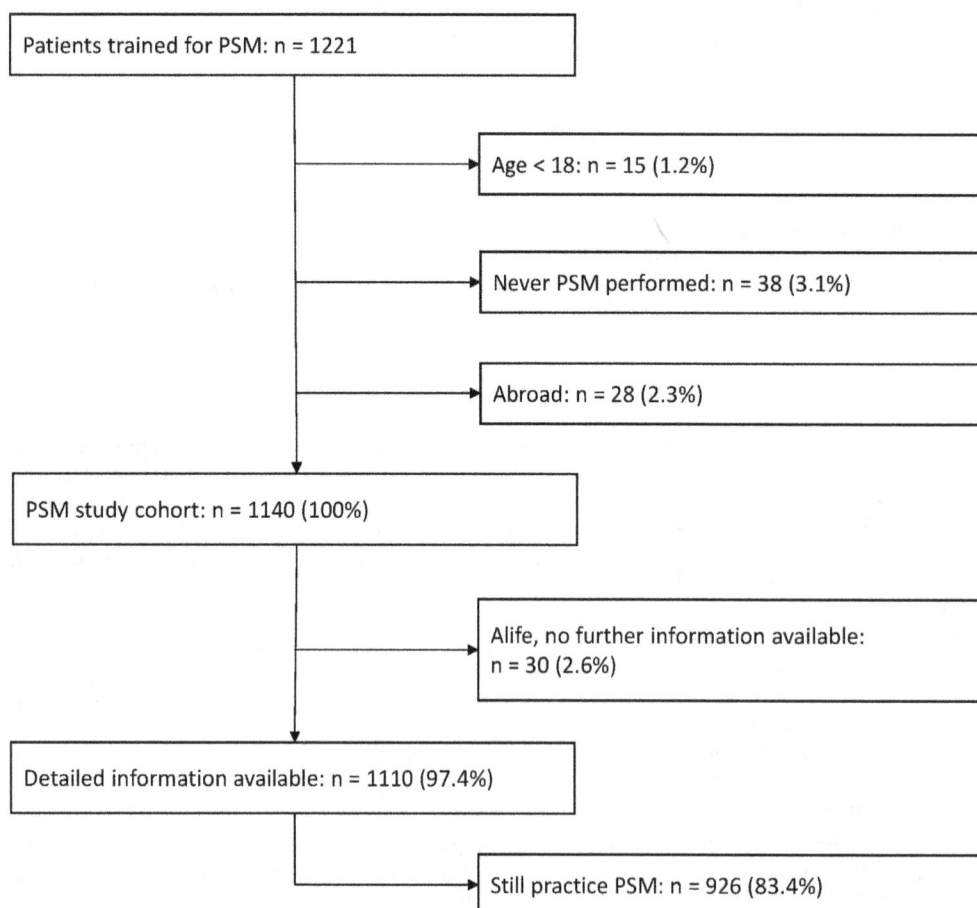

Figure 1. PSM study cohort.

Table 1. Baseline characteristics of the study cohort.

	Patients	Age	Female sex	Observation period	
	n (%)	median (range)	n (%)	patient-years	median (range)
Overall	1140 (100)	54.2 (18.2–85.2)	394 (34.6)	5818.9	4.3 (0.2–12.8)
Venous thromboembolism	463 (40.6)	48.5 (19.0–82.4)	199 (43.0)	2315.9	4.0 (0.2–12.7)
Prosthetic heart valve	365 (32.0)	55.0 (18.7–82.5)	104 (28.5)	2040.1	5.3 (0.8–12.8)
Atrial fibrillation	203 (17.8)	64.8 (18.2–85.2)	53 (26.1)	926.4	3.8 (0.2–12.6)
Arterial thromboembolism	54 (4.7)	57.3 (21.3–83.3)	19 (35.2)	319.8	5.5 (1.0–12.7)
Others	55 (4.8)	47.6 (20.9–82.2)	19 (34.5)	216.7	3.3 (0.4–11.3)

adjustment under supervision. A typical training package is illustrated in Table S2.

Participants were advised to do INR testing at least every two weeks and to get parallel measurements with the family physician two times a year. INR measurements were performed using the portable coagulometer CoaguChek XS (CoaguChek S until 2005 and CoaguChek until 2000; Roche Diagnostics, Basel, Switzerland), showing adequate accuracy, also in the hands of patients [27,28].

Definition of Outcomes

The following events were defined as primary outcome parameters: (i) any death, (ii) venous and arterial thromboembolic events (TE) (including deep vein thrombosis, pulmonary embolism, myocardial infarction, ischemic stroke or transient ischemic attack, systemic embolic events, other thromboembolic events), and (iii) major bleeding (defined as lethal bleeding, clinical overt bleeding, bleeding in critical organs, bleeding that needs transfusions, and any bleeding that necessitates medical consultation with diagnostic or prophylactic interventions). Secondary outcome parameters were (iv) event-related death, (v) event-related death and death of unknown cause, (vi) composite of TE and unknown death, (vii) intracranial bleeding events, and (viii) time in therapeutic range (%TIR). Death was regarded as event-related in case of a thromboembolic event (including myocardial

infarction) or bleeding event. Death was regarded as not event-related in case of infection, cancer or perioperative death.

Data Acquisition

At the time of inclusion, the following data were recorded: age, sex, indication for oral anticoagulation, starting date of anticoagulation and data regarding health insurance. As long as first patients were included in 1998 and risk assessment regarding thromboembolic and bleeding complications were not done regularly at this time, the presence of heart failure, hypertension, diabetes, previous stroke or bleedings, renal failure, or vascular disease were not recorded.

For follow-up, data on TE, bleeding events or deaths were obtained by a standardized questionnaire. In case of deaths, complications or hospitalisations, medical records and additional information were requested by contact with the family physician, hospitals, the relatives and the authorities. Three separate investigators controlled data recording. Two scientists, who are physicians treating PSM patients regularly (M.N. and W.A.W.), discussed unclear cases. In absence of an agreement, classifications were made for the disadvantage of the treatment. Patients were requested and reminded to send their INR- and dosage-documentation to the study centre.

Table 2. Mortality of PSM study cohort.

		All cause mortality	Event-related mortality	Not event-related mortality	Event-related + unknown cause
		n; deaths per 100 patient-years (95% CI)			
	Overall n = 1140	80; **1.4** (1.1–1.7)	5; **0.1** (0.02–0.2)	43; **0.7** (0.5–1.0)	37; **0.6** (0.4–0.9)
Indication	Venous thromboembolism n = 463	25; **1.1** (0.7–1.6)	2; **0.1** (0.01–0.3)	14; **0.6** (0.3–1.0)	11; **0.5** (0.2–0.8)
	Prosthetic heart valve n = 365	21; **1.0** (0.6–1.6)	1; **0.1** (0.001–0.3)	13; **0.6** (0.3–1.1)	8; **0.4** (0.2–0.8)
	Atrial fibrillation n = 203	23; **2.5** (1.6–3.7)	2; **0.2** (0.03–0.8)	10; **1.1** (0.5–2.0)	13; **1.4** (0.7–2.4)
	Arterial thromboembolism n = 54	4; **1.3** (0.3–3.2)	0; **0.0** (0.0–1.1)	3; **0.9** (0.2–2.7)	1; **0.3** (0.01–1.7)
	Others n = 55	7; **3.2** (1.3–6.7)	0; **0.0** (0.0–1.7)	3; **1.4** (0.3–4.0)	4; **1.8** (0.5–4.7)
Age	<50 years n = 464	13; **0.5** (0.3–0.9)	0; **0.0** (0.0–0.2)	10; **0.4** (0.2–0.7)	3; **0.1** (0.03–0.4)
	≥50 years n = 676	67; **2.0** (1.6–2.6)	5; **0.1** (0.04–0.3)	33; **0.9** (0.6–1.3)	34; **0.9** (0.6–1.3)
Sex	Female n = 394	21; **1.0** (0.6–1.5)	2; **0.1** (0.01–0.3)	14; **0.7** (0.4–1.1)	19; **0.9** (0.5–1.4)
	Male n = 746	59; **1.6** (1.2–2.1)	3; **0.1** (0.02–0.2)	29; **0.8** (0.5–1.1)	30; **0.8** (0.5–1.2)

CI, confidence interval.

A

B

C

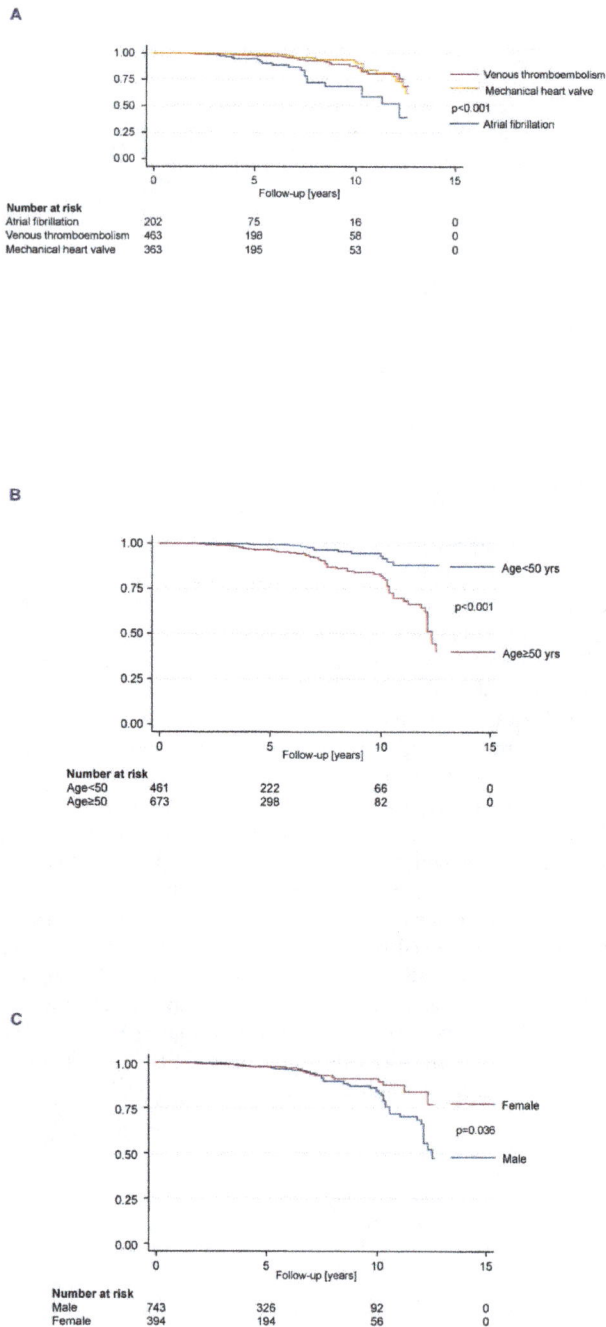

Figure 2. Survival estimates with regard to indications of oral anticoagulation, age, and sex.

Statistical Analysis

For determination of complications, only patients aged 18 or more were considered. We calculated the percentage of time in therapeutic range according using linear interpolation (Rosendaal method) [29,30].

For each of the three outcome parameters (overall mortality, TE, and major bleedings) we performed a univariate survival analysis and estimated differences in survival by indications of oral anticoagulation (atrial fibrillation, venous thromboembolism and mechanical heart valve), age (<50 vs.≥50 years), or sex (male vs. female). Differences in survival were tested using the logrank test if

appropriate. Analyses were performed using the Stata 11.2 statistics software package. (StataCorp. 2009. Stata Statistical Software: Release 11. College Station, TX: StataCorp LP).

Network Meta-analysis

To set our results into context, we performed a network meta-analysis comparing efficacy of PSM with other important anticoagulation schemes. We selected six major studies, investigating the efficacy of Rivaroxaban 20 mg, Apixaban 10 mg, Warfarin or another VKA and Dabigatran 150 mg to reduce the occurrence of recurrent thromboembolism and enrolling 9,872 patients were used for the analysis [31–36]. Dabigatran 150 mg was chosen for comparison, because it has demonstrated a superior efficacy than 110 mg. Whenever possible we used results from intention to treat analysis. Data were abstracted into 2 by 2 tables. A network meta-analysis was performed applying a recently published method [37]. In brief, a logistic regression model was used. Drug and dosage, creating a unique code for each treatment, were entered as covariates. To preserve randomization within each trial, we included an indicator variate for each study. This variate adjusted for all differences in risk profiles and study setup between trials. The event outcome for each single treatment arm was used as the dependent variable. From this regression model we estimated the odds ratio (OR) and 95% confidence intervals between placebo and all other treatment options. To compare the efficacy parameter with the results from our PSM study, we summarized the frequency of occurrence of the outcome in the placebo arms and calculated the corresponding OR and confidence interval.

Results

Patients and Follow-up

Between 1998 and 2009, 1221 patients were trained for PSM (Fig. 1). Fifteen patients were excluded because of age<18 years (1.2%), 38 patients never performed PSM (3.1%), and 28 patients moved abroad (2.3%). The remaining 1140 patients constituted the PSM study cohort, representing 5818.9 patient-years. Survival status was available for all patients. Detailed information on complications was available for 97.4% of the patients, representing 5636.5 patient-years. Median follow-up was 4.3 years (range 0.2–12.8 years). Baseline characteristics of the study cohort and indications for oral anticoagulation are displayed in Table 1. Median age at the time of PSM training was 54.2 years (range 18.2–85.2) and 34.6% were women. Phenprocoumon was used as VKA almost exclusively (95.3%), and acenocoumarol or warfarin in the remaining cases.

Mortality

Eighty patients died during the study period, constituting 1.4 deaths per 100 patient-years (Table 2). Kaplan-Meier survival estimates with regard to relevant subgroups are shown in Fig. 2. Mortality was higher among patients with atrial fibrillation (2.5 per 100 patient-years) compared with venous thromboembolism (1.1 per 100 patient-years) and prosthetic heart valve (1.0 per 100 patient-years; p<0.001). Mortality was higher in patients above 50 years (2.0 vs. 0.5 per 100 patient-years; p<0.001) and higher in men (1.6 vs. 1.0 per 100 patient-years; p = 0.036). However, when adjusting for differences in age between female and male using Cox regression, this effect was reduced and became non-significant. (Hazard Ratio (95% CI) 1.33 (0.79 to 2.24); p-value = 0.277).

Table 3. Thromboembolic and bleeding events.

		Thromboembolic events	Thromboembolic events + unclear deaths	Major bleeding events	Intracranial bleeding events
		numbers per 100 patient-years (95% CI)			
	Overall n = 1110	0.4 (0.2–0.6)	0.9 (0.7–1.2)	1.1 (0.9–1.5)	0.2 (0.1–0.3)
Indication	**Venous thromboembolism** n = 451	0.5 (0.2–0.9)	0.5 (0.3–0.9)	0.9 (0.6–1.4)	0.1 (0.01–0.3)
	Prosthetic heart valve n = 356	0.4 (0.2–0.8)	0.7 (0.4–1.2)	1.5 (1.0–2.2)	0.3 (0.1–0.7)
	Atrial fibrillation n = 198	0.1 (0.002–0.6)	1.3 (0.7–2.3)	1.1 (0.5–2.0)	0.1 (0.003–0.6)
	Arterial thromboembolism n = 51	0.3 (0.01–1.8)	0.6 (0.1–2.3)	1.7 (0.5–3.9)	0 (0–1.2)
	Others n = 54	0 (0–1.7)	1.8 (0.5–4.7)	0 (0–1.7)	0 (0–1.7)
Age	**<50 years** n = 451	0.4 (0.2–0.7)	0.5 (0.3–0.9)	0.7 (0.4–1.1)	0.04 (0.0–0.2)
	≥50 years n = 659	0.4 (0.2–0.7)	1.3 (0.9–1.8)	1.5 (1.1–2.0)	0.2 (0.1–0.5)
Sex	**Female** n = 382	0.5 (0.2–0.9)	0.7 (0.4–1.2)	1.3 (0.9–1.9)	0.2 (0.1–0.5)
	Male n = 728	0.3 (0.2–0.6)	1.1 (0.8–1.5)	1.1 (0.8–1.5)	0.1 (0.05–0.3)

CI, confidence interval.

Thromboembolic Complications

Twenty-two venous and arterial thromboembolic complications were documented during the observation period, leading to a rate of 0.4 per 100 patient-years (95% CI 0.2–0.6; see Table 3). If unclear deaths were counted as thromboembolic complication, the rate would be 0.9 per 100 patient-years (95% CI 0.7–1.2). No differences could be found between the different subgroups (see Fig. 3).

Major Bleedings

Sixty-six major bleedings were reported during the study period, corresponding to a rate of 1.1 per 100 patient-years (95% CI 0.9–1.5; Table 3). The rate was higher among patients older 50 years (1.5 per 100 patient-years; 95% CI 1.1–2.0) than in younger patients (0.7; 95% CI 0.4–1.1; Fig. 4). No differences were found between the established indications and between male and female patients. Nine intracranial bleedings were documented (0.2 per 100 patient-years; 95% CI 0.1–0.3) with a trend towards a higher rate in patients older 50 years (0.2 vs. 0.04 per 100 patient-years; 95% CI 0.1–0.5 vs. 0.0–0.2).

Quality of Anticoagulation

INR data of 653 patients were available for analysis, corresponding to an observation period of 1743 patient-years (74,665 data points; 59% of the patients). Median observation period was 2.19 years (interquartile range [IQR] 0.98–3.97). The median time within the intended therapeutic range was 80% (IQR 66–89%). Median time in a safety range of 2.0 to 4.5 was 96% (IQR 89–99).

Comparison with VKA Standard Care, and New Oral Anticoagulants

Occurrence of recurrent thromboembolism, as observed in a network meta-analysis, was at least comparable to mentioned treatments (Fig. 5). OR of PSM against placebo was 0.16 (0.10–0.26; p<0.001), for warfarin standard care 0.23(0.13–0.39; p<0.001), for rivaroxaban 0.18 (0.08–0.38; p<0.001), for dabigatran 0.24 (0.12–0.50; p<0.001) and for apixaban, 0.19 (0.10–0.36; p<0.001).

Discussion

Key Findings

Our results indicate that PSM of properly trained patients is safe and effective in a long-term real-life setting and robust across different clinical subgroups. Mortality is low, both overall and with regard to different indications of anticoagulation, sex and age. Thromboembolic events are very uncommon and the rate of major bleedings as well as intracranial bleedings is moderate. Furthermore, quality of anticoagulation therapy is high. Efficacy is comparable to VKA standard care and new oral anticoagulants.

Comparison with other Studies

Randomized controlled trials, systematic reviews and individual patient data meta-analyses [4–6] consistently showed that PSM with VKA is effective. Nevertheless, many authors doubted that these results can be transferred to clinical practice straightforwardly because the experimental set-up within trials does not reflect daily routine [4,5,7–10,14,16] and study groups are prone being heavily selected [21,22]. Moreover they criticised that follow-up periods within randomised studies are too short to extrapolate long-term consequences of PSM and called for population-based cohort studies to address these important points.

We are aware of two smaller observational studies investigating the efficacy and safety in patients with PSM. A retrospective analysis of 160 patients on PSM after implantation of a mechanical heart valve revealed a reduction in mortality and severe adverse events if compared with 260 patients on usual care (mean follow-up 8.6±2.1 years) [38]. In another investigation, 116 PSM patients out of 178 patients of a randomised controlled trial were re-analysed after 5 years [39]. Major bleedings were observed with a rate of 0.6 per 100 patient-years as well as 1.1 thromboembolic events per 100 patient-years. However, no mortality data and only few details of the study cohort were provided. Our study expands on their work reporting long-term efficacy and safety of PSM in real-life clinical practice, in a large prospective cohort and with regard to relevant outcome parameters and salient clinical subgroups.

A

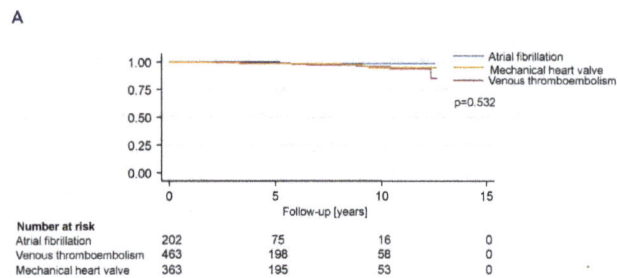

B

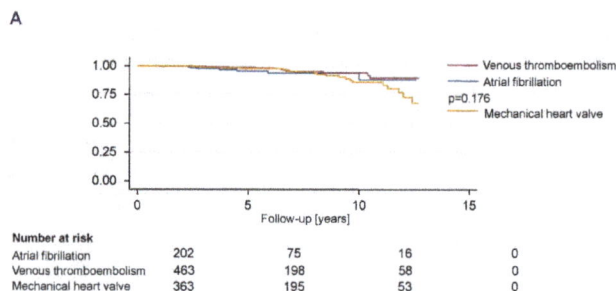

C

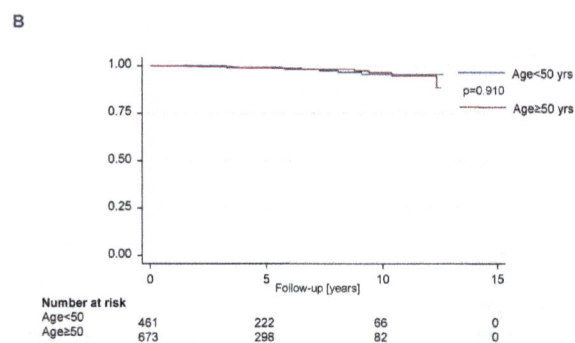

Figure 3. Thromboembolic complications by indications of oral anticoagulation, age, and sex.

A

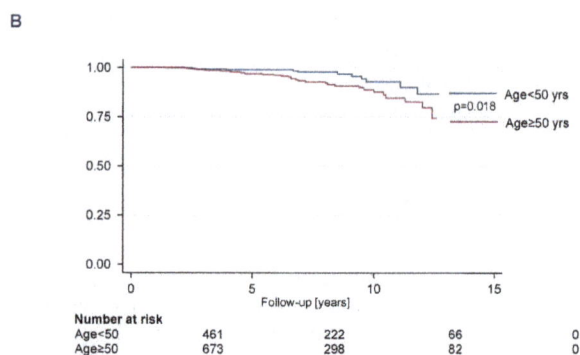

B

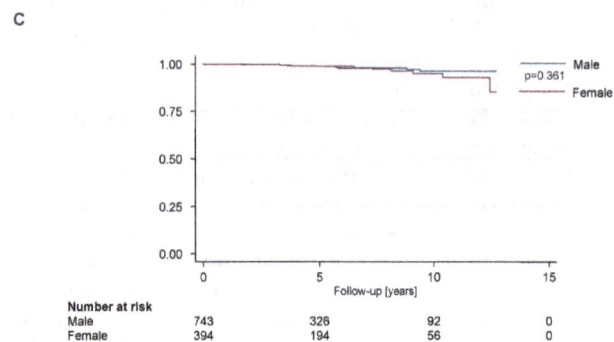

C

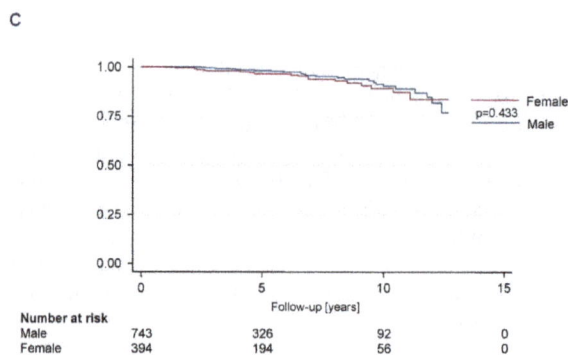

Figure 4. Major bleedings by indications of oral anticoagulation, age, and sex.

Strengths and Limitations

The strength of our investigation is the design of a prospective cohort study of all patients trained for PSM. The nationwide initiative "coagulationcare" covers about 90% of all trained patients in Switzerland and not one single patient was lost to follow-up. This makes any selection bias at the study level unlikely. Our study has several limitations. First, we cannot fully exclude that motivational or other factors may have influenced the referring decision of physicians and thus lead to a selected study group (selection at referral level). However, we believe that a systematic selection – if any – is unlikely. Second, we included patients from one country only, trained by one training program,

using mostly phenprocoumon as anticoagulant. Although the training program was established according to current guidelines [18,19], our results may need confirmation from other countries, using other training programs and anticoagulants such as warfarin. Finally, a direct comparison of death and survival rates with the general population on one hand and with other treatment schemes on the other hand was impossible. To overcome this limitation, we performed a network meta-analysis including PSM as well as VKA standard care and new oral anticoagulants. Furthermore, we put the results of our investigation into context with the results of large thromboembolism trials for different indications (Table S1).

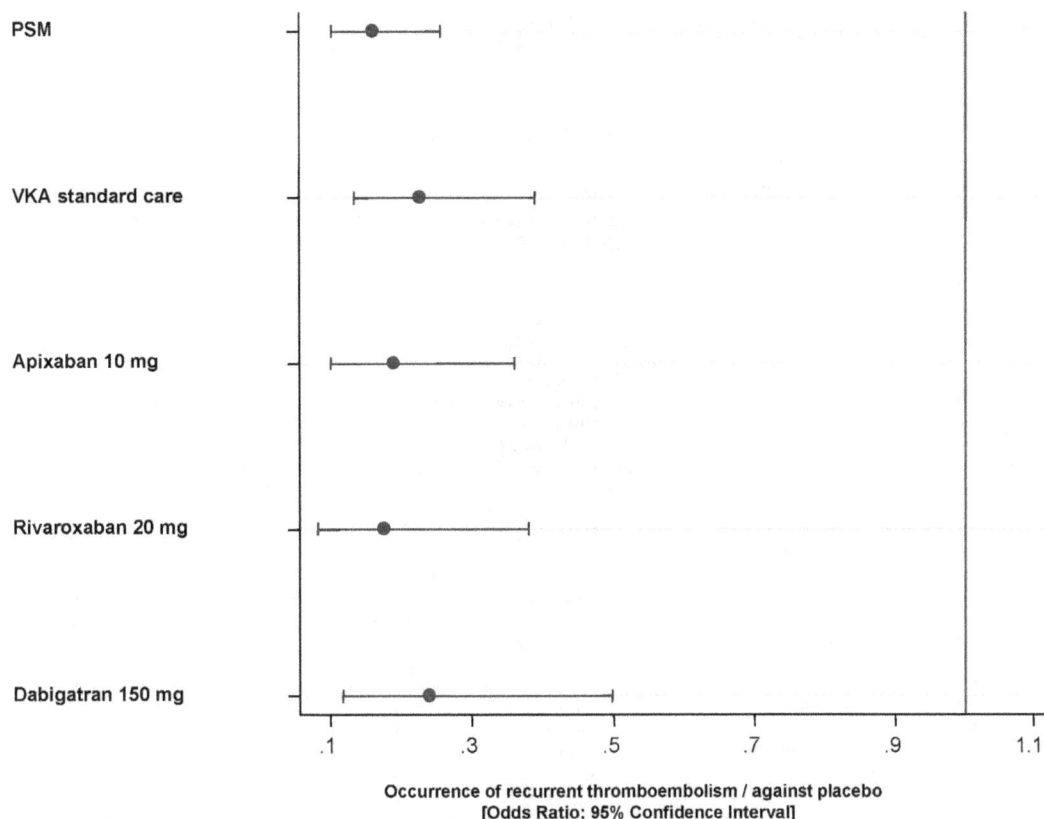

Figure 5. Efficacy of PSM in comparison to VKA standard care and new oral anticoagulants.

Who should Perform PSM?

In 2006, Douketis and Singh identified four requirements that patients qualifying for anticoagulant self-monitoring should fulfill; patients should necessitate long-term treatment, have no vision impairment that precludes appropriate testing, should have the cognitive ability to receive training and should be willing to take an active role in their illness [40]. Down these lines, today, a selection strategy based on existing guidelines targets at motivated patients who represent an important socio-economic group. In this group adherence to therapy, patient satisfaction and quality of life is very high. PSM also represents a rational treatment option in settings with limited access to (para-) medical care and thus qualifies for a variety of healthcare settings. PSM also has the potential to overcome well-known barriers of anticoagulant treatment prescription surveyed in the general practitioner setting [41–44]. We therefore call for efficient implementation strategies promoting PSM in clinical practice.

Is there a Role for PSM in the Era of New Oral Anticoagulants?

In search of drugs with a more predictable effect lacking the need for routine monitoring, new, direct factor Xa and thrombin inhibitors have become available. A recent systematic review concluded that these drugs are a viable option, but benefits compared to warfarin are small and depend on the quality of anticoagulation, that is achieved with warfarin [45]. Ultimately, whether or not these new drugs are worth their money depends on the outcome of randomized controlled trials comparing PSM with new oral anticoagulants and cost effectiveness analyses considering changing costs and reimbursements. To date, efficacy and safety of

new oral anticoagulants in real-life practice is largely unknown. Benefits may be reduced due to a lack of antidote, impaired adherence, and application to patients that would be excluded in clinical trials. Furthermore, new anticoagulants are not applicable in patients with mechanical heart valves and a relevant renal impairment [46].

What are Implications for Research?

Unlike in other chronic clinical conditions such as asthma, arthritis or diabetes, evidence on the usefulness of PSM in oral anticoagulation remains less well established. When developing the research agenda for patient self-management of oral anticoagulation now, several lessons from other experiences can be learned. In the case of chronic obstructive pulmonary disease for instance, a Cochrane review recently concluded that heterogeneity in interventions, study populations, follow-up time, and outcome measures impeded from drawing firm recommendations [3]. Another recent review examining the usefulness of self-measured blood pressure in hypertension concluded that long-term benefits remained uncertain [2]. Besides replications of our study in other countries and using other anticoagulants, we call for systematic investigations specifying those patient profiles benefitting most from PSM. Finally, cost effectiveness analyses considering changing costs and reimbursements in the context of new anticoagulants are needed.

In conclusion, PSM of properly trained patients is effective and safe in a real-life setting and robust across clinical subgroups. It represents a rational strategy to provide high quality anticoagulation therapy in many service settings including those with limited access to (para) medical care or rural areas, where patients need travelling greater distances for healthcare and thus deserves being broadly promoted.

Acknowledgments

We would like to thank Madeleine Bossard and Markus Umiker who collected and cleaned the data. Furthermore, we would like to thank all physicians, who looked for the patients all the years. And first of all, we would like to thank all patients who attended the training courses and provided us with clinical information.

Author Contributions

Conceived and designed the experiments: WAW PR. Performed the experiments: WAW PR MN. Analyzed the data: MN LMB PS. Contributed reagents/materials/analysis tools: WAW. Wrote the paper: MN LMB PS PR WAW.

References

1. Bodenheimer T, Lorig K, Holman H, Grumbach K (2002) Patient self-management of chronic disease in primary care. JAMA 288: 2469–2475.
2. Uhlig K, Patel K, Ip S, Kitsios GD, Balk EM (2013) Self-measured blood pressure monitoring in the management of hypertension: a systematic review and meta-analysis. Ann Intern Med 159: 185–194.
3. Effing T, Monninkhof EM, van der Valk PD, van der Palen J, van Herwaarden CL, et al. (2007) Self-management education for patients with chronic obstructive pulmonary disease. Cochrane Database Syst Rev: CD002990.
4. Garcia-Alamino JM, Ward AM, Alonso-Coello P, Perera R, Bankhead C, et al. (2010) Self-monitoring and self-management of oral anticoagulation. Cochrane database of systematic reviews: CD003839.
5. Heneghan C, Ward A, Perera R, Bankhead C, Fuller A, et al. (2012) Self-monitoring of oral anticoagulation: systematic review and meta-analysis of individual patient data. Lancet 379: 322–334.
6. Bloomfield HE, Krause A, Greer N, Taylor BC, MacDonald R, et al. (2011) Meta-analysis: effect of patient self-testing and self-management of long-term anticoagulation on major clinical outcomes. Ann Intern Med 154: 472–482.
7. Kyrle PA, Eichinger S (2012) Vitamin K antagonists: self-determination by self-monitoring? Lancet 379: 292–293.
8. Siebenhofer A, Jeitler K, Rakovac I (2011) Effect of patient self-testing and self-management of long-term anticoagulation on major clinical outcomes. Ann Intern Med 155: 336; author reply 336–337.
9. Anaya P, Moliterno DJ (2011) Patient, heal thyself: the ongoing evolution of patient self-directed care and hand-held technology. Ann Intern Med 154: 500–501.
10. Li Wan Po A (2012) Self-monitoring of anticoagulation. Lancet 379: 1788–1789; author reply 1789.
11. Siebenhofer A, Rakovac I, Kleespies C, Piso B, Didjurgeit U, et al. (2008) Self-management of oral anticoagulation reduces major outcomes in the elderly. A randomized controlled trial. Thromb Haemost 100: 1089–1098.
12. Soliman Hamad MA, van Eekelen E, van Agt T, van Straten AH (2009) Self-management program improves anticoagulation control and quality of life: a prospective randomized study. Eur J Cardiothorac Surg 35: 265–269.
13. Sidhu P, O'Kane HO (2001) Self-managed anticoagulation: results from a two-year prospective randomized trial with heart valve patients. Ann Thorac Surg 72: 1523–1527.
14. Gardiner C, Williams K, Longair I, Mackie IJ, Machin SJ, et al. (2006) A randomised control trial of patient self-management of oral anticoagulation compared with patient self-testing. Br J Haematol 132: 598–603.
15. Christensen TD, Johnsen SP, Hjortdal VE, Hasenkam JM (2007) Self-management of oral anticoagulant therapy: a systematic review and meta-analysis. Int J Cardiol 118: 54–61.
16. Fitzmaurice DA, Murray ET, McCahon D, Holder R, Raftery JP, et al. (2005) Self management of oral anticoagulation: randomised trial. BMJ 331: 1057.
17. Ageno W, Gallus AS, Wittkowsky A, Crowther M, Hylek EM, et al. (2012) Oral anticoagulant therapy: Antithrombotic Therapy and Prevention of Thrombosis, 9th ed: American College of Chest Physicians Evidence-Based Clinical Practice Guidelines. Chest 141: e44S–88S.
18. Fitzmaurice DA, Gardiner C, Kitchen S, Mackie I, Murray ET, et al. (2005) An evidence-based review and guidelines for patient self-testing and management of oral anticoagulation. Br J Haematol 131: 156–165.
19. Ansell J, Jacobson A, Levy J, Voller H, Hasenkam JM, et al. (2005) Guidelines for implementation of patient self-testing and patient self-management of oral anticoagulation. International consensus guidelines prepared by International Self-Monitoring Association for Oral Anticoagulation. Int J Cardiol 99: 37–45.
20. Lip GY, Rudolf M, Kakar P (2007) Management of atrial fibrillation: the NICE guidelines. Int J Clin Pract 61: 9–11.
21. Levi M, Hovingh GK, Cannegieter SC, Vermeulen M, Buller HR, et al. (2008) Bleeding in patients receiving vitamin K antagonists who would have been excluded from trials on which the indication for anticoagulation was based. Blood 111: 4471–4476.
22. van Walraven C, Jennings A, Oake N, Fergusson D, Forster AJ (2006) Effect of study setting on anticoagulation control: a systematic review and metaregression. Chest 129: 1155–1166.
23. Sawicki PT (1999) A structured teaching and self-management program for patients receiving oral anticoagulation: a randomized controlled trial. Working Group for the Study of Patient Self-Management of Oral Anticoagulation. JAMA 281: 145–150.
24. Fitzmaurice DA, Machin SJ, British Society of Haematology Task Force for Haemostasis and Thrombosis (2001) Recommendations for patients undertaking self management of oral anticoagulation. BMJ 323: 985–989.
25. Murray E, Fitzmaurice D, McCahon D, Fuller C, Sandhur H (2004) Training for patients in a randomised controlled trial of self management of warfarin treatment. BMJ 328: 437–438.
26. Fritschi J, Raddatz-Muller P, Schmid P, Wuillemin WA (2007) Patient self-management of long-term oral anticoagulation in Switzerland. Swiss Med Wkly 137: 252–258.
27. Nagler M, Raddatz-Muller P, Schmid P, Bachmann LM, Wuillemin WA (2013) Accuracy of the point-of-care coagulometer CoaguChek XS in the hands of patients. J Thromb Haemost 11: 197–199.
28. Christensen TD, Larsen TB (2012) Precision and accuracy of point-of-care testing coagulometers used for self-testing and self-management of oral anticoagulation therapy. J Thromb Haemost 10: 251–260.
29. Rosendaal FR, Cannegieter SC, van der Meer FJ, Briet E (1993) A method to determine the optimal intensity of oral anticoagulant therapy. Thrombosis and haemostasis 69: 236–239.
30. Biss TT, Avery PJ, Walsh PM, Kamali F (2011) Comparison of 'time within therapeutic INR range' with 'percentage INR within therapeutic range' for assessing long-term anticoagulation control in children. Journal of thrombosis and haemostasis: JTH 9: 1090–1092.
31. Kearon C, Gent M, Hirsh J, Weitz J, Kovacs MJ, et al. (1999) A comparison of three months of anticoagulation with extended anticoagulation for a first episode of idiopathic venous thromboembolism. N Engl J Med 340: 901–907.
32. Ridker PM, Goldhaber SZ, Danielson E, Rosenberg Y, Eby CS, et al. (2003) Long-term, low-intensity warfarin therapy for the prevention of recurrent venous thromboembolism. N Engl J Med 348: 1425–1434.
33. Palareti G, Cosmi B, Legnani C, Tosetto A, Brusi C, et al. (2006) D-dimer testing to determine the duration of anticoagulation therapy. N Engl J Med 355: 1780–1789.
34. Schulman S, Kearon C, Kakkar AK, Mismetti P, Schellong S, et al. (2009) Dabigatran versus warfarin in the treatment of acute venous thromboembolism. N Engl J Med 361: 2342–2352.
35. Bauersachs R, Berkowitz SD, Brenner B, Buller HR, Decousus H, et al. (2010) Oral rivaroxaban for symptomatic venous thromboembolism. N Engl J Med 363: 2499–2510.
36. Agnelli G, Buller HR, Cohen A, Curto M, Gallus AS, et al. (2013) Apixaban for extended treatment of venous thromboembolism. N Engl J Med 368: 699–708.
37. Kessels AGH, ter Riet G, Puhan MA, Kleijnen J, Bachmann LM, et al. (2013) A simple regression model for network meta-analysis. OA Epidemiology 1: 7.
38. Mair H, Sachweh J, Sodian R, Brenner P, Schmoeckel M, et al. (2012) Long-term self-management of anticoagulation therapy after mechanical heart valve replacement in outside trial conditions. Interact Cardiovasc Thorac Surg 14: 253–257.
39. Sawicki PT, Glaser B, Kleespies C, Stubbe J, Schmitz N, et al. (2003) Self-management of oral anticoagulation: long-term results. J Intern Med 254: 515–516.
40. Douketis JD, Singh D (2006) Self-monitoring and self-dosing of oral anticoagulation improves survival. Evid Based Cardiovasc Med 10: 124–126.
41. Pisters R, de Vos CB, Nieuwlaat R, Crijns HJ (2009) Use and underuse of oral anticoagulation for stroke prevention in atrial fibrillation: old and new paradigms. Semin Thromb Hemost 35: 554–559.
42. Ogilvie IM, Newton N, Welner SA, Cowell W, Lip GY (2010) Underuse of oral anticoagulants in atrial fibrillation: a systematic review. Am J Med 123: 638–645 e634.
43. Baczek VL, Chen WT, Kluger J, Coleman CI (2012) Predictors of warfarin use in atrial fibrillation in the United States: a systematic review and meta-analysis. BMC Fam Pract 13: 5.

18

Origin and Characteristics of High Shannon Entropy at the Pivot of Locally Stable Rotors: Insights from Computational Simulation

Anand N. Ganesan[1]*[ ], Pawel Kuklik[2,3][ ], Ali Gharaviri[2], Anthony Brooks[1], Darius Chapman[1], Dennis H. Lau[1], Kurt C. Roberts-Thomson[1], Prashanthan Sanders[1]

1 Centre for Heart Rhythm Disorders (CHRD), South Australian Health and Medical Research Institute (SAHMRI), University of Adelaide and Royal Adelaide Hospital, Adelaide, Australia, 2 Department of Physiology, Maastricht University Medical Center, Maastricht, The Netherlands, 3 Department of Cardiology, Electrophysiology, University Heart Center, Hamburg, Germany

Abstract

Background: Rotors are postulated to maintain cardiac fibrillation. Despite the importance of bipolar electrograms in clinical electrophysiology, few data exist on the properties of bipolar electrograms at rotor sites. The pivot of a spiral wave is characterized by relative uncertainty of wavefront propagation direction compared to the periphery. The bipolar electrograms used in electrophysiology recording encode information on both direction and timing of approaching wavefronts.

Objective: To test the hypothesis that bipolar electrograms from the pivot of rotors have higher Shannon entropy (ShEn) than electrograms recorded at the periphery due to the spatial dynamics of spiral waves.

Methods and Results: We studied spiral wave propagation in 2-dimensional sheets constructed using a simple cell automaton (FitzHugh-Nagumo), atrial (Courtemanche-Ramirez-Nattel) and ventricular (Luo-Rudy) myocyte cell models and in a geometric model spiral wave. In each system, bipolar electrogram recordings were simulated, and Shannon entropy maps constructed as a measure of electrogram information content. ShEn was consistently highest in the pivoting region associated with the phase singularity of the spiral wave. This property was consistently preserved across; (i) variation of model system (ii) alterations in bipolar electrode spacing, (iii) alternative bipolar electrode orientation (iv) bipolar electrogram filtering and (v) in the presence of rotor meander. Directional activation plots demonstrated that the origin of high ShEn at the pivot was the directional diversity of wavefront propagation observed in this location.

Conclusions: The pivot of the rotor is consistently associated with high Shannon entropy of bipolar electrograms despite differences in action potential model, bipolar electrode spacing, signal filtering and rotor meander. Maximum ShEn is co-located with the pivot for rotors observed in the bipolar electrogram recording mode, and may be an intrinsic property of spiral wave dynamic behaviour.

Editor: Alexander V. Panfilov, Gent University, Belgium

Funding: The authors have no support or funding to report.

Competing Interests: The authors have declared that no competing interests exist.

* Email: anand.ganesan@adelaide.edu.au

[ ] These authors contributed equally to this work.

Introduction

Localized re-entrant circuits known as rotors have been postulated as the drivers of cardiac fibrillation. [1,2,3] Recently, rotor-guided ablation has emerged as a therapeutic strategy in atrial fibrillation (AF). [4,5] Specifically, ablation at the rotor's pivot point (also called the *phase singularity*) has been shown to lead to acute AF termination [4,5] and improved clinical outcome. [4] To date, there is a paucity of information on bipolar electrogram (EGM) properties at rotor sites, which are relevant to the current mapping techniques and application of these emerging technologies.

Recently, we observed high bipolar EGM Shannon entropy (ShEn), a statistical measure of information uncertainty, at the pivoting region of rotors in animal experimental models. [6] The present study aimed to go further and explore the origin and characteristics of this phenomenon, using a computational simulation approach. We also aimed to explore the effects of model spiral wave system, bipolar electrode spacing, signal filtering, and rotor meander on ShEn distribution in the vicinity of spiral waves, which are relevant practical issues in the application of ShEn for rotor mapping. The hypothesis of the study was that high Shannon entropy of bipolar EGMs occurs because of directional diversity of wavefront propagation at the rotor pivot, and may therefore represent an intrinsic property of spiral wave dynamic behavior.

Methods

Computer Simulation of Spiral Wave

Simulations and EGM analysis were performed in a custom designed C++ software package and MATLAB (The MathWorks, Natick, MA, USA). We investigated bipolar EGM formation in simulated two-dimensional sheets based on (i) FitzHugh Nagumo [7], (ii) Luo-Rudy guinea-pig ventricular myocyte [8], and (iii) modified Courtemanche-Ramirez-Nattel (CRN) human atrial action potential models. [9].

Computer Simulations. Computations were carried out on two-dimensional, isotropic, square grids. Details of model implementation can be found in File S1. Extracellular unipolar electrograms were calculated at each mesh node as previously described [10]:

$$u_{i,j}(t) = c \sum_{k,l=0}^{k,l=N} \frac{\vec{r}_{k,l} \nabla v_{k,l}(t)}{r_{k,l}^3} \qquad (1)$$

where $u_{i,j}(t)$ is unipolar voltage at node i,j, c is a scaling coefficient (assumed to be one for simplicity), $v_{k,l}$ is transmembrane voltage at node k,l and $r_{k,l}$ is a distance between nodes. Bipolar electrogram was calculated as a difference of unipolar electrograms at fixed spatial distance:

$$w_{i,j}(t) = u_{i,j}(t) - u_{i+s,j}(t) \qquad (2)$$

where $w_{i,j}$ is a bipolar voltage at node (i,j) and s is a parameter controlling the inter-electrode spacing.

Spiral waves were initiated in the system by setting the spatial distribution of the model's kinetic variables to a distribution mimicking propagating spiral wave. For each element of the simulation grid, phase was calculated as:

$$\theta = \frac{r - k\varphi - 2\pi kn}{2\pi k} \qquad (3)$$

where r and φ are polar coordinates of a given point with respect to the center of the spiral wave, k is its winding number and n is an integer set so as to obtain a phase between 0 and 1. Kinetic variables for a given element of the grid were set depending on the phase. $\theta = 0$ corresponded to the resting state and $\theta = 1$ corresponded to the wave front depolarization. All intermediate values of the variables were copied from the stationary distribution of the variables within the action potential cycle. The spiral wave tip was localized as the intersection point of line defined as $v = 0$ and $dv/dt = 0$ where v is transmembrane voltage variable in the model.

Wave Direction Plots

To examine the hypothesis that underlying high ShEn at the pivot of the rotor occurs because of directional variation of the bipolar EGM, we created directional activation plots. These plots demonstrate the directions of wave propagation at given locations in the system. In order to investigate directional variability of the propagation direction at the pivot of the spiral wave, we calculated directions along the line running from one edge of the sample to the opposite edge. The wavefront was defined as region with voltage in range specified by $(v_{max}-v_{min})/2 \pm 10\%$, during the period where $dv/dt > 0$. The direction of propagation was

computed using gradient of the transmembrane at the half-maximal voltage of phase 0 of the action potential:

$$\psi(x,y,t) = \arctan\left(\frac{\partial v/\partial y}{\partial v/\partial x}\right) \qquad (4)$$

where ψ is a direction of wave propagation at position (x,y) and time instance t, and v is spatial distribution of transmembrane voltage.

Shannon Entropy Map Construction

Shannon entropy measures the distribution of signal values within the signal histogram, and provides a measure of information content. [6,11,12] ShEn was calculated based on histogram of EGM amplitude. In this study, the bin size of the histogram was set at 1% of maximum EGM amplitude. The relative probability density p_i was defined as the number of counts in an amplitude bin i divided by the sum of bin counts in all bins. The Shannon entropy was defined then as:

$$ShEn = -\sum_{i=0}^{N-1} p_i \log_2 p_i \qquad (5)$$

where N is the number of amplitude bins, and p_i is the probability of any sample falling within a particular amplitude bin i. EGMs in which the signal has few states (i.e. narrow deflections) have a narrow distribution in the voltage histogram, and low ShEn values. EGMs in which the signal adopts a broad distribution of states have a wide distribution in the voltage histogram, and high ShEn values. We constructed ShEn maps during spiral waves with a number of cell models and recording conditions to determine the impact on ShEn maps of:

(i)   **action potential model** - by studying ShEn maps of spiral waves created in the FitzHugh-Nagumo, Courtemanche-Ramirez-Nattel and Luo-Rudy models,

(ii)   **electrode spacing** - by varying the number of mesh elements between simulated bipole locations in the CRN model spiral wave.

(iii)   **direction-dependence** - by creation of ShEn maps for bipoles constructed in the horizontal and vertical directions.

(iv)   **electrogram filtering** - to simulate the effect of filtering in the electrophysiology laboratory, Butterworth third order infinite impulse response (IIR) low-pass and high-pass filters were applied to simulated bipolar signals from the CRN model,

(v)   **simulated local rotor meander** – meander is defined as the spontaneous change in the location of a spiral wave related to internal or external instabilities. To study the influence of meander on ShEn distribution, we systematically varied the conductance of slow-inward Ca^{2+} in the Luo-Rudy model spiral wave as previously described. [13,14]

To maximise color resolution of the high ShEn region around the pivot, color maps were drawn with the dynamic range from the median to maximum ShEn.

Geometric Model of Spiral Wave

To extend these observations, we examined ShEn maps in the case of an ideal, rigidly rotating spiral wave in Cartesian coordinate system in parametric form (Figure S1). The aim of this representation is to explore the effects of the spiral wave geometry on ShEn maps, eliminating effects related to action potential model. The mathematical details of the construction of this model are provided in File S1.

Results

Influence of action potential model system on ShEn distribution

We first investigated the effect of action potential model system on bipolar EGM Shannon entropy maps. Figure 1A presents data for spiral waves in the FHN model. The left panels (i)–(iv) shows the position of electrode locations (white stars) in relation to snapshots from action potential. The trajectory of the spiral wave tip is shown in black, and shows a rigid spiral for the FHN model. Electrograms are shown in the right panels for each of the positions (i)–(iv). At the pivot location (i), local unipolar EGMs are low amplitude and regular. Local unipolar EGMs have a broad morphology, with slow dV/dt. The bipolar electrogram is broad but has a regular morphology. This corresponds to a region of high ShEn on the map at the lower left. At the peripheral EGM positions away from the spiral pivot (iii,iv), local EGMs show clean sharp local deflections, and correspond to regions of low ShEn (blue) on the ShEn map. The ShEn map shows the highest entropy regions in red overlaying with the region of the pivot.

Similar patterns were observed in CRN (atrial myocyte model) and LR (ventricular myocyte model) spiral waves. Clean, local bipolar EGMs were observed at peripheral locations, associated with low ShEn regions on corresponding ShEn maps. The highest ShEn EGMs were found to correspond to the region of the spiral wave trip trajectory. In contrast to the FHN which had a rigid spiral, these models demonstrated local meander of the spiral wave tip trajectory. The region of this meander corresponded to the regions of maximum ShEn (Figure 1B, 1C-ShEn maps for atrial and ventricular action potential models).

Influence of wavefront propagation direction on ShEn at the pivot and periphery of the rotor

To examine the influence of propagation direction on ShEn, we created plots of ShEn vs. wave direction at different regions of the rotor for the FHN, CRN, and LR models. In these plots, the angle (ψ) of the approaching wavefront to a chosen meridian line is plotted for a series of activations of the spiral. Each point in the scatter plots in Figure 2 represents the wavefront angle for an individual activation, plotted against position on the x-axis along the meridian line. In these plots, we examined the distribution of wave propagation (ψ) along meridian lines passing through the pivot and periphery of the spiral wave. In Figure 2A, it can be seen that the maximum values of ShEn occur in the region of the lines passing through the pivot (L2) (red bars, Figs 2A). The region of maximum ShEn corresponds to the region showing the broadest distribution in wavefront direction. In Figure 2B, meridian lines through the pivot are shown for the Luo-Rudy spiral wave, in the cases of a rigid and meandering spiral wave. Again, it can be seen that the region of maximum ShEn corresponds to the region showing the broadest distribution in wavefront direction (red bars, Fig. 2B).

Influence of bipolar electrode spacing on ShEn maps

Figure 3 shows color maps of ShEn in the CRN model rotor constructed at increasing bipolar inter-electrode distance, which was assessed by constructing bipoles at increasing distances between mesh elements. The region with highest values for ShEn

(corresponding to the red region on ShEn map) is localized to the region of the spiral wave tip trajectory across the full range of bipolar EGM spacings. With increasing bipolar EGM distance, the maximum ShEn increases slightly from 6.43 at d = 1 to at 6.59 d = 12. The minimum ShEn increases with increasing bipolar spacing from 5.20 at d = 1 to 6.26 at d = 12. The range of ShEn values (maximum-minimum) decreases at high bipolar spacing.

Dependence of ShEn on bipolar electrode orientation

To assess the role of the direction dependence of the bipolar EGM in contributing to the high entropy EGMs at the pivot zone, we evaluated ShEn maps for orthogonally constructed bipoles. Figure 4(left panel) shows a ShEn map and corresponding bipolar EGMs from the pivot zone of a CRN model rotor for bipoles constructed in the horizontal direction. Figure 4(right panel) shows a ShEn for the same CRN rotor with bipoles constructed in the vertical direction. The effect of changing the bipole orientation is equivalent to rotation of ShEn maps by 90°. The area of maximum ShEn in red corresponds to that of the tip trajectory in both examples.

Influence of Bipolar Signal Filtering on ShEn distribution

To assess the influence of signal filtering, we constructed ShEn maps from rotors in each of the model systems under conditions of low-pass and high-pass filtering. In Fig. 5, it can be seen that low-pass filtering at 500 Hz has relatively little impact on ShEn distribution near the pivot of the rotor. We also evaluated ShEn distribution at a variety of high-pass filter cut-offs from 0.5, 5, 10 and 30 Hz. The highest region of ShEn remained localized to the pivot of the rotor under conditions of high-pass filtering(Figure 5 upper left panels). The range of ShEn (maximum ShEn-minimum ShEn) was similar over a range of high pass filter settings. (Figure 5-graph panel).

Influence of spiral wave meander on ShEn distribution

Figure 6 presents the effect of rotor meander on ShEn distribution in an LR model rotor. The diameter of the tip trajectory was modulated by the change in the slow inward Ca^{2+} channel conductance. At low Ca^{2+} channel conductance (Gsi = 0, Gsi = 0.02), the diameter of the trajectory of the spiral wave is narrow in the form of a circle. The spatial extent of the region of high ShEn corresponds to the region of this circle. At higher levels Ca^{2+} conductance (Gsi = 0.03, Gsi = 0.043), the tip trajectory takes on a rosette shape. The maximum ShEn remains co-located with the central region of the tip trajectory.

ShEn distribution in the case of a geometrically perfect spiral wave

To further evaluate ShEn distribution in spiral waves, we studied the ShEn map for a perfect spiral constructed with constant voltage gradient across the wavefront (see File S1 for mathematical details). The aim was to create a pure system to eliminate the effects of specific ionic channel kinetics on the construction of ShEn maps. Bipolar EGMs and ShEn maps in this model system are shown in Figures S1–S3. Broad multi-component potentials are observed at the central bipoles, corresponding to a region of high ShEn. More narrow local deflections are seen at the peripheral bipole electrode locations, corresponding to regions of lower ShEn on the map. The highest ShEn regions are observed at the pivot of the spiral wave.

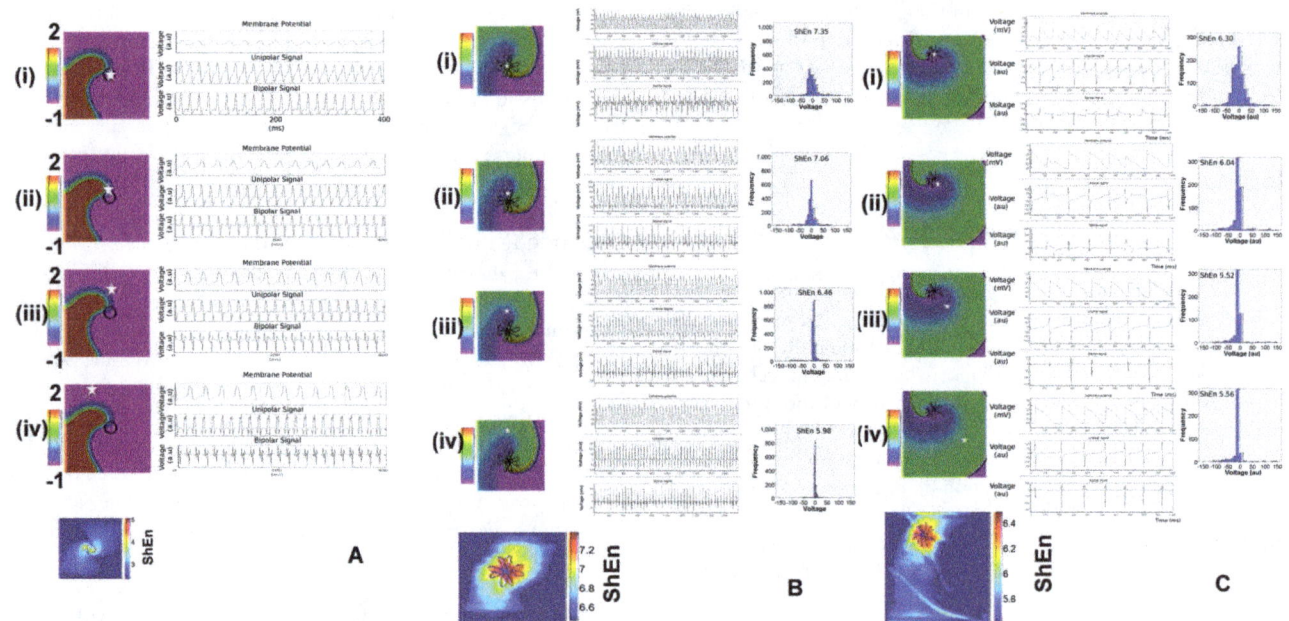

Figure 1. Effect of Model System. A. Electrograms shown from FitzHugh-Nagumo (FHN) Model Rotor. The left panels show action potential movie snapshots of a FHN rotor. The white stars indicate the position of electrodes shown in right panels. Local action potentials, unipolar electrograms and bipolar electrograms are shown in the right panels. At the central bipoles, in panels (i) and (ii), broad deflections are seen, associated with high Shannon entropy (ShEn) seen in the ShEn map (lowest left panel). At the periphery, in panels (iii) and (iv), sharp local bipolar deflections are seen associated with low ShEn. The trajectory of the spiral wave tip is shown in the left panels in black, and on the ShEn map as a blue circle. The area of maximum ShEn overlies the pivot of the rotor. **B. Electrograms from the Luo-Rudy Ventricular Myocyte Model Spiral Wave.** A similar pattern of high ShEn associated with the pivot zone is seen. The left panels show action potential movie snapshots of a LRD rotor. At the central bipoles, position (i), (ii) multi-component EGMs are seen, associated with high ShEn (lowest left panel). At the periphery (panels iii, iv), sharp local bipolar deflections are seen which are associated with low ShEn in the corresponding region on the map. The meandering trajectory of the spiral wave tip is shown in the left panels in black, and on the ShEn map in blue. The area of maximum ShEn overlies the pivot. Histograms are shown on the right panels. These show a broad distribution in the pivot zone bipole (panel (i)) associated with high ShEn, and a narrow distribution bipoles (iii), (iv) and lower ShEn at the periphery. **C. Electrograms from the Courtemanche Ramirez-Nattel-Atrial Myocyte Model Spiral Wave.** A similar pattern of high ShEn associated with the pivot zone is seen. The left panels show action potential movie snapshots of a CRN rotor. The white star indicates the position of electrodes. At the central bipoles, positions (i),(ii) multi-component EGMs are seen, associated with broad amplitude distribution and high ShEn. At the periphery (panels iii, Iv), sharp local bipolar deflections are seen which are associated with narrow amplitude distribution and low ShEn. The meandering trajectory of the spiral wave tip is shown in the left panels in black, and on the ShEn map in blue. The area of maximum Shannon entropy overlies the pivot.

Discussion

In the current study, we studied Shannon entropy distribution in in a variety of model systems with different ionic channel kinetics and conditions. The principal finding of our study is that high ShEn is associated with the phase singularity of spiral waves recorded with bipolar electrograms, occurring as a result of the directional diversity of wavefront propagation direction at the pivot. Specifically, highest Shannon entropy occurs at the pivot zone of the rotor because of maximal directional uncertainty of wavefronts, leading to a broad amplitude distribution of the direction-dependent bipolar electrograms (Fig. 1, Fig. 2). In contrast, low ShEn occurs at the periphery, because in this region of the spiral wave there is less variation in wavefront direction, and consequently a reduced distribution in the amplitude histogram. These specific findings are manifest in spiral waves simulated in a variety of conditions and model systems.

Bipolar electrogram recording and the origin of high ShEn at the pivot

Bipolar recording is the standard method for recording electrical activity in clinical electrophysiology. [15] This technique maximises the contribution of local electrical activity near the exploring electrodes, and minimizes the contribution of non-local "far-field" electrical activity. [16] Because the bipolar electrogram is recorded as the difference between two electrodes, the signal amplitude is influenced by the direction of the approaching wavefront. [15,16].

In our study, high ShEn at the pivot zone was associated with bipolar electrograms in a variety of model systems producing spiral waves, as well as in geometrically perfect spiral waves. The mechanism responsible for high ShEn at the pivot is the broad distribution of wavefront direction at the pivot zone, leading to a broad distribution of possible bipolar EGM morphologies, and therefore high entropy. Since pivoting waves result in varying direction with respect to the bipole orientation, bipolar EGMs from the pivot of the spiral wave exhibit a richer morphology than bipolar electrograms recorded in case of waves passing in a relatively stable direction at the periphery of the spiral. This differences in EGM morphology are reflected in broader amplitude histogram and higher Shannon entropy at the pivot zone. (Figure 1A–C, Figure 2A–B) ShEn remained high in the pivot zone under varying conditions of EGM filtering. During local rotor meander, the region of highest ShEn was colocalized with the trajectory of the pivoting spiral wave. The stability of this finding across action potential model, variation of bipole recording direction, EGM filtering and meander suggests that this is an intrinsic dynamic spatial property spiral waves.

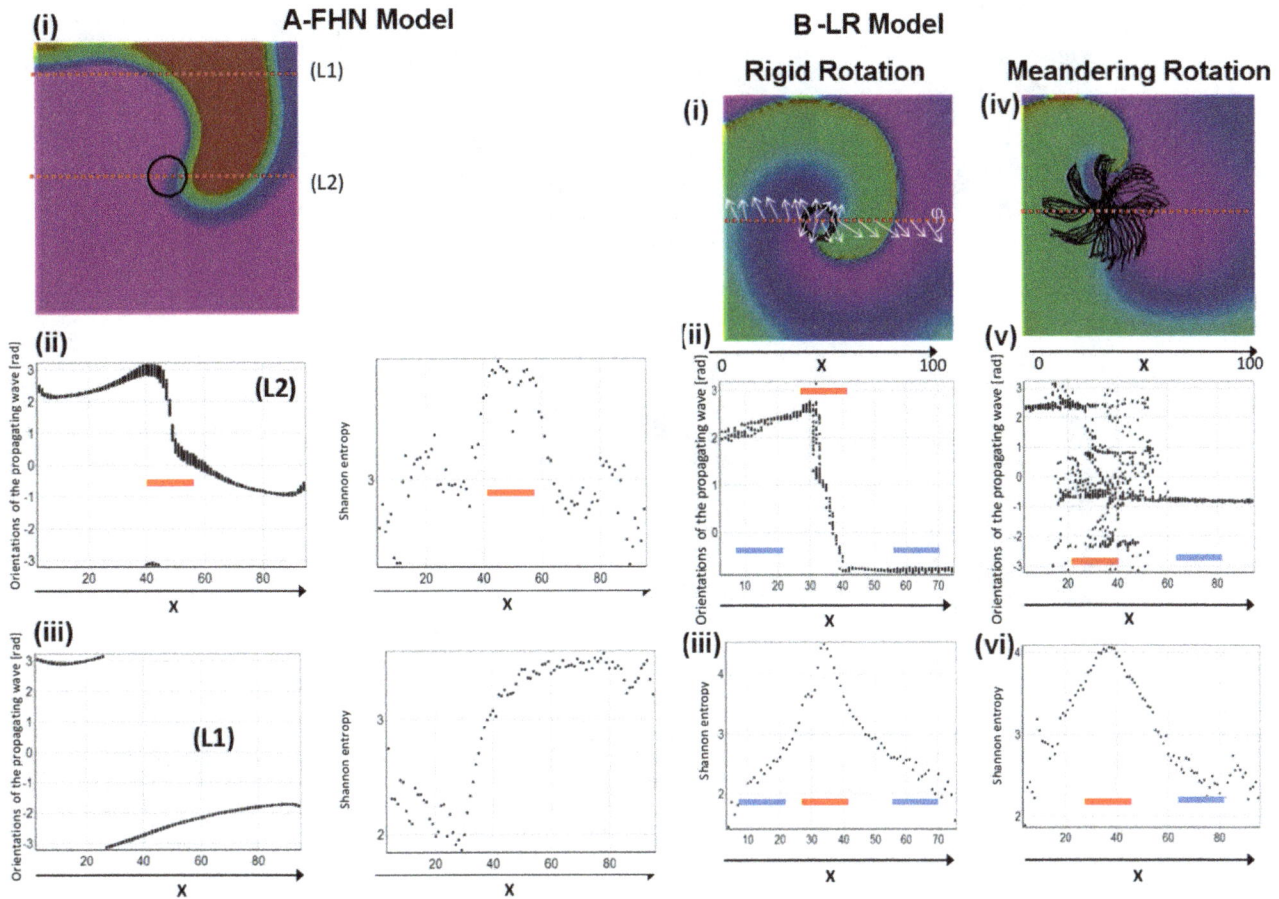

Figure 2. High ShEn at the pivot occurs as a consequence of variable wavefront direction. A. FHN model spiral wave. Panel (i) shows a snapshot from a FHN spiral wave. The trajectory of the spiral wave tip (circle) is shown. The location of meridian lines L1 (which passes through the periphery) and L2 which is at the pivot are shown. In Panel (ii), (iii) left the orientation of wavefront angle (ψ) in radians are shown along L1 and L2. It can be seen that there is a narrow distribution of wavefront angles at the periphery (blue bars), but at the pivot a broad distribution of angles is seen (red bar). This broad distribution of wavefront angles leads to high ShEn at the corresponding region of the pivot (red bar, right upper panel). B. LR spiral wave shown for rigid rotation (where Gsi = 0.00) and meandering rotor (Gsi = 0.43). In the rigid rotation case, it can be seen that at the periphery (blue bars), there is a narrow distribution of wavefront directions, and low ShEn at the periphery. In contrast, at the pivot, there is a broad distribution of wavefront angles (red bar), and high ShEn. Similarly, in the meandering case, there is a broad distribution of wavefront angles (red bars), corresponding to the region of high ShEn.

The role of rotors in cardiac fibrillation

Rotors have long been recognised in a variety of natural and artificial systems, including cardiac muscle. [17] The critical role of rotors as the drivers of cardiac fibrillation is a concept pioneered by the Jalifé group. [2,3,18] The existence of stable rotors in clinical cardiac fibrillation has been a matter of some controversy, with a diversity of viewpoints.[19–21] Recently, ablation at the phase singularity of mapped rotors identified by computational endocardial and epicardial panoramic mapping has been associated with AF termination and improved clinical outcome. [4].

Previous Theoretical Studies of EGMs from the Phase Singularity Region

Few studies have specifically examined the quantitative information properties of EGMs from the pivoting region of rotors. Umapathy et al. qualitatively demonstrated that pseudo-bipolar EGMs from the pivot were associated with qualitative "irregularity" in locally meandering spiral waves. [22] Similarly, Zlochiver et al. demonstrated an increased "residual component"

spectral peak in pseuo-unipolar EGMs from meandering spiral waves. [23].

Bipolar EGM Information Content Distinguishes the Phase Singularity

In our study, utilised ShEn as a quantitative measure to distinguish the pivot region of the rotor. The phase singularity (or pivot, in the terminology of Winfree [17]) of the rotor is defined as any point in a phase map surrounded by neighbors taking on all possible values of phase. [17] A mathematical approach to mapping of the phase singularity in the experimental setting has been to take the line integral of change of phase around each point in the mapped field of the rotor, with the singularity defined as the point where this integral equals to $\pm 2\pi$ (Eq1, File S1). [24] Therefore, localization of rotors with phase integration is enhanced by mapping of the widest possible area, using a "panoramic" approach.

The phase integration technique is not directly possible with bipolar electrograms, because the typical EGM deflection has multiple positive and negative components (as opposed to the *monophasic* deflections seen with voltage-sensitive dye based

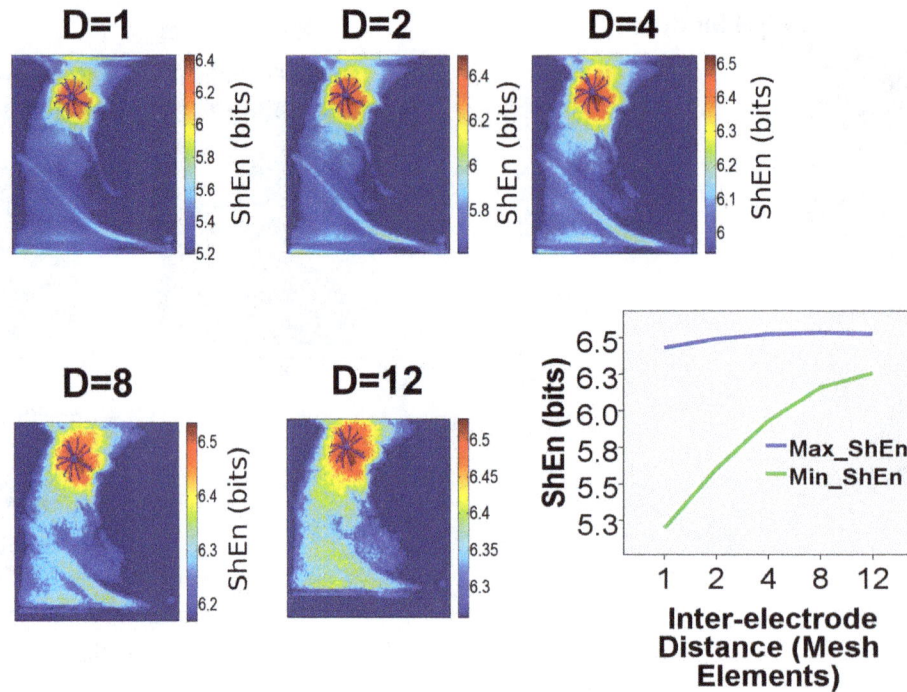

Figure 3. Effect of Bipolar Electrode Spacing. The effect of increasing bipolar electrode spacing on the ShEn distribution is shown in ShEn contour maps constructed with increasing bipolar electrode spacing for the same CRN model rotor shown in Figure 1C. In each map, D is the number of mesh nodes between bipoles, so D = 1 represents a very closely spaced bipole, and D = 12 represents a widely spaced bipole. The highest ShEn values are consistently associated with the pivoting region of the rotor, however, the range of values is narrower at widely spaced bipoles, suggesting the ability to localize the pivot of the rotor will be maximised by relatively more closely spaced bipoles.

optical mapping, or monophasic action potential recordings). The variable components of the bipolar electrogram prevent the direct assignment of phase to these signals.

ShEn based mapping is an alternative technique that utilises differences in bipolar EGM information content to assist localization of the pivot region. ShEn may have an advantage in practical implementations over phase mapping because it avoids the step of assigning phase or activation timing, which can be very difficult with complex irregular bipolar EGMs seen during cardiac fibrillation.

Clinical Implications

Our study has implications for contemporary efforts to map rotors in cardiac fibrillation, using computational endocardial and body surface ECG mapping. At the current time, detailed descriptions of the methodologies utilised to generate these maps are awaited. Our study adds to the theoretical framework, enabling understanding of the mechanisms generating bipolar EGMs in the vicinity of rotors, and therefore will assist interpretation of other rotor mapping approaches. Further, ShEn-based mapping of the rotors could be an adjunctive technique enabling precise localization of rotors identified by wide-field mapping, or as an independent standalone technique to assist rotor mapping.

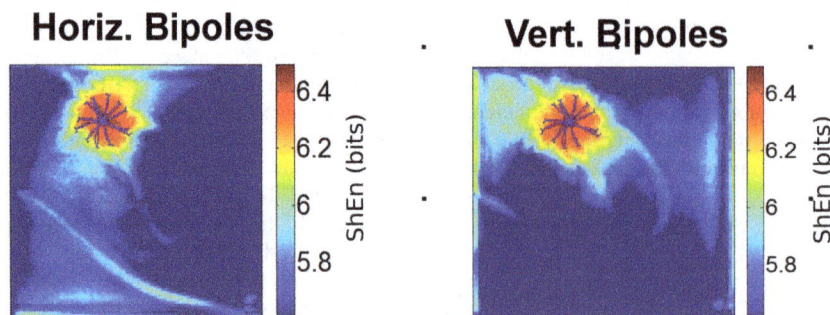

Figure 4. Effect of Bipole Orientation. The effect of bipole EGM orientation is shown. The left panel shows a ShEn map for the CRN model rotor with bipoles in the horizontal orientation (bipole distance = 2 mesh elements). ShEn maps are shown with the trajectory of the spiral wave tip annotated in blue. The right panel shows a ShEn map with bipoles in the vertical orientation.

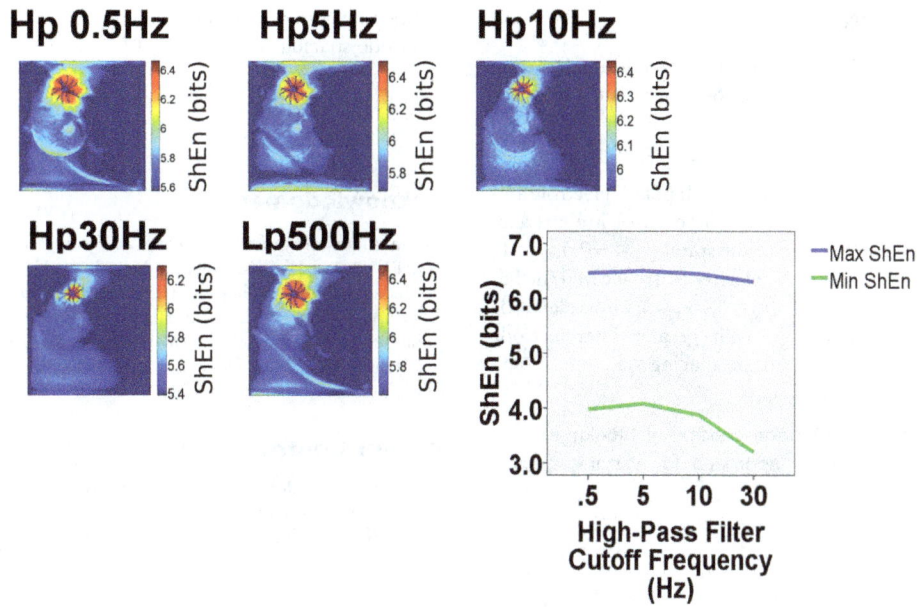

Figure 5. Effect of Filtering on ShEn maps of the CRN rotor. EGMs in the electrophysiology laboratory typically undergo high-pass and low-pass filtering. The effects of simulated Butterworth high-pass (hp) and low-pass (lp) are shown. ShEn maps in the CRN model rotor are shown simulating high pass filters with at 0.5Hz, 5 Hz, 10 Hz and 30 (typically used in the electrophysiology laboratory). It can be seen that the common area of maximum ShEn occurs in each map, in the area overlying the tip of the spiral wave trajectory. Low-pass filtering at 500 Hz has minimal effect on the distribution of ShEn.

Study Limitations

This is a theoretical study aimed at to provide insights into the origin and characteristics of high bipolar EGM ShEn at the pivot of rotors. The study uses a simulation approach. However, the results presented are consistent with our previous experimental evidence. It is likely that other forms of activation could lead to high entropy, although these forms of activation would less likely to be repetitively present during sustained AF recordings. Further, in practical implementations of ShEn it would be essential to minimize noise or baseline wander, as these signal artifacts could influence local ShEn. Finally, it is unclear if ablation at regions of high ShEn would lead to AF slowing or termination, and this is a subject of ongoing investigation.

Conclusions

Bipolar EGM ShEn provides novel framework to analyse bipolar EGMs at rotor sites, with potentially significant translational implications for clinical AF mapping and ablation.

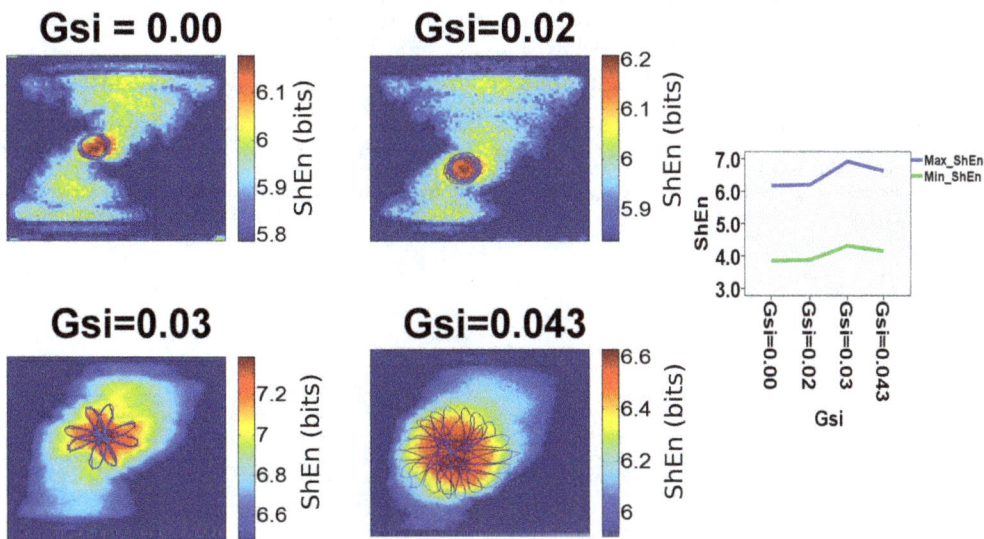

Figure 6. Effect of Rotor Meander. The effects of rotor meander are studied in LRd model rotors, by variation of the conductance of the slow-inward Ca2+ channel (Gsi). [14] When Gsi = 0.00, the spiral wave trajectory follows a narrow circle. The ShEn map shows high entropy associated with the area of rotor meander (shown as a blue line). As Gsi increases, the area of rotor meander increases. The area of high entropy in red corresponds to the region of meander of the spiral wave tip.

Supporting Information

Figure S1 A schematic illustrating elements used in calculation of unipolar electrogram at point (x_e, y_e). See Equation 2 and text and for description.

Figure S2 Examples of unipolar and bipolar electrograms calculated using geometric approach. Three cases are present: electrodes are located at the centre of the spiral ($x_e = -0.5$, $y_e = 0$; interelectrode spacing $= 1$) (panel A), electrodes are located further from the centre of the spiral ($x_e = 5$, $y_e = 5$; interelectrode spacing $= 1$) (panel B) and a case with greater interelectrode spacing ($x_e = -0.5$, $y_e = 0$; interelectrode spacing $= 5$).

Figure S3 Distribution of Shannon entropy of bipolar electrograms obtained using geometric approach for varying spacing

between electrodes d. Distributions were calculated for interelectrode spacing of 1, 2, 4, 8, 12 and 16 units.

File S1

Acknowledgments

The authors acknowledge the kind advice regarding presentation of Dr Sonia Cortassa, Division of Cardiology, Johns Hopkins University School of Medicine. Presented in part by Dr Ganesan who was awarded the Heart Rhythm Society Young Investigator Award (Clinical), May 2012, published in abstract form in *Heart Rhythm* 2012 **9:5** *SUPPL. 1* (S494–S495), and Asia Pacific Heart Rhythm Society Young Investigator Award (Basic Science), October 2012.

Author Contributions

Conceived and designed the experiments: ANG PK. Performed the experiments: ANG PK. Analyzed the data: ANG PK. Wrote the paper: ANG PK. Modeling: AG. Editorial Review: AB DC DHL KRT PS.

References

1. Gray RA, Pertsov AM, Jalife J (1998) Spatial and temporal organization during cardiac fibrillation. Nature 392: 75–78.
2. Skanes AC, Mandapati R, Berenfeld O, Davidenko JM, Jalife J (1998) Spatiotemporal periodicity during atrial fibrillation in the isolated sheep heart. Circulation 98: 1236–1248.
3. Mandapati R, Skanes A, Chen J, Berenfeld O, Jalife J (2000) Stable microreentrant sources as a mechanism of atrial fibrillation in the isolated sheep heart. Circulation 101: 194–199.
4. Narayan SM, Krummen DE, Shivkumar K, Clopton P, Rappel WJ, et al. (2012) Treatment of atrial fibrillation by the ablation of localized sources: CONFIRM (Conventional Ablation for Atrial Fibrillation With or Without Focal Impulse and Rotor Modulation) trial. J Am Coll Cardiol 60: 628–636.
5. Haissaguerre M, Hocini M, Shah AJ, Derval N, Sacher F, et al. (2013) Noninvasive Panoramic Mapping of Human Atrial Fibrillation Mechanisms: A Feasibility Report. J Cardiovasc Electrophysiol.
6. Ganesan AN, Kuklik P, Lau DH, Brooks AG, Baumert M, et al. (2013) Bipolar electrogram shannon entropy at sites of rotational activation: implications for ablation of atrial fibrillation. Circ Arrhythm Electrophysiol 6: 48–57.
7. Kuklik P, Szumowski L, Sanders P, Zebrowski JJ (2010) Spiral wave breakup in excitable media with an inhomogeneity of conduction anisotropy. Comput Biol Med 40: 775–780.
8. Luo CH, Rudy Y (1991) A model of the ventricular cardiac action potential. Depolarization, repolarization, and their interaction. Circ Res 68: 1501–1526.
9. Courtemanche M, Ramirez RJ, Nattel S (1998) Ionic mechanisms underlying human atrial action potential properties: insights from a mathematical model. Am J Physiol 275: H301–321.
10. Maalmivuo JPR (1995) Bioelectromagnetism. New York: Oxford University Press.
11. Shannon C (1948) A Mathematical Theory of Communication. Bell System Technical Journal 27: 379–423, 623–656.
12. Ng J, Borodyanskiy AI, Chang ET, Villuendas R, Dibs S, et al. (2010) Measuring the complexity of atrial fibrillation electrograms. J Cardiovasc Electrophysiol 21: 649–655.

13. Qu Z, Xie F, Garfinkel A, Weiss JN (2000) Origins of spiral wave meander and breakup in a two-dimensional cardiac tissue model. Ann Biomed Eng 28: 755–771.
14. Alonso S, Panfilov AV (2007) Negative filament tension in the Luo-Rudy model of cardiac tissue. Chaos 17: 015102.
15. Stevenson WG, Soejima K (2005) Recording techniques for clinical electrophysiology. J Cardiovasc Electrophysiol 16: 1017–1022.
16. de Bakker JM, Wittkampf FH (2010) The pathophysiologic basis of fractionated and complex electrograms and the impact of recording techniques on their detection and interpretation. Circ Arrhythm Electrophysiol 3: 204–213.
17. Winfree AT (1990) Excitable Kinetics and Excitable Media. The Geometry of Biological Time. Berlin: Springer Verlag. pp. p440.
18. Davidenko JM, Pertsov AV, Salomonsz R, Baxter W, Jalife J (1992) Stationary and drifting spiral waves of excitation in isolated cardiac muscle. Nature 355: 349–351.
19. Allessie MA, de Groot NM, Houben RP, Schotten U, Boersma E, et al. (2010) Electropathological substrate of long-standing persistent atrial fibrillation in patients with structural heart disease: longitudinal dissociation. Circ Arrhythm Electrophysiol 3: 606–615.
20. de Groot NM, Houben RP, Smeets JL, Boersma E, Schotten U, et al. (2010) Electropathological substrate of longstanding persistent atrial fibrillation in patients with structural heart disease: epicardial breakthrough. Circulation 122: 1674–1682.
21. Jalife J (2011) Deja vu in the theories of atrial fibrillation dynamics. Cardiovasc Res 89: 766–775.
22. Umapathy K, Masse S, Kolodziejska K, Veenhuyzen GD, Chauhan VS, et al. (2008) Electrogram fractionation in murine HL-1 atrial monolayer model. Heart Rhythm 5: 1029–1035.
23. Zlochiver S, Yamazaki M, Kalifa J, Berenfeld O (2008) Rotor meandering contributes to irregularity in electrograms during atrial fibrillation. Heart Rhythm 5: 846–854.
24. Iyer AN, Gray RA (2001) An experimentalist's approach to accurate localization of phase singularities during reentry. Ann Biomed Eng 29: 47–59.

19

Attenuation of Acetylcholine Activated Potassium Current (I_{KACh}) by Simvastatin, Not Pravastatin in Mouse Atrial Cardiomyocyte: Possible Atrial Fibrillation Preventing Effects of Statin

Kyoung-Im Cho[1], Tae-Joon Cha[1]*, Su-Jin Lee[1], In-Kyeung Shim[1], Yin Hua Zhang[2], Jung-Ho Heo[1], Hyun-Su Kim[1], Sung Joon Kim[2], Kyoung-Lyoung Kim[3], Jae-Woo Lee[1]

1 Cardiovascular Research Institute, Department of Internal Medicine, Kosin University College of Medicine, Busan, South Korea, 2 Department of Physiology, Seoul National University College of Medicine, Seoul, South Korea, 3 Department of Molecular Biology, Kosin University College of Medicine, Busan, South Korea

Abstract

Statins, 3-hydroxy-3-methyl-glutaryl-CoA reductase inhibitors, are associated with the prevention of atrial fibrillation (AF) by pleiotropic effects. Recent clinical trial studies have demonstrated conflicting results on anti-arrhythmia between lipophilic and hydrophilic statins. However, the underlying mechanisms responsible for anti-arrhythmogenic effects of statins are largely unexplored. In this study, we evaluated the different roles of lipophilic and hydrophilic statins (simvastatin and pravastatin, respectively) in acetylcholine (100 µM)-activated K^+ current (I_{KACh}, recorded by nystatin-perforated whole cell patch clamp technique) which are important for AF initiation and maintenance in mouse atrial cardiomyocytes. Our results showed that simvastatin (1–10 µM) inhibited both peak and quasi-steady-state I_{KACh} in a dose-dependent manner. In contrast, pravastatin (10 µM) had no effect on I_{KACh}. Supplementation of substrates for the synthesis of cholesterol (mevalonate, geranylgeranyl pyrophosphate or farnesyl pyrophosphate) did not reverse the effect of simvastatin on I_{KACh}, suggesting a cholesterol-independent effect on I_{KACh}. Furthermore, supplementation of phosphatidylinositol 4,5-bisphosphate, extracellular perfusion of phospholipase C inhibitor or a protein kinase C (PKC) inhibitor had no effect on the inhibitory activity of simvastatin on I_{KACh}. Simvastatin also inhibits adenosine activated I_{KACh}, however, simvastatin does not inhibit I_{KACh} after activated by intracellular loading of GTP gamma S. Importantly, shortening of the action potential duration by acetylcholine was restored by simvastatin but not by pravastatin. Together, these findings demonstrate that lipophilic statins but not hydrophilic statins attenuate I_{KACh} in atrial cardiomyocytes via a mechanism that is independent of cholesterol synthesis or PKC pathway, but may be via the blockade of acetylcholine binding site. Our results may provide important background information for the use of statins in patients with AF.

Editor: Thomas Hund, The Ohio State University, United States of America

Funding: This study was supported by grants from the Korea Heart Rhythm Society (KHRS 2011-1) and Kosin University College of Medicine (2011). The funders had no role in study design, data collection and analysis, decision to publish, or preparation of the manuscript.

Competing Interests: The authors have declared that no competing interests exist.

* Email: chatjn@gmail.com

Introduction

Atrial fibrillation (AF) is the most common type of chronic cardiac arrhythmia [1,2], and the pathophysiology of AF is complex [3–5]. Statins have pleiotropic effects which are independent of their cholesterol-lowering effects [5,6]. Furthermore, it has been shown that statins can modulate the activities of L-type calcium channels and transient outward potassium channels, which are altered by rapid atrial pacing [7]. These properties can partially explain ionic mechanisms of the anti-arrhythmic effect of statins.

However, clinical trials have shown conflicting results regarding the anti-arrhythmic effects of statins [6,8–11]. In particular, the GISSI Heart Failure (GISSI-HF) trial showed that the hydrophilic statin, rosuvastatin, did not affect clinical outcome and exerted

little benefit with regard to AF occurrence [10,11]. In contrast, simvastatin, a lipophilic statin, has been shown to prevent the occurrence of AF in a rapid atrial pacing animal model [12]. According to the Sarr et al. [13], hydrophilic pravastatin exhibited the lowest association with the lipid monolayer, and lipophilic simvastatin showed a strong membrane elution ability, which can be explained by hydrophobicity of statin molecule [14]. These findings suggest that lipophilic and hydrophilic statins may differ with respect to effects on the myocardium as a result of different ion channel binding affinity. For example, simvastatin may reduce susceptibility to ventricular fibrillation mainly by reducing sympathetic hyperinnervation and electrical remodeling induced by hypercholesterolemia [15]. So, we can hypothesize that simvastatin may modulate membrane ion channel more effectively than hydrophilic pravastatin.

Although simultaneous sympathetic and parasympathetic (sympathovagal) activation may facilitate the onset of paroxysmal AF [16], effects of statins on the neurohormonal imbalances are not known yet [17]. A plausible link between sympathovagal and neurohormonal interactions in cardiac myocytes is the acetylcholine-activated K$^+$ current (I_{KACh}). I_{KACh} is involved in tachycardia-induced electrical remodeling and participates in AF initiation and maintenance. In atrial cardiomyocytes, I_{KACh} is constitutively active, and atrial tachycardia may further increase its activity. Considering the evidence that statins may suppress AF, we hypothesized that statins influence I_{KACh} in atrial myocytes, and that the effects may vary with the lipophilicity of the statin. To test this hypothesis, we compared the effects of the lipophilic simvastatin with effects of the hydrophilic pravastatin on I_{KACh} and acetylcholine-induced action potential duration (APD) in atrial cardiomyocytes.

Materials and Methods

Experimental design

Imprinting Control Region mice weighing 20~30 g were used for animal experiments. The protocols for animal care and use were in accordance with the NIH Guide for the Care and Use of Laboratory Animals and were approved by the Animal Research Committee at Kosin University Gospel Hospital. To isolate mouse atrial myocytes, the hearts were rapidly excised and mounted onto a Langendorff apparatus at 37°C and perfused with a Ca^{2+}-free normal Tyrode solution containing collagenase (0.14 mg/ml). The I_{KACh} current was recorded using a nystatin-perforated whole cell patch-clamp technique following activation by acetylcholine (100 μM for 2 min). After measurement of the baseline I_{KACh} current, atrial myocytes were perfused with lipophilic statins (simvastatin 10 μM for 10 min), after which the I_{KACh} current was re-measured. The I_{KACh} currents were compared with those measured in the presence of a hydrophilic statin (pravastatin 10 μM for 10 min). We also evaluated the underlying mechanism of simvastatin-induced I_{KACh} inhibition.

Isolation of single cardiomyocytes

Ten mice in each group were anesthetized with pentobarbital sodium (50 mg/kg, intraperitoneally). Hearts were removed by thoracotomy and quickly mounted onto a modified Langendorff perfusion system. To ensure coronary circulation, hearts were sequentially perfused with four solutions (all at 37°C) as follows: (1) normal Tyrode's solution containing (in mM): NaCl 143, KCl 5.4, CaCl$_2$ 1.8, MgCl$_2$ 0.5, NaH$_2$PO$_4$ 0.33, HEPES 5 and glucose 10, adjusted with NaOH to pH 7.4, for 4–5 min; (2) Ca^{2+}-free normal Tyrode's solution for 5 min; (3) Ca^{2+}-free normal Tyrode's solution supplemented with collagenase (type II, 15 mg/35 ml, Worthington, USA) for 15–20 min; and (4) a high K$^+$, low-Cl$^-$ solution (modified Kraft-Brühe [KB] solution) containing (in mM): KOH 70, L-glutamic acid 50, KCl 55, taurine 20, KH$_2$PO$_4$ 20, MgCl$_2$ 3, EGTA 0.5, HEPES 10 and glucose 20, adjusted to pH 7.2 with KOH, for 5 min. The atrium was then dissected from the heart and placed in a dish. Individual cardiomyocytes were released by mechanical agitation and stored at 4°C in KB solution.

Electrophysiological measurements

Acetylcholine-activated K$^+$ currents (I_{KACh}) in the whole-cell configuration were recorded using the perforated patch clamp technique [18]. Single atrial cells were placed in a recording chamber attached to an inverted microscope (IMT-2; Olympus, Tokyo) and superfused with normal Tyrode's solution at a rate of 3 ml/min. All experiments were performed at room temperature.

Patch pipettes were made from glass capillaries with a diameter of 1.5 mm using a microelectrode puller (Sutter Instruments, P-97) and were filled with solution to a resistance of 2–3 MΩ. The I_{KACh} was recorded from single isolated myocytes in a perforated patch configuration using nystatin (200 μg/ml; ICN) at room temperature. The composition of the pipette solutions for perforated patches contained (in mM): KCl 140, MgCl$_2$ 1, NaH2PO$_4$ 0.5, HEPES 10 and EGTA 5, adjusted to pH 7.2 with KOH. I_{KACh} was activated by extracellular application of acetylcholine (Ach, 100 μM for 2 min), and peak I_{KACh} was measured as the difference between the peak and the steady-state current at the end of the pulse. After the baseline I_{KACh} current was measured, varying concentrations of simvastatin or pravastatin were applied for 10 minutes, and a second I_{KACh} current was recorded. The peak and quasi-steady-state I_{KACh} recordings (taken before and after 10 minutes of statin treatment, respectively) were then compared. Current signals were recorded using Clampfit 6.0 software (Axon Instruments, Inc., Foster City, CA, USA).

Materials

Simvastatin, pravastatin, mevalonic acid lactone, and all other chemicals were from Sigma Chemical Co. (St. Louis, MO, USA). Simvastatin was dissolved in dimethyl sulfoxide (DMSO, Amresco), and pravastatin was dissolved in distilled water. Simvastatin was prepared fresh for each experiment from a stock solution (10 mM in DMSO, stored at −20°C) and diluted a final concentration of 10 μM, and added in the bath solution. For each experiment, small aliquots of the HMG-CoA reductase inhibitor stock solutions were added to normal Tyrode's solution. The final concentration of DMSO was 0.1% and had no effecton I_{KACh} in atrial cardiomyocytes [20].

Statistical analysis

Statistical analyses were performed using SPSS for Windows, ver. 15.0, (SPSS, Inc., Chicago, IL, USA). Numeric data were expressed as the mean ± SD, and electrophysiological data were presented as the mean ± standard error of the mean (SEM). The statistical differences among the nominal variables of the groups were analyzed using the one-way ANOVA test, and the differences between the subgroups were assessed with the post-hoc Tukey test. A P value of <0.05 was considered statistically significant for all the tests.

Results

Effect of simvastatin on I_{KACh} in mouse atrial cells

Application of acetylcholine (100 μM) to the bath solution promptly activated I_{KACh} in mouse atrial myocytes (Fig. 1A). Re-application of acetylcholine after washout for >10 min induced I_{KACh} to a similar amplitude (Fig. 1A), indicating reproducibility of I_{KACh} during the investigation period. We next examined the effects of simvastatin on I_{KACh}. After baseline I_{KACh} measurement (I1), simvastatin (10 μM) was applied for 10 minutes, and I_{KACh} in the presence of simvastatin (I2) was compared to baseline I_{KACh} (I1). As shown in Fig. 1B, treatment with simvastatin for 10 min significantly reduced peak I_{KACh} current. After 10 minutes washout of simvastatin, I_{KACh} was partially recovered 76.4±11.3% of baseline current (Fig. 1D). On average, peak I2 (I2, peak) was 35.5±13.6% of I1 (I1, peak), while the quasi-steady-state amplitude of I2 (I2, qss) was 19.9±11.8% of I1 (I1, qss) (p<0.001 for the I2 peak and p<0.001 for the I2 qss (each n = 10, Figs. 1E–F). Current–voltage (I–V) curves were obtained from the current response induced by voltage ramps between −120 and +60 mV from the holding potential of −40 mV. Corresponding

I–V curves were plotted in Fig. 1 G, H and I–V relationships demonstrated that simvastatin inhibited the net I_{KACh} over the whole tested voltage range. In addition, simvastatin inhibited I_{KACh} in a dose-dependent manner between 1 and 10 μM (1 μM, n=6; 91.5±9.0%, 3 μM, n=6; 80.8±9.9%, 5 μM, n=6; 68.7±15.7%, 10 μM, n=10; 35.5±13.6%, p<0.001, Fig. 2), which was also shown in I-V relationships (Fig. 1H). When we tested the effect of simvastatin on the I_{KAch} without acetylcholine administration, simvastatin had no influence on the I_{KAch} over the whole tested voltage range (n=3, Fig. S1A). When we test a time dependent effect for achieving steady-state block of I_{KACh}, there were no significant differences in achieving steady-state block of I_{KAch} among 5 min, 10 min, and 15 min after simvastatin application (each n=5, p=NS, Fig. S2). The percent inhibition in the presence of simvastatin was calculated with respect to the amplitude of peak ($Ipeak$) and quasi-steady-state ($Iqss$) in the presence of simvastatin and plotted in Fig. 2F and 2H. The data were fitted with the Hill equation, showing that the concentration for half-maximal inhibition (IC50) was 5.80 μM for the $Ipeak$ and 5.27 μM for the $Iqss$ (n=3 in every points, total n=21). Importantly, acetylcholine significantly shorted APD at 90% repolarization (APD$_{90}$, from 27.3±2.2 ms to 7.2±1.6 ms, p< 0.01), while treatment with simvastatin recovered levels to those of vehicle treatment (vehicle, n=7; 27.3±2.2 ms, simvastatin, n=7; 19.3±3.3 ms, p=0.34, Figs. 3A, C). When we tested the effect of

simvastatin on the APD$_{90}$ without acetylcholine, simvastatin had no influence on the APD$_{90}$ (n=3, Fig. S1B).

Effect of pravastatin on I_{KACh} in mouse atrial cells

We next investigated the effects of pravastatin on I_{KACh} using the same experimental protocol. Addition of pravastatin in a bath solution for 10 minutes did not significantly alter peak amplitude or quasi-steady-state of the currents compared to controls (n=10, p=0.48 for peak I_{KACh} and n=10, p=0.19 for qss I_{KACh}, Figs. 1C, E, F) and did not restore the acetylcholine-induced shortening of APD (acetylcholine, n=6; 8.5±3.7 ms, pravastatin, n=6; 9.1±4.3 ms, p=0.85, Figs. 3B, C).

Mechanism of simvastatin-induced I_{KACh} inhibition in mouse atrial cells

To investigate the association between simvastatin-induced I_{KACh} inhibition and inhibition of cholesterol synthesis, substrates for cholesterol synthesis consisting of mevalonate (MVA, Fig. 4A), geranylgeranyl pyrophosphate (GGPP, Fig. 4B), or farnesyl pyrophosphate (FPP, Fig. 4C) were added with simvastatin in the bath solution. However, the reductions in peak amplitude and quasi-steady-state current of I_{KACh} by simvastatin were not prevented by supplementation with any of these substrates (p=0.28, p=0.37 and p=0.41 for MVA, GGPP and FPP, respectively, each n=7, Figs. 4D,E). Moreover, to investigate if

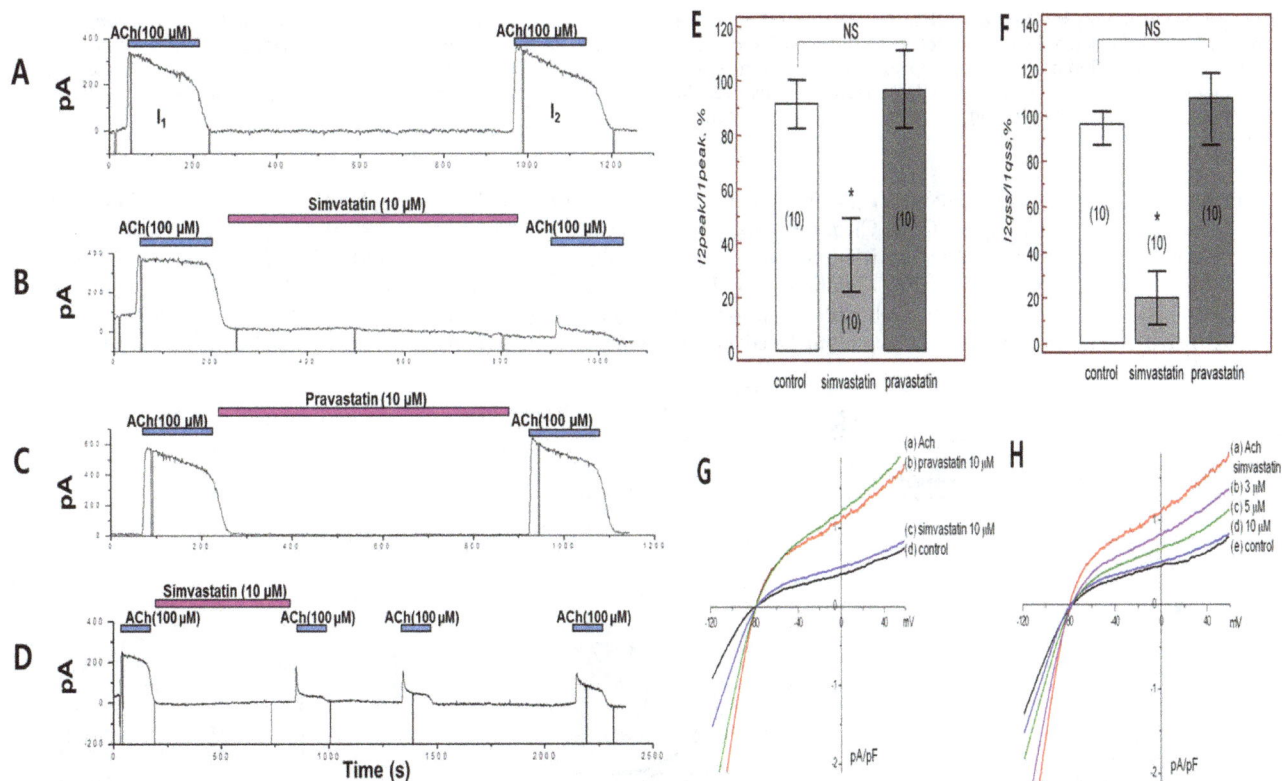

Figure 1. Acetylcholine-activated K⁺ currents (I_{KACh}) were recorded using a nystatin-perforated whole cell patch clamp technique. A. Acetylcholine (100 μM) was applied to the bath solution, and I_{KACh} was promptly activated. B. Simvastatin (10 μM) treatment for 10 minutes significantly reduced the peak and quasi-steady-state I_{KACh} amplitudes. C. Pravastatin (10 μM) treatment for 10 minutes did not change peak or quasi-steady-state I_{KACh} amplitude. D. After 10 minutes washout of simvastatin, I_{KAch} was partially recovered. E. Peak amplitude at baseline I_{KACh} (I1, peak) and the second I_{KACh} peak (I2, peak), after statin application. F. Quasi-steady state amplitude of baseline I_{KACh} (I1, qss) and second qss I_{KACh} (I2, qss) after statin application. G. Current–voltage (I–V) curves were plotted. The ramps were applied before (d) and after acetylcholine 100 μM application (a), in the presence of pravastatin 10 μM (b) and simvastatin 10 μM (c). H. The ramps were applied before (e) and after acetylcholine 100 μM application (a), in the presence of simvastatin 3 μM (b), 5 μM (c) and 10 μM (d). NS; no significant change, *; p<0.05 compared to controls.

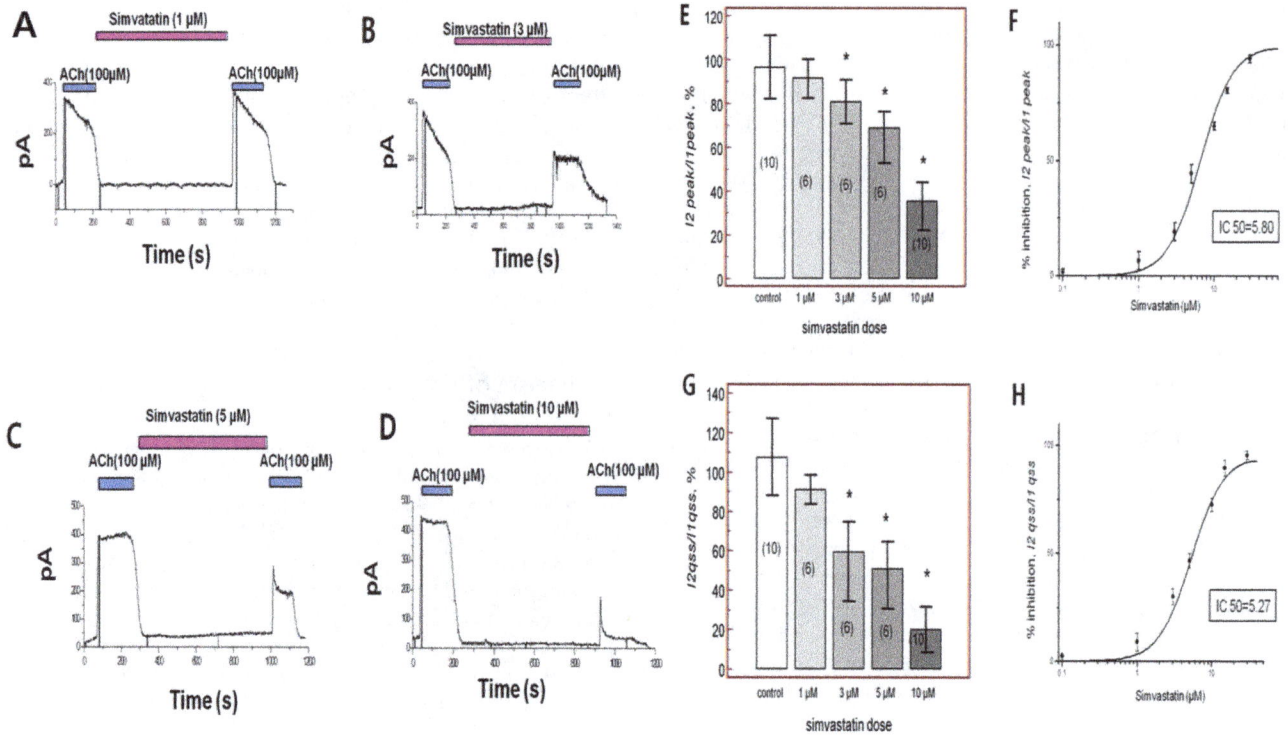

Figure 2. Simvastatin inhibits acetylcholine-activated K$^+$ current (I_{KACh}) in a dose-dependent manner at A. 1 μM, B. 3 μM, C. 5 μM and D. 10 μM. E. Peak amplitude of baseline I_{KACh} (I1, peak) and second I_{KACh} peak (I2, peak) after application of simvastatin. F. Dose response curve for the percent inhibition of peak I_{KACh} amplitude in the presence of simvastatin. G. Quasi-steady state amplitudes of baseline I_{KACh} (I1, qss) and the second I_{KACh} (I2, qss) after simvastatin. H. Dose response curve for the percent inhibition of quasi-steady state I_{KACh} amplitude in the presence of simvastatin. NS; no significant change, *; p<0.05 compared to controls.

the modulation of simvastatin-induced I_{KACh} inhibition may happen through the phospholipase C (PLC), protein kinase C (PKC) pathway or depletion of phosphatidylinositol 4,5-bisphosphate (PIP$_2$) [19,20], PLC inhibitor, PKC inhibitor, and PIP2 were tested. Loading the patch pipette with PIP$_2$ via whole cell ruptured patch clamp did not alter simvastatin-mediated inhibi-

tion of I_{KACh} (Fig. 5A), implying that simvastatin did not limit the availability of these agents. Similarly, application of the PLC inhibitor neomycin (50 μM, Fig. 5B) or the PKC inhibitor calphostin C extracellular solution (1 μM, Fig. 5C) failed to alter simvastatin-inhibition of I_{KACh} (each n = 7, Figs. 5D,E). When we activate I_{KACh} by intracellular loading of GTP gamma S

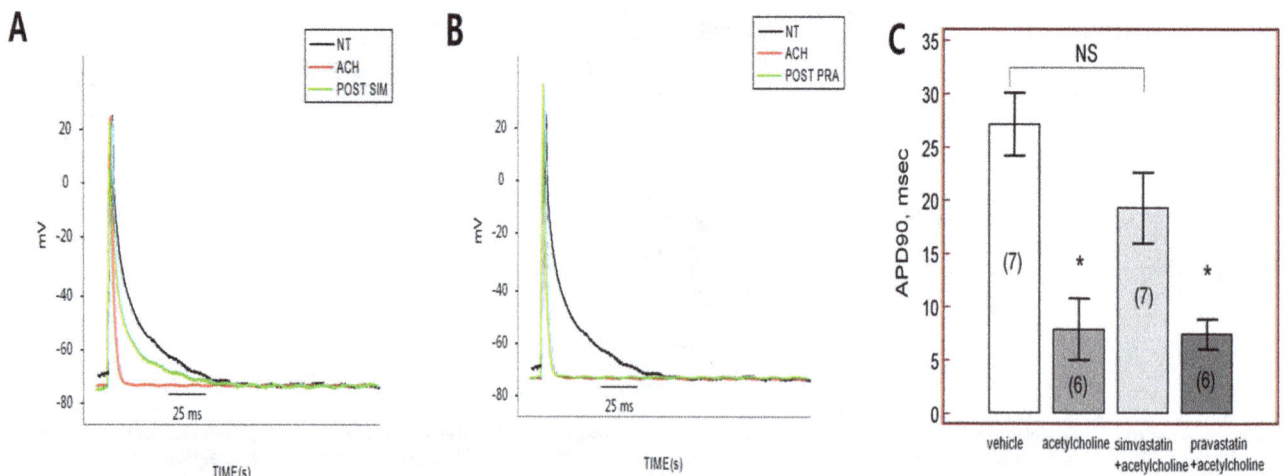

Figure 3. Change of action potential duration (APD) after acetylcholine application with or without statins. A. Acetylcholine significantly shortened APD at 90% repolarization, while simvastatin restored APD to vehicle level (NT, normal tyrode). B. Pravastatin did not restore the shortened APD induced by acetylcholine. C. Comparison of APD at 90% repolarization after acetylcholine application with simvastatin or pravastatin. NS; no significant change, *; p<0.05 compared to controls.

(100 µM/L) via whole cell patch, simvastatin did not inhibit I_{KACh} (n = 5, Figs. 5F,H). However, when we activate I_{KACh} by extracellular application of adenosine, simvastatin also inhibit adenosine activated I_{KACh} (n = 5, Figs. 5G,H), which suggest that simvastatin influence on the adenosine binding site as well as acetylcholine binding sites. This result suggests that acute administration of simvastatin may inhibit the I_{KACh} by blockade of acetylcholine binding site.

Discussion

The results of this study indicated that lipophilic simvastatin but not hydrophilic pravastatin suppressed I_{KACh} in mouse atrial myocytes. These effects were not dependent on cholesterol biosynthesis or PIP$_2$ pathway, suggesting the involvement of direct inhibition of I_{KACh}. In addition, simvastatin significantly attenuated acetylcholine-induced APD shortening. Importantly, these results provided the first direct evidence that the lipophilic HMG CoA reductase inhibitor simvastatin facilitates its potent anti-

arrhythmic effect by inhibiting I_{KAch} and suppressing electrical remodeling in mammalian atrial myocytes.

Effects of statins on I_{KACh} in mouse atrial cells

Statins exert pleiotropic effects in part by reducing the availability of intermediary metabolites in cholesterol synthesis (isoprenoids), which in turn mediate regulatory signaling through activation of guanosine nucleotide-binding proteins (G-proteins). Through G-protein inhibition, treatment with statins may induce rapid and significant improvement in endothelial function [21], in part by reversing the suppression of endothelial nitric oxide synthase [23] associated with hypercholesterolemia [21,22].

The effectiveness of statins in both primary and secondary prevention of AF implies that multiple mechanisms may be involved in their anti-arrhythmic activity. The capacity of statins to reduce inflammation, thereby reducing the risk of AF [24], may reflect the pleiotropic properties of these drugs, in part because they are independent of the lipid-lowering effects. Although a direct causative relationship between inflammation and AF has not been established [25], inflammation may induce autonomic

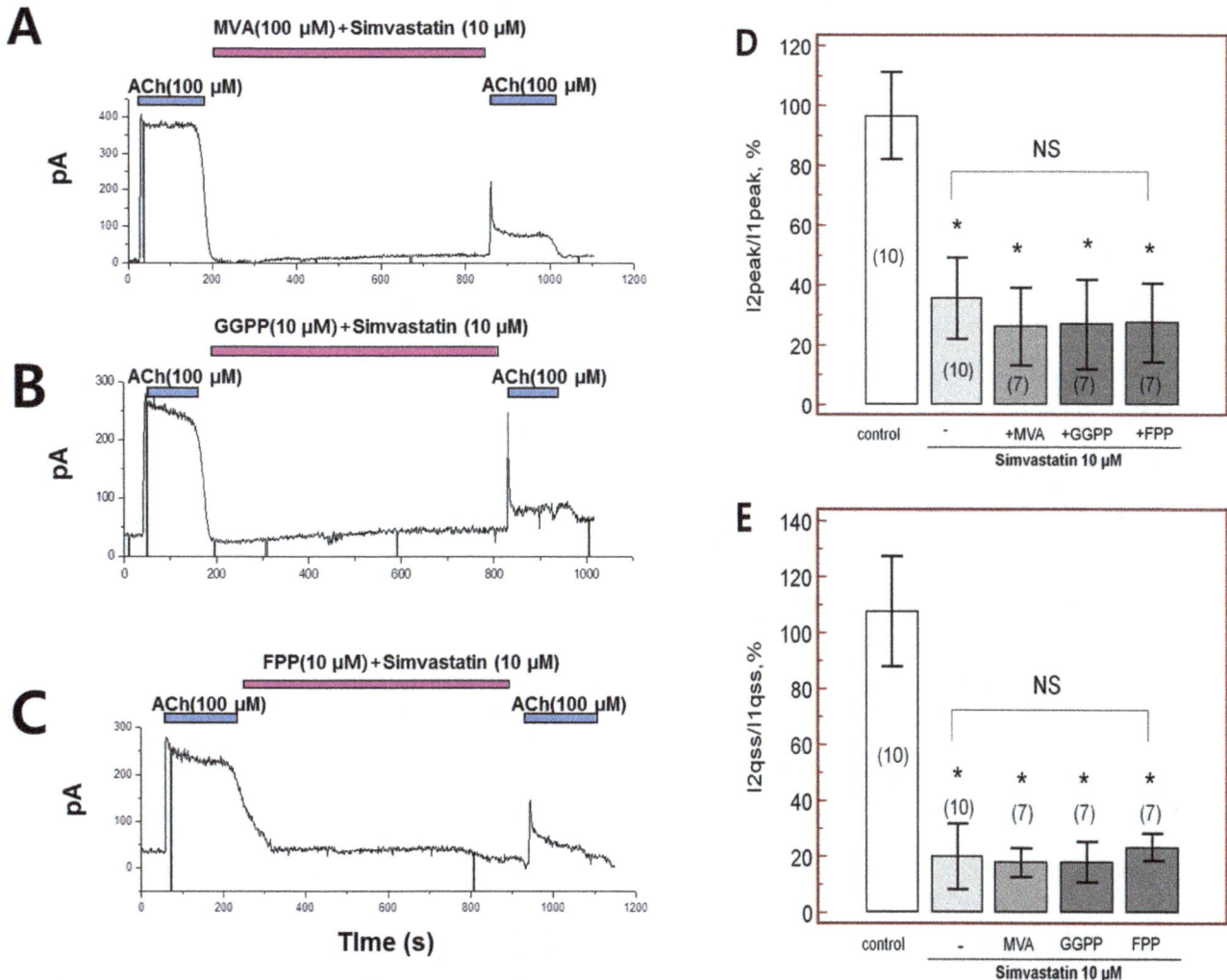

Figure 4. Acetylcholine-activated K⁺ current (I_{KACh}) after simvastatin in the presence of substrates and intermediary metabolites in cholesterol synthesis; A. mevalonate (MVA), B. geranylgeranyl pyrophosphate (GGPP), and C. farnesyl pyrophosphate (FPP). D. Peak amplitudes at baseline I_{KACh} ($I1$, peak) and the second I_{KACh} peak ($I2$, peak) after simvastatin with various cholesterol biosynthetic intermediates. E. Quasi-steady state amplitude of baseline I_{KACh} ($I1$, qss) and second I_{KACh} ($I2$, qss) after simvastatin with various cholesterol biosynthetic intermediates. NS; no significant change, *; p<0.05 compared to controls.

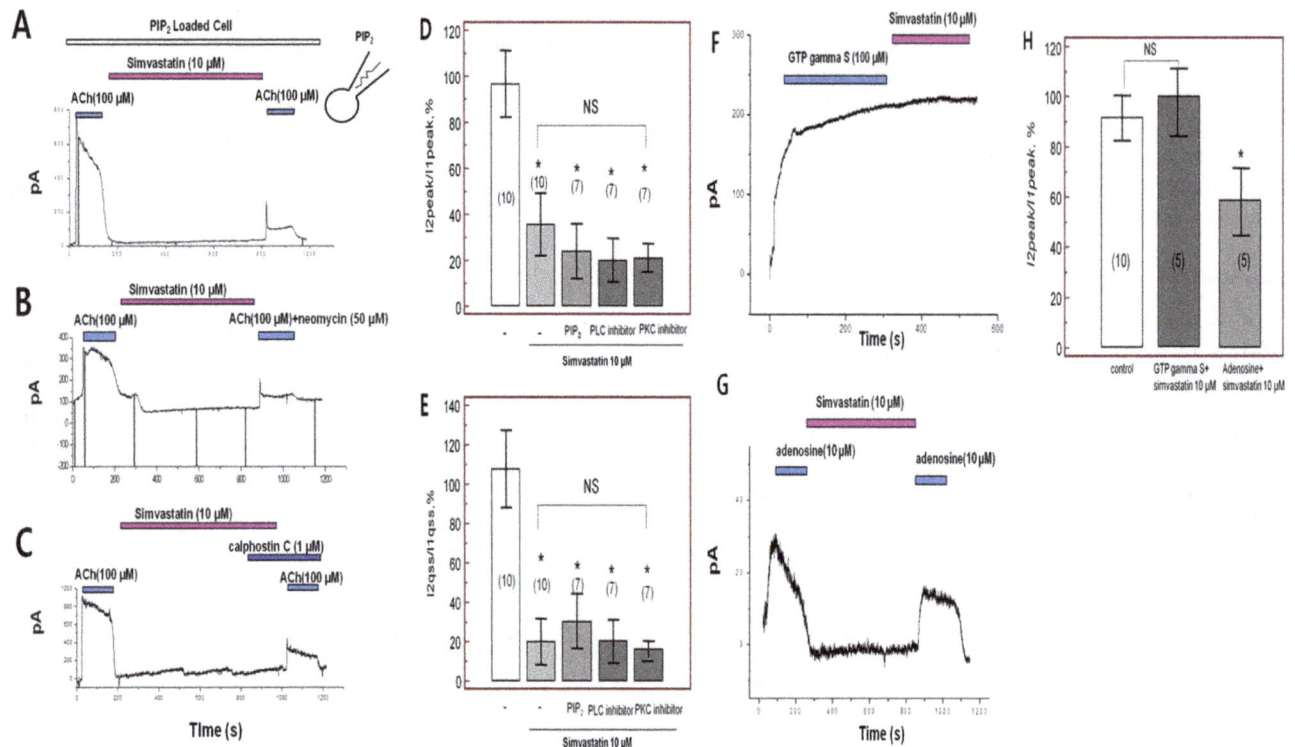

Figure 5. Acetylcholine-activated K$^+$ current (I_{KACh}) after simvastatin with A. phosphatidylinositol 4,5-bisphosphate (PIP$_2$), B. phospholipase C inhibitor (PLC inhibitor, neomycin 50 μM), and C. protein kinase C inhibitor (PKC inhibitor, calphostin C 1 μM). D. Peak amplitudes of baseline I_{KACh} (*I1*, peak) and the second I_{KACh} (*I2*, peak) after treatment with PIP$_2$, PLC inhibitor, and PKC inhibitor. E. Quasi-steady state amplitudes of baseline I_{KACh} (qss *I1*) and second I_{KACh} (qss *I2*) after treatment with PIP$_2$, PLC inhibitor, and PKC inhibitor. F. Simvastatin did not inhibit the activated I_{KACh} by intracellular loading of GTP gamma S (100 μM/L). G. Simvastatin inhibit activated I_{KACh} by adenosine. H. Peak amplitudes of baseline I_{KACh} (qss *I1*) and second I_{KACh} (qss *I2*) activated by GTP gamma S and adenosine after treatment with simvastatin. NS; no significant change, *; $p < 0.05$ compared to controls.

remodeling, providing a substrate for initiation and maintenance of AF [26]. In addition to indirect anti-arrhythmic effects, statins may also act directly by modulating fatty acid composition and physiochemical properties of cell membranes, resulting in alterations of the properties of transmembrane ion channels [7,27]. The established role of atrial tachycardia–induced electrical remodeling in AF [28,29] implies that changes in ion channel function ("ionic remodeling") are involved in this pathophysiological process [28–30], and thus statins may in turn influence ion channel activities. Seto et al. [31] reported that simvastatin inhibits Ca^{2+}-activated K$^+$ channels in arterial smooth muscle cells, while Bergdahl *et al.* [32] showed that lovastatin inhibits L-type Ca^{2+} currents in rat basilar artery smooth muscle cells. Atorvastatin and simvastatin produce a concentration-dependent blockade of hKv1.5 channels *in vitro* [33]. In addition, simvastatin attenuates cerebrovascular remodeling in the hypertensive rat through inhibition of vascular smooth muscle cell proliferation by suppression of volume-regulated chloride channels [13].

Upregulation of inwardly rectifying potassium channels is an important contribution to the electrical remodeling underlying AF. Accordingly, inhibition of these currents may be a potential anti-arrhythmic target devoid of ventricular side effects [34]. We previously demonstrated that the constitutively active I_{KACh} substantially contributes to the repolarization phase of atrial action potential in AF. Further, as a potential ionic determinant of AF, I_{KACh} represents a plausible target for therapy [35–37]. The results of the present study confirmed our hypothesis that treatment with the lipophilic statin simvastatin but not with

hydrophilic pravastatin attenuates I_{KACh} as a component of the anti-arrhythmic effect of statins.

Contrasting effects of simvastatin and pravastatin on I_{KACh} in mouse atrial cells

Clinical trials of statins in the prevention of AF recurrence have reported mixed results. Although atorvastatin and simvastatin reduced AF recurrence after electrical cardioversion (EC) [6], use of pravastatin before EC did not decrease AF recurrence [9] and rosuvastatin did not affect clinical outcome and AF occurrence [10,11]. Lipophilic statins improve cardiac sympathetic activity by reducing oxidative stress [38,39], and an active metabolite of atorvastatin displays stronger antioxidant activity than rosuvastatin [40]. Simvastatin but not pravastatin significantly reduces angiotensin II-induced calcium mobilization [41], and simvastatin may exert direct anti-arrhythmic effect by suppressing events that trigger AF [42]. Accordingly, our results indicate that the inhibition of I_{KACh} may represent another important anti-arrhythmic mechanism of simvastatin. This inhibitory action on the I_{KACh} current was not reversed by addition of mevalonate (MVA), GGPP, or FPP, implying that simvastatin may suppress I_{KACh} independently from signaling proteins activated by isoprenylation. Moreover, PLC/PKC inhibition and PIP$_2$ supplementation did not change simvastatin induced I_{KACh} inhibition, implicating that statin-induced I_{KACh} inhibition is independent of PKC pathway. Interestingly, simvastatin also inhibit adenosine activated I_{KACh}, which suggest that simvastatin influence on the adenosine binding site as well as acetylcholine binding sites.

However, intracellular application of gamma GTP 100 μM/L induced I_{KACh} activation was not suppressed by simvastatin, which possibly suggest that simvastatin induced I_{KACh} inhibition may be done by interference of acetylcholine ligand binding pocket. We observed the inhibition of I_{KACh} as soon as 10 ± 20 sec after administration of simvastatin, which suggested that inhibition of I_{KACh} does not involve metabolism of the drug but occurs through direct interaction of the drug with K^+ channels within the membrane. The highly lipophilic simvastatin has a strong affinity for the cell membrane [13] and, consequently, it may has easy access to the intracellular space; this may explain the ability of simvastatin to effectively inhibit I_{KACh} in atrial myocytes. In contrast, hydrophilic pravastatin has limited access to the plasma membrane and intracellular space [13], which may explain the absence of immediate effect on I_{KACh}. In accordance with our results, Matsuda et al. [43] showed that the inhibitory effect of simvastatin on catecholamine secretion induced by acetylcholine does not involve its inhibition of mevalonate-derived isoprenoid synthesis, and that pravastatin does not inhibit acetylcholine-induced catecholamine secretion in cultured adrenal medullary cells. Pravastatin significantly increases parasympathetic modulation of heart rate by stimulation of Gα (i2) expression [44] and protects against ventricular arrhythmias [45], while parasympathetic stimulation is known to promote AF through shortening of atrial refractory periods.

It should be noted that we studied acute exposure rather than chronic treatment, which should be taken into consideration in addition to the extreme caution that must be taken when extrapolating results from mouse atrial cardiomyocytes to human disease. Moreover, we did not manipulate membrane cholesterol and did not study the gating kinetics, and these will be interesting future research themes. In conclusion, we found that the lipophilic statin simvastatin suppressed acetylcholine-activated I_{KACh}, while the hydrophilic statin pravastatin did not. These results provide important background information for using lipophilic statins in the clinical treatment of AF.

Supporting Information

Figure S1   A. Simvastatin had no influence on the I_{KACh} over the whole tested voltage range without acetylcholine. B. Simvastatin had no influence on the APD_{90} without acetylcholine.

Figure S2   To investigate a time dependent effect, steady-state block of I_{KACh} were achieved at the 5 minute, 10 minute, and 15 minutes after simvastatin application. There were no significant differences in achieving "steady-state" block of I_{KACh} among 5 min, 10 min, and 15 min (each n = 5, total n = 15, p = NS). NS = no significant change.

Author Contributions

Conceived and designed the experiments: TJC KIC. Performed the experiments: SJL IKS. Analyzed the data: YHZ JHH HSK. Contributed reagents/materials/analysis tools: SJK KLK JWL. Wrote the paper: TJC KIC.

References

1. Naccarelli GV, Varker H, Lin J, Schulman KL (2009) Increasing prevalence of atrial fibrillation and flutter in the united states. Am J Cardiol 104:1534–1539.
2. Tsadok MA, Jackevicius CA, Essebag V, Eisenberg MJ, Rahme E, et al. (2012) Rhythm versus rate control therapy and subsequent stroke or transient ischemic attack in patients with atrial fibrillation. Circulation 126:2680–2687.
3. Korantzopoulos P, Kolettis T, Siogas K, Goudevenos J (2003) Atrial fibrillation and electrical remodeling: The potential role of inflammation and oxidative stress. Med Sci Monit 9:RA225–229.
4. Cai H, Li Z, Goette A, Mera F, Honeycutt C, et al. (2002) Downregulation of endocardial nitric oxide synthase expression and nitric oxide production in atrial fibrillation: potential mechanisms for atrial thrombosis and stroke. Circulation 106:2854–2858.
5. Riesen WF, Engler H, Risch M, Korte W, Noseda G (2002) Short-term effects of atorvastatin on C-reactive protein. Eur Heart J 23:794–799.
6. Siu CW, Lau CP, Tse HF (2003) Prevention of atrial fibrillation recurrence by statin therapy in patients with lone atrial fibrillation after successful cardioversion. Am J Cardiol 92:1343–1345.
7. Laszlo R, Menzel KA, Bentz K, Schreiner B, Kettering K, et al. (2010) Atorvastatin treatment affects atrial ion currents and their tachycardia-induced remodeling in rabbits. Life Sci 87: 507–513.
8. Ozaydin M, Varol E, Aslan SM, Kucuktepe Z, Dogan A, et al. (2006) Effect of atorvastatin on the recurrence rates of atrial fibrillation after electrical cardioversion. Am J Cardiol 97:1490–1493.
9. Tveit A, Grundtvig M, Gundersen T, Vanberg P, Semb AG, et al. (2004) Analysis of pravastatin to prevent recurrence of atrial fibrillation after electrical cardioversion. Am J Cardiol 93:780–782.
10. Maggioni AP, Fabbri G, Lucci D, Marchioli R, Franzosi MG, et al. (2009) Effects of rosuvastatin on atrial fibrillation occurrence: ancillary results of the GISSI-HF trial. Eur Heart J 30:2327–2336.
11. GISSI-HF investigators, Tavazzi L, Maggioni AP, Marchioli R, Barlera S, et al. (2008) Effect of rosuvastatin in patients with chronic heart failure (the GISSI-HF trial): a randomised, double-blind, placebo-controlled trial. Lancet 372: 1231–1239.
12. Shiroshita-Takeshita A, Brundel BJ, Burstein B, Leung TK, Mitamura H, et al. (2007) Effects of simvastatin on the development of the atrial fibrillation substrate in dogs with congestive heart failure. Cardiovasc Res 74: 75–84.
13. Sarr FS, André C, Guillaume YC (2008) Statins (HMG-coenzyme A reductase inhibitors)-biomimetic membrane binding mechanism investigated by molecular chromatography J Chromatogr B Analyt Technol Biomed Life Sci 868:20–27.
14. Davidson MH, Toth PP (2004) Comparative effects of lipid-lowering therapies. Prog Cardiovasc Dis 47:73–104.

15. Liu YB, Lee YT, Pak HN, Lin SF, Fishbein MC, et al. (2009) Effects of simvastatin on cardiac neural and electrophysiologic remodeling in rabbits with hypercholesterolemia. Heart Rhythm 6: 69–75.
16. Sharifov OF, Fedorov VV, Beloshapko GG, Glukhov AV, Yushmanova AV, et al. (2004) Roles of adrenergic and cholinergic stimulation in spontaneous atrial fibrillation in dogs. J Am Coll Cardiol 43: 483–490.
17. Chen PS, Tan AY (2007) Autonomic nerve activity and atrial fibrillation. Heart Rhythm 4:S61–S64.
18. Hamil OP, Marty A, Neher E, Sakmann B, Sigworth FJ (1981) Improved patch-clamp techniques for high-resolution current recording *from cells and cell*-free membrane patches. Pflugers Arch 391:85–100.
19. Cho H, Nam GB, Lee SH, Earm YE, Ho WK (2001) Phosphatidylinositol 4,5-bisphosphate is acting as a signal molecule in alpha(1)-adrenergic pathway via the modulation of acetylcholine-activated K(+) channels in mouse atrial myocytes. J Biol Chem 276:159–164.
20. Cho H, Youm JB, Ryu SY, Earm YE, Ho WK (2001) Inhibition of acetylcholine-activated K^+ currents by U73122 is mediated by the inhibition of PIP(2)-channel interaction. Br J Pharmacol 134:1066–1072.
21. Maron DJ, Fazio S, Linton MF (2000) Current perspectives on statins. Circulation 101:207–213.
22. Ludmer PL, Selwyn AP, Shook TL, Wayne RR, Mudge GH, et al. (1986) Paradoxical vasoconstriction induced by acetylcholine in atherosclerotic coronary arteries. N Engl J Med 315:1046–1051.
23. Laufs U, Liao JK (1998) Post-transcriptional regulation of endothelial nitric oxide synthase mrna stability by rho gtpase. J Biol Chem 273:24266–24271.
24. Ganotakis ES, Mikhailidis DP, Vardas PE (2006) Atrial fibrillation, inflammation and statins. Hellenic J Cardiol 47:51–53.
25. Patel P, Dokainish H, Tsai P, Lakkis N (2010) Update on the association of inflammation and atrial fibrillation. J Cardiovasc Electrophysiol 21: 1064–1070.
26. Zhu W, Saba S, Link MS, Bak E, Homoud MK, et al. (2005) Atrioventricular nodal reverse facilitation in connexion 40-deficient mice. Heart Rhythm 2: 1231–1237.
27. Pound EM, Kang JX, Leaf A (2001) Partitioning of polyunsaturated fatty acids, which prevent cardiac arrhythmias, into phospholipid cell membranes. J Lipid Res 42:346–351.
28. Allessie M, Ausma J, Schotten U (2002) Electrical, contractile and structural remodeling during atrial fibrillation. Cardiovasc Res 54:230–246.
29. Nattel S (2002) New ideas about atrial fibrillation 50 years on. Nature 415:219–226.
30. Dobrev D, Ravens U (2003) Remodeling of cardiomyocyte ion channels in human atrial fibrillation. Basic Res Cardiol 98:137–148.

31. Seto SW, Au AL, Lam TY, Chim SS, Lee SM, et al. (2007) Modulation by simvastatin of iberiotoxin-sensitive, Ca2+-activated K+ channels of porcine coronary artery smooth muscle cells. Br J Pharmacol 151:987–997.

32. Bergdahl A, Persson E, Hellstrand P, Swärd K (2003) Lovastatin induces relaxation and inhibits L-type Ca2+ current in the rat basilar artery. Pharmacol Toxicol 93:128–134.

33. Vaquero M, Caballero R, Gómez R, Núñez L, Tamargo J, et al. (2007) Effects of atorvastatin and simvastatin on atrial plateau currents. J Mol Cell Cardiol 42:931–945.

34. Ehrlich JR. Inward rectifier potassium currents as a target for atrial fibrillation therapy (2008) Cardiovasc Pharmacol 52:129–135.

35. Ehrlich JR, Cha TJ, Zhang L, Chartier D, Villeneuve L, et al. (2004) Characterization of a hyperpolarization-activated time-dependent potassium current in canine cardiomyocytes from pulmonary vein myocardial sleeves and left atrium. J Physiol 557:583–597.

36. Cha TJ, Ehrlich JR, Zhang L, Chartier D, Leung TK, et al. (2005) Atrial tachycardia remodeling of pulmonary vein cardiomyocytes: comparison with left atrium and potential relation to arrhythmogenesis. Circulation 111:728–735.

37. Cha TJ, Ehrlich JR, Chartier D, Qi XY, Xiao L, et al. (2005) Kir3-based inward rectifier potassium current: potential role in atrial tachycardia remodeling effects on atrial repolarization and arrhythmias. Circulation 111:728–735.

38. Gomes ME, Tack CJ, Verheugt FW, Smits P, Lenders JW (2010) Sympathoinhibition by atorvastatin in hypertensive patients. Circ J 74: 2622–2626.

39. Tsutamoto T, Sakai H, Ibe K, Yamaji M, Kawahara C, et al. (2011) Effect of Atorvastatin vs. Rosuvastatin on Cardiac Sympathetic Nerve Activity in Non-Diabetic Patients With Dilated Cardiomyopathy. Circ J 75: 2160–2166.

40. Mason RP, Walter MF, Day CA, Jacob RF (2006) Active metabolite of atorvastatin inhibits membrane cholesterol domain formation by an antioxidant mechanism. J Biol Chem 281: 9337–9345.

41. Escobales N, Crespo MJ, Altieri PI, Furilla RA (1996) Inhibition of smooth muscle cell calcium mobilization and aortic ring contraction by lactone vastatins. J Hypertens 14:115–121.

42. Sicouri S, Gianetti B, Zygmunt AC, Cordeiro JM, Antzelevitch C (2011) Antiarrhythmic effects of simvastatin in canine pulmonary vein sleeve preparations. J Am Coll Cardiol 57:986–993.

43. Matsuda T, Toyohira Y, Ueno S, Tsutsui M, Yanagihara N (2008) Simvastatin inhibits catecholamine secretion and synthesis induced by acetylcholine via blocking Na+ and Ca2+ influx in bovine adrenal medullary cells. J Pharmacol Exp Ther 327:130–136.

44. Welzig CM, Shin DG, Park HJ, Kim YJ, Saul JP, et al. (2003) Lipid lowering by pravastatin increases parasympathetic modulation of heart rate: Galpha(i2), a possible molecular marker for parasympathetic responsiveness. Circulation 108:2743–2746.

45. Welzig CM, Park HJ, Naggar J, Confalone D, Rhofiry J, et al. (2010) Differential effects of statins (pravastatin or simvastatin) on ventricular ectopic complexes: Galpha(i2), a possible molecular marker for ventricular irritability. Am J Cardiol 105:1112–1117.

20

Calcium-Activated Potassium Current Modulates Ventricular Repolarization in Chronic Heart Failure

Ingrid M. Bonilla[1,2], Victor P. Long, III[1,2], Pedro Vargas-Pinto[3¤], Patrick Wright[2], Andriy Belevych[2], Qing Lou[2], Kent Mowrey[4], Jae Yoo[1], Philip F. Binkley[2], Vadim V. Fedorov[2], Sandor Györke[2], Paulus M. L. Janssen[2], Ahmet Kilic[2], Peter J. Mohler[2], Cynthia A. Carnes[1,3]*

1 College of Pharmacy, The Ohio State University, Columbus, Ohio, United States of America, **2** Dorothy M. Davis Heart and Lung Research Institute, The Ohio State University Wexner Medical Center, Columbus, Ohio, United States of America, **3** College of Veterinary Medicine, The Ohio State University, Columbus, Ohio, United States of America, **4** St Jude Medical, Sylmar, California, United States of America

Abstract

The role of I_{KCa} in cardiac repolarization remains controversial and varies across species. The relevance of the current as a therapeutic target is therefore undefined. We examined the cellular electrophysiologic effects of I_{KCa} blockade in controls, chronic heart failure (HF) and HF with sustained atrial fibrillation. We used perforated patch action potential recordings to maintain intrinsic calcium cycling. The I_{KCa} blocker (apamin 100 nM) was used to examine the role of the current in atrial and ventricular myocytes. A canine tachypacing induced model of HF (1 and 4 months, n = 5 per group) was used, and compared to a group of 4 month HF with 6 weeks of superimposed atrial fibrillation (n = 7). A group of age-matched canine controls were used (n = 8). Human atrial and ventricular myocytes were isolated from explanted end-stage failing hearts which were obtained from transplant recipients, and studied in parallel. Atrial myocyte action potentials were unchanged by I_{KCa} blockade in all of the groups studied. I_{KCa} blockade did not affect ventricular myocyte repolarization in controls. HF caused prolongation of ventricular myocyte action potential repolarization. I_{KCa} blockade caused further prolongation of ventricular repolarization in HF and also caused repolarization instability and early afterdepolarizations. SK2 and SK3 expression in the atria and SK3 in the ventricle were increased in canine heart failure. We conclude that during HF, I_{KCa} blockade in ventricular myocytes results in cellular arrhythmias. Furthermore, our data suggest an important role for I_{KCa} in the maintenance of ventricular repolarization stability during chronic heart failure. Our findings suggest that novel antiarrhythmic therapies should have safety and efficacy evaluated in both atria and ventricles.

Editor: Blanca Rodriguez, University of Oxford, United Kingdom

Funding: Pacemakers and leads provided by St. Jude Medical, Sylmar, CA as an in-kind donation (Carnes). Research supported in part by NIH grants (R01-HL115580 to CAC and VVF; R01-HL089836 to CAC; HL074045 to SG; HL084583, HL083422, HL114383 to PJM) and the American Heart Association (PJM). The funders had no role in study design, data collection and analysis, decision to publish or preparation of the manuscript.

Competing Interests: The authors have declared that no competing interests exist.

* Email: carnes.4@osu.edu

¤ Current address: University of LaSalle, Bogota, Columbia

Introduction

Heart failure (HF) is a chronic disease that develops over months to years, and is defined by insufficient cardiac output to meet the physiologic and metabolic needs of the body. Atrial fibrillation (AF) and HF are common coexisting disease states, and HF results in a 4.5 to 5.9 fold increase in the risk of developing AF. [1] Moreover, in patients with HF, the development of AF significantly increases the risk of death. [2] Thus, identifying and elucidating pharmacological targets to treat AF may significantly reduce mortality and morbidity in HF.

Small-conductance Ca^{2+}- activated K^+ (SK) channels are expressed in multiple tissues such as skeletal and smooth muscle, the central and peripheral nervous system and the heart.[3–5] Cardiac myocytes express SK1, SK2 and SK3 gene products. [6] SK- encoded current is voltage-independent and activated by intracellular calcium. [7] All three members of the SK family have similar calcium sensitivity for activation (0.6–0.7 μM) [8]. SK-

encoded current is blocked by apamin, a constituent of bee venom, which appears to be highly selective for I_{KCa}. [7,9,10].

I_{KCa}, the potassium current conducted by SK channels, contributes to repolarization, [3,11] but the importance of I_{KCa} in repolarization remains poorly elucidated. For example, ventricular I_{KCa} shortens repolarization and promotes peri-infarct arrhythmias in rats. [12] Conversely, blockade of I_{KCa} promotes ventricular arrhythmias in human HF and a non-ischemic rabbit HF model, suggesting a protective role for I_{KCa}. [13,14] The contribution of I_{KCa} to *atrial* repolarization is also unclear as some reports demonstrate that I_{KCa} is proarrhythmic while others suggest it is protective. [15,16].

We measured the impact of I_{KCa} block on action potentials in intact myocytes using perforated patch recordings to maintain intrinsic Ca^{2+} cycling. We utilized a well-validated canine model that emulates all key features of human HF including chamber dilatation, impaired contractility, impaired functional capacity, repolarization abnormalities, dysregulated myocyte calcium

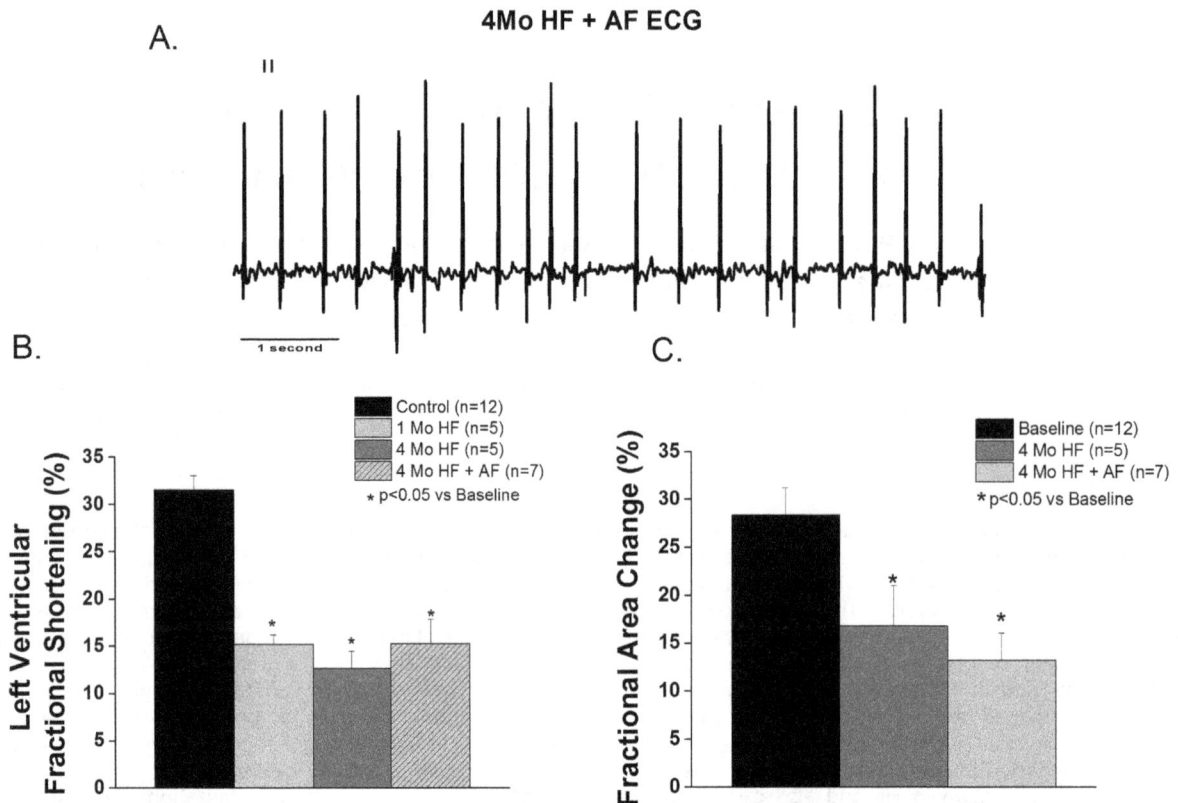

Figure 1. In vivo data from 1 month (1 Mo), 4 month (4 Mo), and 4 month HF with sustained AF (4 Mo HF+AF) canine groups. A. Representative ECG recording from a 4 month HF+AF dog showing the absence of P waves and irregularly irregular QRS complexes characteristic of AF. **B.** LVFS was similarly decreased in the 1 month HF, 4 month HF and the 4 month HF+AF groups compared to baseline. ($p < 0.05$ vs baseline). **C.** Atrial contractility was decreased in 4 month HF and 4 month HF+AF groups compared to baseline. ($p < 0.05$, N = 5–7 per group).

handling, increased predisposition to AF and increased myocardial fibrosis. [17,18] Complementary experiments were conducted in end-stage human HF. The role of I_{KCa} in AF was evaluated in atrial myocytes from a canine model of chronic HF with sustained AF.

Methods

Heart failure and atrial fibrillation animal models

All animal procedures conformed to the Guide for the Care and Use of Laboratory Animals of the National Institutes of Health, and were approved by the Ohio State University Institutional Animal Care and Use Committee (Protocol: 2010A00000103-R1). Canine heart failure was induced by right ventricular (RV) tachypacing as previously described. [19] Animals were assigned to one or four months of RV tachypacing to induce heart failure.

Atrial fibrillation was induced in dogs with HF using a customized pacemaker (St Jude Medical, Sylmar, CA). One pacing lead was implanted in the right atria (RA) and the second lead was implanted in the RV, with HF induced as previously described. [20] After 10 weeks of RV tachypacing, RA tachypacing was initiated, with the RA stimulated at 10 Hz for 60 seconds, followed by a 10 second pause for automated interrogation of atrial rhythm. This cycle of RA tachypacing was repeated every 70 seconds until AF was detected. Subsequent detection of normal atrial rhythm resulted in resumption of the atrial tachypacing. The total HF duration in the HF+AF group was 4 months. Ventricular pacing was stopped during atrial stimulation, and the ventricular rate was 150–200 BPM during atrial pacing or AF. Serial echocardiograms and ECGs were performed as previously reported. [17,21] Serial pacemaker interrogations were used to monitor cardiac rhythm.

Myocyte Isolation and Tissue Collection

On the day of the terminal procedure, the dogs were anesthetized with pentobarbital sodium (50 mg/kg intravenously; Nembutal, Abbott Laboratories). The heart was rapidly removed and perfused with cold cardioplegia solution containing the following (mM): NaCl 110, $CaCl_2$ 1.2, KCl 16, $MgCl_2$ 16 and $NaHCO_3$ 10. Cannulation of the left circumflex artery was used to perfuse left atria and ventricle following removal of the right atrium and right ventricle, as previously described. [22] Adjacent tissue samples were collected and snap frozen for protein analyses. Tyrode's solution (mM) containing NaCl 130, KCl 5.4, $MgCl_2$ 3.5, NaH_2PO_4 0.5, Glucose 10, HEPES 5 and taurine 20, was used as the initial perfusate. During the cell isolation process the heart was perfused with three different solutions (36°C). The heart was initially perfused for 10 minutes with Tyrode's solution with 0.1 mM EGTA; this was followed by perfusion with Tyrode's solution containing 0.3 mM Calcium, 0.12 mg/ml of Trypsin Inhibitor (NIBCO) and 1.33 mg/ml of collagenase (Type II, Worthington) for a maximum of 45 minutes. Then following enzymatic digestion, the heart was perfused with normal Tyrode's solution for five minutes to remove residual enzyme. Subsequently, left ventricular mid-myocardial and left atrial myocytes were obtained through secondary digestion, as previously described. [22] After secondary digestion the cells were re-suspended in

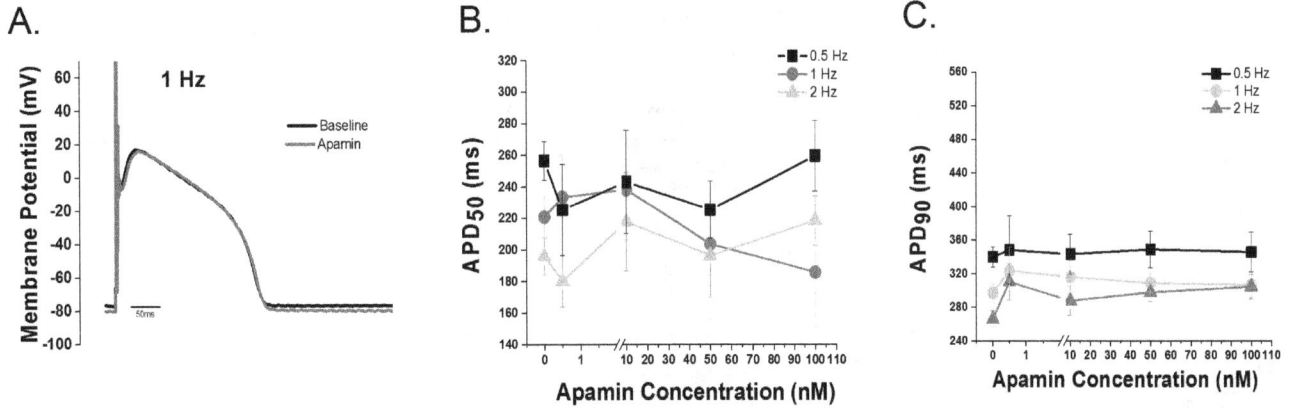

Figure 2. I_{KCa} inhibition does not alter repolarization in control ventricular cells. A. Representative action potential tracing before and after 100 nM apamin recorded at 1 Hz. **B.** APD_{50} and **C.** APD_{90} dose response data (0–100 nM apamin) recorded at stimulation rates of 0.5, 1 and 2 Hz. (p = NS, n = 5–11 cells per group; 8 animals). The Grubb's test for outlier data was applied and one cell was rejected and is not included in the summary data.

incubation buffer. [23] This isolation procedure typically yields 70–90% and 40–60% rod shaped ventricular and atrial myocytes, respectively. All myocyte electrophysiology experiments were conducted within 10 hours of isolation.

In parallel experiments, failing human cardiac tissue was obtained after written informed consent with the documentation of consent securely stored as approved by the Institutional Review Board approval of The Ohio State University (IRB 2008H0113

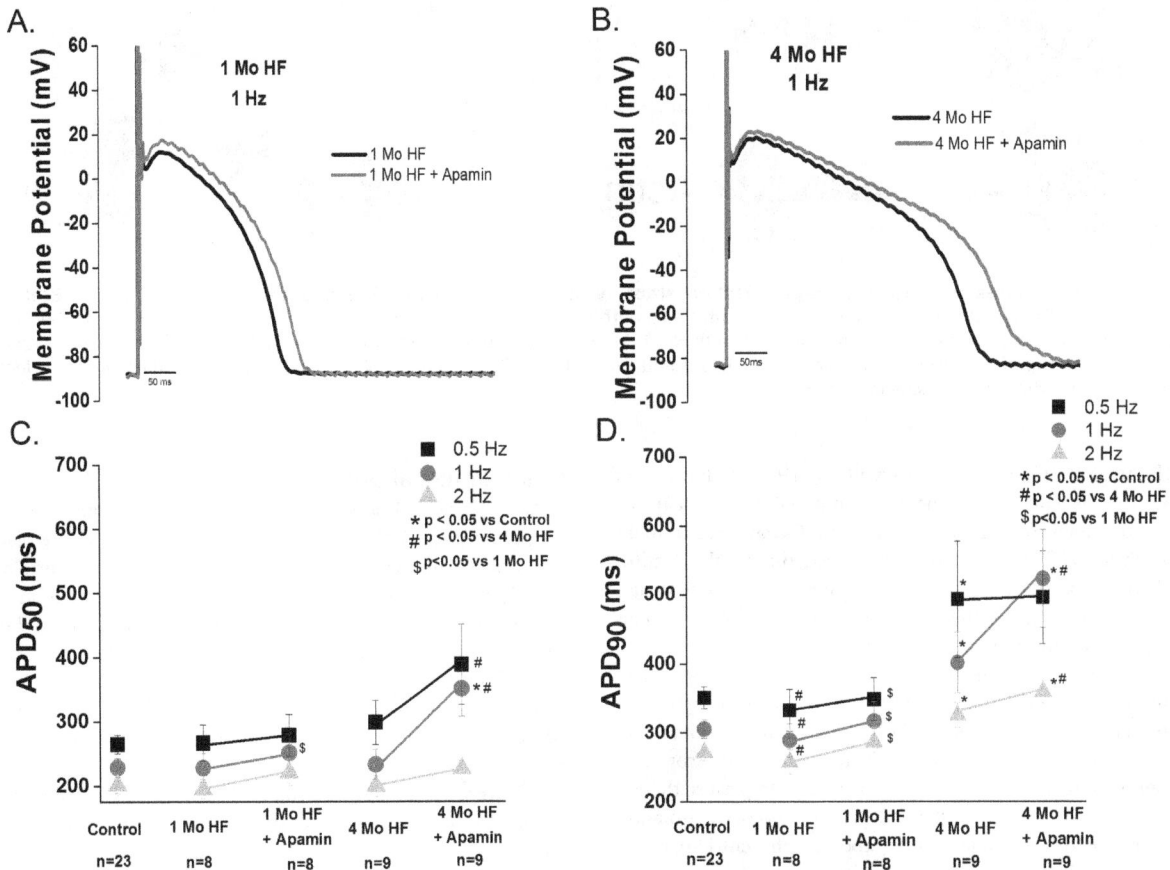

Figure 3. Apamin modulates ventricular repolarization during HF. Representative action potential of a 1 month (**A**) HF and 4 month HF (**B**) ventricular cell before and after apamin superfusion. **C.** Summary data of APD_{50} in control, 1 month and 4 month HF before and after apamin treatment. No difference between 1 month HF, 4 month HF and control is observed (2–8 animals per group). Apamin treatment of 1 month HF cells causes a prolongation only at 2 Hz(p<0.05), likewise apamin treatment of 4 month HF cells causes a prolongation at 0.5 Hz (p<0.05) and 1 Hz (p< 0.05). **D.** Apamin prolongs APD_{90} in both 1 and 4 month HF (p<0.05).

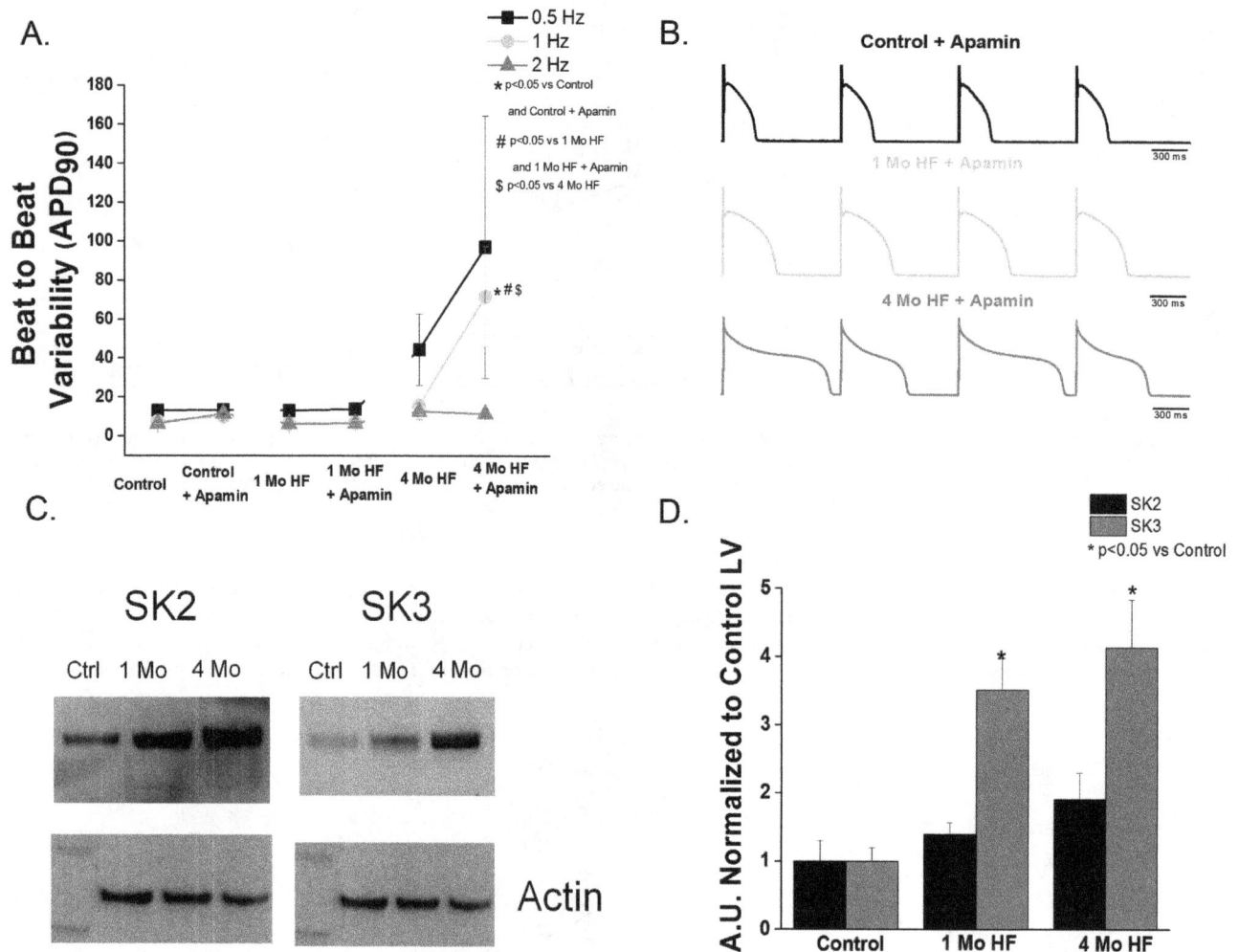

Figure 4. I_{Kca} contributes to ventricular repolarization stability in canine HF, and HF increases SK3 expression. A. Beat to beat variability of APD_{90} (BTBV, ms) is unchanged in both 1 month or 4 month HF vs. controls. I_{KCa} block increases the BTBV in the 4 month, but not the 1 month HF group (p<0.05 vs control, 1 month HF and 4 month HF; 2–8 animals per group). **B.** Representative AP tracings of control, 1 month HF and 4 month HF during superfusion with 100 nm apamin. **C.** Representative blots of SK2 and SK3. **D.** SK3 in the 1 and 4 month HF groups is increased (p<0.05 vs control) while SK2 is unchanged (N=4–5).

and IRB 2012H0197), in accordance with the 1964 Declaration of Helsinki and its later amendments. Additional human cardiac tissue was obtained from the Lifeline of Ohio Organ Procurement program (http://lifelineofohio.org). For these tissues, the Institutional Review Board waived the need for consent and these tissues were used according to the Ohio State University guidelines regarding the use of data and/or specimens.

Left ventricular mid-myocardial and left atrial appendage myocytes were isolated and adjacent tissues were collected from explanted end-stage failing hearts (n = 6; obtained from the Ohio State University Wexner Medical Center transplant program). After cannulation of a superficial coronary artery to perfuse the left atrium and/or left ventricle, the methods for myocyte isolation were as described for canine samples above. Left ventricular mid myocardium and left atrial appendege tissues were collected from non-failing heart for Western blotting purposes (n = 8 obtained from Lifeline of Ohio). Non-HF status was confirmed in these tissues by lack of CaMKII pS286 hyperphosphorylation.

Action Potential (AP) Measurements

Amphotericin-B perforated patch clamp techniques with a bath temperature of $36 \pm 0.5°C$ were used. The myocytes were placed in a laminin-coated cell chamber (Cell Microcontrols, Norfolk, VA) and superfused (~ 1 mL/min) with bath solution containing (mM): 135 NaCl, 5 $MgCl_2$, 5 KCl, 10 glucose, 1.8 $CaCl_2$, and 5 HEPES with pH adjusted to 7.40 with NaOH. Borosilicate glass micropipettes with tip resistance of 1.5–3 $M\Omega$, were filled with pipette solution containing the following (mM): 100 K-aspartate, 40 KCl, 5 MgCl, 5 EGTA, 5 HEPES, pH adjusted to 7.2 with KOH.

APs were recorded in a train of 25 traces at 0.5, 1 and 2 Hz at baseline and after apamin perfusion. The average of the last 10 traces (i.e. from trace 16–25) was used to calculate the action potential duration (APD). APD was calculated at 50 and 90 percent of repolarization (APD_{50} and APD_{90}).

To evaluate repolarization instability, beat to beat variability (BTBV) of APD_{90} was assessed as the standard deviation of the APD_{90}, as previously described. [24,25] Early afterdepolarization (EAD) propensity was assessed as the percentage of cells exhibiting

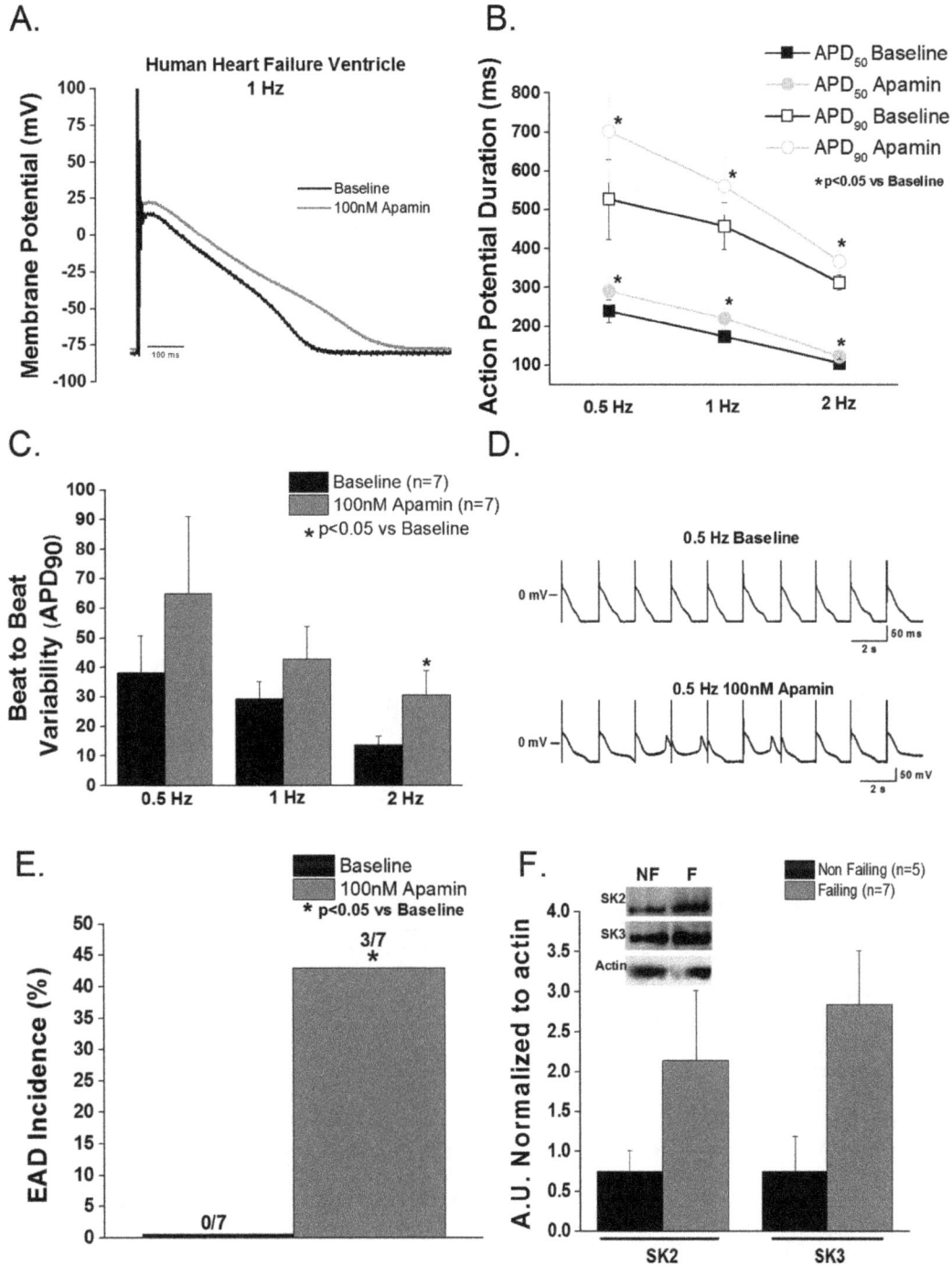

Figure 5. Apamin modulates ventricular repolarization in end-stage human HF. A. Representative action potential recorded at 1 Hz from an end-stage human HF ventricular myocyte before and after apamin. **B.** Apamin superfusion prolongs APD_{50} and APD_{90} in end-stage human HF ventricular myocytes at all rates ($p<0.05$ vs baseline, $n=7$). **C.** Apamin superfusion increases ($p<0.05$ vs baseline) BTBV (ms) at 2 Hz. **D.** Representative action potential showing late phase 3 EADs after apamin superfusion. **E.** Apamin treatment increases EAD incidence in failing human ventricular myocytes. ($p<0.05$ vs baseline) **F.** Representative blots of control and end-stage human HF SK2 and SK3 proteins (SK2 $p=0.556$ and SK3 $p=0.141$ vs. control). HF: $N=7$ (4 male/3 female); age $=52\pm13$ years and LV ejection fraction of $14.5\pm5.2\%$; non-failing controls: $n=5$ (2 male/3 female); age $=47\pm12$ years.

EADs. Recordings exhibiting EADs were excluded from APD and BTBV measurements.

Data collection was done at baseline and after superfusion with the I_{KCa} blocker apamin (100 nM), a concentration known to block SK1, SK2 and SK3 encoded-current.[26–28] An Axopatch 200A amplifier with Digidata 1440A (Molecular devices, Sunnyvale, CA) and Clampex 10.2 software was used for data acquisition. At the initiation of each recording the resting potential was examined. For canine cells, atrial cells with a resting membrane potential of ≥ -55 mV were recorded; for ventricular

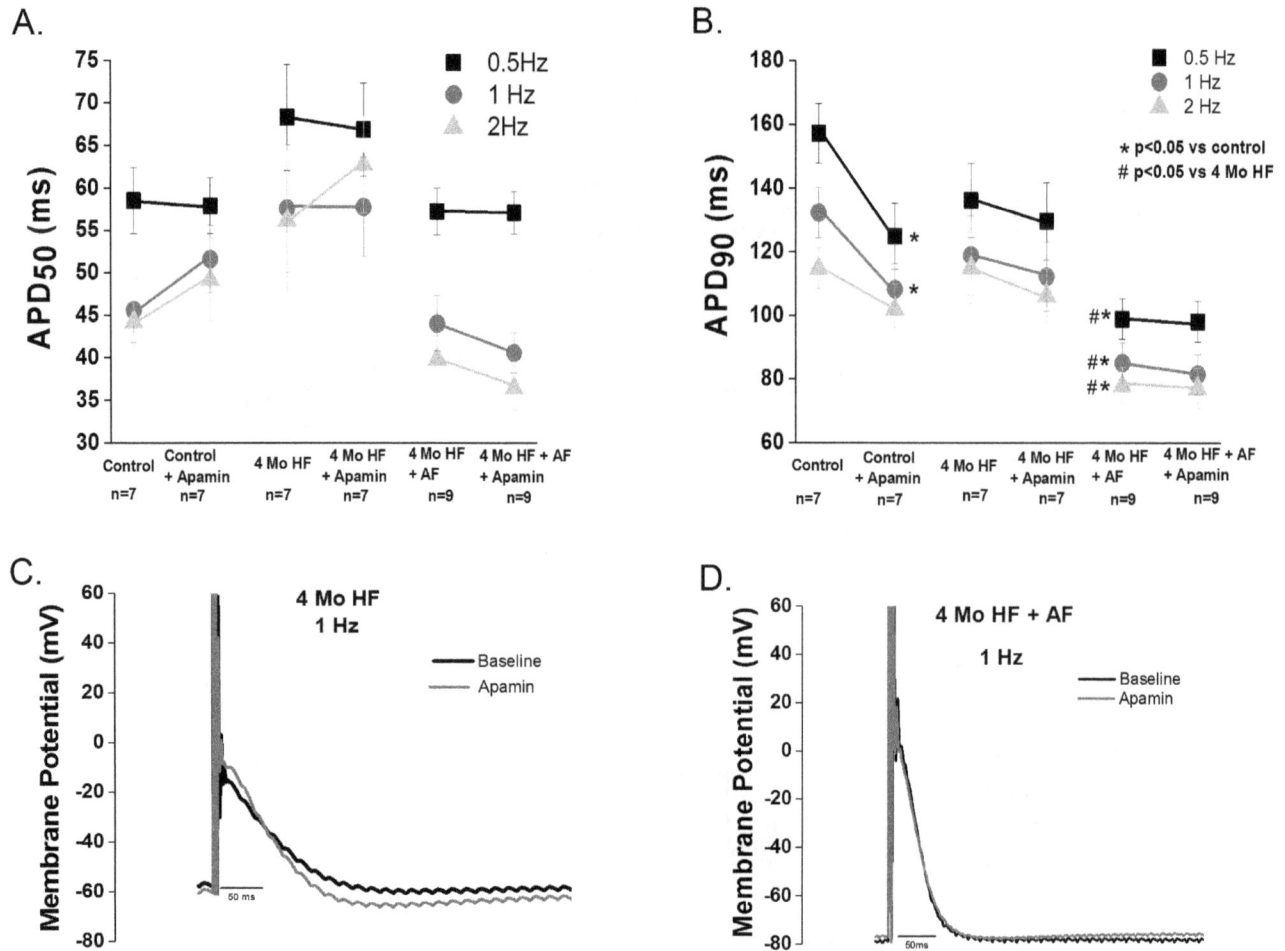

Figure 6. I_{KCa} block does not affect repolarization in normal or diseased atrial myocytes. A. 100 nM apamin does not affect atrial APD_{50} in any of the studied groups (i.e. control, 4 month HF and 4 month HF+AF, n = 7–9 cells per group) **B.** 100 nM apamin shortened the APD_{90} in controls at 0.5 and 1 Hz. (p<0.05). HF+AF had a shorter baseline APD_{90} compared to control and HF (p<0.05), however no change in APD_{90} was observed after apamin treatment in either 4 month HF or 4 month HF+AF groups. (n = 7–9 cells per groups) **C and D.** Atrial action potential tracings before and after apamin treatment from the 4 month HF group and the 4 month HF+ AF group (2–6 animals per group).

cells those with a resting membrane potential of ≥ -70 mV were recorded. For the human cells, every cell with complete baseline and apamin-treatment data was included. One apamin-treated ventricular canine cell action potential recording was excluded as an outlier.

Calcium transient Measurements

Calcium transients were recorded using Ca^{2+} sensitive dye Fluo-4AM (10 μM) and an Olympus Fluoview 1000 confocal microscope in line scan mode. Myocytes were loaded with dye for 25 minutes at room temperature. Fluo-4 was excited with a 488 nm argon laser and fluorescence collected at wavelength 500–600 nm. Myocytes were paced by extracellular stimulation at 1 Hz with platinum electrodes. External solution contained (mM): 140 NaCl, 5.4 KCl, 2 $CaCl_2$, 0.5 $MgCl_2$, 10 HEPES and 5.6 glucose (pH 7.3).

Immunoblots

Following protein quantification, tissue lysates were analyzed on Mini-PROTEAN tetra cell (BioRad) on a 4–15% precast TGX gel (BioRad) in Tris/Glycine/SDS Buffer (BioRad). Gels were transferred to a nitrocellulose membrane using the Mini-

PROTEAN tetra cell (BioRad) in Tris/Glycine buffer with 20% methanol (v/v, BioRad). Membranes were blocked for 1 hour at room temperature using a 3% BSA solution and incubated with primary antibody overnight at 4°C. Antibodies included: SK2 (Alomone, Santa Cruz), SK3 (Alomone, Santa Cruz), GAPDH (Fitzgerald), and actin (Sigma). Secondary antibodies included donkey anti-mouse-HRP and donkey anti-rabbit-HRP (Jackson Laboratories). Densitometry was performed using Image lab software and all data was normalized to GAPDH or actin levels present in each sample.

Data Analysis

Cellular electrophysiology and Ca^{2+} imaging data were analyzed using Clampfit 10.3 software (Axon Instruments) and Origin 9.0 software (OriginLab, Northampton, MA, USA). APD data was examined for outliers by application of the Grubb's test, which rejected one control ventricular myocyte (GraphPad). All APD paired data were compared by paired student t-test. Unpaired data and comparisons between groups were analyzed by one-way ANOVA with post hoc least significant difference testing. Differences in EADs incidence were tested with Pearson's Chi-Square test. For protein experiments, differences were

A.

B.

C.

D.

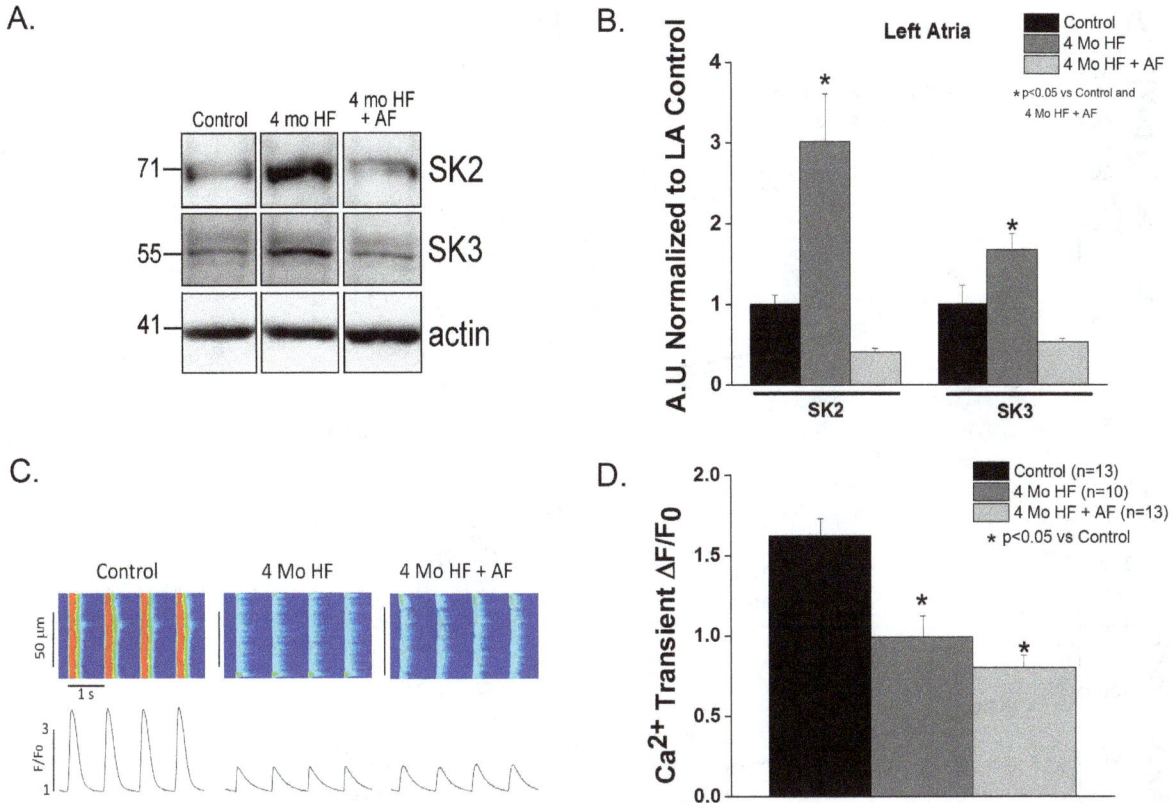

Figure 7. Atrial SK expression and calcium transients in chronic HF with and without AF. A. Representative Western blots of SK2 and SK3. **B.** SK2 and SK3 are increased 3- and 2-fold, respectively in the 4 month HF atria. ($p < 0.05$ vs control and 4 month HF+AF) No differences between control and 4 month HF+AF were found in any of the subunits. (N = 3) **C.** Representative calcium transient line scans. **D.** Calcium transient amplitude was decreased in the 4 month HF and 4 month HF+AF groups compared to control ($p < 0.05$ vs control; 3–8 animals per group).

assessed with a paired Student's t test (2-tailed) or ANOVA, as appropriate, for continuous data. The Bonferroni test was used for post-hoc testing. All data are presented as mean ± SE and $p < 0.05$ was the criterion for statistical significance for all comparisons.

Chemicals

All chemicals were purchased from Sigma-Aldrich (St. Louis, MO, USA) and Fisher Scientific (Pittsburg, PA, USA), unless otherwise noted. All buffers and solutions were prepared daily.

Results

In vivo cardiac remodeling

Left ventricular fractional shortening (LVFS) was similarly reduced in the 1 month HF, 4 month HF and 4 month HF+AF groups (Figure 1B), consistent with HF. Electrocardiograms (ECGs) in all canines assigned to the HF+ AF group demonstrated sustained atrial tachyarrhythmias, evident as the absence of P waves and the irregularly irregular ventricular rate characteristic of AF (Figure 1A). Additionally, atrial contractility, measured as left atrial fractional area change (FAC), was significantly reduced in both the 4 month HF and 4 month HF+AF groups compared to baseline ($p < 0.05$) as shown in Figure 1C. Notably, the presence of sustained AF did not cause a further decrement in atrial contractility compared to HF alone.

I_{KCa} inhibition in control ventricular myocytes

Action potentials before and after apamin treatment were recorded from control canine ventricular myocytes. Varying apamin concentrations (0.5–100 nM) were tested in order to generate a concentration response curve. Apamin did not alter APD_{50} or APD_{90} in control ventricular myocytes (Figure 2A).

I_{KCa} inhibition and SK expression in failing ventricle

Canine. We observed no HF-induced difference in APD_{50} or APD_{90} in the 1 month HF myocytes compared with control myocytes. However, apamin (100 nM) caused a significant prolongation of the APD_{90} in one month HF ($p < 0.05$; Figure 3 A–D). In contrast to 1 month HF, 4 month HF significantly increased APD_{90} relative to control ventricular myocytes ($p < 0.05$ vs control). Furthermore, when I_{KCa} was blocked in 4 month HF ventricular myocytes (100 nM apamin), there was a significant prolongation of the APD_{50} at lower rates (i.e. $p < 0.05$ vs control at 0.5 and 1 Hz) and a further prolongation in the APD_{90} ($p < 0.05$ vs control and baseline 4 month HF).

In order to assess repolarization instability induced by block of I_{KCa}, we measured the beat to beat variability (BTBV) of $APD_{90} \pm$ apamin. HF alone did not increase the BTBV in either HF group compared to controls. Block of I_{KCa} significantly increased BTBV in the 4 month, but not one month, HF group. (Figure 4A,B).

Canine cardiac I_{KCa} encoding proteins SK2 and SK3 were measured in control, 1 month HF and 4 month HF ventricular tissues. No significant change in SK2 protein expression in either HF group ($p > 0.05$ vs control) was found. An ~4-fold increase in

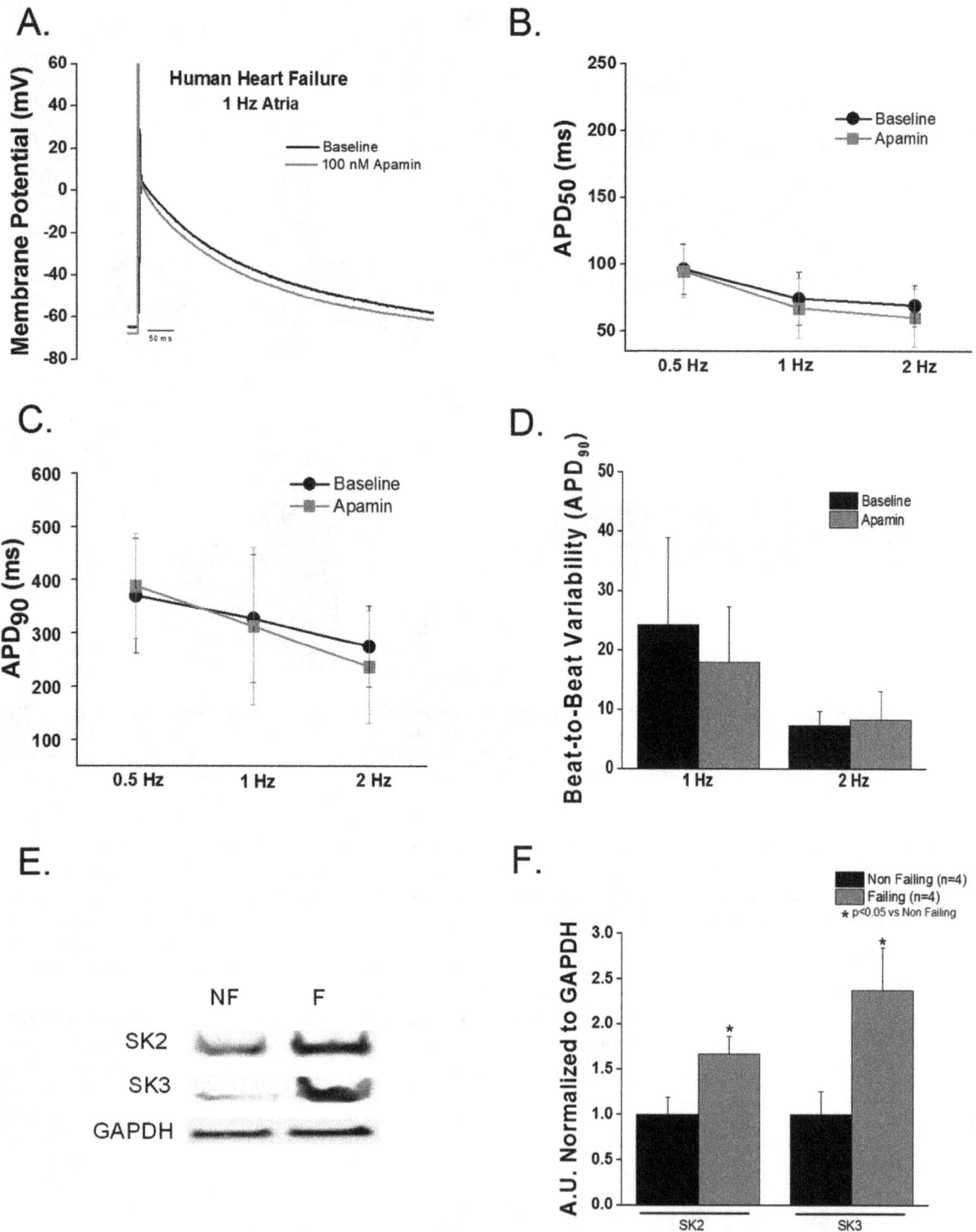

Figure 8. Apamin does not modulate repolarization in end-stage human HF atrial myocytes. A. Representative atrial action potential tracing recorded at 1 Hz. **B and C.** Apamin did not change APD_{50} or APD_{90} in human atrial myocytes. (n = 3) **D.** Apamin superfusion did not increase BTBV (ms). **E.** Representative SK2 and SK3 Western blots. **F.** HF increased SK2 and SK3 expression in left atrial tissue (p<0.05 vs non-failing). HF: N = 4 (2 male/2 female); age = 56±4 years and LV ejection fraction of 14.5±1.1%; non-failing controls: n = 4 (2 male/2 female); age = 46±14 years.

SK3 expression was found in both 1 month and 4 month HF groups. (p<0.05 vs control) (Figure 4C,D).

End-stage human heart failure. In end-stage human HF, inhibition of I_{KCa} (100 nM apamin) caused a significant prolongation of both APD_{50} and APD_{90} compared to baseline (p<0.05,

Figure 5 A, B). In addition to AP prolongation, BTBV was significantly increased at 2 Hz in end-stage human HF ventricular cells compared to baseline (Figure 5C). I_{KCa} blockade induced late phase 3 early afterdepolarizations (EADs) in ~40% of myocytes; while no EADs were observed at baseline (Figure 5D,E).

Human cardiac I_{KCa} encoding proteins SK2 and SK3 were measured in control and end-stage human HF ventricular tissue lysate (Figure 5F). While there was a trend toward increased SK2 expression in HF, this did not achieve statistical significance. SK3 protein also showed a tendency to increase in human end-stage HF compared to control ($p = 0.14$).

I_{KCa} inhibition and SK expression in atrial myocytes

Canine. Neither HF nor AF caused any change in APD_{50} compared to control. HF with superimposed AF caused significant APD_{90} shortening compared to control and 4 month HF ($p<0.05$ vs control and 4 Mo HF). I_{KCa} blockade (100 nM apamin) in control atrial myocytes did not change APD_{50} (Figure 6A) but caused an unexpected shortening of the APD_{90} at 0.5 and 1 Hz ($p<0.05$ vs baseline) as shown in Figure 6B. I_{KCa} blockade in the 4 month HF and 4 month HF+AF atrial cells did not cause any change in the APD_{50} or the APD_{90} (Figure 6). In further contrast to what we observed in the ventricle, no change in the BTBV of repolarization was observed in either the control, 4 month HF or the 4 month HF+AF groups after I_{KCa} blockade (data not shown). Thus, contrary to what we observed in the ventricle, I_{KCa} does not modulate repolarization in the atria in our chronic HF model.

The cardiac I_{KCa} encoding proteins SK2 and SK3 were measured in left atrial appendage tissue from the three groups (i.e. Control, 4 month HF and 4 month HF+AF). A 3-fold and 2-fold increase in SK2 and SK3, respectively in the 4 month HF group was observed compared to both control and 4 month HF+AF groups ($p<0.05$, Figure 7A, B); while the 4 month HF+AF group did not differ from control. HF, with or without sustained AF, caused a similar significant decrease in calcium transient amplitude compared to controls ($p<0.05$ vs control, Figure 7C, D).

End-stage human heart failure. Human end-stage HF atrial myocytes showed no significant change in either APD_{50} or APD_{90} when treated with apamin (100 nM). Contrary to what we observed in the ventricular cells no difference was observed in BTBV or afterdepolarizations after apamin treatment in human HF atrial cells (Figure 8). SK2 and SK3 were significantly increased in atrial human HF samples compared with atrial samples from non-failing individuals ($p<0.05$, Figure 8).

Discussion

It is well known that HF is a substrate for AF and these are common co-existing disease states. [1,20] HF patients are at an increased risk for both atrial and ventricular arrhythmias, which contribute to morbidity and mortality. [2] Our main findings were two-fold: first, we did not find any modulation of atrial myocyte repolarization by I_{KCa} in the settings of normal, failing or sustained AF hearts. Secondly, I_{KCa} is activated during HF contributing to stability of ventricular repolarization. Thus, block of I_{KCa} in chronic HF ventricular myocytes prolonged repolarization and increased repolarization instability; these effects have been shown to predict proarrhythmia. [29] Consistent with our findings, I_{KCa} has been previously suggested to play a protective role in the human ventricle during HF. [14].

One interesting question is how I_{KCa} becomes an important modulator of ventricular repolarization during heart failure. Potential explanations for this finding include 1) increased channel expression; 2) altered channel sensitivity to calcium; 3) increased calcium concentrations; or 4) loss of other repolarizing current(s), thereby unmasking the role of I_{KCa}.

In considering these possibilities, we observed an increase in SK3, but not SK2 in our canine HF model. However, we did not observe a statistically significant increase in either SK2 or SK3 in human HF, although there was a trend toward an increase in SK3 ($p = 0.14$); our findings are in contrast to a previous report where SK2 expression was increased in human HF. [14] While the expression was not significantly increased in human HF, the inter-species differences we observed may be explained by the intrinsic enhanced variability in explanted human end-stage heart failure samples resulting from inhomogeneities in etiology, comorbidities and drug treatments.

Other possible explanations for our findings are altered channel sensitivity to calcium, altered calcium cycling, or altered repolarization. Recently it was reported in human end-stage HF that SK channel sensitivity to calcium was increased in ventricular myocytes, [14] which could contribute in part to our findings. Of note, other proteins such as: protein kinase, calmodulin and protein phosphatase A, [7,30] are also known to contribute to the regulation of SK channels, and thus may modulate I_{KCa} during HF.

Since I_{KCa} is a calcium-activated potassium current, HF-induced changes in ventricular calcium handling should directly affect the current. We have previously reported that in our HF model, there is a significant reduction in SR calcium release and calcium transient amplitude, which would reduce rather than augment I_{KCa}. [31] In support of this interpretation, a recent report indicates that SR release is necessary and sufficient for I_{KCa} activation. [32] Considering the HF-induced reduction in calcium cycling, and the lack of apamin effect in control cells where calcium cycling is robust, this suggests that altered calcium cycling is not responsible for the protective role of I_{KCa} in heart failure.

Reduced ventricular repolarization reserve may unmask the role of small currents such as I_{KCa}. [33] Decreased repolarization reserve is well-described in the ventricle during HF and attributed to reductions in repolarizing currents such as I_{K1}, I_{Kr} and I_{Ks}. These changes predispose to repolarization instability and/or arrhythmias.[33–35] Since I_{KCa} blockade prolonged the AP only during HF and not in controls, we suggest that the contribution of I_{KCa} becomes evident only in settings of decreased repolarization reserve. Thus we suggest that increased channel expression, altered calcium sensitivity of SK channels, or altered repolarization reserve may contribute to the stabilizing role of I_{KCa}.

I_{KCa} has been suggested as a therapeutic target for AF. [36] I_{KCa} is defined pharmacologically as apamin-sensitive current, as apamin blocks SK1, SK2 and SK3-encoded channels [9]. One potential problem with this approach is non-selective effects on other ion currents. However, a recent paper surveying apamin effects on human ion channel protein function has demonstrated a high degree of specificity for SK-encoded I_{KCa}, even at a concentration five-fold higher than in the present study. [10] A potential limitation of previous studies evaluating I_{KCa} blockade has been a focus on primarily one cardiac chamber; this is limiting since electrical remodeling during HF is chamber-dependent. Specifically during chronic HF, the atrial action potential is shortened [20,37,38] while the ventricular action potential is prolonged. [39].

Interest in I_{KCa} as a therapeutic target for atrial arrhythmias followed reports of a genetic predisposition to lone AF attributed to a single nucleotide mutation in the gene KCNN3, which encodes for SK3. [40,41] The exact mechanism(s) by which a single mutation affects SK channel function remains unclear. Data supporting both loss of function and gain of function as possible mechanisms for AF have been reported in multiple models. [15,16] Additionally, SK2 and SK3 down regulation have been associated with human AF. [42]

One goal of this study was to elucidate the role of I_{KCa} in atrial electrophysiology during HF and HF with superimposed AF. Considering HF alone, contrary to previous reports, [15,16] I_{KCa} blockade failed to prolong the atrial action potential in either control or HF atrial myocytes, at physiologic rates. Our findings are different from a recent report where I_{KCa} blockade prolonged the atrial action potential in a whole atrial preparation in a reverse rate-dependent fashion; however this only occurred at rates slower than those used in the present study. [16].

The atrial action potential was not prolonged with I_{KCa} block in HF despite increased both SK2 and SK3 expression. Possible explanations include altered protein trafficking, altered channel calcium sensitivity or altered myocyte calcium handling. We previously reported that HF causes a decrease in calcium current in our 4 months HF tachypacing induced canine model, [20,43] and in the present study we report reduced calcium transient amplitude. Surprisingly, even in control myocytes where the calcium transient and current are normal, apamin failed to prolong the action potential.

Since a role for I_{KCa} blockers in the treatment of AF has been suggested [11,36] we also evaluated a HF model with superimposed AF. In a recent report in a canine atrial tachypacing AF model, with preserved LV function, I_{KCa} reduction via a drug which reduced calcium sensitivity of the channel caused a significant prolongation of left atrial action potentials. [15] This contrasts with our AF results in the setting of chronic HF, where I_{KCa} blockade failed to prolong the action potential. Notably, we observed that atrial HF myocytes had similar calcium transient amplitudes whether or not AF was superimposed, suggesting that calcium cycling in HF may be insufficient to activate the current.

In agreement with a previous study of patients with chronic AF who had decreased expression of SK proteins, we found that AF superimposed on HF caused a decrease in the SK2 and SK3 protein expression relative to HF alone. [42] Thus, the lack of apamin effect in the 4 months HF+AF atrial cells may be explained by a decrease in protein expression and/or a decrease in the calcium available for current activation. Since I_{KCa} is a very small current ($\sim$14 pS) [44] and repolarization is accelerated in AF (AP is shortened [45]), it may be less likely that a change in I_{KCa} would affect the overall AP duration. The same logic might apply in chronic HF, where atrial repolarization is also accelerated. [20,37].

While we did not find a beneficial role for I_{KCa} block in HF or AF, I_{KCa} blockade might have utility in disease states where atrial repolarization is prolonged, or if there is spatial dispersion of atrial repolarization. Additionally, a recent study shows that I_{KCa} blockade in pulmonary veins terminates AF suggesting a potential role for I_{KCa} blockers in paroxysmal AF. [15].

Limitations

Several studies have shown a gradient of SK channel expression and I_{KCa} current density across the human ventricular wall. [14] However, our experiments used only mid-myocardial myocytes. A similar limitation occurred in the atria, where we only studied cells from the left atrial appendage, and there may be a difference in I_{KCa} between free wall and appendage. [16] Additionally, we used only single cells which may differ in response compared to coupled cells or intact tissue.

References

1. Kannel WB, Wolf PA, Benjamin EJ, Levy D (1998) Prevalence, incidence, prognosis, and predisposing conditions for atrial fibrillation: population-based estimates. Am J Cardiol 82: 2N–9N.

One confounding variable in studying I_{KCa} is that the activity varies during the cardiac cycle in a calcium concentration-dependent manner. [32] To assess the role of I_{KCa} in an integrated system, we used perforated patch action potential recordings to permit maintenance of intrinsic calcium cycling, rather than conducting voltage clamp studies to assess the current.

We relied on a pharmacologic approach to define I_{KCa}. As with any pharmacologic approach there is a concern about non-specific effects. A recent report evaluated apamin selectivity in multiple human cardiac ion channels including L-type calcium channels, and confirmed the selectivity of apamin for I_{KCa} at 500 nM which is 5-fold higher than the concentration in the present study. [10] However, it has also been reported that apamin inhibits calcium current in neonatal chick and fetal cells. [46] These reported differences of apamin on calcium current may reflect maturation-dependent differences in channel subunit expression. [47] We did not directly evaluate the effects of apamin on calcium current, but our experimental system is closest to that in the recent report by Yu et al. [10], suggesting that block of calcium current was unlikely to mediate the observed effects of apamin in the present study.

Conclusions

These experiments highlight the need to evaluate novel therapeutic targets for arrhythmias in both atria and ventricles. In chronic HF, I_{KCa} plays a protective role in the ventricle and currrent block is proarrhythmic. Notably, in early HF (1 month canine HF), I_{KCa} blockade is not proarrhythmic, perhaps reflecting a relatively preserved repolarization reserve with a diminished dependence on I_{KCa} for repolarization stability compared to chronic HF.

We found that I_{KCa} does not play a role in repolarization in the atria as current block does not prolong the action potential in either human or canine HF. Similarly, I_{KCa} does not play a role in repolarization of the atrial AP during sustained AF with concurrent chronic HF, despite increased protein expression.

Collectively, our data do not support a role for I_{KCa} blockers for the treatment of atrial arrhythmias. Rather, our findings suggest that therapeutic strategies to reduce I_{KCa} may be unsafe in the setting of atrial arrhythmias with concurrent HF due to potential proarrhythmic effects in the ventricles.

Acknowledgments

Technical support provided by Jeanne Green and Destiny Allen. Human cardiac tissue was obtained through IRB approved protocols and also through collaboration of the Dorothy Davis Heart and Lung Research Institute of the Ohio State University Wexner Medical Center with the Lifeline of Ohio Organ Procurement program.

Author Contributions

Conceived and designed the experiments: IMB SG PJM CC. Performed the experiments: IMB VPL PVP PW AB QL. Analyzed the data: IMB VPL PVP PW AB JY PJM CC. Contributed reagents/materials/analysis tools: KM PFB PMLJ AK PJM. Contributed to the writing of the manuscript: IMB PVP VVF SG PJM CC.

2. Wang TJ, Larson MG, Levy D, Vasan RS, Leip EP, et al. (2003) Temporal relations of atrial fibrillation and congestive heart failure and their joint influence on mortality: the Framingham Heart Study. Circulation 107: 2920–2925. doi: 10.1161/01.CIR.0000072767.89944.6E.

3. Xu Y, Tuteja D, Zhang Z, Xu D, Zhang Y, et al. (2003) Molecular identification and functional roles of a Ca(2+)-activated K+ channel in human and mouse hearts. J Biol Chem 278: 49085–49094. doi: 10.1074/jbc.M307508200.

4. Vergara C, Latorre R, Marrion NV, Adelman JP (1998) Calcium-activated potassium channels. Curr Opin Neurobiol 8: 321–329. doi: 10.1016/S0959-4388(98)80056-1.

5. Ro S, Hatton WJ, Koh SD, Horowitz B (2001) Molecular properties of small-conductance Ca2+-activated K+ channels expressed in murine colonic smooth muscle. Am J Physiol Gastrointest Liver Physiol 281: G964–G973.

6. Tuteja D, Xu D, Timofeyev V, Lu L, Sharma D, et al. (2005) Differential expression of small-conductance Ca2+-activated K+ channels SK1, SK2, and SK3 in mouse atrial and ventricular myocytes. Am J Physiol Heart Circ Physiol 289: H2714–H2723. doi: 10.1152/ajpheart.00534.2005.

7. Xia XM, Fakler B, Rivard A, Wayman G, Johnson-Pais T, et al. (1998) Mechanism of calcium gating in small-conductance calcium-activated potassium channels. Nature 395: 503–507. doi: 10.1038/26758.

8. Wei AD, Gutman GA, Aldrich R, Chandy KG, Grissmer S, et al. (2005) International Union of Pharmacology. LII. Nomenclature and molecular relationships of calcium-activated potassium channels. Pharmacol Rev 57: 463–472. doi: 10.1124/pr.57.4.9.

9. Grunnet M, Jensen BS, Olesen SP, Klaerke DA (2001) Apamin interacts with all subtypes of cloned small-conductance Ca2+-activated K+ channels. Pflugers Arch 441: 544–550.

10. Yu CC, Ai T, Weiss JN, Chen PS (2014) Apamin does not inhibit human cardiac Na+ current, L-type Ca2+ current or other major K+ currents. PLoS One 9: e96691. doi: 10.1371/journal.pone.0096691 [doi];PONE-D-14-01991 [pii].

11. Li N, Timofeyev V, Tuteja D, Xu D, Lu L, et al. (2009) Ablation of a Ca2+-activated K+ channel (SK2 channel) results in action potential prolongation in atrial myocytes and atrial fibrillation. J Physiol 587: 1087–1100. doi: 10.1113/jphysiol.2008.167718.

12. Gui L, Bao Z, Jia Y, Qin X, Cheng ZJ, et al. (2013) Ventricular tachyarrhythmias in rats with acute myocardial infarction involves activation of small-conductance Ca2+-activated K+ channels. Am J Physiol Heart Circ Physiol 304: H118–H130. doi: 10.1152/ajpheart.00820.2011.

13. Chua SK, Chang PC, Maruyama M, Turker I, Shinohara T, et al. (2011) Small-conductance calcium-activated potassium channel and recurrent ventricular fibrillation in failing rabbit ventricles. Circ Res 108: 971–979. doi: 10.1161/CIRCRESAHA.110.238386.

14. Chang PC, Turker I, Lopshire JC, Masroor S, Nguyen BL, et al. (2013) Heterogeneous upregulation of apamin-sensitive potassium currents in failing human ventricles. J Am Heart Assoc 2: e004713. doi: 10.1161/JAHA.112.004713.

15. Qi XY, Diness JG, Brundel B, Zhou XB, Naud P, et al. (2013) Role of Small Conductance Calcium-Activated Potassium Channels in Atrial Electrophysiology and Fibrillation in the Dog. Circulation 430–440. doi: 10.1161/CIRCULATIONAHA.113.003019.

16. Hsueh CH, Chang PC, Hsieh YC, Reher T, Chen PS, et al. (2013) Proarrhythmic effect of blocking the small conductance calcium activated potassium channel in isolated canine left atrium. Heart Rhythm 10: 891–898. doi: 10.1016/j.hrthm.2013.01.033.

17. Nishijima Y, Feldman DS, Bonagura JD, Ozkanlar Y, Jenkins PJ, et al. (2005) Canine nonischemic left ventricular dysfunction: a model of chronic human cardiomyopathy. J Card Fail 11: 638–644. doi: 10.1016/j.cardfail.2005.05.006.

18. Terentyev D, Gyorke I, Belevych AE, Terentyeva R, Sridhar A, et al. (2008) Redox modification of ryanodine receptors contributes to sarcoplasmic reticulum Ca2+ leak in chronic heart failure. Circ Res 103: 1466–1472. doi: 10.1161/CIRCRESAHA.108.184457.

19. Nishijima Y, Feldman DS, Bonagura JD, Ozkanlar Y, Jenkins PJ, et al. (2005) Canine nonischemic left ventricular dysfunction: a model of chronic human cardiomyopathy. J Card Fail 11: 638–644.

20. Sridhar A, Nishijima Y, Terentyev D, Khan M, Terentyeva R, et al. (2009) Chronic heart failure and the substrate for atrial fibrillation. Cardiovasc Res 84: 227–236. doi: 10.1093/cvr/cvp216.

21. Nishijima Y, Sridhar A, Viatchenko-Karpinski S, Shaw C, Bonagura JD, et al. (2007) Chronic cardiac resynchronization therapy and reverse ventricular remodeling in a model of nonischemic cardiomyopathy. Life Sci 81: 1152–1159. doi: 10.1016/j.lfs.2007.08.022.

22. Bonilla IM, Sridhar A, Nishijima Y, Gyorke S, Cardounel AJ, et al. (2013) Differential effects of the peroxynitrite donor, SIN-1, on atrial and ventricular myocyte electrophysiology. J Cardiovasc Pharmacol 61: 401–407. doi: 10.1097/FJC.0b013e31828748ca.

23. Bonilla IM, Sridhar A, Gyorke S, Cardounel AJ, Carnes CA (2012) Nitric oxide synthases and atrial fibrillation. Front Physiol 3: 105. doi: 10.3389/fphys.2012.00105.

24. Thomsen MB, Volders PG, Beekman JD, Matz J, Vos MA (2006) Beat-to-Beat variability of repolarization determines proarrhythmic outcome in dogs susceptible to drug-induced torsades de pointes. J Am Coll Cardiol 48: 1268–1276. doi: 10.1016/j.jacc.2006.05.048.

25. Bonilla IM, Vargas-Pinto P, Nishijima Y, Pedraza-Toscano A, Ho HT, et al. (2013) Ibandronate and Ventricular Arrhythmia Risk. J Cardiovasc Electrophysiol. doi: 10.1111/jce.12327.

26. Weatherall KL, Seutin V, Liegeois JF, Marrion NV (2011) Crucial role of a shared extracellular loop in apamin sensitivity and maintenance of pore shape of small-conductance calcium-activated potassium (SK) channels. Proc Natl Acad Sci U S A 108: 18494–18499. doi: 10.1073/pnas.1110724108.

27. Weatherall KL, Goodchild SJ, Jane DE, Marrion NV (2010) Small conductance calcium-activated potassium channels: from structure to function. Prog Neurobiol 91: 242–255. doi: 10.1016/j.pneurobio.2010.03.002.

28. Grunnet M, Jespersen T, Angelo K, Frokjaer-Jensen C, Klaerke DA, et al. (2001) Pharmacological modulation of SK3 channels. Neuropharmacology 40: 879–887. doi: 10.1016/S0028-3908(01)00028-4.

29. Thomsen MB, Oros A, Schoenmakers M, van Opstal JM, Maas JN, et al. (2007) Proarrhythmic electrical remodelling is associated with increased beat-to-beat variability of repolarisation. Cardiovasc Res 73: 521–530. doi: 10.1016/j.cardiores.2006.11.025.

30. Bildl W, Strassmaier T, Thurm H, Andersen J, Eble S, et al. (2004) Protein kinase CK2 is coassembled with small conductance Ca(2+)-activated K+ channels and regulates channel gating. Neuron 43: 847–858. doi: 10.1016/j.neuron.2004.08.033.

31. Belevych AE, Terentyev D, Terentyeva R, Nishijima Y, Sridhar A, et al. (2011) The relationship between arrhythmogenesis and impaired contractility in heart failure: role of altered ryanodine receptor function. Cardiovasc Res 90: 493–502. doi: 10.1093/cvr/cvr025.

32. Terentyev D, Rochira JA, Terentyeva R, Roder K, Koren G, et al. (2013) Sarcoplasmic reticulum Ca2+ release is both necessary and sufficient for SK channel activation in ventricular myocytes. Am J Physiol Heart Circ Physiol In Press. doi: 10.1152/ajpheart.00621.2013.

33. Roden DM (1998) Taking the "idio" out of "idiosyncratic": predicting torsades de pointes. Pacing Clin Electrophysiol 21: 1029–1034.

34. Winslow RL, Rice J, Jafri S, Marban E, O'Rourke B (1999) Mechanisms of altered excitation-contraction coupling in canine tachycardia-induced heart failure, II: model studies. Circ Res 84: 571–586. doi: 10.1161/01.RES.84.5.571.

35. Kaab S, Nuss HB, Chiamvimonvat N, O'Rourke B, Pak PH, et al. (1996) Ionic mechanism of action potential prolongation in ventricular myocytes from dogs with pacing-induced heart failure. Circ Res 78: 262–273. doi: 10.1161/01.RES.78.2.262.

36. Nattel S (2009) Calcium-activated potassium current: a novel ion channel candidate in atrial fibrillation. J Physiol 587: 1385–1386. doi: 10.1113/jphysiol.2009.170621.

37. Workman AJ, Pau D, Redpath CJ, Marshall GE, Russell JA, et al. (2009) Atrial cellular electrophysiological changes in patients with ventricular dysfunction may predispose to AF. Heart Rhythm 6: 445–451. doi: 10.1016/j.hrthm.2008.12.028.

38. Schreieck J, Wang Y, Overbeck M, Schomig A, Schmitt C (2000) Altered transient outward current in human atrial myocytes of patients with reduced left ventricular function. J Cardiovasc Electrophysiol 11: 180–192.

39. Glukhov AV, Fedorov VV, Kalish PW, Ravikumar VK, Lou Q, et al. (2012) Conduction remodeling in human end-stage nonischemic left ventricular cardiomyopathy. Circulation 125: 1835–1847. doi: 10.1161/CIRCULATIONAHA.111.047274.

40. Chang SH, Chang SN, Hwang JJ, Chiang FT, Tseng CD, et al. (2012) Significant association of rs13376333 in KCNN3 on chromosome 1q21 with atrial fibrillation in a Taiwanese population. Circ J 76: 184–188. doi: 10.1253/circj.CJ-11-0525.

41. Ellinor PT, Lunetta KL, Glazer NL, Pfeufer A, Alonso A, et al. (2010) Common variants in KCNN3 are associated with lone atrial fibrillation. Nat Genet 42: 240–244. doi: 10.1038/ng.537.

42. Yu T, Deng C, Wu R, Guo H, Zheng S, et al. (2012) Decreased expression of small-conductance Ca2+-activated K+ channels SK1 and SK2 in human chronic atrial fibrillation. Life Sci 90: 219–227. doi: 10.1016/j.lfs.2011.11.008.

43. Kubalova Z, Terentyev D, Viatchenko-Karpinski S, Nishijima Y, Gyorke I, et al. (2005) Abnormal intrastore calcium signaling in chronic heart failure. Proc Natl Acad Sci U S A 102: 14104–14109. doi: 10.1073/pnas.0504298102.

44. Park YB (1994) Ion selectivity and gating of small conductance Ca(2+)-activated K+ channels in cultured rat adrenal chromaffin cells. J Physiol 481 (Pt 3): 555–570.

45. Van Wagoner DR, Pond AL, Lamorgese M, Rossie SS, McCarthy PM, et al. (1999) Atrial L-type Ca2+ currents and human atrial fibrillation. Circ Res 85: 428–436. doi: 10.1161/01.RES.85.5.428.

46. Bkaily G, Sculptoreanu A, Jacques D, Economos D, Menard D (1992) Apamin, a highly potent fetal L-type Ca2+ current blocker in single heart cells. Am J Physiol 262: H463–H471.

47. Brillantes AM, Bezprozvannaya S, Marks AR (1994) Developmental and tissue-specific regulation of rabbit skeletal and cardiac muscle calcium channels involved in excitation-contraction coupling. Circ Res 75: 503–510.

21

Intravenous Thrombolysis with Recombinant Tissue Plasminogen Activator for Ischemic Stroke Patients over 80 Years Old: The Fukuoka Stroke Registry

Ryu Matsuo[1,2], Masahiro Kamouchi[2,3]*, Haruhisa Fukuda[2,3], Jun Hata[1,3], Yoshinobu Wakisaka[1], Junya Kuroda[1], Tetsuro Ago[1], Takanari Kitazono[1,3], on behalf of the FSR Investigators

1 Department of Medicine and Clinical Science, Graduate School of Medical Sciences, Kyushu University, Fukuoka, Japan, 2 Department of Health Care Administration and Management, Graduate School of Medical Sciences, Kyushu University, Fukuoka, Japan, 3 Center for Cohort Studies, Graduate School of Medical Sciences, Kyushu University, Fukuoka, Japan

Abstract

Objectives: The benefit of intravenous recombinant tissue plasminogen activator (rt-PA) therapy for very old patients with acute ischemic stroke remains unclear. The aim of this study was to elucidate the efficacy and safety of intravenous rt-PA therapy for patients over 80 years old.

Methods: Of 13,521 stroke patients registered in the Fukuoka Stroke Registry in Japan from June 1999 to February 2013, 953 ischemic stroke patients who were over 80 years old, hospitalized within 3 h of onset, and not treated with endovascular therapy were included in this study. Among them, 153 patients were treated with intravenous rt-PA (0.6 mg/kg). For propensity score (PS)-matched case-control analysis, 148 patients treated with rt-PA and 148 PS-matched patients without rt-PA therapy were selected by 1:1 matching with propensity for using rt-PA. Clinical outcomes were neurological improvement, good functional outcome at discharge, in-hospital mortality, and hemorrhagic complications (any intracranial hemorrhage [ICH], symptomatic ICH, and gastrointestinal bleeding).

Results: In the full cohort of 953 patients, rt-PA use was associated positively with neurological improvement and good functional outcome, and negatively with in-hospital mortality after adjustment for multiple confounding factors. In PS-matched case-control analysis, patients treated with rt-PA were still at lower risk for unfavorable clinical outcomes than non-treated patients (neurological improvement, odds ratio 2.67, 95% confidence interval 1.61–4.40; good functional outcome, odds ratio 2.23, 95% confidence interval 1.16–4.29; in-hospital mortality, odds ratio 0.30, 95% confidence interval 0.13–0.65). There was no significant association between rt-PA use and risk of hemorrhagic complications in the full and PS-matched cohorts.

Conclusions: Intravenous rt-PA therapy was associated with improved clinical outcomes without significant increase in risk of hemorrhagic complications in very old patients (aged>80 years) with acute ischemic stroke.

Editor: Jens Minnerup, University of Münster, Germany

Funding: This study was supported by JSPS KAKENHI Grant Numbers 22249069 for MK, 24310024 for MK and TK, and 26293158 for MK, and Coordination, Support and Training Program for Translational Research from the Japanese Ministry of Education, Culture, Sports, Science and Technology for TK. The funders had no role in study design, data collection and analysis, decision to publish, or preparation of the manuscript.

Competing Interests: The authors read the journal's policy and stated the following competing interests: Takanari Kitazono received honoraria and grants from Mitsubishi Tanabe Pharma Corporation and Kyowa Hakko Kirin Co., Ltd.

* Email: kamouchi@hcam.med.kyushu-u.ac.jp

Introduction

Thrombolysis with intravenous recombinant tissue plasminogen activator (rt-PA) is currently the most effective therapy to improve clinical outcomes in patients with acute ischemic stroke [1]. However, the efficacy and safety of the therapy for very old patients are still controversial.

A large number of studies have reported that functional outcome and in-hospital mortality are unfavorable after throm-bolytic therapy in very old patients compared with those in younger patients [2]–[13]. Regarding the safety, it remains unclear whether thrombolysis is associated with an increased risk of adverse events, such as intracranial hemorrhage (ICH), in older patients. Although most previous studies have shown no significant difference in the occurrence of ICH after rt-PA therapy between very old and young patients [2]–[10], [12]–[18], a recent study using the National Impatient Sample Database revealed a significantly higher risk of ICH after thrombolysis in very old versus younger patients [11].

Because of the poor prognosis and hemorrhagic complications after thrombolysis in older adults, randomized controlled trials have typically excluded patients>80 years old [1]. Therefore, evidence for the benefit of thrombolytic therapy in very old individuals remains scarce and the therapy is currently withheld in very old patients with acute ischemic stroke. Recently, the Third International Stroke Trial (IST-3) enrolled ischemic stroke patients up to 6 h from onset without upper age limit to determine whether intravenous thrombolysis with rt-PA is beneficial to a wider range of patients [19]. Consequently, the effect of thrombolysis within 6 h of onset in elderly patients seemed to be at least as large as that in younger patients [20]. As life expectancy is increasing worldwide, data regarding whether to treat very old stroke patients with thrombolysis are important.

Since Asians are more likely to suffer intracranial hemorrhage than non-Asians [21], the effect of rt-PA in very old patients should be validated in different cohorts including an Asian population. In this study, we investigated the association between rt-PA use and clinical outcomes among Japanese patients over 80 years old who were hospitalized within 3 h of onset using a database of acute stroke in the overall cohort and a propensity score (PS)-matched cohort. The aim of this study was to elucidate whether intravenous thrombolysis with rt-PA is efficacious and safe even in very old patients in an Asian setting.

Methods

The Fukuoka Stroke Registry

The Fukuoka Stroke Registry (FSR) is a multicenter hospital-based registry in which acute stroke patients within 7 days of onset were enrolled (UMIN Clinical Trial Registry 000000800) [22], [23]. Kyushu University Hospital, National Hospital Organization Kyushu Medical Center, National Hospital Organization Fukuoka-Higashi Medical Center, Fukuoka Red Cross Hospital, St. Mary's Hospital, Steel Memorial Yawata Hospital, and the Japan Labor Health and Welfare Organization Kyushu Rosai Hospital in Fukuoka, Japan participate in this registry (Text S1). Standardized instruments were used to collect demographic characteristics, co-morbidities, laboratory data, and medical histories of the patients.

Study subjects

Stroke was defined as sudden onset of focal neurological deficits persisting for more than 24 h and classified into ischemic stroke, brain hemorrhage, subarachnoid hemorrhage, or other types of stroke by means of brain imaging (computed tomography [CT] and/or magnetic resonance imaging). In a total of 13,521 patients registered in the FSR retrospective (7387 patients from June 1999 to May 2007) and prospective (6134 patients from June 2007 to February 2013) databases, 11,432 patients were diagnosed as having ischemic stroke. Among them, 972 patients who were aged older than 80 years and hospitalized within 3 h after onset were selected. After excluding 19 patients who underwent endovascular therapy, we included 953 patients (506 patients in retrospective and 447 patients in prospective cohorts) as the full cohort of this study.

Patients in the full cohort were further divided into two groups according to whether they were admitted before or after approval of intravenous administration of rt-PA (alteplase in Japan). Accordingly, 336 patients were included in the pre-marketing phase (June 1999 to September 2005) and 617 patients in the post-marketing phase (October 2005 to February 2013). In the post-

marketing phase, 153 cases were treated with intravenous administration of rt-PA. Patient eligibility for alteplase was determined in accordance with a Japanese guideline [24], and alteplase was administered in 25.9% of patients of all ages who were hospitalized within 3 h from onset in the post-marketing phase. Each patient received alteplase (0.6 mg/kg) intravenously with 10% given as a bolus within 3 h of stroke onset and the remainder was delivered through continuous intravenous infusion over 1 h. PS-matched controls were selected from ischemic stroke patients who were aged older than 80 years and hospitalized within 3 h of onset during the pre-marketing phase. After calculating PS, 148 cases and 148 PS-matched controls were selected for PS-matched analysis (Figure 1).

Clinical assessment

Hypertension was defined as systolic blood pressure ≥140 mm Hg or diastolic blood pressure ≥90 mm Hg in the chronic stage, or as a previous history of treatment with antihypertensive drugs. Dyslipidemia was defined as a low-density lipoprotein-cholesterol level ≥3.62 mmol/L, high-density lipoprotein-cholesterol level ≤ 1.03 mmol/L, triglyceride level ≥1.69 mmol/L, or a previous history of treatment with a lipid-lowering drug. Diabetes mellitus was determined by either the diagnostic criteria of the Japan Diabetes Society in the chronic stage or based on a medical history of diabetes. Atrial fibrillation was diagnosed based on electrocardiographic findings on admission or during hospitalization, or a

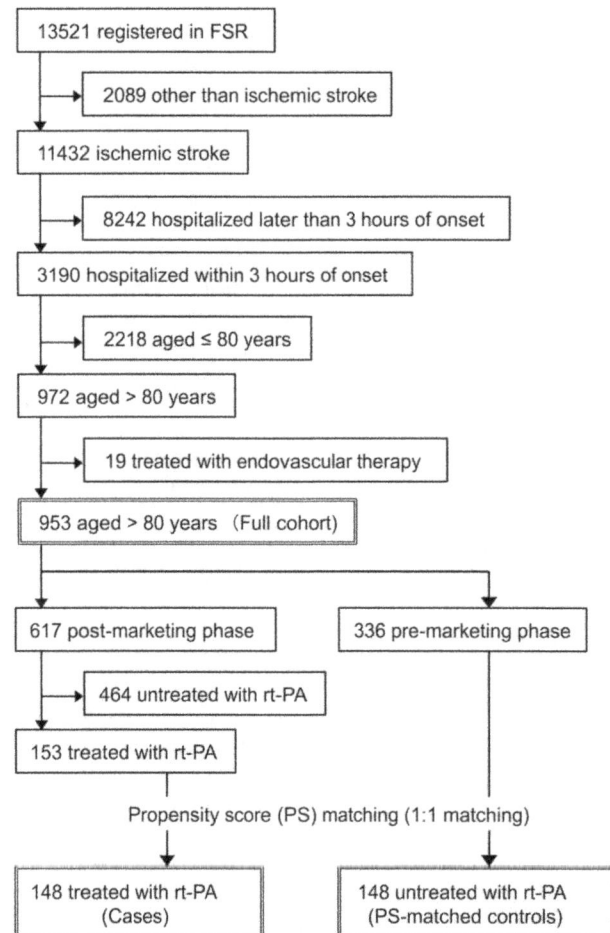

Figure 1. Flow chart of patient selection.

Table 1. Baseline characteristics in rt-PA-treated and non-treated patients in the full cohort.

	rt-PA treated	rt-PA non-treated	P
	n = 153	n = 800	
Age, years, median (IQR)	86 (84–89)	85 (83–88)	0.09
Female, n (%)	96 (62.7)	489 (61.1)	0.71
Risk factors, n (%)			
Hypertension	117 (76.5)	602 (75.3)	0.75
Dyslipidemia	47 (30.7)	200 (25.0)	0.15
Diabetes	28 (18.3)	187 (23.4)	0.16
Atrial fibrillation	94 (61.4)	396 (49.5)	0.007
Smoking	41 (26.8)	198 (24.8)	0.59
Drinking	26 (17.0)	125 (15.6)	0.67
Chronic kidney disease, n (%)	83 (54.2)	446 (55.8)	0.73
Pre-stroke independency, n (%)	108 (70.6)	474 (59.3)	0.007
Previous stroke, n (%)	29 (19.0)	243 (30.4)	0.003
Previous ischemic heart disease, n (%)	38 (24.8)	165 (20.6)	0.25
Pre-stroke antithrombotic therapy, n (%)	76 (49.7)	352 (44.0)	0.20
Cardioembolic stroke, n (%)	108 (70.6)	406 (50.8)	<0.001
Admission within 2 hours from onset, n (%)	136 (88.9)	586 (73.3)	<0.001
Systolic blood pressure, mmHg, mean ± SD	156±27	161±31	0.045
NIHSS on admission, median (IQR)	16 (9.5–21)	9 (3–16.75)	<0.001
Length of hospital stay, days, mean ± SD	31.8±17.6	33.1±25.1	0.53

IQR: interquartile range. Pre-stroke independency was defined as mRS 0–1 before onset.

previous history of atrial fibrillation. Smoking was defined as current or former cigarette smoking, and alcohol intake was defined as habitual consumption of alcohol beverages before onset of stroke. Chronic kidney disease was defined as an estimated glomerular filtration rate (eGFR) <60 mL/min per 1.73 m^2, in which eGFR was determined using the equation proposed by the Japanese Society of Nephrology as follows: eGFR (mL/min per 1.73 m^2) = 194×(serum creatinine [mg/dL])$^{1.094}$×age [year])$^{-0.287}$×0.739 (if female) [25]. Ischemic heart disease was defined as a previous history of angina pectoris, myocardial infarction, and percutaneous coronary intervention or coronary artery bypass graft surgery. Pre-stroke independency was defined as a modified Rankin Scale (mRS) score of 0–1 before stroke onset.

Study outcomes

Neurological severity was scaled by the National Institutes of Health Stroke Scale (NIHSS) score on admission and at discharge. The average length of stay was 32.9±22.3 days. Neurological improvement was defined as a ≥4 point decrease in the NIHSS score during hospitalization or a NIHSS score of 0 at discharge [26]. In-hospital mortality was defined as all causes of death during hospitalization. To evaluate the short-term functional outcome, post-stroke functional impairment at discharge was graded using an mRS. A good outcome was defined as functional independence (mRS score of 0–2). To evaluate the safety of rt-PA, three types of hemorrhagic complications were assessed during hospitalization: any ICH, symptomatic ICH, and gastrointestinal bleeding. ICH was determined by using CT irrespective of neurological worsening, and symptomatic ICH was defined as any type of CT-documented hemorrhage either within the infarct area or in other areas, concomitant with any neurological worsening.

Gastrointestinal bleeding was defined as any episodes of hematemesis or melena during hospitalization.

PS matching and statistical analysis

Baseline characteristics were compared by the χ^2 test or the McNemar-Bowker test, the unpaired or paired t test, and the Wilcoxon rank sum test or the Wilcoxon signed rank test, as appropriate. In the full cohort model, logistic regression analyses were used to estimate multivariable-adjusted odds ratios and 95% confidence intervals for study outcomes. Statistical analyses were performed using JMP software ver. 11 (SAS Institute, Cary, NC, USA). The probability of receiving rt-PA therapy (PS) was calculated for the rt-PA-treated and the non-treated patients using a logistic regression model. Eighteen covariates, including age, sex, hypertension, dyslipidemia, diabetes, atrial fibrillation, smoking, drinking, ischemic heart disease, chronic kidney disease, pre-stroke independency, previous stroke, antithrombotic therapy before onset, cardioembolic stroke, NIHSS on admission, admission within 2 h from onset, systolic blood pressure, and length of hospital stay were used to generate PS. After PS generation, patients treated with rt-PA and those untreated with rt-PA underwent 1:1 nearest neighbor (Greedy-type) matching of the standard deviation of the logit of the PS with a caliper width of 0.25. Matching was performed without replacement, and unpaired cases and controls not meeting matching criteria were excluded. Each PS-derived matched pair was assigned a unique pair ID. A total of 148 matched pair IDs were selected. Calculation of PS and 1:1 matching were performed using STATA13 (StataCorp LP, College Station, TX, USA). In the PS-matched cohort model, odds ratios of clinical outcomes were calculated after matching using conditional logistic regression analysis. Probability values of <0.05 were considered statistically significant.

Table 2. Association between rt-PA and clinical outcomes in the full cohort.

	Events (%)		Age- and sex-adjusted			Multivariable-adjusted		
	rt-PA-treated n = 153	rt-PA non-treated n = 800	OR	95% CI	P	OR	95% CI	P
Neurological improvement	95 (62.1)	295 (36.9)	2.90	2.03–4.18	<0.001	2.60	1.77–3.84	<0.001
Good functional outcome	39 (25.5)	199 (24.9)	1.12	0.74–1.69	0.58	3.09	1.66–5.83	<0.001
In-hospital mortality	13 (8.5)	97 (12.1)	0.66	0.34–1.17	0.16	0.31	0.15–0.61	<0.001
Any ICH	19 (12.4)	49 (6.1)	2.20	1.23–3.81	0.009	1.75	0.96–3.09	0.07
Symptomatic ICH	8 (5.2)	23 (2.9)	1.95	0.80–4.29	0.13	1.82	0.73–4.16	0.19
Gastrointestinal bleeding	4 (2.6)	13 (1.6)	1.72	0.48–4.97	0.37	1.56	0.42–3.46	0.48

OR: odds ratio, CI: confidence interval, ICH: intracranial hemorrhage. Neurological improvement was defined as a ≥4 point decrease in the NIHSS score during hospitalization or a NIHSS score of 0 at discharge. Good functional outcome was defined as an mRS score of 0–2 at discharge. Multivariable logistic model for neurological improvement, good functional outcome, and in-hospital mortality included age, sex, hypertension, dyslipidemia, diabetes, atrial fibrillation, smoking, drinking, chronic kidney disease, pre-stroke independency, previous stroke, previous ischemic heart disease, pre-antithrombotic therapy, cardioembolic stroke, admission within 2 h of onset, and NIHSS on admission. Multivariable logistic model for ICH, symptomatic ICH, and gastrointestinal bleeding included age, sex, systolic blood pressure, diabetes, chronic kidney disease, and NIHSS on admission.

Ethics Statement

The study design was approved by the institutional review boards and ethics committees of all hospitals (Kyushu University Hospital Institutional Review Board, National Hospital Organization Kyushu Medical Center Institutional Review Board, National Hospital Organization Fukuoka-Higashi Medical Center Institutional Review Board, Fukuoka Red Cross Hospital Institutional Review Board, St. Mary's Hospital Institutional Review Board, Steel Memorial Yawata Hospital Institutional Review Board, and the Japan Labor Health and Welfare Organization Kyushu Rosai Hospital Institutional Review Board). The study was conducted according to the principles expressed in the Declaration of Helsinki. For the retrospective database, we reviewed medical records of all consecutive patients with acute stroke who were hospitalized in participating hospitals within 24 h of onset. The institutional review boards waived the requirement for obtaining informed consent from patients in retrospective database, because medical information had been collected as part of routine clinical care and processed into anonymized database. In prospective database, written informed consent was obtained from each patient or his/her proxy [22], [23].

Results

Background characteristics in the full cohort

Background characteristics of ischemic stroke patients who were over 80 years old and hospitalized within 3 h of onset are shown according to treatment with or without intravenous administration of rt-PA (Table 1). The frequency of atrial fibrillation, pre-stroke independency, cardioembolic stroke, and admission within 2 h from onset was significantly higher, but the prevalence of previous stroke was less frequent, in rt-PA-treated versus rt-PA non-treated patients. Systolic blood pressure on admission was lower and neurological symptoms were more severe in rt-PA treated patients compared with those without rt-PA. The numbers of patients aged 81–85 years, 86–90 years, 91–95 years and ≥96 years were 478 (50.2%), 326 (34.2%), 119 (12.5%), and 30 (3.1%), respectively. In the post-marketing period, 307 (49.8%), 206 (33.4%), 78 (12.6%), and 26 (4.2%) patients were aged 81–85 years, 86–90 years, 91–95 years and ≥96 years, respectively, and the frequencies of patients treated with rt-PA therapy were 23.4%, 25.7%, 25.6%, and 30.8% in each age range, respectively.

Treatment with rt-PA and clinical outcomes in the full cohort

Without adjustment for background characteristics, the severity of neurological symptoms at discharge was comparable between rt-PA treated (NIHSS score: median 7, interquartile range [IQR] 1–16) and non-treated (NIHSS score: median 6, IQR 1–15.75; P = 0.73) patients. Further, mRS at discharge was not different between patients with (median 4, IQR 2–5) and without (median 4, IQR 3–5; P = 0.27) intravenous rt-PA.

Next, we performed multivariable logistic regression analysis to adjust for possible confounding factors. Age- and sex- or multivariable-adjusted odds ratios for each clinical outcome are shown in Table 2. Consequently, use of rt-PA was positively associated with neurological improvement and good functional outcome and inversely with in-hospital mortality after adjustment for confounders. The age- and sex-adjusted risk of any ICH was higher in the rt-PA treated group than the rt-PA non-treated group, but this association failed to reach significance after adjustment for multiple confounding factors. rt-PA treatment was not associated with risk of symptomatic ICH and gastrointestinal bleeding.

Table 3. Baseline characteristics in rt-PA-treated and non-treated patients in the PS-matched cohort.

	rt-PA treated	rt-PA non-treated	P
	n = 148	n = 148	
Age, years, median (IQR)	86 (84–89)	86 (83–90)	0.88
Female, n (%)	93 (62.8)	99 (66.9)	0.47
Risk factors, n (%)			
Hypertension	112 (75.7)	112 (75.7)	1.00
Dyslipidemia	43 (29.1)	42 (28.4)	0.90
Diabetes	28 (18.9)	33 (22.3)	0.47
Atrial fibrillation	91 (61.5)	85 (57.4)	0.48
Smoking	39 (26.4)	38 (25.7)	0.89
Drinking	24 (16.2)	25 (16.9)	0.88
Chronic kidney disease, n (%)	81 (54.7)	84 (56.8)	0.73
Pre-stroke independency, n (%)	103 (69.6)	105 (70.9)	0.80
Previous stroke, n (%)	29 (19.6)	27 (18.2)	0.77
Previous ischemic heart disease, n (%)	34 (23.0)	38 (25.7)	0.59
Pre-stroke antithrombotic therapy, n (%)	72 (48.6)	66 (44.6)	0.48
Cardioembolic stroke, n (%)	105 (70.9)	96 (64.9)	0.26
Admission within 2 hours from onset, n (%)	131 (88.5)	127 (85.8)	0.49
Systolic blood pressure, mmHg, mean ± SD	156±28	157±30	0.87
NIHSS on admission, median (IQR)	16 (9.25–21)	16 (9–21)	0.86
Length of hospital stay, days, mean ± SD	31.8±17.8	31.8±23.0	0.98

IQR: interquartile range. Pre-stroke independency was defined as an mRS score of 0–1 before onset.

Background characteristics in the PS-matched cohort

To control confounding factors by indication, we calculated PS of rt-PA-treated cases and randomly selected one control that had a similar PS to each case. The mean standardized difference in covariates decreased from 19.1% (range 1.2–75.7%) before matching to 4.3% (range 0–12.7%) after matching (Figure S1). After 1:1 matching, covariates were statistically indistinguishable between rt-PA-treated cases and PS-matched rt-PA-non-treated controls (Table 3).

Treatment with rt-PA and clinical outcomes in the PS-matched cohort

In the PS-matched cohort, neurological symptoms were less severe at discharge in rt-PA-treated (NIHSS score: median 7, IQR 1–16) compared with PS-matched non-treated (NIHSS score: median 13, IQR 4–26; P<0.001) patients. Further, mRS at discharge was significantly lower in rt-PA-treated (median 4, IQR 2.25–5) compared with non-treated (median 5, IQR 4–5; P< 0.001) patients. Incident rates and odds ratios of clinical outcomes and hemorrhagic complications are shown in Table 4. Intravenous rt-PA therapy was associated positively with neurological improvement and good functional outcome, and negatively with in-hospital mortality. The frequencies of hemorrhagic complications, including any ICH, symptomatic ICH, and gastrointestinal bleeding were not statistically different between rt-PA-treated and PS-matched non-treated patients.

Table 4. Association between rt-PA and clinical outcomes in the PS-matched cohort.

	Events (%)		Unadjusted		
	rt-PA-treated, n = 148	rt-PA non-treated, n = 148	OR	95% CI	P
Neurological improvement	91 (61.5)	56 (37.8)	2.67	1.61–4.40	<0.001
Good functional outcome	37 (25.0)	21 (14.2)	2.23	1.16–4.29	0.02
In-hospital mortality	13 (8.8)	32 (21.6)	0.30	0.13–0.65	0.003
Any ICH	17 (11.5)	12 (8.1)	1.45	0.68–3.13	0.34
Symptomatic ICH	7 (4.7)	6 (4.1)	1.17	0.39–3.47	0.78
Gastrointestinal bleeding	4 (2.7)	3 (2.0)	1.33	0.30–5.96	0.71

OR: odds ratio, CI: confidence interval, ICH: intracranial hemorrhage. Neurological improvement was defined as a ≥4 point decrease in the NIHSS score during hospitalization or a NIHSS score of 0 at discharge. Good functional outcome was defined as an mRS score of 0–2 at discharge.

Discussion

The main findings of the present study were that in patients aged over 80 years, (1) rt-PA was associated positively with neurological improvement and good functional outcome, and negatively with in-hospital mortality, and (2) there was no association between rt-PA use and hemorrhagic complications, including any ICH, symptomatic ICH, and gastrointestinal bleeding. These data support the idea that thrombolytic therapy using intravenous rt-PA is efficacious without increasing risk of harmful hemorrhagic complications in Japanese patients over 80 years old.

A number of studies have investigated the benefit of thrombolytic therapy in very old patients (aged>80 years) compared with younger patients. However, the majority of studies suggest that clinical outcomes are unfavorable after thrombolytic therapy in very old compared with younger patients [2]–[13]. Recently, we have also reported that poor functional outcome and in-hospital mortality were more prevalent after thrombolytic therapy in older patients compared with younger ones [27]. Because the prognosis is generally poor in older versus younger patients, further understanding of the benefit of thrombolytic therapy among elderly patients is required. Therefore, in the present study, we compared the efficacy and safety of intravenous thrombolysis among patients over 80 years old in the overall cohort and a PS-matched cohort to control confounding factors by indication.

There are few studies that have investigated the efficacy of rt-PA therapy among patients aged>80 years. Alshekhlee et al. reported that the odds ratio of in-hospital mortality was increased to 1.38 (95% confidence interval 1.22–1.58) in patients>80 years old treated with thrombolysis compared with non-treated patients [11]. Sung et al. found no difference in the frequency of home discharges and mRS $\leq$2 between rt-PA-treated and rt-PA-non-treated patients $\geq$80 years with acute ischemic stroke [17]. However, a recent study using the database of Safe Implementation of Treatment in Stroke-International Stroke Thrombolysis Registry (SITS-ISTR, December 2002 to November 2009) and Virtual International Stroke Trials Archive (VISTA, 1998–2007) showed that improved outcome was maintained in very old patients [28]. Additionally, IST-3 enrolled acute ischemic stroke patients up to 6 h of stroke onset without upper age limit from non-Asian countries. Though 53% were older than 80 years of age and 72% were treated between 3 h and 6 h of onset in IST-3, intravenous thrombolytic therapy seemed to have favorable effects on functional outcome in very old patients [20]. Therefore, age alone may not be a barrier to treatment. In this study, approximately half of patients were distributed in their early eighties. However, intravenous thrombolysis with rt-PA was performed equally throughout all age ranges. Thus, in the clinical setting rt-PA therapy is performed even in extremely old patients irrespective of age. We found that intravenous rt-PA therapy was significantly associated with favorable outcomes after adjustment for possible confounding factors in the full cohort of patients aged over 80 years. Moreover, PS-matched analysis revealed that the relative risk of poor functional outcome and in-hospital mortality was reduced by 13% and 59%, respectively, after intravenous thrombolysis. Our results support the idea that clinical outcomes are improved by thrombolysis even in older patients in an Asian setting.

We also investigated the frequency of hemorrhagic complications to evaluate the safety of thrombolysis using intravenous alteplase. Most previous studies report that the risk of hemorrhagic complications after thrombolysis was not higher in very older patients than in younger subjects [2]–[10], [12]–[18]. By contrast, Alshekhlee et al. reported that use of thrombolysis was associated with increased risk of ICH (odds ratio 9.69, 95% confidence interval 6.25–15.02) in older patients after adjustment for multiple confounding factors [11]. In our study, there was no difference in the incidence of hemorrhagic complications such as symptomatic ICH and gastrointestinal bleeding, suggesting that intravenous thrombolysis may not cause significant harm to very old patients.

In October 2005, the use of intravenous alteplase was approved as a treatment for acute ischemic stroke in Japan. As the Asian population has a higher risk for spontaneous brain hemorrhage [21], the dose of alteplase approved for Japanese patients was as low as 0.6 mg/kg based on data from the Japan Alteplase Clinical Trial (J-ACT) [29]. Nonetheless, the frequency of symptomatic ICH in J-ACT (17%) was comparable to that in elderly patients reported in other observational studies from Europe or North America (3–14%). Low-dose rt-PA might reduce the risk of hemorrhagic complications, but not improve clinical outcomes due to thrombus lysis. Our data suggest that low-dose intravenous alteplase (0.6 mg/kg) provides greater benefit than harm in Japanese patients aged>80 years. The optimal dose and benefit of intravenous rt-PA in very old patients should be validated in other cohorts.

The present study has strengths. The benefit of intravenous thrombolysis in very old patients was evaluated using PS matching. To avoid confounding by indication, controls were selected from those enrolled before approval of intravenous alteplase. Patients in the registry were consecutively enrolled based on the standardized measurement. There are also limitations in our study. First, the number of patients over 80 years old was still small and hemorrhagic events rarely occurred. Second, background characteristics could not be completely adjusted for. A progress in stroke care may have affected the results, although possible confounders were included in multivariable adjustment or PS. Third, the generalizability is problematic, because patients were selected from those admitted to one university hospital and six community hospitals in the restricted region of Japan. Additionally, the dose of rt-PA was lower than that in other countries. External validation is required to confirm our findings.

Acknowledgments

We thank all FSR investigators and their hospitals for participating in this study, and all clinical research coordinators (Hisayama Research Institute for Lifestyle Diseases) for help in obtaining informed consent and collecting clinical data.

Author Contributions

Conceived and designed the experiments: RM MK HF JH YW JK TA TK. Performed the experiments: RM MK JH YW JK TA TK. Analyzed the data: RM MK HF JH. Wrote the paper: RM MK. Contributed to interpretation of data: RM MK HF JH YW JK TA TK. Critically revised the manuscript: HF JH YW JK TA TK. Approved the final version: RM MK HF JH YW JK TA TK.

References

1. The National Institute of Neurological Disorders and Stroke rt-PA Stroke Study Group (1995) Tissue plasminogen activator for acute ischemic stroke. N Engl J Med 333: 1581–1587.

2. Berrouschot J, Rother J, Glahn J, Kucinski T, Fiehler J, et al. (2005) Outcome and severe hemorrhagic complications of intravenous thrombolysis with tissue plasminogen activator in very old (≥80 years) stroke patients. Stroke 36: 2421–2425.

3. Engelter ST, Reichhart M, Sekoranja L, Georgiadis D, Baumann A, et al. (2005) Thrombolysis in stroke patients aged 80 years and older: Swiss survey of IV thrombolysis. Neurology 65: 1795–1798.

4. Mouradian MS, Senthilselvan A, Jickling G, McCombe JA, Emery DJ, et al. (2005) Intravenous rt-PA for acute stroke: Comparing its effectiveness in younger and older patients. J Neurol Neurosurg Psychiatry 76: 1234–1237.

5. Engelter ST, Bonati LH, Lyrer PA (2006) Intravenous thrombolysis in stroke patients of ≥80 versus <80 years of age-a systematic review across cohort studies. Age Ageing 35: 572–580.

6. Sylaja PN, Cote R, Buchan AM, Hill MD (2006) Thrombolysis in patients older than 80 years with acute ischaemic stroke: Canadian Alteplase for Stroke Effectiveness Study. J Neurol Neurosurg Psychiatry 77: 826–829.

7. van Oostenbrugge RJ, Hupperts RM, Lodder J (2006) Thrombolysis for acute stroke with special emphasis on the very old: experience from a single Dutch centre. J Neurol Neurosurg Psychiatry 77: 375–377.

8. Ringleb PA, Schwark C, Kohrmann M, Kulkens S, Juttler E, et al. (2007) Thrombolytic therapy for acute ischaemic stroke in octogenarians: selection by magnetic resonance imaging improves safety but does not improve outcome. J Neurol Neurosurg Psychiatry 78: 690–693.

9. Zeevi N, Chhabra J, Silverman IE, Lee NS, McCullough LD (2007) Acute stroke management in the elderly. Cerebrovasc Dis 23: 304–308.

10. Toni D, Lorenzano S, Agnelli G, Guidetti D, Orlandi G, et al. (2008) Intravenous thrombolysis with rt-PA in acute ischemic stroke patients aged older than 80 years in Italy. Cerebrovasc Dis 25: 129–135.

11. Alshekhlee A, Mohammadi A, Mehta S, Edgell RC, Vora N, et al. (2010) Is thrombolysis safe in the elderly? Analysis of a national database. Stroke 41: 2259–2264.

12. Ford GA, Ahmed N, Azevedo E, Grond M, Larrue V, et al. (2010) Intravenous alteplase for stroke in those older than 80 years old. Stroke 41: 2568–2574.

13. Bhatnagar P, Sinha D, Parker RA, Guyler P, O'Brien A (2011) Intravenous thrombolysis in acute ischaemic stroke: a systematic review and meta-analysis to aid decision making in patients over 80 years of age. J Neurol Neurosurg Psychiatry 82: 712–717.

14. Tanne D, Gorman MJ, Bates VE, Kasner SE, Scott P, et al. (2000) Intravenous tissue plasminogen activator for acute ischemic stroke in patients aged 80 years and older: the tPA stroke survey experience. Stroke 31: 370–375.

15. Chen CI, Iguchi Y, Grotta JC, Garami Z, Uchino K, et al. (2005) Intravenous TPA for very old stroke patients. Eur Neurol 54: 140–144.

16. Gomez-Choco M, Obach V, Urra X, Amaro S, Cervera A, et al. (2008) The response to IV rt-PA in very old stroke patients. Eur J Neurol 15: 253–256.

17. Sung PS, Chen CH, Hsieh HC, Fang CW, Hsieh CY, et al. (2011) Outcome of acute ischemic stroke in very elderly patients: is intravenous thrombolysis beneficial? Eur Neurol 66: 110–116.

18. Koga M, Shiokawa Y, Nakagawara J, Furui E, Kimura K, et al. (2012) Low-dose intravenous recombinant tissue-type plasminogen activator therapy for patients with stroke outside European indications: Stroke Acute Management with Urgent Risk-factor Assessment and Improvement (SAMURAI) rtPA Registry. Stroke 43: 253–255.

19. Sandercock P, Lindley R, Wardlaw J, Dennis M, Lewis S, et al. (2008) Third international stroke trial (IST-3) of thrombolysis for acute ischaemic stroke. Trials 9: 37.

20. Sandercock P, Wardlaw JM, Lindley RI, Dennis M, Cohen G, et al. (2012) The benefits and harms of intravenous thrombolysis with recombinant tissue plasminogen activator within 6 h of acute ischaemic stroke (the third international stroke trial [IST-3]): a randomised controlled trial. Lancet 379: 2352–2363.

21. Toyoda K (2009) Pharmacotherapy for the secondary prevention of stroke. Drugs 69: 633–647.

22. Kamouchi M, Matsuki T, Hata J, Kuwashiro T, Ago T, et al. (2011) Prestroke glycemic control is associated with the functional outcome in acute ischemic stroke: the Fukuoka Stroke Registry. Stroke 42: 2788–2794.

23. Kumai Y, Kamouchi M, Hata J, Ago T, Kitayama J, et al. (2012) Proteinuria and clinical outcomes after ischemic stroke. Neurology 78: 1909–1915.

24. Shinohara Y, Yamaguchi T (2008) Outline of the Japanese Guidelines for the Management of Stroke 2004 and subsequent revision. Int J Stroke 3: 55–62.

25. Matsuo S, Imai E, Horio M, Yasuda Y, Tomita K, et al. (2009) Revised equations for estimated GFR from serum creatinine in Japan. Am J Kidney Dis 53: 982–992.

26. Yong M, Kaste M (2008) Dynamic of hyperglycemia as a predictor of stroke outcome in the ECASS-II trial. Stroke 39: 2749–2755.

27. Matsuo R, Kamouchi M, Ago T, Hata J, Shono Y, et al. (2013) Thrombolytic therapy with intravenous recombinant tissue plasminogen activator in Japanese older patients with acute ischemic stroke: Fukuoka Stroke Registry. Geriatr Gerontol Int DOI: 10.1111/ggi.12205. In press.

28. Mishra NK, Ahmed N, Andersen G, Egido JA, Lindsberg PJ, et al. (2010) Thrombolysis in very elderly people: controlled comparison of SITS International Stroke Thrombolysis Registry and Virtual International Stroke Trials Archive. BMJ 341: c6046.

29. Yamaguchi T, Mori E, Minematsu K, Nakagawara J, Hashi K, et al. (2006) Alteplase at 0.6 mg/kg for acute ischemic stroke within 3 hours of onset: Japan Alteplase Clinical Trial (J-ACT). Stroke 37: 1810–1815.

22

Impact of Body Mass Index on Plasma N-Terminal ProB-Type Natriuretic Peptides in Chinese Atrial Fibrillation Patients without Heart Failure

Li-hui Zheng, Ling-min Wu, Yan Yao*, Wen-sheng Chen, Jing-ru Bao, Wen Huang, Rui Shi, Kui-jun Zhang, Shu Zhang

State Key Laboratory of Cardiovascular Disease, Clinical EP Lab & Arrhythmia Center, Fuwai Hospital, National Center for Cardiovascular Diseases, Chinese Academy of Medical Sciences and Peking Union Medical College, Beijing, China

Abstract

Background: An inverse relationship between body mass index (BMI) and circulating levels of N-terminal proB-type natriuretic peptide (NT-proBNP) has been demonstrated in subjects with and without heart failure. Obesity also has been linked with increased incidence of atrial fibrillation (AF), but its influence on NT-proBNP concentrations in AF patients remains unclear. This study aimed to investigate the effect of BMI on NT-proBNP levels in AF patients without heart failure.

Methods: A total of 239 consecutive patients with AF undergoing catheter ablation were evaluated. Levels of NT-proBNP and clinical characteristics were compared in overweight or obese (BMI$\geq$25 kg/m^2) and normal weight (BMI$<$25 kg/m^2) patients.

Results: Of 239 patients, 129 (54%) were overweight or obese. Overweight or obese patients were younger, more likely to have a history of nonparoxysmal AF, hypertension, and diabetes mellitus. Levels of NT-proBNP were significantly lower in overweight or obese than in normal weight subjects (P$<$0.05). The relationship of obesity and decreased NT-proBNP levels persisted in subgroup of hypertension, both gender and both age levels ($\geq$65 yrs and $<$65 yrs).Multivariate linear regression identified BMI as an independent negative correlate of LogNT-proBNP level.

Conclusions: An inverse relationship between BMI and plasma NT-proBNP concentrations have been demonstrated in AF patients without heart failure. Overweight or obese patients with AF appear to have lower NT-proBNP levels than normal weight patients.

Editor: Marta Letizia Hribal, University of Catanzaro Magna Graecia, Italy

Funding: The authors have no support or funding to report.

Competing Interests: The authors have declared that no competing interests exist.

* Email: ianyao@263.net.cn

Introduction

B-type natriuretic peptide (BNP) is synthesized as preproBNP in response to the stretch and pressure overload of the cardiac myocyte. After enzymatic cleavage, it is released into the circulation system in equimolar proportions as the hormonally active BNP and the inactive N-terminal fragment (N-terminal-pro-B-type natriuretic peptide, NT-proBNP).The expression of NT-proBNP is affected by several variations, such as age, gender, hypertension, renal function and thyroid function [1].

Several recent reports suggest that obesity, as indexed by elevated body mass index (BMI), may also affect NT-proBNP levels, with lower circulating levels in those with higher BMI in subjects with acute or chronic heart failure [2,3], significant coronary artery disease or acute myocardial infarction [4,5] and healthy general populations [6]. However, isolated study showed that obesity is not statistically associated with NT-proBNP in asymptomatic patients with hypertension [7].

Atrial fibrillation (AF) is the most common cardiac arrhythmia in the clinical practice. NT-proBNP levels are increased in AF [8], and have proven their potential utility in the risk stratification, prognostication, and therapeutic decision-making in AF [9–11]. However, the effect of obesity on NT-proBNP in AF patients has yet to be clarified. We aimed to explore this relationship in the present study. Because AF has been linked with congestive heart failure, we hypothesized that a similar relationship might exist in AF.

Methods

Patients

Two hundred and thirty-nine consecutive patients with AF undergoing radiofrequency catheter ablation in our institution between January 2007 and January 2009 were included in this study. Exclusion criteria included chronic heart failure or left ventricular ejection fraction (LVEF) $\leq$50%, cardiomyopathy, valvular heart disease, hepatic or renal failure, acute coronary

Table 1. Characteristics of patients with body mass index (BMI)≥25 or <25 kg/m^2.

	Overweight or obese: BMI≥25 kg/m^2 (n = 129)	Normal weight: BMI<25 kg/m^2 (n = 110)	P value
BMI(kg/m^2)	26.9±1.9	22.0±1.6	<0.05
Age (yrs)	55±12	58±9	<0.05
Men (%)	94/129(72.9%)	85/110(77.3%)	NS
AF duration (yrs)	6.4±7.1	6.7±5.6	NS
Nonparoxysmal AF	50/129(38.8%)	29/110(26.4%)	<0.05
Smoking	50/129(38.8%)	41/110(37.2%)	NS
Diabetes mellitus(%)	20/129(15.5%)	7/110(6.4%)	<0.05
Hypertension(%)	76/129(58.9%)	45/110(40.9%)	<0.05
CHD(%)	6/129(4.7%)	5/110(4.5%)	NS
Serum creatinine (umol/L)	81±15	81±13	NS
Systolic blood pressure (mmHg)	130±16	126±15	NS
Diastolic blood pressure (mmHg)	79±13	77±11	NS
Heart rate (bpm)	79±18	76±15	NS
LAD (mm)	43±7	41±8	<0.05
LVEDD (mm)	50±4	49±5	<0.05
LVEF (%)	62±7	62±7	NS
Medications			
Warfarin(%)	6/129(4.7%)	4/110(3.6%)	NS
Aspirin(%)	24/129(18.6%)	21/110(19.1%)	NS
ACEI/ARB(%)	47/129(36.4%)	24/110(21.8%)	<0.05
Statin(%)	9/129(7.0%)	6/110(5.5%)	NS
CCB(%)	16/129(12.4%)	5/110(4.5%)	<0.05
βblocker(%)	42/129(32.6%)	33/110(30%)	NS
Profenanone(%)	19/129(14.7%)	17/110(15.5%)	NS
Amiodarone(%)	23/129(17.8%)	18/110(16.4%)	NS
NT-proBNP(fmol/ml)	437(324–550)	501(447–638)	<0.05
Log NT-proBNP	2.62±0.18	2.75±0.15	<0.001

CHD = Coronary heart disease; LAD = Left atrial diameter; LVEDD = Left ventricular end diastolic diameter; LVEF = Left ventricular ejection fraction; ACEI = Angiotensin-converting enzyme inhibitor; ARB = Angiotensin receptor blocker; CCB = Calcium channel blocker; NT-proBNP = N-terminal proB-type natriuretic peptide; NS = No significant.

syndrome, acute pulmonary embolism, chronic obstructive pulmonary disease, rheumatic heart disease, and thyroid dysfunction. Informed written consent was obtained from all patients, and this study was approved by the Ethics Committee of Fuwai Hospital and clinical investigations are conducted according to the principles expressed in the Declaration of Helsinki.

Clinical characteristics

Patients were interviewed and records were reviewed to determine past medical history, medications, and pertinent laboratory values. Left atrial diameter (LAD), left ventricular end diastolic diameter (LVEDD), and LVEF was determined within 3 days before the ablation procedure by echocardiography. Blood pressure and heart rate were measured in the morning upon admission, prior to the procedure. The BMI was calculated as body weight (kg) divided by the square of the height (m) at the time of the admission.

According to the World Health Organization/National Institutes of Health classification scheme, BMI groups were divided into 2 categories: overweight or obesity (BMI≥25 kg/m^2) and normal weight (BMI<25 kg/m^2) [12].

Measurement of NT-proBNP concentrations

Venous blood samples were collected from the antecubital vein in the morning upon admission, prior to the procedure. For each NT-proBNP measurement, 5 ml of whole blood was collected into tubes containing potassium EDTA (1 mg/ml blood) as anticoagulant to produce plasma. Specimens were centrifuged at 3000 r/min within 1 hour of collection. The resulting serum or plasma was aliquoted into respective storage vials and then frozen and maintained at −70°C until analysis. All testing and system operation were in accordance with manufacturer's recommendations. The serum specimen was used for NT-proBNP measurements using the assay kits (BIOMEDICA Medizinpordukte GmbH & Co KG, Wein, Australia). Assays were performed in a single run and normalized to a standard curve. Inter-assay coefficients of variation for NT-proBNP were <9%.

Statistical analysis

All statistical analyses were performed in SPSS 13.0 (SPSS, Inc., Chicago, Illinois). Continuous data are presented as mean ± SD or median plus interquartile ranges, as appropriate. Because of the large range in NT-proBNP, analysis and results of its log are also

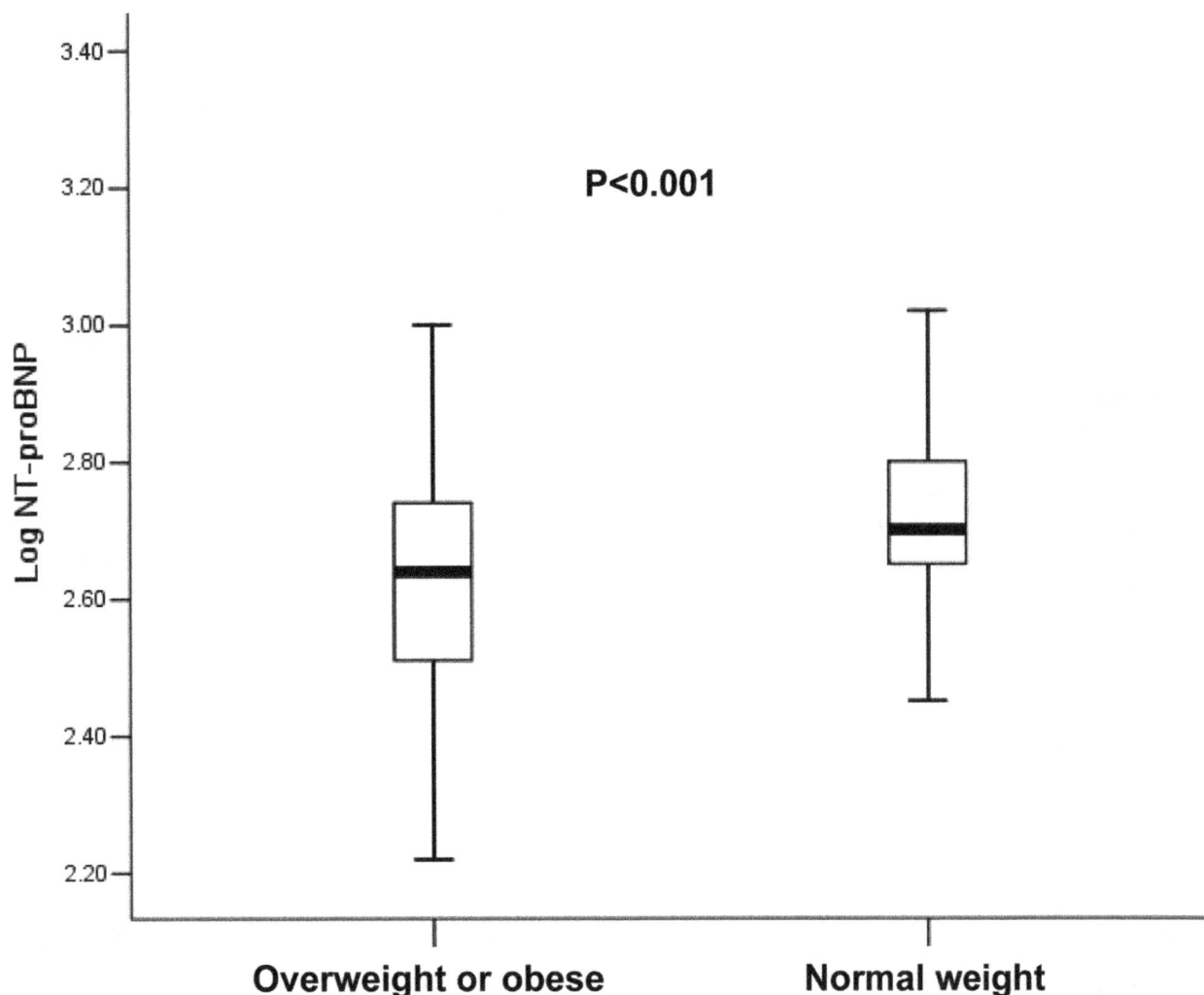

Figure 1. Comparison of LogNT-proBNP between overweight or obese patients and normal weight patients. Box plots of log of circulating N-terminal proB-type natriuretic peptide (NT-proBNP) levels showing medians with interquartile ranges. Overweight or obese patients have lower levels of Log NT-proBNP (2.62±0.18) compared with that of normal weight patients (2.75±0.15) with atrial fibrillation (P<0.001).

reported. Categorical variables were compared using the Pearson's χ^2 test. With continuous variables, group mean values were compared using the Student t test or analysis of variants, as appropriate. If the data distribution did not follow the normality assumption, the Wilcoxon rank-sum test was used. P<0.05 is considered statistically significant.

Further linear regression was performed to determine the independent relationship of BMI and LogNT-proBNP. In addition to BMI, the following covariates were also analyzed by multivariate linear regression: age, gender, AF duration, nonparoxysmal AF, smoking, diabetes mellitus, hypertension, coronary heart disease, serum creatinine, systolic blood pressure, diastolic blood pressure, LAD, LVEDD, LVEF, heart rate, using of warfarin, aspirin, angiotensin-converting enzyme inhibitor (ACEI)/angiotensin receptor blocker (ARB), statin, calcium channel block, β-blocker, propafenone, and amiodarone. The models were fit by a stepwise backward-selection algorithm, where all variables were entered into the original model and then variables with probability values of >0.05 were removed.

Results

Patients

The study included 239 consecutive patients (age 56±11 yrs; 75% men) with AF. Of these, the mean LVEF was 62±7%, the mean LAD was 41±8 mm, and the mean LVEDD was 50±4 mm. The mean serum creatinine was 81±14 umol/L. Of these, 121 (50.6%) had hypertension, 27 (11.3%) had diabetes mellitus, and 11(4.6%) had a history of coronary heart disease. The total population's BMI was 24.7±3.0 kg/m², 129 (54%) were overweight or obese (≥25 kg/m²), and 110 (46%) normal weight (<25 kg/m²). Overweight or obese patients were younger, and more likely to have a history of nonparoxysmal AF, hypertension, and diabetes mellitus (Table 1).

Comparison of NT-proBNP levels in overweight or obese and normal weight patients

Levels of NT-proBNP were significantly lower in overweight or obese patients than in normal weight patients (Table 1) (Figure 1). The median NT-proBNP in overweight or obese patients were

Table 2. Relationships of BMI and NT-proBNP levels in the subgroups.

	Overweight or obese: BMI≥25 kg/m² (fmol/ml)	Normal weight: BMI<25 kg/m² (fmol/ml)	P value
Male (n = 179)			
NT-proBNP	431(316–552)	489(436–638)	<0.001
Log NT-proBNP	2.69±0.18	2.74±0.15	<0.001
Female(n = 60)			
NT-proBNP	436(346–549)	513(468–686)	0.004
Log NT-proBNP	2.63±0.19	2.77±0.16	0.003
Age<65 yrs(n = 188)			
NT-proBNP	417(314–537)	495(437–603)	<0.001
Log NT-proBNP	2.60±0.17	2.72±0.13	0.005
Age≥65 yrs(n = 51)			
NT-proBNP	490(363–661)	795(490–1097)	0.003
Log NT-proBNP	2.69±0.20	2.88±0.18	0.001
Hypertension(n = 121)			
NT-proBNP	437(306–543)	490(447–617)	0.001
Log NT-proBNP	2.62±0.19	2.75±0.15	<0.001

NT-proBNP = N-terminal proB-type natriuretic peptide; BMI = body mass index.

437 fmol/ml, compared to 501 fmol/ml in the normal weight patients. The higher concentrations occurred despite similar LVEF and higher LVEDD and LAD.

To further evaluate the influence of age and its possible interaction with NT-proBNP levels in the context of obesity, we divided the cohort into elderly (≥65 yrs) and nonelderly (<65 yrs), and found that the relationship of obesity and decreased NT-proBNP levels persisted in both nonelderly and elderly (P<0.05), respectively. Similarly, the relationship of obesity and decreased NT-BNP concentrations persisted in patients with hypertension (P<0.001), and over the different gender (P<0.05), respectively (Table 2).

An inverse relationship between the LogNT-proBNP and BMI was found in the total study population (r = −0.306, P<0.001) (Figure 2), and for the two BMI groups, respectively (normal weight r = −0.276, P<0.001; overweigh or obese r = −0.273, P< 0.001) and for both genders, respectively (male r = −0.275, P< 0.001; female r = −0.381; P<0.001).

Multivariate predictors of NT-proBNP levels

Multivariate regressions analysis revealed BMI as an independent negative correlate of LogNT-BNP level (t = −10.063, P< 0.001). Other independent factors included age (t = 3.415, P = 0.001),using of ACEI/ARB (t = −2.080, P = 0.039), and LAD (t = 7.098, P<0.001). Particularly, we did not find any significant independent influence of hypertension and diabetes mellitus on NT-proBNP levels (Table 3).

Discussion

Major Findings

This study demonstrates an inverse relationship between higher BMI and lower NT-proBNP levels in AF patients; overweight or obese patients with AF have lower NT-proBNP levels compared to normal weight AF subjects. The validity of this observation is supported by its consistency in subgroup of hypertension, both gender and both age levels (≥65 yrs and <65 yrs).

Average level and distribution of BMI

In this study, the average level (around 24.7 kg/m²) and distribution of BMI was comparable with other Asian studies [4,13], but it was much lower in comparison with the western populations (around 28 kg/m²) [2,3,5,7]. Of this study populations, 46% was normal weight (BMI<25 kg/m²), 51% overweight (BMI = 25–29.9 kg/m²), and 3% obese (BMI≥30 kg/m²). Therefore, in the present study, the actual obese patients were rare, and we divided the study patients into overweight or obese group and normal weight group. The difference of average level and distribution of BMI may be due to an ethnic difference.

AF and NT-proBNP

Recently, the relationship between AF and NT-proBNP has been intensely studied. NT-proBNP is increased in AF [8]. In a community-based population, increased NT-proBNP levels at baseline independently predicted newly detected AF [8]. Deftereos et al demonstrated that NT-proBNP levels could predict the presence of left atrial thrombus in AF patients of unknown onset and no heart failure [10]. Furthermore, baseline NT-proBNP levels could predict risk of new-onset AF after cardiac surgery [11] or non-cardiac surgery [14], and predict AF recurrence after successful electrical cardioversion [15] or catheter ablation [9]. Thus, NT-proBNP has proven their diagnostic usefulness in the risk stratification, prognostication, and guiding therapy in patients with AF.

Obesity and NT-proBNP

Many studies have evaluated the relationship between plasma NT-proBNP and obesity. An inverse relationship between BMI and NT-proBNP levels has been demonstrated in subjects with acute or chronic heart failure [2,3], significant coronary artery disease or acute myocardial infarction [4,5] and healthy general populations in Framingham Heart study [6]. However, in asymptomatic patients with essential hypertension, with or without left ventricular hypertrophy, the inverse association was not observed [7]. In addition, two recent studies showed that NT-proBNP is closely associated with lean mass than with fat mass [6],

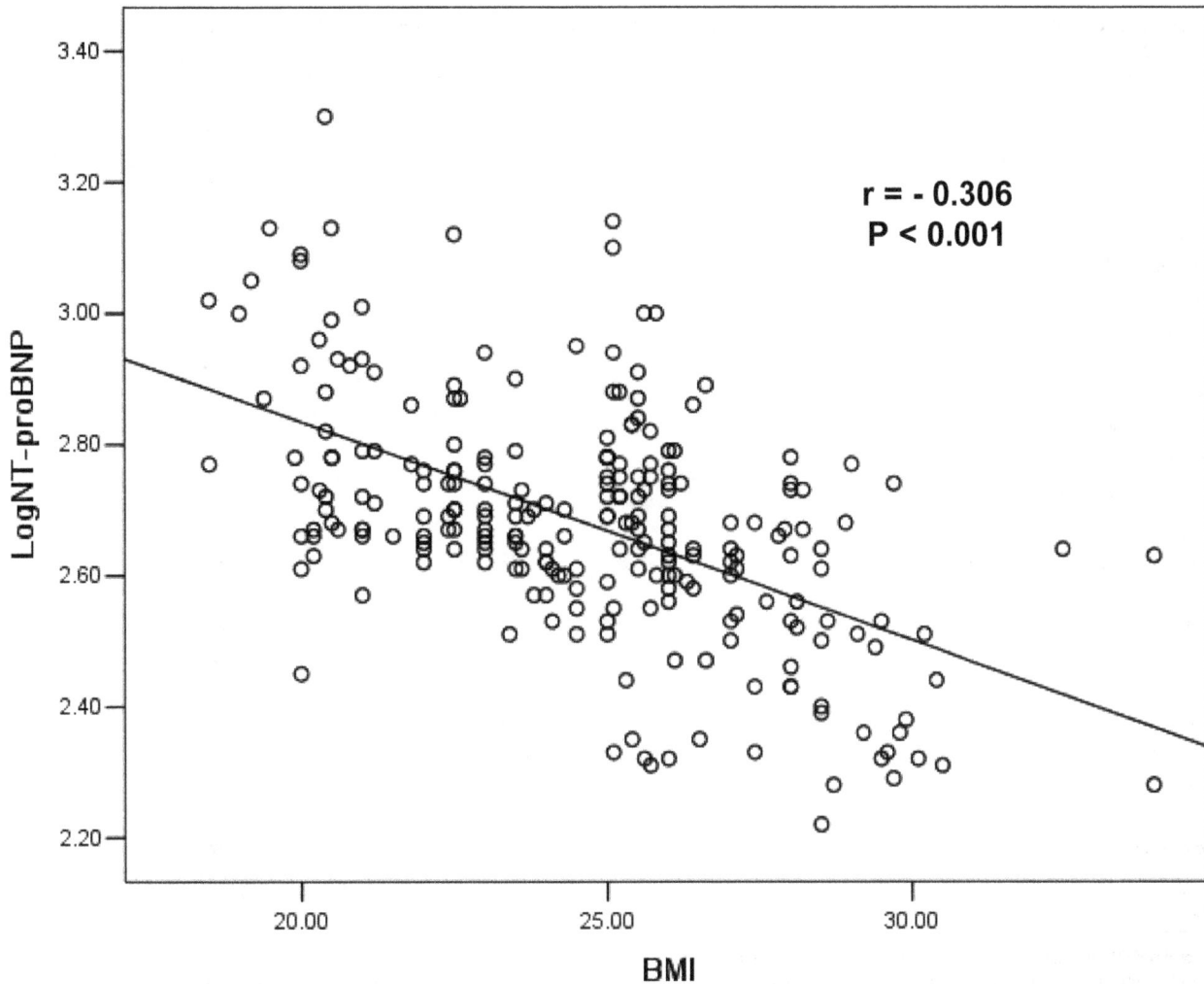

Figure 2. Inverse relationship between LogNT-proBNP and BMI in atrial fibrillation. This figure depicts the raw data demonstrating a significant inverse correlation between log of circulating N-terminal proB-type natriuretic peptide (NT-proBNP) levels and body mass index (BMI) in patients with atrial fibrillation ($r = -0.306$, $P<0.001$).

and is related with visceral adipose tissue than subcutaneous adipose tissue [16]. Nevertheless, the relationship between plasma NT-proBNP levels and BMI in AF patients has not been analyzed. In one study from the Framingham Heart study [17], Wang et al reported that higher BMI was associated with decreased BNP and N-terminal proatrial natriuretic peptides (NT-proANP) levels. In that study, only a small number of AF patients were included, and accounted for 0.5%, 1% and 2% of the normal, overweight and obese group. Furthermore, the BNP levels of AF patients were not compared among different BMI groups.

In this study, although the patient average BMI level was much lower than the general western populations, the association between higher BMI and lower NT-proBNP levels were observed in AF patients. Furthermore, the validity of our findings is supported by its consistency across both genders, by the adjustment methods with numerous covariates. The present results therefore extend previous studies from heart failure, coronary artery disease to atrial fibrillation, at least in selected patients.

The exact mechanisms for the inverse relationship between NT-proBNP levels and BMI remain uncertain. Natriuretic peptide clearance receptors (NPR-C) are abundant in adipose tissue, and it is suggested that lipolysis is driven partly by natriuretic peptides, leading

to the lower levels of natriuretic peptides in obese individuals [18]. However, the structure of NT-proBNP is distinct from natriuretic peptides and thus unlikely to be cleared via NPR-C, suggesting that the inverse relationship may be due to non-clearance mechanisms. A previous study reported that NT-proBNP decreased with increasing BMI in a manner nearly parallel to the decrease of BNP [3]. In addition, in the Framingham Heart study, NT-proANP levels were also lower in the obese subjects [17]. Because both NT-proANP and NT-proBNP are not cleared by NPR-C in adipose tissue, thus, decreased release or impaired synthesis of natriuretic peptides from the heart may at least partly underlie the possible mechanism. In addition, natriuretic peptides itself may exert potential lipolytic effects in human adipose tissue, leading to lipolysis and weight loss [19]. Further studies are required to explore the associated mechanisms.

Pathophysiological implications

Several studies have demonstrated that obesity is a major risk factor for the development of AF [20,21]. The potential mechanism may be that eccentric and concentric left ventricular hypertrophy with resultant progressive atrial enlargement [22,23]. The elevated circulating volume and enhanced neurohormonal activation (obliged by a larger body mass) may also contribute to

Table 3. Multivariate linear regression results for detecting independent factors on log-transformed plasma NT-proBNP in AF patients.

Variable	t	P value
Age	3.415	0.001
Gender	1.763	0.079
AF duration	0.721	0.471
Nonparoxysmal AF	0.026	0.979
Smoking	1.559	0.120
Diabetes mellitus	0.987	0.325
Hypertension	0.221	0.826
CHD	0.062	0.951
Serum creatinine	0.810	0.419
Systolic blood pressure	−0.149	0.881
Diastolic blood pressure	1.546	0.124
LAD	7.098	0.000
LVEDD	0.938	0.349
LVEF	−0.423	0.672
Heart rate	−0.358	0.720
Warfarin	0.234	0.815
Aspirin	−0.785	0.433
ACEI/ARB	−2.080	0.039
Statin	1.045	0.297
CCB	1.801	0.069
βblocker	0.916	0.361
Profenanone	0.290	0.772
Amiodarone	1.132	0.259
BMI	−10.063	0.000

NT-proBNP = N-terminal proB-type natriuretic peptide; AF = Atrial fibrillation; CHD = Coronary heart disease; LAD = Left atrial diameter; LVEDD = Left ventricular end diastolic diameter; LVEF = Left ventricular ejection fraction; ACEI = Angiotensin-converting enzyme inhibitor; ARB = Angiotensin receptor blocker; CCB = Calcium channel blocker; BMI = body mass index.

the left atrium dilation and electrical instability [21,24]. Although the exact significance of decreased NT-proBNP levels in overweight or obese state of AF patients are not yet understood, it at least raises the possibility that there may be lesser natriuretic-mediated vasodilation and antagonism of the rennin-angiotensin system, or loss of natriuretic ability in overweight or obese patients, which may also play a role in the development of the AF in overweight or obese patients.

Study limitations

The present study has several limitations. First, this study included Chinese populations, which may be different with those from western countries. As discussed previously, the average level and distribution of BMI in the present study was much lower than that reported in previous western studies. In addition, the use of warfarin for stroke prevention among AF patients was low in this study, although it is similar to other Chinese study [25]. This may reflect the current medical system pattern in China. Thus, our results must be extended to other populations with caution.

Second, this study involved a population of patients referred for catheter ablation of AF. Thus, due to the patients not eligible for ablation have been excluded, therefore, the conclusions may be possibly not extrapolated to the general population of patients with AF. However, with the increasing numbers of patients receiving ablation, we believe that the results of this study remains valuable, at least in selected patients, which could be millions.

Third, the usual dosage of NT-proBNP is based on pg/ml. In this study, the plasma NT-proBNP level was quantitatively determined using competitive enzyme immunoassay from BIOMEDICA; results are given in fmol/ml. In order to convert the results of NT-proBNP from fmol/ml to pg/ml, results should be multiplied by 8.457 [26]. However, we think that the results using fmol/ml did not affect our conclusions between BMI and NT-proBNP.

Conclusions

In the present study, we demonstrated an inverse association between higher BMI and lower NT-proBNP levels in AF patients. Overweigh or obese patients have reduced levels of NT-proBNP compared to lean patients. In the clinical practice, it should be considered the effect of the obesity on the NT-proBNP levels for the AF patients.

Author Contributions

Conceived and designed the experiments: LHZ LMW YY. Performed the experiments: LHZ LMW. Analyzed the data: LHZ RS WH. Contributed reagents/materials/analysis tools: LMW. Wrote the paper: LHZ. Acquisition of data: WSC JRB. Final review and correction of the version to be published: YY KJZ SZ.

References

1. Raymond I, Groenning BA, Hildebrandt PR, Nilsson JC, Baumann M, et al. (2003) The influence of age, sex and other variables on the plasma level of N-terminal pro brain natriuretic peptide in a large sample of the general population. Heart 89: 745–751.

2. Rivera M, Cortés R, Salvador A, Bertomeu V, de Burgos FG, et al. (2005) Obese subjects with heart failure have lower N-terminal pro-brain natriuretic peptide plasma levels irrespective of aetiology. Eur J Heart Fail 7: 1168–1170.

3. Krauser DG, Lloyd-Jones DM, Chae CU, Cameron R, Anwaruddin S, et al. (2005) Effect of body mass index on natriuretic peptide levels in patients with acute congestive heart failure: a ProBNP Investigation of Dyspnea in the Emergency Department (PRIDE) substudy. Am Heart J 149: 744–750.

4. Hong SN, Ahn Y, Yoon NS, Moon JY, Kim KH, et al. (2008) N-terminal pro-B-type natriuretic peptide level is depressed in patients with significant coronary artery disease who have high body mass index. Int Heart J 49: 403–412.

5. Lorgis L, Cottin Y, Danchin N, Mock L, Sicard P, et al. (2011) Impact of obesity on the prognostic value of the N-terminal pro-B-type natriuretic peptide (NT-proBNP) in patients with acute myocardial infarction. Heart 97: 551–956.

6. Das SR, Drazner MH, Dries DL, Vega GL, Stanek HG, et al. (2005) Impact of body mass and body composition on circulating levels of natriuretic peptides: results from the Dallas Heart Study. Circulation 112: 2163–2168.

7. Cortés R, Otero MR, Morillas P, Roselló-Lletí E, Grigorian L, et al. (2008) Obese and nonobese patients with essential hypertension show similar N-terminal proBNP plasma levels. Am J Hypertens 21: 820–825.

8. Patton KK, Ellinor PT, Heckbert SR, Christenson RH, DeFilippi C, et al. (2009) N-terminal pro-B-type natriuretic peptide is a major predictor of the development of atrial fibrillation: the Cardiovascular Health Study. Circulation 120: 1768–1774.

9. den Uijl DW, Delgado V, Tops LF, Ng AC, Boersma E, et al. (2011) Natriuretic peptide levels predict recurrence of atrial fibrillation after radiofrequency catheter ablation. Am Heart J 161: 197–203.

10. Deftereos S, Giannopoulos G, Kossyvakis C, Raisakis K, Kaoukis A, et al. (2011) Estimation of atrial fibrillation recency of onset and safety of cardioversion using NTproBNP levels in patients with unknown time of onset. Heart 97: 914–917.

11. Gibson PH, Croal BL, Cuthbertson BH, Rae D, McNeilly JD, et al. (2009) Use of preoperative natriuretic peptides and echocardiographic parameters in predicting new-onset atrial fibrillation after coronary artery bypass grafting: a prospective comparative study. Am Heart J 158: 244–251.

12. National Heart, Lung, and Blood Institute Expert Panel (1998) Clinical Guidelines on the Identification, Evaluation, and Treatment of Overweight and Obesity in Adults: Evidence Report. Bethesda, Md: National Heart, Lung, and Blood Institute; June.

13. Sugisawa T, Kishimoto I, Kokubo Y, Makino H, Miyamoto Y, et al. (2010) Association of plasma B-type natriuretic peptide levels with obesity in a general urban Japanese population: the Suita Study. Endocr J 57: 727–733.

14. Karthikeyan G, Moncur RA, Levine O, Heels-Ansdell D, Chan MT, et al. (2009) Is a pre-operative brain natriuretic peptide or N-terminal pro-B-type natriuretic peptide measurement an independent predictor of adverse cardiovascular outcomes within 30 days of noncardiac surgery? A systematic review and meta-analysis of observational studies. J Am Coll Cardiol 54: 1599–1606.

15. Mollmann H, Weber M, Elsasser A, Nef H, Dill T, et al. (2008) NT-ProBNP predicts rhythm stability after cardioversion of lone atrial fibrillation. Circ J 72: 921–925.

16. Malavazos AE, Morricone L, Marocchi A, Ermetici F, Ambrosi B, et al. (2006) N-terminal pro-B-type natriuretic peptide and echocardiographic abnormalities in severely obese patients: correlation with visceral fat. Clin Chem 52: 1211–1213.

17. Wang TJ, Larson MG, Levy D, Benjamin EJ, Leip EP, et al. (2004) Impact of obesity on plasma natriuretic peptide levels. Circulation 109: 594–600.

18. Sengenès C, Berlan M, De Glisezinski I, Lafontan M, Galitzky J (2000) Natriuretic peptides: a new lipolytic pathway in human adipocytes. FASEB J 14: 1345–1351.

19. Sarzani R, Dessi-Fulgheri P, Paci VM, Espinosa E, Rappelli A (1996) Expression of natriuretic peptide receptors in human adipose and other tissues. J Endocrinol Invest 19: 581–585.

20. Benjamin EJ, Levy D, Vaziri SM, D'Agostino RB, Belanger AJ, et al. (1994) Independent risk factors for atrial fibrillation in a population-based cohort. The Framingham Heart Study. JAMA 271: 840–844.

21. Wang TJ, Parise H, Levy D, D'Agostino RB Sr, Wolf PA, et al. (2004) Obesity and the risk of new-onset atrial fibrillation. JAMA 292: 2471–2477.

22. Hense HW, Gneiting B, Muscholl M, Broeckel U, Kuch B, et al. (1998) The associations of body size and body composition with left ventricular mass: impacts for indexation in adults. J Am Coll Cardiol 32: 451–457.

23. de Simone G, Daniels SR, Devereux RB, Meyer RA, Roman MJ, et al. (1992) Left ventricular mass and body size in normotensive children and adults: assessment of allometric relations and impact of overweight. J Am Coll Cardiol 20: 1251–1260.

24. Abed HS, Samuel CS, Lau DH, Kelly DJ, Royce SG, et al. (2013) Obesity results in progressive atrial structural and electrical remodeling: implications for atrial fibrillation. Heart Rhythm 10: 90–100.

25. Zhou ZQ, Hu DY, Chen J, Zhang RH, Li KB, et al. (2003) An epidemiological survey of atrial fibrillation in China. Chin J Intern Med (Chin) 43: 491–494.

26. Rutten FH, Gramer MJM, Zuithoff NPA, Lammers JWJ, Verweij W, et al. (2007) Comparison of B-type natriuretic peptide assays for identifying heart failure in stable elderly patients with a clinical diagnosis of chronic obstructive pulmonary disease. Eur J Heart Fail 9: 651–659.

23

Defining Disease Phenotypes Using National Linked Electronic Health Records: A Case Study of Atrial Fibrillation

Katherine I. Morley[1,2,3]*[9], Joshua Wallace[1][9], Spiros C. Denaxas[1], Ross J. Hunter[4], Riyaz S. Patel[1,5], Pablo Perel[1,6], Anoop D. Shah[1], Adam D. Timmis[4], Richard J. Schilling[4], Harry Hemingway[1]

1 Farr Institute of Health Informatics Research, University College London, London, United Kingdom, and Clinical Epidemiology, Department of Epidemiology and Public Health, University College London, London, United Kingdom, 2 Institute of Psychiatry, Psychology and Neuroscience, King's College London, London, United Kingdom, 3 Melbourne School of Global and Population Health, The University of Melbourne, Melbourne, Australia, 4 Barts NIHR Biomedical Research Unit, Queen Mary University London, London, United Kingdom, 5 The Heart Hospital, University College London NHS Trust, London, United Kingdom, 6 London School of Hygiene and Tropical Medicine, London, United Kingdom

Abstract

Background: National electronic health records (EHR) are increasingly used for research but identifying disease cases is challenging due to differences in information captured between sources (e.g. primary and secondary care). Our objective was to provide a transparent, reproducible model for integrating these data using atrial fibrillation (AF), a chronic condition diagnosed and managed in multiple ways in different healthcare settings, as a case study.

Methods: Potentially relevant codes for AF screening, diagnosis, and management were identified in four coding systems: Read (primary care diagnoses and procedures), British National Formulary (BNF; primary care prescriptions), ICD-10 (secondary care diagnoses) and OPCS-4 (secondary care procedures). From these we developed a phenotype algorithm via expert review and analysis of linked EHR data from 1998 to 2010 for a cohort of 2.14 million UK patients aged ≥30 years. The cohort was also used to evaluate the phenotype by examining associations between incident AF and known risk factors.

Results: The phenotype algorithm incorporated 286 codes: 201 Read, 63 BNF, 18 ICD-10, and four OPCS-4. Incident AF diagnoses were recorded for 72,793 patients, but only 39.6% (N = 28,795) were recorded in primary care and secondary care. An additional 7,468 potential cases were inferred from data on treatment and pre-existing conditions. The proportion of cases identified from each source differed by diagnosis age; inferred diagnoses contributed a greater proportion of younger cases (≤60 years), while older patients (≥80 years) were mainly diagnosed in SC. Associations of risk factors (hypertension, myocardial infarction, heart failure) with incident AF defined using different EHR sources were comparable in magnitude to those from traditional consented cohorts.

Conclusions: A single EHR source is not sufficient to identify all patients, nor will it provide a representative sample. Combining multiple data sources and integrating information on treatment and comorbid conditions can substantially improve case identification.

Editor: Stefan Kiechl, Innsbruck Medical University, Austria

Funding: This study was carried out on behalf of the ClinicAL research using LInked bespoke studies and Electronic health Records (CALIBER) programme. This study was supported by National Institute for Health Research (ADT, HH, RP-PG-0407-10314), Wellcome Trust (ADT, HH, 086091/Z/08/Z), and the Medical Research Council Prognosis Research Strategy (PROGRESS) Partnership (PP, ADT, HH, G0902393/99558; www.progress-partnership.org), and by awards to establish the Farr Institute of Health Informatics Research at UCL Partners (HH, SCD, ADT), from the Medical Research Council, Arthritis Research UK, British Heart Foundation, Cancer Research UK, Chief Scientist Office, Economic and Social Research Council, Engineering and Physical Sciences Research Council, National Institute for Health Research, National Institute for Social Care and Health Research, and Wellcome Trust (ADT, HH, grant MR/K006584/1). KIM and JW were supported by the PROGRESS Partnership while undertaking this research. SCD was supported by a UCL Provost's Strategic Development Fund Fellowship. ADS was supported by a clinical research training fellowship from the Wellcome Trust (0938/30/Z/10/Z). ADT was supported by Barts and The London NIHR Cardiovascular Biomedical Research Unit, funded by the National Institute for Health Research. The funders had no role in study design, data collection and analysis, decision to publish, or preparation of the manuscript.

Competing Interests: The authors have declared that no competing interests exist.

* Email: katherine.morley@ucl.ac.uk

[9] These authors contributed equally to this work.

Introduction

One of the major challenges presented by the increasing use of electronic health record (EHR) data for research is the development of strategies for reliably identifying disease cases [1–4]. Hripcsak and Albers [5] argue that in order to improve the extraction of disease information from this type of data:

...[W]e need a better understanding of the EHR. The EHR is not a direct reflection of the patient and physiology, but a reflection of the recording process inherent in healthcare with noise and feedback loops. We must study the EHR as an object in itself, as if it were a natural system.(p. 119)

This recommendation is particularly relevant to identification of chronic conditions in which patients may have multiple interactions with primary and secondary care, and undergo assessments and diagnostic tests, before ultimately receiving a diagnosis. Even after diagnosis, patients may receive follow-up care such as monitoring, prescriptions, or other medical interventions [6]. Consequently, one EHR data source rarely covers the full patient journey; usually data from different record sources (e.g. primary, secondary, and tertiary care; medication prescription and dispensing; mortality data) must be integrated to obtain a complete picture [7]. However, these data also encompass variation in patient measurement that may be context-dependent and thus effective integration requires an exploration of what is recorded in the EHR in relation to a particular condition, and how this compares to expectations based upon guidelines and preconceptions about clinical practice [4,8,9].

To highlight the challenges and complexities of identifying onset of a chronic condition in linked national EHR data, and how these can inform the development of strategies for identifying patients, we present a case study of atrial fibrillation (AF) using national linked EHR and administrative health data from the English National Health Service (NHS). AF is the most common cardiac arrhythmia, associated with increased risk of stroke, heart failure (HF), and premature mortality [10,11]. It presents many important challenges that may be encountered when developing strategies for case identification, or phenotypes, in EHR data including variability in symptoms and signs, different coding strategies and treatment options, and changes in clinical practice (for more in-depth discussion see [12]).

Clinical context of atrial fibrillation

Onset of AF often precedes diagnosis considerably; patients may be asymptomatic or experience paroxysmal AF (characterized by irregular, sudden symptoms) and clinical signs, such as irregular pulse, may be episodic. AF may also be diagnosed when a patient is admitted to hospital for another, potentially unrelated, condition. UK diagnostic guidelines and those from the European Society of Cardiology (ESC) recommend pulse palpation followed by an electrocardiogram if an irregular pulse is detected [13,14]. Opportunistic screening of patients over the age of 65 is recommended by the ESC, but not by North American organisations [15].

Confirming an AF diagnosis does not necessarily simplify documentation as recording and treatment may differ between primary and secondary care, which use different coding systems with different levels of granularity. Read codes, a subset of the Systematic Nomenclature Of Medicine - Clinical Terms (SNOMED-CT) clinical terminology, are used in primary care

and permit specification of disease subtypes and differentiation of AF from atrial flutter. In contrast, the International Classification of Disease – 10th revision (ICD-10) terminology used in secondary care has one term for all categories. Treatment varies between patients depending upon symptoms, age and other clinical characteristics, and clinical context. Currently, most patients receive anti-thrombotic treatment to reduce stroke risk, although drugs for rate or rhythm control, and procedures such as cardioversion or catheter ablation, may also be used [14].

AF diagnostic and treatment practices have changed substantially over the last 10–15 years. This is due to increasing awareness of AF and recognition that, at least in the UK, it is more likely to be subject to under, rather than over, diagnosis [16,17]. Policy initiatives have been introduced in the UK to address this including: the 2004 Quality and Outcomes Framework (QOF), which financially rewards general practitioners for implementing treatment plans for chronic conditions, including AF [18]; the 2006 UK National Institute for Health and Care Excellence guidelines for AF diagnosis and management [19]; the English NHS Commissioning for Quality and Innovation (CQUIN) scheme, introduced in 2009 to provide financial incentives for quality improvements. Thus there may be temporal differences in coding practices for AF.

Identification of patients with atrial fibrillation

A consistent approach to integrating EHR and administrative health data to identify AF will facilitate transparent and reproducible research, but currently no universal method exists. Previous UK EHR studies have focused on primary care [20–23], but other studies used secondary care data. We reviewed research on AF risk factors and found substantial variation in the data sources used to identify AF cases; 21 of 27 studies identified used EHR data, with two using primary care [24,25], 15 using secondary care [26–40], and four using both [41–44]. However, many researchers are developing strategies for integrating EHR data for research and defining EHR phenotypes [2,45–51]. The USA-based eMERGE Consortium have developed an AF phenotype algorithm [52], but this was created for data from nine health care providers actively participating in research and focuses on clinical notes and electrocardiogram impressions. As these data are not available on a large scale to researchers in the UK, and elsewhere, using data from nationalised health services, our aims were to develop an understanding of EHR data relating to AF, and to use this to develop a phenotype algorithm applicable to linked, nationally collected data.

Thus we describe the development of the ClinicAl disease research using Linked Bespoke studies and Electronic Records (CALIBER) AF phenotype and use this to demonstrate how exploration of recording patterns in multiple data sources can inform the development of disease case identification strategies for EHR data. We investigated whether EHR data beyond diagnosis codes could be leveraged to refine date of disease onset; whether cases could be inferred on the basis of medical treatment; and whether changes in health care policy may have affected data collection. We evaluated the face validity of the phenotype by testing for associations with known risk factors. The strategies used and lessons learned are broadly applicable to all EHR phenotype development, particularly where the aim is to identify disease cases for longitudinal research.

Materials and Methods

Study population and linked electronic records

Anonymised patients were selected from the CALIBER cohort, which includes linked data from: (1) primary care EHR data: diagnoses coded using the Read system by general practitioners during consultation or by practice administrators from hospital discharge letters (from the Clinical Practice Research Datalink) and prescriptions; (2) secondary care administrative records: diagnoses and procedures recorded using the ICD terminology and Office of Population Censuses and Surveys Classification of Interventions and Procedures (OPCS-4, comparable to the American Medical Association Current Procedural Terminology medical classification system) by audit nurses after patient admission by abstracting data from hospital records (from Hospital Episode Statistics); (3) administrative mortality data from death certificates where cause(s) of death are recorded by a doctor and ICD-9 and ICD-10 codes added by trained non-clinical coders (from UK Office of National Statistics; ONS); (4) small-area patient social deprivation information from multiple administrative data sets (from ONS) [12]. CALIBER was approved by the Lewisham Local Research Ethics Committee (ref:09/H0810/16 date: 08/04/2009) and the Ethics and Confidentiality Committee (ECC) (ref: ECC 2-06(b)/2009 CALIBER dataset). CALIBER has been registered with the University College London Data Protection Officer (ref: Z6364106/2009/2/26). CALIBER EHR data are anonymized; individual informed consent was not sought from study participants.

Inclusion criteria were: age greater than 30, minimum one year of validated data prior to entry, and registration at a primary care provider with up-to-standard data. This defined a base cohort of 2,128,151 individuals in which to identify AF. Exclusion criteria were any records of AF diagnosis prior to cohort entry, or the first record of AF after entry being a term indicating monitoring of existing AF or a historical diagnosis of AF. Patients were included and followed-up from the date they met all inclusion criteria or January 1st, 1998, whichever was later. Follow-up ended on: the first of the administrative censoring date for primary care data (March 26th, 2010); last data collection date for a particular primary care provider; a patient leaving their primary care provider; or patient death as recorded in ONS. Risk factor analyses excluded patients with missing data for blood pressure (BP) measurements, body mass index (BMI), ethnicity or index of multiple deprivation score.

Strategy for EHR phenotype development

The CALIBER approach to EHR phenotype development iteratively cycles between expert discussion, review of codes and their semantic relations, and analysis of data (see Figure 1). An initial case definition listing codes, or combinations of codes, indicating diagnosis of a condition is drafted based on discussion with experts in the clinical phenotype, epidemiology, computer science, and bioinformatics. For AF, this preliminary definition only included diagnosis codes directly related to AF from primary or secondary care (extraction of data from free text or image processing is currently limited), but we also identified codes for medications and procedures used in AF treatment for further investigation (lists of all identified codes are available online on the CALIBER Data Portal at www.caliberresearch.org).

Initial examination of code usage. A test data set of 100,000 patients was used to investigate how frequently codes were used in practice, and the relationship between diagnosis codes and those for medications and procedures. We found, as have others [53], that although codes for AF subtypes exist within the Read system, they are infrequently used and most patients simply have an all-encompassing diagnosis of AF recorded. Codes indicating an existing condition (e.g. when taking a new patient's history) and monitoring of AF are used, but the main codes recorded relate to a diagnosis of AF. We examined procedure and prescription codes to see if they could assist in identifying additional cases. For procedure codes, the overall frequency was low and they were almost always recorded for patients with a pre-existing AF diagnosis. However, many patients had prescription records for warfarin or digoxin (medications used almost exclusively to treat AF during the time frame of the available data), but no AF diagnosis code.

Review of these results by the expert group led to three decisions: (i) due to the infrequent coding of AF subtypes in primary care, and the single ICD-10 code in secondary care, we should develop an AF phenotype algorithm combining all subtypes; (ii) the case definition should not include procedure codes; (iii) where AF-related prescriptions were made without recorded diagnoses, we should investigate whether a diagnosis of AF could be reasonably inferred. To pursue the latter aim, we developed case definitions based on clinical knowledge of treatment patterns strongly indicative of AF; warfarin prescriptions in the absence of prior deep vein thrombosis (DVT) or pulmonary embolism (PE), or digoxin prescriptions in the absence of heart failure (HF) were taken as evidence to support an "inferred" diagnosis of AF. These conditions were identified using previously defined CALIBER phenotype algorithms for DVT, PE, and HF (see CALIBER Data Portal at www.caliberresearch.org for details).

Exploration of the EHR

Refining disease onset. We investigated the time elapsed between incident AF diagnoses recorded using ICD-10 or Read codes in multiple data sources to see if combing data improved estimation of disease onset. We also investigated the utility of further refining onset using an indicator marker (irregular pulse), examining the frequency of these codes and the time that elapsed between the relevant code(s) being recorded and a subsequent coded diagnosis of AF.

Disease case identification. We investigated whether combining multiple sources of EHR data increased the overall number of disease cases identified by permitting us to infer AF diagnoses on the basis of patterns of medication use and comorbid conditions.

Characteristics of diagnosed patients

As the phenotype algorithm we developed was used to identify diagnoses from different data sources over an extended time period, we wanted to explore whether there were context-level and/or patient-level differences in the cases identified. We quantified the unique and non-unique AF cases identified in each source. We then investigated the relationship between the data source and (i) diagnosis context, specifically the year of diagnosis and whether AF was the primary or secondary reason for admission for secondary care diagnoses (HES provides up 15 secondary diagnosis codes); and (ii) individual patient characteristics at diagnosis including sex, age, and important comorbid conditions (HF, myocardial infarction, hypertension, stroke, diabetes, thyroid disease, renal failure, and chronic obstructive pulmonary disease).

Association with known risk factors

The face validity of the CALIBER AF phenotype was evaluated by conducting a pre-specified analysis of the association between AF diagnosis and factors for which there is strong prior evidence of

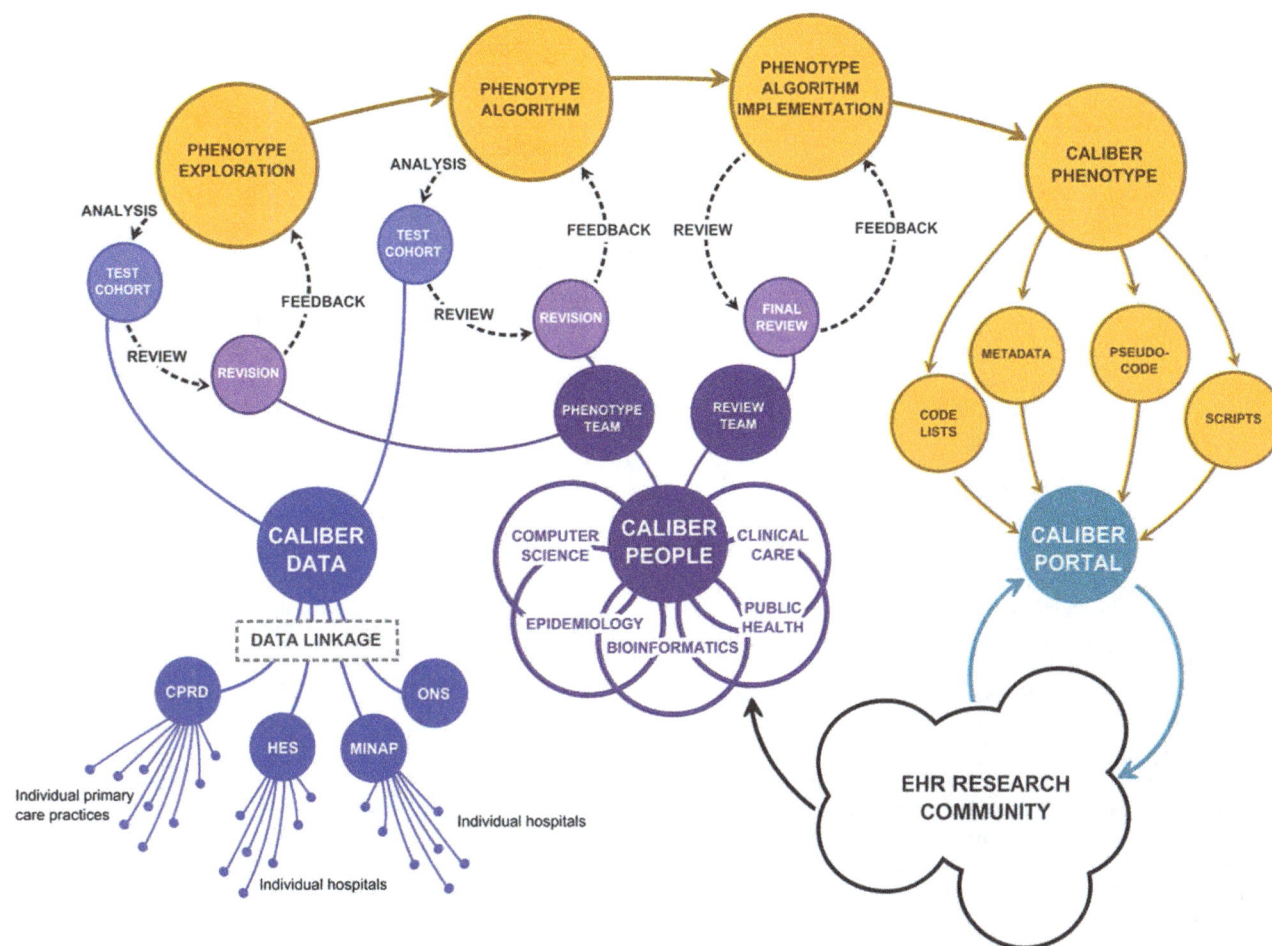

Figure 1. Illustration of phenotype algorithm developing using the Clinical Research Using Linked Bespoke Studies and Electronic health records (CALIBER) programme. CPRD represents the Clinical Practice Research Data link; HES represents Hospital Episode Statistics; MINAP is the Myocardial Ischaemia National Audit Registry; ONS is the UK Office of National Statistics (mortality and social deprivation data).

association with AF diagnosis from both clinical observations and multiple epidemiological studies: HF, hypertension, and myocardial infarction (MI) [11]. Cause specific Cox proportional hazards models were used to estimate hazard ratio and 95% confidence intervals for incident AF diagnosis associated with baseline measures of risk factors, adjusted for age, sex, and primary care practice [54,55]. All analyses excluded patients diagnosed with AF prior to study baseline. All statistical analyses were conducted in R version 15.2 for Mac and Linux [56].

Results

Sample characteristics

We identified 24 codes (23 Read codes and one ICD-10 code) relating to AF diagnosis. Ten codes refer to monitoring of pre-existing AF, three confirm a prior diagnosis of AF, and the remaining 11 indicate diagnosis by a current care provider. The CALIBER cohort of 2,128,151 participants included 33,383 individuals with an AF code in their record indicating diagnosis prior to cohort entry. Thus, at baseline, approximately 1.6% of the sample had already received a diagnosis of AF, which is similar to prevalence estimate of 2.0% (95% C.I. 1.6–2.4%) provided by the recent UK-based general population ECHOES study [57]. Of the remaining 2,094,768 patients without an AF diagnosis at baseline,

72,793 received their first recorded AF diagnosis code during the study period. A total of 22,939 (45.2%) of patients were initially diagnosed in primary care, with the remaining 39,863 (54.8%) initially diagnosed in secondary care (those diagnosed on the same date in two sources were attributed to secondary care).

Exploration of the EHR

Refining disease onset: Timeframe for diagnosis. To investigate whether combining data from primary and secondary care improved resolution of disease onset, we examined the data for 28,795 individuals with incident diagnoses recorded in both primary and secondary care. The time elapsed between AF diagnoses in the two sources depended on the source of the initial diagnosis. An AF diagnosis was first recorded in primary care for 13,707 individuals, and in secondary care for 10,380 individuals (for 4,708 individuals the dates were the same). The median time from primary care diagnosis to secondary care diagnosis was just over one year (367.0 days), while the mean was almost two years (724.4 days). In contrast, the median time from secondary to primary care AF diagnosis was 20 days (mean 212.6 days).

Refining disease onset: Irregular pulse. The primary care Read code system includes five codes for pulse palpation: two indicate a normal or "regular" pulse, and three indicate an "irregular" pulse. Only 1,252 (1.78%) of the 72,793 participants with an incident AF diagnosis had any pulse palpation recorded between study entry and AF diagnosis, with irregular pulse the record closest to AF diagnosis for 964 patients (77.1% of those with any pulse palpation recorded). The median time from first irregular pulse to AF diagnosis in patients where both were recorded after study entry was 71 days. Less than half (40.1%) of patients were diagnosed with AF by 30 days after the irregular pulse code, with 65.8% diagnosed by 12 months.

Disease case identification: Inferred diagnosis. Inferred diagnoses were identified based on a combination of 262 codes: 63 relating to prescriptions (36 for warfarin, 27 for digoxin) and 199 excluding conditions (97 for prior HF, 60 for prior DVT, 22 for prior PE) and procedures (20 for heart valve replacement). A total of 39,527 patients met the criteria for an inferred diagnosis of AF during the study period. Warfarin prescriptions accounted for 18,714 (47%) patient diagnoses, digoxin prescriptions for 10,592 (28%), and the remaining 10,221 (26%) had both prescription patterns. A small percentage of patients with an inferred diagnosis (3,754; 9.5%) received coded or historical diagnoses of AF prior to cohort entry. Of the remaining 35,773 individuals, 28,305 (71.6%) had an AF diagnosis code recorded during follow-up and 7,468 (18.9%) had no codes relating to AF diagnosis in their record.

Of the 28,305 individuals who met the inferred AF diagnosis criteria and had an AF diagnosis code within the study window, the majority (75.7%; 21,420 individuals) received the diagnosis code before meeting the criteria for an inferred diagnosis, and for a further 11.2% (3,167 individuals) this occurred on the same day. Thus only 13% of patients (3,718 individuals) met the inferred diagnosis criteria before an AF diagnosis was recorded. For these 3,718 individuals, the average time between an inferred diagnosis and receiving a diagnosis code was 19.8 months (median 6.54 months). Within 30 days of meeting inferred diagnosis criteria, 21.1% of these patients received a diagnosis code; 59.7% received a diagnosis code within one year. However, the temporal relationship between these diagnoses varied depending on the year of the initial inferred diagnosis; the proportion receiving a diagnosis code within 12 months increased gradually over time from 37.1% in 1998 to 92.3% in 2009. The proportion of AF cases based on inferred criteria also decreased over the study period, from just over 15% of cases in 1998 to less than 10% of cases from 2006 onwards.

EHR phenotype algorithm

The results above informed the development of the AF phenotype algorithm in two ways. First, as pulse palpation was only recorded for a small minority of patients we concluded it did not provide enough additional information to warrant inclusion in our current AF case definition. Second, although examining the pattern of treatments and co-existing conditions did identify additional disease cases, without additional information (e.g. review of free text) we could not confidently conclude that patients without a recorded AF diagnosis code should be considered as cases, or that medication prescriptions represent a diagnosis date. Consequently, we included individuals with only an inferred diagnosis in our EHR case definition as a separate category, and used date of recoded AF diagnosis code in preference to date of meeting inferred criteria.

The case definition for AF using the phenotype algorithm thus had three categories:

1. Historical: first recorded AF code indicates monitoring of an existing condition, or reference to a previous AF diagnosis.

2. Diagnosed: first record is a diagnosis code for AF; preference given to the earliest dated record rather than diagnosis source (i.e. no preference for primary *versus* secondary care).

3. Inferred: no diagnosis code is present, but the patient record includes a warfarin prescription in the absence of prior DVT or PE, or a digoxin prescription in the absence of HF.

The phenotype algorithm incorporates these definitions in a hierarchical, mutually exclusive manner (see **Figure 2**). If the earliest recorded AF codes relate to a historical diagnosis or monitoring, the patient is in category 1 which precludes inclusion in other categories. If these codes are absent, then the presence of a coded diagnosis from primary or secondary care places a patient in category 2. Finally, in the absence of a coded diagnosis, a patient may be allocated to category 3, depending on the combination of prescriptions and diagnoses in their record. Otherwise a participant is treated as undiagnosed.

Characteristics of diagnosed patients

Using the phenotype algorithm we identified 80,261 individuals with an incident coded or inferred AF diagnosis in the CALIBER cohort. Of these, 7,468 had no diagnosis code but met the inferred diagnosis criteria. Almost half the patients with a diagnosis code (39.6%; 28,795 individuals) had diagnoses recorded in both primary and secondary care (see **Figure 3**). All sources provided unique diagnoses, but substantially more were identified from secondary care, which provided almost three times the number of unique cases (32,930 cases compared to 11,068 from primary care). The proportion of AF cases identified in primary care or by inferred diagnosis decreased by year of diagnosis, whereas the proportion identified in secondary care increased, but no threshold effect was identified around the introduction of the QOF in 2004.

The proportion of cases contributed by each source differed by age at diagnosis; individuals identified by inferred diagnosis criteria made up a greater proportion of cases diagnosed at younger ages (≤60 years), while cases diagnosed at older ages (≥ 80 years) were mostly identified from secondary care data (see **Figure 4**). The proportion of cases identified in primary care was highest for ages 60–80 years, but for all age groups primary care contributed fewer cases than secondary care. For patients diagnosed in secondary care, AF was more likely to be the main diagnosis for the hospital episode when individuals were younger (≤50 years), whereas amongst those diagnosed at older ages AF was much more likely to be a secondary diagnosis made during admission for another condition. Patients with diagnoses recorded only in secondary care were slightly more likely to be female compared to those with diagnoses in both data sources, primary care only, or inferred diagnoses (51.3%, 48.2%, 48.8% and 47.6% female respectively).

The percentage of patients with comorbid conditions at the time that their AF diagnosis was recorded differed by source of diagnosis (see **Table 1**). Patients for which an AF diagnosis was drawn only from secondary care were more likely to have already received a diagnosis for all the conditions examined, with the exception of hypertension, than those with a diagnosis drawn from primary care or meeting the inferred diagnosis criteria. The difference between data sources was largest for renal failure; the percentage of patients with renal failure amongst those diagnosed with AF in secondary care only was twice that of patients with AF diagnoses recorded in the other data sources (22.4% *versus* 10.9%, 11.0%, and 10.0%). A similar, although less extreme, pattern was also observed for HF, MI, stroke, and diabetes (Type 2). This does not appear to be completely due to differences in the age of patients from each source as even within age groups the

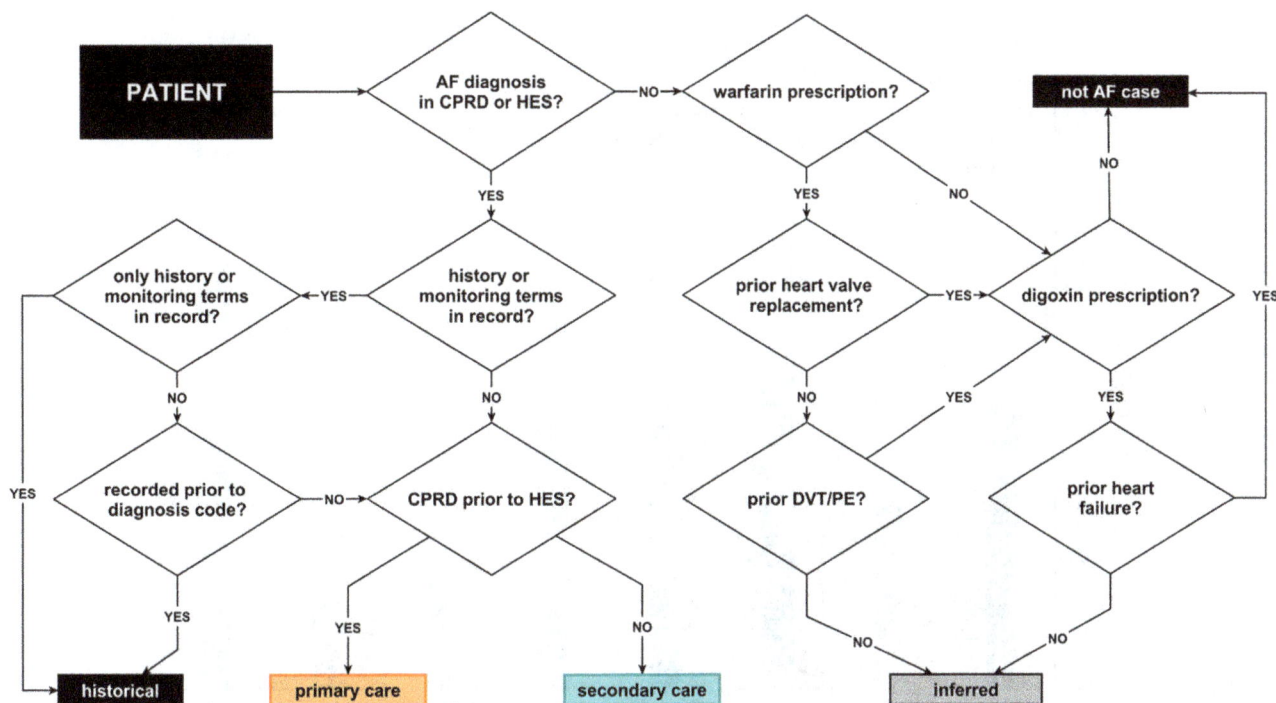

Figure 2. Flow diagram illustrating CALIBER phenotype for atrial fibrillation.

percentages of patients with pre-existing conditions were still higher for those diagnosed in secondary care, particularly for HF and diabetes. In contrast, the percentage of AF patients with hypertension was highest amongst those with a primary care diagnosis (86.0% for primary and secondary, 86.2% for primary only, compared to 83% for secondary only and 78% for inferred).

Associations with known risk factors

The associations between pre-specified risk factors and incident AF were consistent in magnitude across EHR sources and with estimates from traditional consented cohorts (see **Figure 5** and **Table S1**). For HF, the hazard ratio estimate was 2.07 (95% CI 1.95–2.19) using only primary care data for AF diagnosis, 2.31 (2.21–2.43) for secondary care data only, and 2.35 (2.25–2.46) for both sources combined (an inferred diagnosis could not be used for

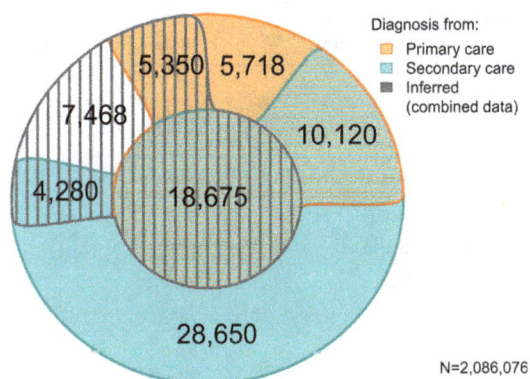

Figure 3. Euler diagram displaying the number of incident cases identified in the different sources, including overlap between multiple sources.

the HF analysis as this diagnosis is incorporated into the case definition). For hypertension, the hazard ratio estimates were 1.74 (95% CI 1.70–1.78) for primary care only, 1.80 (1.76–1.84) for secondary care only, 1.72 (1.68–1.77) for inferred diagnoses, and 1.80 (1.77–1.84) for the composite endpoint. The hazard ratio estimates for MI were 1.53 (1.46–1.60) for primary care only, 1.75 (1.68–1.82) for secondary care only, 1.69 (1.61–1.77) for inferred diagnoses, and 1.70 (1.64–1.76) for the composite endpoint.

The estimates for hypertension and MI were comparable to age and sex adjusted results from traditional cohort studies such as the Framingham Heart Study [58] (HR 1.80, 95% C.I. 1.48–2.18 for hypertension; HR 1.44, 95% C.I. 1.02–2.03 for MI) as well as those from the other EHR studies (see **Table S1**). The estimates for heart failure were towards the lower bound of those obtained from the Framingham Heart Study (HR 3.2, 95% C.I. 1.99–5.16) and EHR studies.

Discussion

We explored the characteristics of the information recorded around the diagnosis of a chronic condition, AF, in multiple linked data sources for a cohort of 2,128,151 individuals from the general population. This exploration highlighted a number of key findings with implications for EHR research on AF, and on chronic conditions more broadly. We found that: (i) refining the timing of disease onset can potentially be improved by the clinically-informed use of data that goes beyond diagnosis codes for the condition in question, but what is recorded as part of routine clinical practice may differ substantially from clinical guidelines; (ii) integrating data from multiple EHR sources and administrative data does improve case detection; (iii) the context in which data are collected may have an impact on the characteristics of the disease cases identified. We used this information to develop an EHR phenotype for identifying AF disease cases that was informed

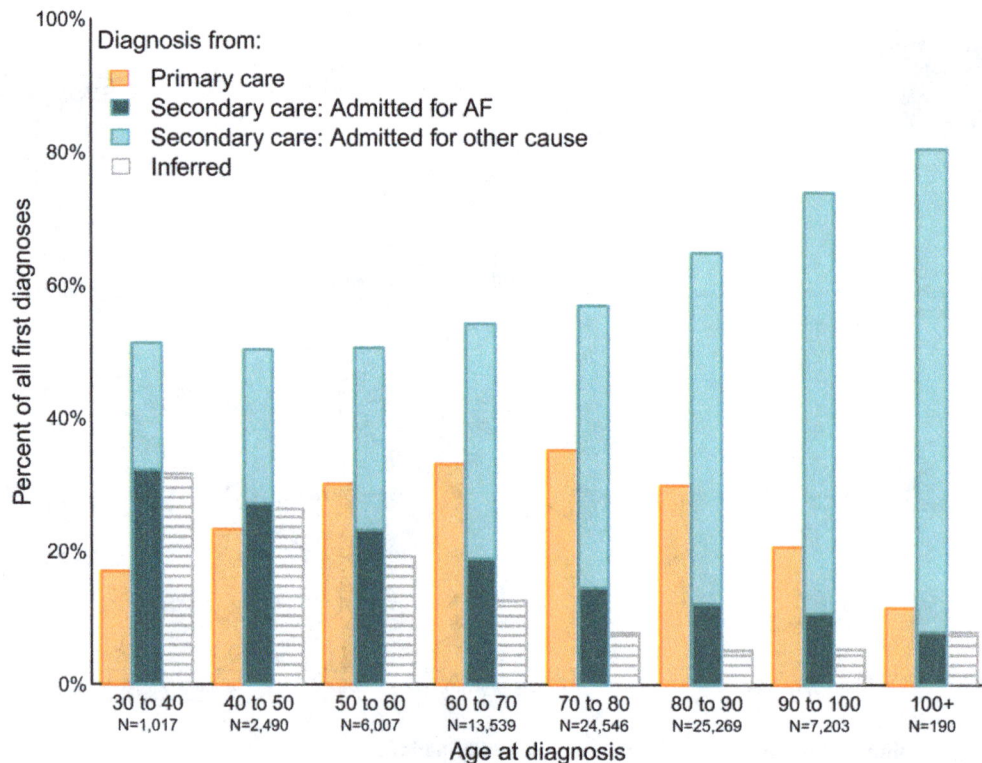

Figure 4. Proportion of incident atrial fibrillation cases identified in each source by age at diagnosis.

by an understanding of the patient record, and evaluated the face validity of it using epidemiological analyses.

Combining data from multiple sources to identify AF cases helped to refine estimates of disease onset in this sample. Using primary care data brought the date of diagnosis forward by one to two years for patients subsequently diagnosed in secondary care. Although there was a slight lag (median 20 days) from a diagnosis being recorded in secondary care to it being recorded in primary

care, this more likely indicates a delay in transfer of diagnosis information from hospital to general practitioner than separate diagnoses. Pulse palpation records were investigated because this is recommended as a screening test for AF in primary care [11,14]. In our cohort, very few AF patients (just over 2%) had a record of pulse palpation prior to diagnosis and therefore these data had limited use for refining disease onset and were not incorporated into the phenotype algorithm. This underlines the importance of

Table 1. Percentage of patients with different comorbid conditions at date of atrial fibrillation diagnosis, by source of diagnosis.

Characteristic	Category	Source of diagnosis			
		Secondary only (N = 32930)	Primary and secondary (N = 28795)	Primary only (N = 11068)	Inferred (N = 7468)
HF		18.8	15.1	12.7	8.5
MI		13.2	10.0	8.3	14.1
Stroke		9.2	6.0	6.2	8.7
Diabetes	Type 1	0.62	0.39	0.49	0.90
	Type 2	14.73	10.79	9.40	9.53
	NOS	1.76	1.13	1.38	1.94
Hypertension		83.0	86.0	86.2	78.0
Thyroid disease	Hyper	1.7	1.5	1.6	1.0
	Hypo	8.5	7.1	6.8	5.6
Renal failure		22.4	10.9	11.0	10.0
COPD		46.9	44.7	40.9	38.7

Practice Research HF indicates heart failure, MI indicates myocardial infarction, COPD indicates chronic obstructive pulmonary disease, NOS indicates not otherwise specified. Note that some conditions may have been recorded on the same date as the atrial fibrillation diagnosis.

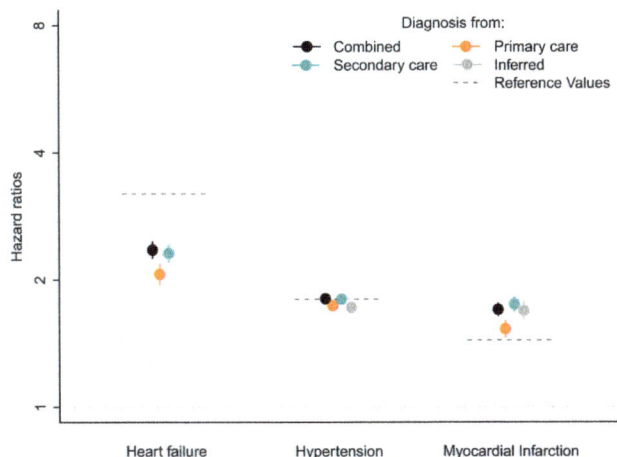

Figure 5. Hazard ratio estimates and 95% confidence intervals for pre-specified risk factors of interest. Results are shown separately for associations between each risk factor and incident AF, defined according to each source of cases and for a composite using all sources. All analyses were adjusted for age, sex, and practice ID. Note that the use of heart failure diagnosis in the algorithm for inferred AF precludes estimation of the hazard ratio. The dashed lines are point estimates of hazard ratios from the Framingham Heart Study for the same risk factors, adjusted for age and sex (see reference [58]).

understanding the EHR; a phenotype algorithm for AF based only on clinical guidelines could have required pulse palpation prior to diagnosis and would have excluded the vast majority of cases drawn from primary care data. However, Nicholson *et al.*, [2] found that "indicator markers" for rheumatoid arthritis in primary care, such as joint signs and symptoms or non-steroidal anti-inflammatory drug prescriptions, were potentially informative so the utility of "indicator markers" and screening tests should be evaluated on a disease-by-disease basis, and may inform further quality of care research as well as EHR research.

Integrating data from multiple sources identified more AF cases than examining any single source, as has been demonstrated for other cardiovascular conditions [7,59]. This was primarily due to the fact that a substantial percentage of cases were unique to each data source (13.8% from primary care, 41.0% from secondary care), but integrating data from both sources to infer diagnoses also identified unique cases (9.3%). This demonstrates that clinically informed combinations of treatment records and diagnoses of other conditions can be useful for interrogating EHR datasets, although this may not be true for all conditions in all contexts. For example, Pascoe *et al.* [60] found that procedure codes (such as mastectomy) and prescriptions (such as tamoxifen) could be combined to improve identification of cancer cases in UK EHR data, but we found that procedure codes (such as direct current cardioversion) did not improve AF case detection because they were almost exclusively recorded in patients with a pre-existing AF diagnosis. Additionally, coding combinations could be so complex for some conditions that this approach is infeasible; the inferred AF diagnosis incorporated not only medications but also whether diagnoses were recorded for another condition for which these medications might be used, namely HF, DVT, and PE. The CALIBER programme facilitated this as case definitions and associated EHR phenotypes had already been developed for these conditions; without access to a resource such as this, use of treatment and/or comorbidity information could be substantially more onerous.

The AF patients we identified differed by data source in regard to age, sex, and comorbid conditions, and also over time. Patients identified in secondary care were comparatively older than those identified in primary care, and in many cases AF was a secondary diagnosis made when the patient was admitted for another condition. These patients were also more likely to have a comorbid diagnosis for another condition such as HF, renal failure, or diabetes. Focusing on only one source of data could, therefore, give misleading results about the age distribution and relative health of the AF patient population; integrating data from multiple sources is important for obtaining a representative sample. Ignoring the temporal context of EHR data could also misrepresent the sample and present challenges for phenotyping. We found, as have others (e.g. [61]), that the impact of clinical guidelines can be investigated using EHR data. In our sample, the proportion of inferred AF cases decreased over the study period, as did the time between meeting the inferred criteria and receiving an AF diagnosis code. This gradual change in diagnostic and coding practices may be due to increasing awareness of AF as a condition warranting specific treatment, and potentially the inclusion in the QOF from 2004, although we did not observe a sharp alteration around this time point. This has broader implications for identification of disease cases in EHR data, particularly where treatment information is incorporated; case definitions and phenotype algorithms may need to allow for temporal changes in clinical practice and recording, and not rely on a single strategy being equally effective for all time points.

Limitations

The work described here has three major limitations relating to the data sources available for use, the strategy used for the AF case definition, and the capacity for external validation. Currently our phenotype algorithm does not use natural language processing (NLP) or imaging data. Use of non-coded data via NLP has been shown to improve detection of other cardiovascular conditions that are difficult to diagnose, such as angina pectoris [62], but although work in this area for application to CALIBER data is ongoing [63,64], it is not currently ready for general use. Ideally, AF cases identified in EHR data would be confirmed by electrocardiogram readings that displayed variability in the R-R intervals [14], but this source of data is also not currently available on a national scale.

As our aim was to develop an AF phenotype that was of use to all researchers using EHR data, regardless of computational resources, we did not employ some of the more sophisticated techniques used in some other EHR phenotyping studies. We interpreted the first diagnosis code in a patient record as a confirmed diagnosis, but in other EHR phenotypes researchers have required multiple diagnosis codes (e.g. [65]), or used more complex analytical methods (e.g. [66]). These strategies are undoubtedly useful for EHR phenotyping, particularly if the probability of false diagnoses is high, but this will be disease- and context-specific. In the case of AF in the UK during the time period considered, under-diagnosis is the more likely clinical scenario [16,17], and thus we deemed one AF diagnosis code sufficient. The inferred AF case definition was developed to capture some patients without a recorded diagnosis, but of course this cannot capture patients for whom no AF-related codes were recorded.

An important aspect of EHR phenotype development is validation, preferably against a "gold standard" (such as a manual review of case notes). We could not validate the AF phenotype in this manner as for the CALIBER programme, the initiation and funding of a separate study is required for re-contacting participants or clinicians to confirm diagnoses or review records. However, previous research has shown that AF diagnoses recorded in NHS primary care have a high degree of reliability even when relying on a single diagnosis code [24], although similar information is not available for secondary care (particularly when AF is not the primary diagnosis). The inferred diagnosis category also requires further validation work, particularly as it incorporates information on multiple diagnoses which may have their own limitations (for example, some HF patients will inadvertently be classified as AF patients if the sensitivity of HF diagnoses is less than perfect). In the near future we will apply CALIBER phenotype algorithms to data from the UK Biobank resource, which provides scope for validation of EHR phenotypes against self-reported data and clinical notes [67]. In the absence of external confirmation of AF diagnoses, we evaluated our phenotype definition by conducting epidemiological analyses of the association between known risk factors for AF onset and disease diagnosis in the CALIBER data set, and comparing our estimates to those from other studies. Our point estimates for the hazard ratios for AF and HF, hypertension, and MI were in the same direction as those obtained from comparable analyses in both traditional cohort [58,68] and EHR studies [26,31], which suggests that our AF identification strategy indexes a similar AF patient population.

Future research

The AF phenotype we have developed has been primarily informed by clinical understanding and interpretation of the EHR data. However, research on EHR phenotypes for other conditions has shown that data-driven approaches, such as using lagged linear correlations, can inform the EHR phenotyping process and facilitate the identification of patient subgroupings [4,69]. Once more sources of data, such as electrocardiogram results and clinical notes, are available on a national scale such approaches may prove useful for improved identification (especially refining

the inferred diagnosis category) and further classification of AF patients.

Conclusion

Overall, we have developed a transparent and reproducible method for identifying AF cases in data from linked EHR sources that detects more cases than using a single data source. We have also highlighted the importance of exploring the patient record prior to developing EHR phenotype algorithms, including a number of challenges that may be encountered and potential strategies for overcoming them. Development of CALIBER phenotype algorithms is an ongoing, iterative process involving researchers within, and outside, the CALIBER network. To facilitate this, the code lists, case definitions, and algorithm for AF are freely available via from the CALIBER website (www. caliberresearch.org), and we encourage feedback from those who make use of this, and other, CALIBER phenotype algorithms.

Acknowledgments

The authors would like to thank the reviewers, S. L. Kristensen and D. Albers, for helpful comments that improved the manuscript.

Author Contributions

Conceived and designed the experiments: KIM JW SCD HH. Performed the experiments: KIM JW SCD RJH RSP PP ADS ADT RJS HH. Analyzed the data: KIM JW. Contributed reagents/materials/analysis tools: KIM JW SCD RJH RSP PP ADS ADT RJS HH. Wrote the paper: KIM JW SCD RJH RSP PP ADS ADT RJS HH.

References

1. Newton KM, Peissig PL, Kho AN, Bielinski SJ, Berg RL, et al. (2013) Validation of electronic medical record-based phenotyping algorithms: results and lessons learned from the eMERGE network. Journal of the American Medical Informatics Association. pp. e147–e154.

2. Nicholson A, Ford E, Davies KA, Smith HE, Rait G, et al. (2013) Optimising Use of Electronic Health Records to Describe the Presentation of Rheumatoid Arthritis in Primary Care: A Strategy for Developing Code Lists. PLoS ONE. pp. e54878.

3. Richesson RL, Hammond WE, Nahm M, Wixted D, Simon GE, et al. (2013) Electronic health records based phenotyping in next-generation clinical trials: a perspective from the NIH Health Care Systems Collaboratory. Journal of the American Medical Informatics Association. pp. 1–7.

4. Hripcsak G, Albers DJ (2013) Correlating electronic health record concepts with healthcare process events. Journal of the American Medical Informatics Association 20: e311–e318.

5. Hripcsak G, Albers DJ (2013) Next-generation phenotyping of electronic health records. Journal of the American Medical Informatics Association: JAMIA 20: 117–121.

6. Weber GM, Mandl KD, Kohane IS (2014) Finding the Missing Link for Big Biomedical Data. JAMA: the journal of the ... 311: 2479–2480.

7. Rapsomaniki E, Timmis A, George J, Pujades-Rodriguez M, Shah AD, et al. (2014) Blood pressure and incidence of twelve cardiovascular diseases: lifetime risks, healthy life-years lost, and age-specific associations in 1.25 million people. Lancet 383: 1899–1911.

8. Albers DJ, Hripcsak G (2010) A statistical dynamics approach to the study of human health data: resolving population scale diurnal variation in laboratory data. Physics Letters A 374: 1159–1164.

9. Albers DJ, Hripcsak G (2012) Using time-delayed mutual information to discover and interpret temporal correlation structure in complex populations. Chaos (Woodbury, NY) 22: 013111–013111.

10. Conen D, Chae CU, Glynn RJ, Tedrow UB, Everett BM, et al. (2011) Risk of death and cardiovascular events in initially healthy women with new-onset atrial fibrillation. JAMA. pp. 2080–2087.

11. Lip GYH, Tse HF, Lane DA (2012) Atrial fibrillation. Lancet. pp. 648–661.

12. Denaxas SC, George J, Herrett E, Shah AD, Kalra D, et al. (2012) Data Resource Profile: Cardiovascular disease research using linked bespoke studies and electronic health records (CALIBER). International Journal of Epidemiology. pp. 1625–1638.

13. Camm AJ, Lip GYH, De Caterina R, Savelieva I, Atar D, et al. (2012) 2012 focused update of the ESC Guidelines for the management of atrial fibrillation: an update of the 2010 ESC Guidelines for the management of atrial fibrillation. Developed with the special contribution of the European Heart Rhythm Association. European heart journal 33: 2719–2747.

14. National Collaborating Centre for Chronic Conditions (2007) Atrial fibrillation: national clinical guidline for management in primary and secondary care. London: Royal College of Physicians. 1–171 p.

15. Kirchhof P, Curtis AB, Skanes AC, Gillis AM, Samuel Wann L, et al. (2013) Atrial fibrillation guidelines across the Atlantic: a comparison of the current recommendations of the European Society of Cardiology/European Heart Rhythm Association/European Association of Cardiothoracic Surgeons, the American College of Cardiology Foundation/American Heart Association/ Heart Rhythm Society, and the Canadian Cardiovascular Society. European heart journal 34: 1471–1474.

16. Fitzmaurice DA, Hobbs FDR, Jowett S, Mant J, Murray ET, et al. (2007) Screening versus routine practice in detection of atrial fibrillation in patients aged 65 or over: cluster randomised controlled trial. BMJ (Clinical research ed) 335: 383–383.

17. Scowcroft ACE, Cowie MR (2014) Atrial fibrillation: improvement in identification and stroke preventive therapy - data from the UK Clinical Practice Research Datalink, 2000–2012. International journal of cardiology 171: 169–173.

18. Gillam S, Steel N (2013) The Quality and Outcomes Framework–where next? BMJ (Clinical research ed) 346: f659–f659.

19. National Institute for Health and Care Excellence (2006) Atrial fibrillation: The management of atrial fibrillation. Available: http://www.nice.org.uk/guidance/ cg36/resources/guidance-atrial-fibrillation-the-management-of-atrial-fibrillation-pdf. Accesssed 2014 Oct 2.

20. De Caterina R, Ruigómez A, Rodríguez LAG (2010) Long-term use of anti-inflammatory drugs and risk of atrial fibrillation. Arch Intern Med. pp. 1450–1455.

21. Gallagher AM, Setakis E, Plumb JM, Clemens A, Van Staa T-P (2011) Risks of stroke and mortality associated with suboptimal anticoagulation in atrial fibrillation patients. Thromb Haemost. pp. 968–977.

22. Grosso A, Douglas I, Hingorani A, MacAllister R, Smeeth L (2009) Oral Bisphosphonates and Risk of Atrial Fibrillation and Flutter in Women: A Self-Controlled Case-Series Safety Analysis. PLoS ONE. pp. e4720.

23. Van Staa TP, Setakis E, Di Tanna GL, Lane DA, Lip GYH (2011) A comparison of risk stratification schemes for stroke in 79884 atrial fibrillation patients in general practice. Journal of Thrombosis and Haemostasis. pp. 39–48.

24. Ruigómez A, Johansson S, Wallander MA, Rodríguez LAG (2002) Incidence of chronic atrial fibrillation in general practice and its treatment pattern. Journal of clinical epidemiology 55: 358–363.

25. Watanabe H, Tanabe N, Makiyama Y, Chopra SS, Okura Y, et al. (2006) ST-segment abnormalities and premature complexes are predictors of new-onset atrial fibrillation: the Niigata preventive medicine study. Am Heart J 152: 731–735.

26. Ahlehoff O, Gislason GH, Jørgensen CH, Lindhardsen J, Charlot M, et al. (2012) Psoriasis and risk of atrial fibrillation and ischaemic stroke: a Danish Nationwide Cohort Study. European heart journal 33: 2054–2064.

27. Alonso A, Agarwal SK, Soliman EZ, Ambrose M, Chamberlain AM, et al. (2009) Incidence of atrial fibrillation in whites and African-Americans: the Atherosclerosis Risk in Communities (ARIC) study. American Heart Journal 158: 111–117.

28. Chiang C-H, Huang C-C, Chan W-L, Huang P-H, Chen Y-C, et al. (2013) Herpes simplex virus infection and risk of atrial fibrillation: A nationwide study. International journal of cardiology 164: 201–204.

29. Emilsson L, Smith JG, West J, Melander O, Ludvigsson JF (2011) Increased risk of atrial fibrillation in patients with coeliac disease: a nationwide cohort study. European heart journal 32: 2430–2437.

30. Fedorowski A, Hedblad B, Engström G, Gustav Smith J, Melander O (2010) Orthostatic hypotension and long-term incidence of atrial fibrillation: the Malmö Preventive Project. Journal of internal medicine 268: 383–389.

31. Friberg J, Buch P, Scharling H, Gadsbphioll N, Jensen GB (2003) Rising rates of hospital admissions for atrial fibrillation. Epidemiology (Cambridge, Mass) 14: 666–672.

32. Frost L, Vestergaard P (2004) Alcohol and risk of atrial fibrillation or flutter: a cohort study. Archives of internal medicine 164: 1993–1998.

33. Grundvold I, Skretteberg PT, Liestøl K, Gjesdal K, Erikssen G, et al. (2012) Importance of physical fitness on predictive effect of body mass index and weight gain on incident atrial fibrillation in healthy middle-age men. The American journal of cardiology 110: 425–432.

34. Nyrnes A, Mathiesen EB, Njølstad I, Wilsgaard T, Løchen M-L (2012) Palpitations are predictive of future atrial fibrillation. An 11-year follow-up of 22,815 men and women: the Tromso Study. European journal of preventive cardiology.

35. Perez MV, Dewey FE, Marcus R, Ashley EA, Al-Ahmad AA, et al. (2009) Electrocardiographic predictors of atrial fibrillation. American heart journal 158: 622–628.

36. Psaty BM, Manolio TA, Kuller LH, Kronmal RA, Cushman M, et al. (1997) Incidence of and risk factors for atrial fibrillation in older adults. Circulation 96: 2455–2461.

37. Schnabel RB, Aspelund T, Li G, Sullivan LM, Suchy-Dicey A, et al. (2010) Validation of an atrial fibrillation risk algorithm in whites and African Americans. Archives of internal medicine 170: 1909–1917.

38. Selmer C, Olesen JB, Hansen ML, Lindhardsen J, Olsen A-MS, et al. (2012) The spectrum of thyroid disease and risk of new onset atrial fibrillation: a large population cohort study. BMJ (Clinical research ed) 345: e7895–e7895.

39. Stewart S, Hart CL, Hole DJ, McMurray JJ (2001) Population prevalence, incidence, and predictors of atrial fibrillation in the Renfrew/Paisley study. Heart (British Cardiac Society) 86: 516–521.

40. Tsang TSM, Gersh BJ, Appleton CP, Tajik AJ, Barnes ME, et al. (2002) Left ventricular diastolic dysfunction as a predictor of the first diagnosed nonvalvular atrial fibrillation in 840 elderly men and women. Journal of the American College of Cardiology 40: 1636–1644.

41. Djoussé L, Levy D, Benjamin EJ, Blease SJ, Russ A, et al. (2004) Long-term alcohol consumption and the risk of atrial fibrillation in the Framingham Study. The American journal of cardiology 93: 710–713.

42. Heeringa J, Kors JA, Hofman A, van Rooij FJA, Witteman JCM (2008) Cigarette smoking and risk of atrial fibrillation: the Rotterdam Study. American heart journal 156: 1163–1169.

43. Lipworth L, Okafor H, Mumma MT, Edwards TL, Roden DM, et al. (2012) Race-specific impact of atrial fibrillation risk factors in blacks and whites in the southern community cohort study. The American journal of cardiology 110: 1637–1642.

44. Maddox TM, Ross C, Ho PM, Magid D, Rumsfeld JS (2009) Impaired heart rate recovery is associated with new-onset atrial fibrillation: a prospective cohort study. BMC cardiovascular disorders 9: 11–11.

45. Gottesman O, Kuivaniemi H, Tromp G, Faucett WA, Li R, et al. (2013) The Electronic Medical Records and Genomics (eMERGE) Network: past, present, and future. Genetics in medicine: official journal of the American College of Medical Genetics 15: 761–771.

46. Kho AN, Pacheco Ja, Peissig PL, Rasmussen L, Newton KM, et al. (2011) Electronic medical records for genetic research: results of the eMERGE consortium. Science translational medicine 3: 79re71–79re71.

47. Köhler S, Doelken SC, Mungall CJ, Bauer S, Firth HV, et al. (2014) The Human Phenotype Ontology project: linking molecular biology and disease through phenotype data. Nucleic acids research 42: D966–974.

48. McCarty Ca, Chisholm RL, Chute CG, Kullo IJ, Jarvik GP, et al. (2011) The eMERGE Network: a consortium of biorepositories linked to electronic medical records data for conducting genomic studies. BMC medical genomics 4: 13–13.

49. Overby CL, Pathak J, Gottesman O, Haerian K, Perotte A, et al. (2013) A collaborative approach to developing an electronic health record phenotyping algorithm for drug-induced liver injury. Journal of the American Medical Informatics Association. pp. 1–11.

50. Perlis RH, Iosifescu DV, Castro VM, Murphy SN, Gainer VS, et al. (2012) Using electronic medical records to enable large-scale studies in psychiatry: treatment resistant depression as a model. Psychol Med. pp. 41–50.

51. Rea S, Pathak J, Savova G, Oniki TA, Westberg L, et al. (2012) Building a robust, scalable and standards-driven infrastructure for secondary use of EHR data: The SHARPn project. Journal of Biomedical Informatics. pp. 763–771.

52. Ritchie MD, Denny JC, Crawford DC, Ramirez AH, Weiner JB, et al. (2010) Robust replication of genotype-phenotype associations across multiple diseases in an electronic medical record. American journal of human genetics 86: 560–572.

53. Hodgkinson JA, Taylor CJ, Hobbs FDR (2011) Treatment pathways for patients with atrial fibrillation. International Journal of Clinical Practice. pp. 44–52.

54. Cox DR (1972) Regression models and life-tables. J R Stat Soc Ser B 34.

55. Andersen PK, Abildstrøm SZ, Rosthøj S (2002) Competing risks as a multi-state model. Statist Med 26: 2389–2430.

56. R Core Team (2013) R: A language and environment for statistical computing. Vienna, Austria: R Foundation for Statistical Computing.

57. Davis RC, Hobbs FDR, Kenkre JE, Roalfe AK, Iles R, et al. (2012) Prevalence of atrial fibrillation in the general population and in high-risk groups: the ECHOES study. Europace 14: 1553–1559.

58. Schnabel RB, Sullivan LM, Levy D, Pencina MJ, Massaro JM, et al. (2009) Development of a risk score for atrial fibrillation (Framingham Heart Study): a community-based cohort study. Lancet 373: 739–745.

59. Herrett E, Shah AD, Boggon R, Denaxas S, Smeeth L, et al. (2013) Completeness and diagnostic validity of recording acute myocardial infarction events in primary care, hospital care, disease registry, and national mortality records: cohort study. BMJ. pp. f2350.

60. Pascoe SW, Neal RD, Heywood PL, Allgar VL, Miles JN, et al. (2008) Identifying patients with a cancer diagnosis using general practice medical records and Cancer Registry data. Family practice 25: 215–220.

61. Pivovarov R, Albers DJ, Hripcsak G, Sepulveda JL, Elhadad N (2014) Temporal trends of hemoglobin A1c testing. Journal of the American Medical Informatics Association: JAMIA: 1–7.

62. Pakhomov SS, Hemingway H, Weston SA, Jacobsen SJ, Rodeheffer R, et al. (2007) Epidemiology of angina pectoris: role of natural language processing of the medical record. Am Heart J 153: 666–673.

63. Shah AD, Martinez C, Hemingway H (2012) The freetext matching algorithm: a computer program to extract diagnoses and causes of death from unstructured text in electronic health records. BMC Medical Informatics & Decision Making 12.

64. Wang Z, Shah AD, Tate AR, Denaxas S, Shawe-Taylor J, et al. (2012) Extracting diagnoses and investigation results from unstructured text in electronic health records by semi-supervised machine learning. PLoS One 7: e30412.

65. Peissig PL, Rasmussen LV, Berg RL, Linneman JG, Mccarty CA, et al. (2012) Importance of multi-modal approaches to effectively identify cataract cases from electronic health records. Journal of the American Medical Informatics Association. pp. 225–234.

66. Perotte A, Hripcsak G (2013) Temporal properties of diagnosis code time series in aggregate. IEEE Journal Biomed Health Inform 17: 477–483.

67. Collins R (2012) What makes UK Biobank special? Lancet 379: 1173–1174.

68. Smith JG, Platonov PG, Hedblad B, Engstrom G, Melander O (2010) Atrial fibrillation in the Malmo Diet and Cancer study: a study of occurrence, risk factors and diagnostic validity. Eur J Epidemiol 25: 95–102.

69. Hripcsak G, Albers DJ, Perotte A (2011) Exploiting time in electronic health record correlations. Journal of the American Medical Informatics Association: JAMIA 18 Suppl 1: i109–115.

24

Association of Sick Sinus Syndrome with Incident Cardiovascular Disease and Mortality: The Atherosclerosis Risk in Communities Study and Cardiovascular Health Study

Alvaro Alonso[1]*, **Paul N. Jensen**[2], **Faye L. Lopez**[1], **Lin Y. Chen**[3], **Bruce M. Psaty**[4,5], **Aaron R. Folsom**[1], **Susan R. Heckbert**[2]

1 Division of Epidemiology and Community Health, School of Public Health, University of Minnesota, Minneapolis, Minnesota, United States of America, **2** Department of Epidemiology, School of Public Health, University of Washington, Seattle, Washington, United States of America, **3** Cardiovascular Division, Department of Medicine, University of Minnesota Medical School, Minneapolis, Minnesota, United States of America, **4** Cardiovascular Health Research Unit, Departments of Medicine, Epidemiology, and Health Services, University of Washington, Seattle, Washington, United States of America, **5** Group Health Research Institute, Group Health Cooperative, Seattle, Washington, United States of America

Abstract

Background: Sick sinus syndrome (SSS) is a common indication for pacemaker implantation. Limited information exists on the association of sick sinus syndrome (SSS) with mortality and cardiovascular disease (CVD) in the general population.

Methods: We studied 19,893 men and women age 45 and older in the Atherosclerosis Risk in Communities (ARIC) study and the Cardiovascular Health Study (CHS), two community-based cohorts, who were without a pacemaker or atrial fibrillation (AF) at baseline. Incident SSS cases were validated by review of medical charts. Incident CVD and mortality were ascertained using standardized protocols. Multivariable Cox models were used to estimate the association of incident SSS with selected outcomes.

Results: During a mean follow-up of 17 years, 213 incident SSS events were identified and validated (incidence, 0.6 events per 1,000 person-years). After adjustment for confounders, SSS incidence was associated with increased mortality (hazard ratio [HR] 1.39, 95% confidence interval [CI] 1.14–1.70), coronary heart disease (HR 1.72, 95%CI 1.11–2.66), heart failure (HR 2.87, 95%CI 2.17–3.80), stroke (HR 1.56, 95%CI 0.99–2.46), AF (HR 5.75, 95%CI 4.43–7.46), and pacemaker implantation (HR 53.7, 95%CI 42.9–67.2). After additional adjustment for other incident CVD during follow-up, SSS was no longer associated with increased mortality, coronary heart disease, or stroke, but remained associated with higher risk of heart failure (HR 2.00, 95%CI 1.51–2.66), AF (HR 4.25, 95%CI 3.28–5.51), and pacemaker implantation (HR 25.2, 95%CI 19.8–32.1).

Conclusion: Individuals who develop SSS are at increased risk of death and CVD. The mechanisms underlying these associations warrant further investigation.

Editor: Carmine Pizzi, University of Bologna, Italy

Funding: The Atherosclerosis Risk in Communities Study is carried out as a collaborative study supported by National Heart, Lung, and Blood Institute (NHLBI) contracts (HHSN268201100005C, HHSN268201100006C, HHSN268201100007C, HHSN268201100008C, HHSN268201100009C, HHSN268201100010C, HHSN268201100011C, and HHSN268201100012C). This Cardiovascular Health Study research was supported by contracts HHSN268201200036C, HHSN268200800007C, N01 HC55222, N01HC85079, N01HC85080, N01HC85081, N01HC85082, N01HC85083, N01HC85086, and grant HL080295 from the NHLBI, with additional contribution from the National Institute of Neurological Disorders and Stroke (NINDS). Additional support was provided by AG023629 from the National Institute on Aging (NIA). A full list of principal CHS investigators and institutions can be found at http://www.chs-nhlbi.org. This study was additionally funded by grant R21 HL109611 from the NHLBI. The funders had no role in study design, data collection and analysis, decision to publish, or preparation of the manuscript.

Competing Interests: The authors have declared that no competing interests exist.

* Email: alonso@umn.edu

Introduction

Sick sinus syndrome (SSS) is a disorder characterized by symptomatic dysfunction of the sinoatrial node. On the electro-cardiogram (ECG), SSS usually manifests as sinus bradycardia, sinus arrest, or sinoatrial block, sometimes accompanied by supraventricular tachyarrhythmias ("tachy-brady" syndrome).

Typical symptoms of SSS include syncope, dizziness, palpitations, exertional dyspnea and easy fatigability from chronotropic incompetence, heart failure, or angina [1–3]. Recent estimates suggest that>75,000 new cases of SSS occur in the US every year and that this number will more than double by 2060 [4].

Despite being relatively frequent and a major indication for pacemaker implantation [5], the impact of SSS on the risk of other cardiovascular outcomes and mortality has received little attention. The existing evidence on this issue is limited to clinical series and randomized trials of pacemaker implantation [6–11]. Overall, these studies show that mortality in patients with SSS can be substantial and potentially explained by the presence of other comorbidities. Most of these reports, however, did not directly compare outcomes in patients with SSS to individuals without this condition and, thus, the association of SSS occurrence with overall survival and risk of cardiovascular disease (CVD) in the general population, independent of other risk factors, remains unclear.

With the general aim of providing current and valid information on the prognosis of SSS, we identified and validated SSS events, and evaluated whether incident SSS was associated with mortality and CVD events in two large community-based cohorts, the Atherosclerosis Risk in Communities (ARIC) study and the Cardiovascular Health Study (CHS).

Methods

Study population

In 1987–89, the ARIC study recruited 15,792 men and women aged 45–64 from 4 US communities (Forsyth Co, NC; Jackson, MS; Minneapolis suburbs, MN; and Washington Co, MD) with the aim of identifying risk factors of atherosclerosis and incidence of CVD in the general population [12]. Participants were mostly white in the Minneapolis and Washington Co field centers, both white and black in Forsyth Co, while only blacks were recruited in Jackson. Study participants completed 4 follow-up visits in 1990–1992, 1993–1995, 1996–1998, and 2011–2013. Since baseline, participants have been called annually to obtain information on vital status, hospitalizations, and occurrence of CVD (response rate>90%).

Between 1989 and 1990, CHS recruited 5201 men and women aged 65 and older selected from Medicare eligibility lists in 4 US counties (Allegheny, PA; Forsyth, NC; Sacramento, CA; Washington, MD). An additional 687 participants, nearly all blacks, were recruited in 1990–1992 [13,14]. Participants had annual exams through 1999, with a follow-up phone call between exams. Since 1999, participants have been contacted semi-annually on the phone to determine vital status, hospitalizations, and occurrence of CVD. Average response rate to follow-up annual contacts was 92%.

For this analysis, we excluded participants who met any of the following criteria at baseline: atrial fibrillation (AF) or presence of a pacemaker, heart rate <50 bpm while not using beta-blockers, missing ECG data or covariates or, in the ARIC study, individuals not reporting white or black race, as well as blacks in the Minneapolis and Washington County field centers (because of small numbers). After exclusions, 14,816 individuals in ARIC and 5077 in CHS were included.

All study participants provided written informed consent at baseline and follow-up exams. The University of Minnesota Institutional Review Board and the University of Washington Institutional Review Board approved the present study.

Ascertainment of SSS

Details of SSS ascertainment and validation have been published elsewhere [4]. Briefly, hospitalizations during follow-up were identified through follow-up telephone calls, surveillance of local hospitals (only in ARIC), and inpatient Medicare claims (only in CHS). In both studies, trained abstractors collected information on all hospitalizations. Possible SSS cases were identified if a hospitalization listed International Classification of Diseases (ICD) 9 code 427.81 [sick sinus syndrome, sinus node dysfunction, tachy-brady syndrome] among the discharge diagnoses. Available medical records were reviewed by at least one study investigator. SSS was considered to be present if the record included a medical diagnosis of SSS and symptoms or signs consistent with SSS (e.g. syncope, dizziness, bradycardia, sinus pauses), without evidence of other conditions responsible for the episode, such as atrioventricular block or medication use. In the ARIC study, 294 individuals had an ICD9 code 427.81 in at least 1 hospitalization. Medical charts at the ARIC study sites were available in 195, and 130 were confirmed as SSS after review (no additional efforts were made to retrieve missing records from hospitals). Of these, 117 occurred among eligible participants. In CHS, the ICD9 code 427.81 was present in 179 individuals and a SSS diagnosis was confirmed in 99 of the 169 individuals with available medical charts, 96 of them in eligible participants. Only confirmed SSS cases were included in the primary analysis.

Outcome ascertainment

The outcomes of interest included coronary heart disease (CHD), stroke, heart failure, atrial fibrillation, pacemaker implantation, and all-cause mortality occurring during the follow-up. In both the ARIC study and CHS, incident CHD and stroke were validated using established criteria with physician review of records [15–17]. Specifically, incident CHD was defined as definite or probable myocardial infarction, or definite coronary death. Angina and subclinical CHD were not included in this definition. Stroke (ischemic or hemorrhagic) was defined as the sudden or rapid onset of neurological symptoms lasting for at least 24 hours or leading to death in the absence of evidence for a non-stroke cause. Incident heart failure in the ARIC study was defined as presence of an ICD code for heart failure (ICD9 428, ICD10 I50) in a hospitalization or death certificate [18]. In CHS, heart failure events were adjudicated based on review of study exams and hospital records [17]. Incident AF was identified from ECGs done during study exams, presence of ICD9 codes 427.31 or 427.32 in any hospitalization, from death certificates including AF as a cause of death (in ARIC only; ICD9 427.3 or ICD10 I48), and when 2 outpatient ICD9 codes 427.31 or 427.32 were present in Medicare claims within a 1-year period (in CHS only) [19–21]. Pacemaker implantation was based on the presence of the following ICD9 codes in any hospitalization: 37.8 (insertion, placement and revision of pacemaker), V45.01 (status post-pacemaker implantation), or V53.31 (fitting and adjustment of cardiac pacemaker). For pacemaker implantation occurring in the same hospitalization as the SSS diagnosis, we defined the length of follow-up as one day. Finally, information on all-cause mortality was obtained from follow-up calls, review of obituaries in local newspapers, and linkage to the National Death Index.

Assessment of other covariates

Measurements followed similar protocols in both ARIC and CHS. At baseline, study participants provided information on education, smoking status, medication use, and prevalence of cardiovascular disease. A physical examination collected information on height and weight, and blood pressure was measured with

Table 1. Baseline characteristics by sick sinus syndrome (SSS) diagnosis during follow-up, Atherosclerosis Risk in Communities (ARIC) study and Cardiovascular Health Study (CHS).

	ARIC		CHS	
	SSS	No SSS	SSS	No SSS
N	117	14699	96	4981
Age, years	57.7 (4.7)	54.1 (5.8)	72.3 (5.2)	72.7 (5.5)
Women, %	53	56	63	59
Non-white, %	13	26	7	16
Completed high school, %	77	77	69	71
Current smoker, %	21	26	8	12
BMI, kg/m^2	29.2 (5.4)	27.7 (5.4)	27.7 (4.8)	26.7 (4.7)
Hypertension, %	47	35	68	58
Diabetes, %	21	12	18	16
Total cholesterol, mg/dL	218 (40)	215 (42)	213 (40)	212 (39)
HDL cholesterol, mg/dL	45.7 (14.3)	51.5 (17.1)	54.3 (15.6)	54.4 (15.9)
Prevalent CHD, %	8	5	20	18
Prevalent HF, %	8	5	5	4
Prevalent stroke, %	1	2	3	4

Values correspond to means (standard deviations) or proportions. BMI: body mass index; CHD: coronary heart disease; HF: heart failure.

a random-zero sphygmomanometer. Fasting glucose and lipids were measured from blood samples obtained during the exam. Diabetes was defined as a fasting glucose level of ≥126 mg/dl, a non-fasting glucose of ≥200 mg/dl, use of an oral hypoglycemic agent or insulin, or, in the ARIC study, self-reported medical diagnosis of diabetes.

Statistical analysis

We calculated age-, sex- and race-specific incidence rates of the different outcomes among those with and without SSS in ARIC and CHS. Person-time for incidence calculations in those with SSS started at the time of SSS diagnosis until the outcome of interest, death, or censoring (December 31, 2009 in ARIC, or June 30, 2008 in CHS). Person-time for event rates during follow-up without SSS was calculated in a similar way, starting at baseline until SSS incidence, incidence of the outcome of interest, death, or censoring. Age, sex, and race-standardized rates were calculated via direct standardization using the pooled ARIC and CHS person-time as the reference. The associations between SSS incidence and each of the outcomes were assessed with Cox proportional hazards model including incident SSS as a time-varying exposure and adjusting for baseline covariates. Separate models were run in each cohort for the different outcomes. Initial models (Model 1) adjusted for age, sex, race, study center, education, smoking, body mass index, hypertension, total cholesterol, HDL cholesterol, diabetes, prevalent CHD, prevalent heart failure, and prevalent stroke. Additional models (Model 2) also adjusted for nonfatal incident CHD, incident HF, incident stroke and incident AF as time-dependent covariates, excluding the corresponding time-dependent incident disease from models in which that specific disease was the outcome. Individuals with prevalent stroke, CHD or heart failure at baseline were excluded from the corresponding analysis of incident disease. To address the impact of pacemaker implantation in the risk of AF and HF in those with SSS, we conducted two additional analyses. First, we included pacemaker implantation as a time-dependent covariate.

Second, in a separate analysis, we subclassified SSS as SSS with a pacemaker and SSS without pacemaker.

Cohort-specific results were meta-analyzed to provide pooled hazard ratios using inverse-of-variance weighting. Between-cohort heterogeneity was assessed with Cochran's Q and I^2 statistics [22]. Because medical records were not available for one third of cases with ICD9 427.81 in the ARIC study, and therefore could not be validated, we conducted a sensitivity analysis in the ARIC cohort including these possible SSS cases (n = 82) in addition to the validated cases. Analyses were conducted using SAS 9.3 (SAS Institute, Cary, NC) and Stata 12 (Stata Corp, College Station, TX).

Results

Among 19,893 eligible participants (14,816 in ARIC, 5077 in CHS), 213 incident SSS events were identified and validated (117 in ARIC, 96 in CHS) during a mean follow up of 17 years. The crude incidence rate of confirmed SSS was 0.4 and 1.5 per 1000 person-years in ARIC and CHS, respectively. In both cohorts, participants who developed SSS had a higher body mass index, were more likely to be white, and had higher prevalence of hypertension, diabetes, heart failure and CHD, compared to those without SSS (Table 1).

Overall, individuals with SSS had higher age, race, and sex-standardized incidence rates of mortality and CVD than those without SSS (Table 2). Standardized mortality rates were 55 per 1000 person-years in those with SSS compared to 22 per 1000 person-years in those without SSS (rate ratio 2.5, 95% confidence interval (CI) 1.4–4.3). Similar rate ratios were observed for heart failure, CHD, and stroke, while rates of AF and pacemaker implantation were more than 10 and 200 times higher for those with SSS compared to those without SSS, respectively. SSS was associated with higher mortality and CVD rates in men and women, whites and non-whites, and across age groups (Figure 1).

SSS was associated with a higher incidence of all outcomes after adjustment for baseline covariates (including sociodemographic

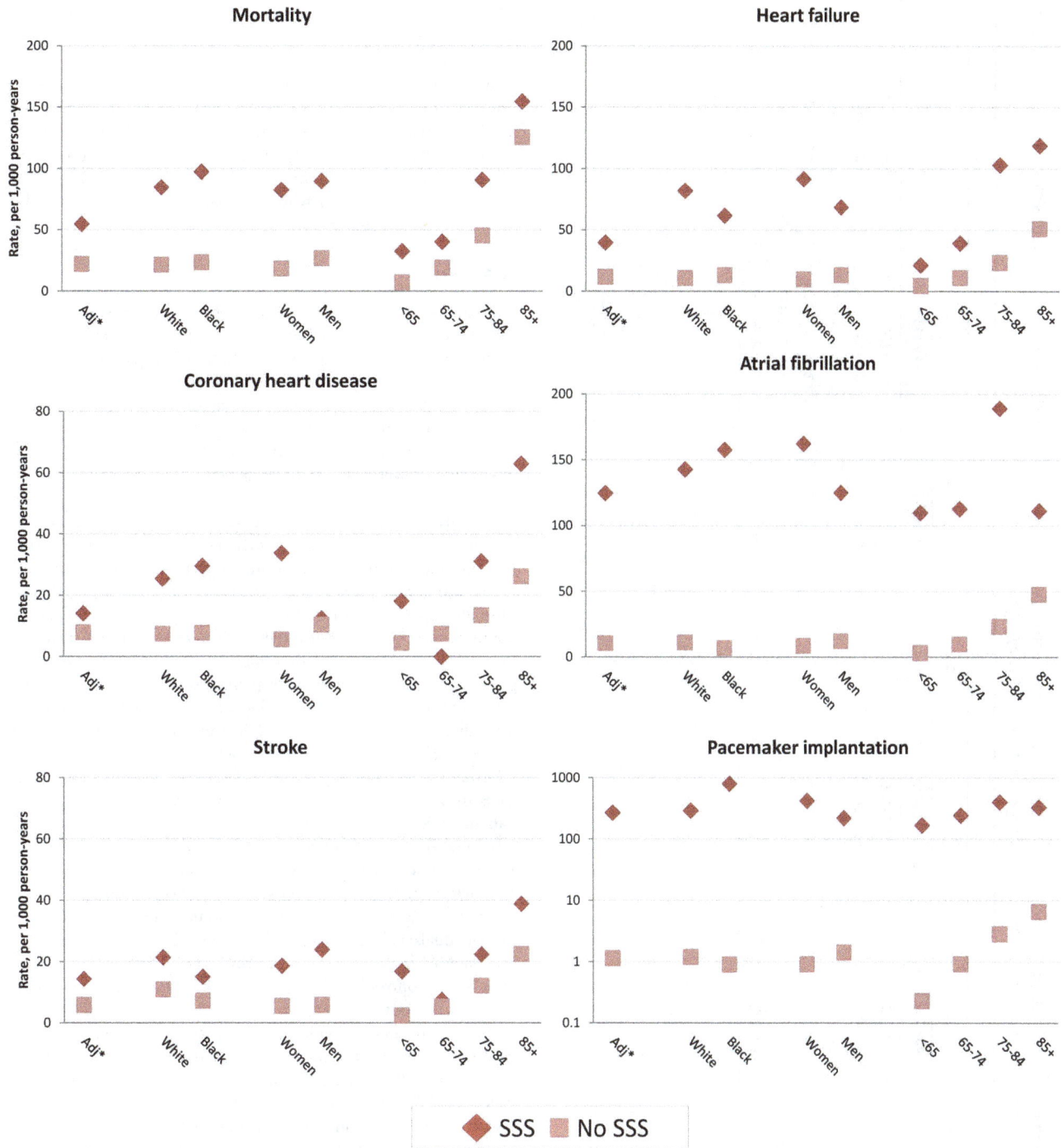

Figure 1. Incidence rates of selected cardiovascular diseases by SSS status, overall and by race, sex and age groups, combined Atherosclerosis Risk in Communities study and Cardiovascular Health Study, 1987–2009. Dark squares correspond to rates in SSS, light diamonds to rates in non SSS. Adj*: Standardized by age, sex and race to the combined ARIC and CHS person-time.

and clinical factors), with hazard ratios ranging from 1.4–1.7 for mortality, stroke and CHD, to 2.9 for heart failure, 5.8 for AF, and 54 for pacemaker implantation (Figure 2, Model 1). The higher risk of AF, heart failure and pacemaker implantation associated with SSS remained after adjusting for incident of other CVD as a time-dependent variable, though increased risk of death and other CVD among participants with SSS no longer were present (Figure 2, Model 2). Analysis restricted to the ARIC cohort that

incorporated possible SSS events without available charts in addition to validated cases yielded similar results (Table S1).

Adjustment for pacemaker implantation as a time-dependent covariate attenuated, but did not eliminate, the association of SSS with increased risk of AF and HF (Table 3). In an additional analysis classifying SSS patients according to pacemaker implantation status, we found that the elevated risk of AF and HF in those

Table 2. Age, race, and sex-standardized rates (per 1000 person-years) of mortality and selected cardiovascular events in individuals with and without sick sinus syndrome (SSS), combined Atherosclerosis Risk in Communities study, 1987–2009, and Cardiovascular Health Study, 1989–2008.

	No SSS			SSS			IRR (95% CI)
	Cases	Person-years	Rate (95%CI)	Cases	Person-years	Rate (95%CI)	
Mortality	7471	341,775	22.0 (21.5–22.5)	97	1135	54.5 (24.6–84.5)	2.5 (1.4–4.3)
Coronary heart disease	2326	309,467	7.9 (7.6–8.2)	22	854	14.2 (0.0–28.1)	1.8 (0.7–4.8)
Stroke	1831	327,396	5.7 (5.5–6.0)	20	955	14.3 (2.7–25.9)	2.5 (1.1–5.6)
Heart failure	3502	311,658	11.6 (11.2–12.0)	54	672	39.5 (22.7–56.3)	3.4 (2.2–5.2)
Atrial fibrillation	3256	327,078	10.5 (10.2–10.8)	60	416	125 (76.2–173)	12 (8.1–18)
Pacemaker implantation	423	340,162	1.1 (1.0–1.3)	132	423	268 (199–338)	235 (178–310)

CI: confidence interval; IRR: incidence rate ratio.

with SSS was lower among those with a pacemaker than among those without one (Table 3).

We observed significant between-cohort heterogeneity for the association between SSS and mortality, AF and pacemaker implantation. In the ARIC study, but not in CHS, SSS was associated with increased mortality after adjustment for cardiovascular risk factors. Similarly, the association of SSS with AF risk was stronger in the ARIC study than in CHS. In contrast, SSS was more strongly associated with pacemaker implantation in CHS than in ARIC (Figure 2).

Discussion

In this analysis of two community-based cohort studies in the US, we observed a higher risk of mortality and incident CVD, particularly AF, in individuals with SSS compared with those without SSS. As expected, SSS occurrence was a strong predictor of pacemaker implantation. Associations between SSS and investigated outcomes were weakened after adjustment for baseline covariates and incident CVD occurring during the follow-up. Between-cohort heterogeneity was observed for some outcomes.

Few prior studies have assessed mortality and CVD risk among patients with SSS compared to unaffected individuals. Most current information derives from clinical series or pacemaker implantation trials. Two studies compared age- and sex-adjusted mortality rates in SSS patients with rates observed in the general population [6,7]. In these studies, SSS patients without structural heart disease experienced mortality rates similar to those in the general population; however, this comparison can be problematic since the general population includes both healthy and sick individuals, potentially masking differences in mortality. Published clinical trials of pacemaker implantation modalities have offered information on mortality and CVD rates in SSS patients. These trials have consistently reported high mortality rates among patients with SSS (in excess of 5%/year), and considerable incidence of AF and other cardiovascular complications [8–11], which may be explained by the high prevalence of cardiovascular risk factors among SSS patients [23–25]. Trials, however, do not clarify the association of SSS with mortality and CVD compared to individuals without the condition. To the best of our knowledge, our analysis is the first to make this comparison in the general population controlling for cardiovascular risk factors and other potential confounding variables.

We found that individuals with SSS had higher mortality, stroke, and CHD rates than those without SSS. These differences disappeared after adjusting for cardiovascular risk factors and incident CVD. In contrast, the risk of heart failure and AF remained elevated in SSS patients compared to non-SSS individuals even after multiple adjustments. Taken together, our results would suggest that SSS patients have elevated mortality and higher risk of stroke and CHD in part through the association of SSS with higher incidence of AF and heart failure. CHD is an established risk factor for AF [26,27] and potentially for SSS [4,28], but recent findings suggest that AF also increases the risk of CHD events, supporting our hypothesis [29]. The relationship between AF and SSS is well-established, as attested by the co-occurrence of the two conditions in the so-called "tachy-brady syndrome", the involvement of the sinoatrial node in the development of atrial tachycardias [30], and the presence of diffuse atrial remodeling in SSS patients [31]. Further, the risk of both SSS and AF is elevated in association with polymorphisms and mutations in the *HCN4* gene [32], which encodes the hyperpolarization-activated ion channel HCN4, key for sponta-

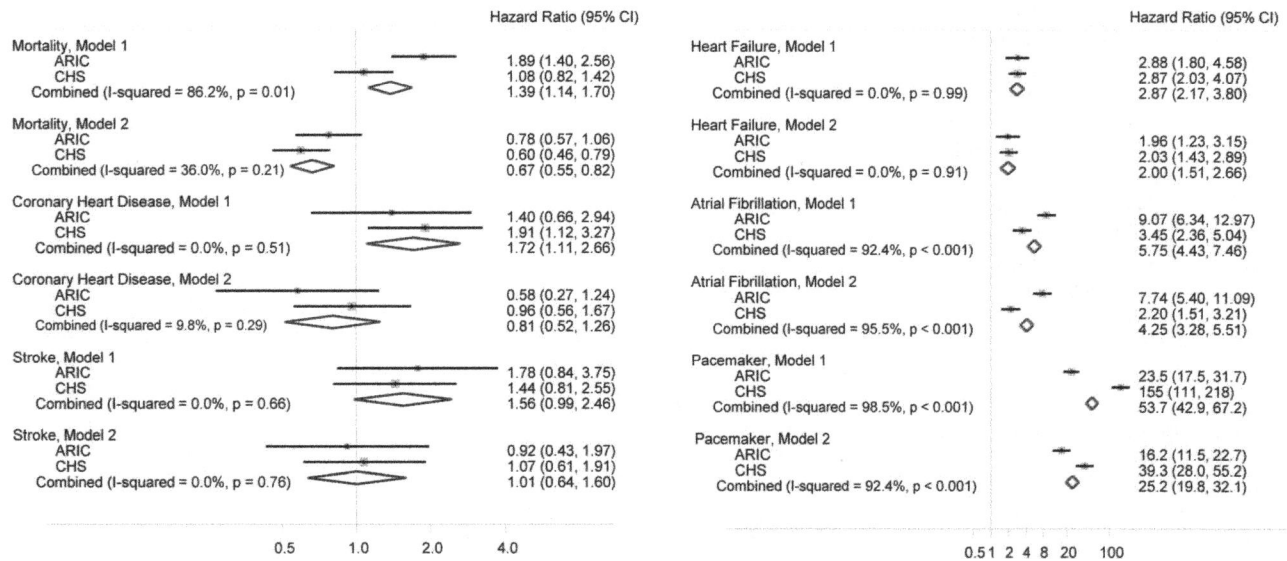

Figure 2. Cohort-specific and pooled hazard ratios (95% confidence intervals) of mortality and selected cardiovascular diseases comparing individuals with and without sick sinus syndrome (SSS), Atherosclerosis Risk in Communities (ARIC) study, 1987–2009, and Cardiovascular Health Study (CHS), 1989–2008. Model 1: Cox proportional hazards model adjusted for age, sex, race, study center, education, smoking, body mass index, hypertension, total cholesterol, HDL cholesterol, diabetes, prevalent coronary heart disease, prevalent heart failure, and prevalent stroke. Model 2: Adjusted as in model 1, and for incident coronary heart disease, incident heart failure, incident stroke and incident atrial fibrillation as time-dependent covariates.

neous pacemaker activity. Similarly, HF can result in dysfunction of the sinoatrial node and development of SSS [33], though no clearly described mechanism explains the increased risk of HF in individuals with SSS in our study. Reverse causation could be partly responsible: in a previous analysis of the ARIC and CHS cohorts, we found that higher levels of NTproBNP–a biomarker of volume overload and heart failure severity–were strongly associated with the subsequent development of SSS [4]. Future research should investigate these mechanisms in order to inform the management of SSS patients.

We observed that SSS patients receiving a pacemaker had a smaller increase of AF and HF risk that those without a device. These findings, however, need to be carefully interpreted given the lack of adequate information on patients' characteristics and, therefore, the potential for confounding by indication (i.e. healthier SSS patients being more likely to receive a pacemaker than those with more comorbidities).

Table 3. Cohort-specific and pooled hazard ratios (95% confidence intervals) for the association of sick sinus syndrome (SSS) with atrial fibrillation and heart failure, adjusting for cardiovascular risk factors and accounting for pacemaker implantation, Atherosclerosis Risk in Communities (ARIC) study, 1987–2009, and Cardiovascular Health Study (CHS), 1989–2008.

Adjustment for pacemaker implantation as a time-dependent covariate		ARIC	CHS	Pooled
Heart failure	No SSS	1 (ref.)	1 (ref.)	1 (ref.)
	SSS[a]	1.55 (0.91–2.65)	1.99 (1.30–3.06)	1.80 (1.29–2.52)
Atrial fibrillation	No SSS	1 (ref.)	1 (ref.)	1 (ref.)
	SSS[a]	5.39 (3.56–8.14)	2.15 (1.42–3.26)	3.40 (2.55–4.57)
Categorization of SSS status by pacemaker implantation				
Heart failure	No SSS	1 (ref.)	1 (ref.)	1 (ref.)
	SSS without pacemaker[b]	2.35 (1.22–4.54)	3.12 (1.85–5.25)	2.80 (1.86–4.21)
	SSS with pacemaker[b]	1.68 (0.87–3.26)	1.60 (1.01–2.53)	1.63 (1.12–2.37)
Atrial fibrillation	No SSS	1 (ref.)	1 (ref.)	1 (ref.)
	SSS without pacemaker[b]	8.01 (4.77–13.4)	2.64 (1.68–4.15)	4.27 (3.03–6.00)
	SSS with pacemaker[b]	7.18 (4.36–11.8)	1.63 (0.84–3.16)	4.20 (2.82–6.26)

[a,b]Results correspond to Cox proportional hazards model adjusted for age, sex, race, center, education, smoking, BMI, hypertension, total cholesterol, HDL cholesterol, diabetes, prevalent and time-dependent CHD, prevalent and time-dependent HF (for the AF analysis only), prevalent and time-dependent stroke, time-dependent AF (for the HF analysis only). Model [a] additionally adjusted for time-dependent pacemaker implantation.

Our study has relevant clinical and public health implications. First, the increased mortality and CVD risk in SSS patients could inform future clinical trials to refine the criteria for SSS treatment, for example evaluating a lower clinical threshold for pacemaker implantation or optimizing pacing modality, which may reduce risk of AF. Second, the higher risk of AF among SSS patients emphasizes the need for increased AF surveillance in this group. Additional studies should assess whether screening for AF in SSS patients could lead to better outcomes by providing adequate anticoagulation, rate, and rhythm control. And, third, because SSS is associated with increased CVD risk, guidelines for the management of SSS patients may need to address comprehensive cardiovascular prevention in addition to symptom relief, as well as a complete evaluation to identify possible substrates of SSS.

Limitations of this study include the partial information on SSS characteristics (such as severity of signs and symptoms), unavailability of outpatient data, where some SSS diagnoses might have been made, lack of detailed data on the management of SSS patients (e.g. type of pacemaker implanted), and the absence of systematic information on medication use at the time of SSS diagnosis and afterwards, which may influence the risk of the studied outcomes. Additionally, the small number of SSS events precluded the study of race, sex, or age differences. We also noticed significant between-cohort heterogeneity for the association of SSS with mortality and some outcomes, which may be due to differences in the age distribution of the cohorts. End-point ascertainment had also some shortcomings. Our definition of CHD included only hard end-points (myocardial infarction and definite coronary death) and, therefore, we could not assess the association of SSS with angina or subclinical CHD. In the ARIC cohort, heart failure was defined based on the presence of ICD codes in the discharge summary or death certificate, which could lead to overascertainment of events [34]. Nonetheless, study strengths include the large number of CVD events in these two community-based populations, the sociodemographic diversity of the study cohorts, the detailed data on cardiovascular risk factors, and the careful ascertainment and adjudication of cardiovascular outcomes and other covariates.

Conclusion

We have shown that individuals who develop SSS are at higher risk of several cardiovascular complications than those without SSS. Our study should provide renewed impetus to understand the pathophysiology of SSS and improve the management of these patients.

Supporting Information

Table S1 Hazard ratios (95% confidence intervals) of mortality and selected cardiovascular diseases comparing individuals with and without sick sinus syndrome (SSS), using alternative SSS definitions, Atherosclerosis Risk in Communities (ARIC) study, 1987–2009. Model 1: Cox proportional hazards model adjusted for age, sex, race, study center, education, smoking, body mass index, hypertension, total cholesterol, HDL cholesterol, diabetes, prevalent coronary heart disease, prevalent heart failure, and prevalent stroke. Model 2: As model 1, additionally adjusted for nonfatal incident coronary heart disease, incident heart failure, incident stroke and incident atrial fibrillation as time-dependent covariates

Acknowledgments

The authors thank the staff and participants of the ARIC study and CHS for their important contributions. Drs. Alvaro Alonso and Susan Heckbert had full access to all of the data in the study and take responsibility for the integrity of the data and the accuracy of the data analysis.

Author Contributions

Conceived and designed the experiments: AA PNJ FLL LYC BMP ARF SRH. Performed the experiments: AA PNJ FLL SRH. Analyzed the data: AA PNJ FLL. Contributed reagents/materials/analysis tools: ARF BMP. Wrote the paper: AA PNJ FLL LYC BMP ARF SRH.

References

1. Ferrer MI (1968) The sick sinus syndrome in atrial disease. JAMA 206: 645–646.
2. Ferrer MI (1973) The sick sinus syndrome. Circulation 47: 635–641.
3. Adán V, Crown LA (2003) Diagnosis and treatment of sick sinus syndrome. Am Fam Physician 67: 1725–1732.
4. Jensen PN, Gronroos NN, Chen LY, Folsom AR, deFilippi C, et al. (2014) The incidence of and risk factors for sick sinus syndrome in the general population. J Am Coll Cardiol 64: 531–538.
5. Bernstein AD, Parsonnet V (1996) Survey of cardiac pacing and defibrillation in the United States in 1993. Am J Cardiol 78: 187–196.
6. Shaw DB, Holman RR, Gowers JI (1980) Survival in sinoatrial disorder (sick-sinus syndrome). BMJ 280: 139–141.
7. Tung RT, Shen W-K, Hayes DL, Hammill SC, Bailey KR, et al. (1994) Long-term survival after permanent pacemaker implantation for sick sinus syndrome. Am J Cardiol 74: 1016–1020.
8. Andersen HR, Nielsen JC, Thomsen PEB, Thuesen L, Mortensen PT, et al. (1997) Long-term follow-up of patients from a randomized trial of atrial versus ventricular pacing for sick sinus syndrome. Lancet 350: 1210–1216.
9. Connolly SJ, Kerr CR, Gent M, Roberts RS, Yusuf S, et al. (2000) Effects of physiologic pacing versus ventricular pacing on the risk of stroke and death due to cardiovascular causes. N Engl J Med 342: 1385–1391.
10. Flaker G, Greenspon A, Tardiff B, Schron E, Goldman L, et al. (2003) Death in patients with permanent pacemakers for sick sinus syndrome. Am Heart J 146: 887–893.
11. Nielsen JC, Thomsen PEB, Højberg S, Møller M, Vesterlund T, et al. (2011) A comparison of single-lead atrial pacing with dual-chamber pacing in sick sinus syndrome. Eur Heart J 32: 686–696.
12. The ARIC Investigators (1989) The Atherosclerosis Risk in Communities (ARIC) study: design and objectives. Am J Epidemiol 129: 687–702.
13. Fried LP, Borhani NO, Enright P, Furberg CD, Gardin JM, et al. (1991) The Cardiovascular Health Study: design and rationale. Ann Epidemiol 1: 263–276.
14. Tell GS, Fried LP, Hermanson B, Manolio TA, Newman AB, et al. (1993) Recruitment of adults 65 years and older as participants in the Cardiovascular Health Study. Ann Epidemiol 3: 358–366.
15. White AD, Folsom AR, Chambless LE, Sharret AR, Yang K, et al. (1996) Community surveillance of coronary heart disease in the Atherosclerosis Risk in Communities (ARIC) Study: Methods and initial two years' experience. J Clin Epidemiol 49: 223–233.
16. Rosamond W, Folsom AR, Chambless LE, Wang CH, McGovern PG, et al. (1999) Stroke incidence and survival among middle-aged adults: 9-year follow-up of the Atherosclerosis Risk in Communities (ARIC) cohort. Stroke 30: 736–743.
17. Ives DG, Fitzpatrick AL, Bild DE, Psaty BM, Kuller LH, et al. (1995) Surveillance and ascertainment of cardiovascular events. The Cardiovascular Health Study. Ann Epidemiol 5: 278–285.
18. Loehr LR, Rosamond WD, Chang PP, Folsom AR, Chambless LE (2008) Heart failure incidence and survival (from the Atherosclerosis Risk in Communities Study). Am J Cardiol 101: 1016–1022.
19. Alonso A, Agarwal SK, Soliman EZ, Ambrose M, Chamberlain AM, et al. (2009) Incidence of atrial fibrillation in whites and African-Americans: the Atherosclerosis Risk in Communities (ARIC) study. Am Heart J 158: 111–117.
20. Psaty BM, Manolio TA, Kuller LH, Kronmal RA, Cushman M, et al. (1997) Incidence of and risk factors for atrial fibrillation in older adults. Circulation 96: 2455–2461.
21. Piccini JP, Hammill BG, Sinner MF, Jensen PN, Hernandez AF, et al. (2012) Incidence and prevalence of atrial fibrillation and associated mortality among Medicare beneficiaries: 1993–2007. Circ Cardiovasc Qual Outcomes 5: 85–93.
22. Higgins JPT, Thompson SG, Deeks JJ, Altman DG (2003) Measuring inconsistency in meta-analyses. BMJ 327: 557–560.
23. Lamas GA, Lee KL, Sweeney MO, Silverman R, Leon A, et al. (2002) Ventricular pacing or dual-chamber pacing for sinus-node dysfunction. N Engl J Med 346: 1854–1862.

24. Sweeney MO, Bank AJ, Nsah E, Koullick M, Zeng QC, et al. (2007) Minimizing ventricular pacing to reduce atrial fibrillation in sinus-node disease. N Engl J Med 357: 1000–1008.

25. Lau C-P, Tachapong N, Wang C-C, Wang J-f, Abe H, et al. (2013) Prospective randomized study to assess the efficacy of site and rate of atrial pacing on long-term progression of atrial fibrillation in sick sinus syndrome: Septal Pacing for Atrial Fibrillation Suppression Evaluation (SAFE) Study. Circulation 128: 687–693.

26. Weijs B, Pisters R, Haest RJ, Kragten JA, Joosen IA, et al. (2012) Patients originally diagnosed with idiopathic atrial fibrillation more often suffer from insidious coronary artery disease compared to healthy sinus rhythm controls. Heart Rhythm 9: 1923–1929.

27. Alonso A, Krijthe BP, Aspelund T, Stepas KA, Pencina MJ, et al. (2013) Simple risk model predicts incidence of atrial fibrillation in a racially and geographically diverse population: the CHARGE-AF Consortium. J Am Heart Assoc 2: e000102.

28. D'Ascenzi F, Iadanza A, Zaca V, Pierli C, Mondillo S (2010) Subocclusion of the sinus node artery during coronary angioplasty: arrhythmological considerations. Clinical Cardiology 33: E35–E37.

29. Soliman EZ, Safford MM, Muntner P, Khodneva Y, Dawood FZ, et al. (2014) Atrial fibrillation and the risk of myocardial infarction. JAMA Intern Med 174: 107–114.

30. Fedorov VV, Chang R, Glukhov AV, Kostecki G, Janks D, et al. (2010) Complex interactions between the sinoatrial node and atrium during reentrant arrhythmias in the canine heart. Circulation 122: 782–789.

31. Sanders P, Morton JB, Kistler PM, Spence SJ, Davidson NC, et al. (2004) Electrophysiological and electroanatomic characterization of the atria in sinus node disease: evidence of diffuse atrial remodeling. Circulation 109: 1514–1522.

32. Duhme N, Schweizer PA, Thomas D, Becker R, Schröter J, et al. (2013) Altered HCN4 channel C-linker interaction is associated with familial tachycardia–bradycardia syndrome and atrial fibrillation. Eur Heart J 34: 2768–2775.

33. Sanders P, Kistler PM, Morton JB, Spence SJ, Kalman JM (2004) Remodeling of sinus node function in patients with congestive heart failure: reduction in sinus node reserve. Circulation 110: 897–903.

34. Schellenbaum GD, Heckbert SR, Smith NL, Rea TD, Lumley T, et al. (2006) Congestive heart failure incidence and prognosis: case identification using central adjudication versus hospital discharge diagnoses. Ann Epidemiol 16: 115–122.

25

Multiple Biomarkers and Atrial Fibrillation in the General Population

Renate B. Schnabel[1]*, **Philipp S. Wild**[2,3], **Sandra Wilde**[1], **Francisco M. Ojeda**[1], **Andreas Schulz**[2], **Tanja Zeller**[1], **Christoph R. Sinning**[1], **Jan Kunde**[4], **Karl J. Lackner**[5], **Thomas Munzel**[2◐], **Stefan Blankenberg**[1◐]

1 Department of General and Interventional Cardiology, University Heart Center Hamburg-Eppendorf, Germany, 2 Department of Medicine 2, University Medical Center of the Johannes Gutenberg-University Mainz, Germany, 3 Center of Thrombosis and Hemostasis University Medical Center of the Johannes Gutenberg-University Mainz, Germany, 4 BRAHMS GmbH, Hennigsdorf/Germany, 5 Institute of Clinical Chemistry and Laboratory Medicine, University Medical Center of the Johannes Gutenberg-University Mainz, Germany

Abstract

Background: Different biological pathways have been related to atrial fibrillation (AF). Novel biomarkers capturing inflammation, oxidative stress, and neurohumoral activation have not been investigated comprehensively in AF.

Methods and Results: In the population-based Gutenberg Health Study (n = 5000), mean age 56±11 years, 51% males, we measured ten biomarkers representing inflammation (C-reactive protein, fibrinogen), cardiac and vascular function (midregional pro adrenomedullin [MR-proADM], midregional pro atrial natriuretic peptide [MR-proANP], N-terminal pro-B-type natriuretic peptide [Nt-proBNP], sensitive troponin I ultra [TnI ultra], copeptin, and C-terminal pro endothelin-1), and oxidative stress (glutathioneperoxidase-1, myeloperoxidase) in relation to manifest AF (n = 161 cases). Individuals with AF were older, mean age 64.9±8.3, and more often males, 71.4%. In Bonferroni-adjusted multivariable regression analyses strongest associations per standard deviation increase in biomarker concentrations were observed for the natriuretic peptides Nt-proBNP (odds ratio [OR] 2.89, 99.5% confidence interval [CI] 2.14–3.90; $P<0.0001$), MR-proANP (OR 2.45, 99.5% CI 1.91–3.14; $P<0.0001$), the vascular function marker MR-proADM (OR 1.54, 99.5% CI 1.20–1.99; $P<0.0001$), TnI ultra (OR 1.50, 99.5% CI 1.19–1.90; $P<0.0001$) and. fibrinogen (OR 1.44, 99.5% CI 1.19–1.75; $P<0.0001$). Based on a model comprising known clinical risk factors for AF, all biomarkers combined resulted in a net reclassification improvement of 0.665 (99.3% CI 0.441–0.888) and an integrated discrimination improvement of >13%.

Conclusions: In conclusion, in our large, population-based study, we identified novel biomarkers reflecting vascular function, MR-proADM, inflammation, and myocardial damage, TnI ultra, as related to AF; the strong association of natriuretic peptides was confirmed. Prospective studies need to examine whether risk prediction of AF can be enhanced beyond clinical risk factors using these biomarkers.

Editor: Jane-Lise Samuel, Inserm, France

Funding: The Gutenberg Health Study is funded through the government of Rheinland-Pfalz ("Stiftung Rheinland Pfalz für Innovation", contract number AZ 961-386261/733), the research programs "Wissenschafft Zukunft" and "Schwerpunkt Vaskuläre Prävention" of the Johannes Gutenberg-University of Mainz and its contract with Boehringer Ingelheim and PHILIPS Medical Systems including an unrestricted grant for the Gutenberg Health Study. This work was further supported by research grants from the Brandenburg Ministry of Economics, Germany, and the European Regional Development Fund (EFRE/ERDF). The test kits for Copeptin, Ct-pro-endothelin-1, MR-proADM, and MR-proANP were provided by B.R.A.H.M.S, Hennigsdorf, and for Nt-proBNP by Roche Diagnostics, Mannheim at no cost. Dr. Schnabel is supported by Deutsche Forschungsgemeinschaft (German Research Foundation) Emmy Noether Program SCHN 1149/3-1. The funders had no role in study design, data collection and analysis, decision to publish, or preparation of the manuscript.

Competing Interests: There are no conflicting interests to disclose by any of the other co-authors. The authors received funding (unrestricted grant) from commercial sources "Boehringer Ingelheim" and "PHILIPS Medical Systems". Co-author Jan Kunde, PhD, is employee of B.R.A.H.M.S GmbH, Hennigsdorf/Germany.

* Email: schnabelr@gmx.de

◐ Both authors contributed equally to the manuscript.

Introduction

With an increasing prevalence atrial fibrillation (AF) and its sequelae have become a significant public health burden not only through rising costs [1,2]. Despite its clinical relevance the pathophysiological background of atrial remodeling and AF is little understood. Several biological pathways have been studied in depth to gain insights into disease susceptibility. Most consistently three pathways have been focused on: inflammation, oxidative stress and neurohumoral activity [3–5]. Inflammatory changes are present in atrial tissue specimens even in lone AF patients without overt cardiovascular disease. [6] Besides inflammation, signs of oxidative stress are omnipresent in AF. Myocardial nicotinamide adenine dinucleotide phosphate oxidase activity and, to a minor extent, uncoupling of the endothelial nitric oxide synthase generate reactive oxygen species in atria of patients with AF. [7]

In experimental studies anti-oxidant ascorbate prevents AF by reducing oxidative stress and consecutive atrial remodeling [5]. Furthermore, autonomous imbalance and enhanced neurohumoral activation are risk factors for AF and perpetuate disease. Atrial and B-type natriuretic peptides and their precursors are cardiac specific markers of cardiovascular stress [4,8].

Recent investigations showed associations of circulating inflammatory biomarkers, oxidative stress and natriuretic peptides with AF risk that have not entered clinical practice yet [9–12]. In the meantime, novel blood biomarkers that reflect the three major pathophysiological pathways of AF have been reported. We hypothesized that newer biomarkers of cardiac and vascular function in normal physiology and during vascular stress (mid-regional pro adrenomedullin [MR-proADM], Copeptin, C-terminal pro endothelin-1) [13], sensitve cardiac troponin I ultra [TnI ultra] [14], and oxidative stress (glutathioneperoxidase-1, myeloperoxidase) [15] may be more strongly correlated with AF in a contemporary population-based cohort in comparison with known markers such as C-reactive protein [CRP], fibrinogen, and the natriuretic peptide precursor N-terminal pro B-type natriuretic peptide [Nt-proBNP] [9–13].

Methods

Ethics statement

Prior to enrolment participants signed written, informed consent. The study has been approved by the local Ethics Committee (Landesaerztekammer Rheinland-Pfalz, 837.020.07).

Study participants

Current analyses are based on the first 5000 individuals of the Gutenberg Health Study. The cohort constitutes a randomly selected population-based sample of European descent incepted in 2007 at the Department of Medicine 2, University Medical Center Mainz. Study participants are enrolled within 10-year age strata from 35–74 years. During a 5-hour clinic visit comprehensive information on cardiovascular risk factors are collected by standardized computer-assisted interview and anthropometric measures. Cardiovascular risk factor definitions comprised the following: smoking status comprised the categories non-smokers (never smokers and former smokers) and smokers. Diabetes mellitus was diagnosed when individuals reported a physician diagnosis of diabetes and/or a fasting blood glucose concentration of ≥126 mg/dL (minimum 8-hour fast) or a blood glucose level of ≥200 mg/dL at any time was measured on site. Dyslipidemia was defined based on a physician's diagnosis of dyslipidemia and/or an LDL/HDL ratio of >3.5. The definition of hypertension comprised anti-hypertensive drug treatment and/or a mean systolic blood pressure of ≥140 mmHg and/or a mean diastolic blood pressure of ≥90 mmHg. A history of cardiovascular disease (CVD) was self-reported myocardial infarction, stroke, prevalent coronary heart disease and heart failure. Heart failure was defined by clinic (New York Heart Association classification, heart failure medication) and echocardiography (left ventricular ejection fraction<55%).

The diagnosis of AF was made on a history of AF reported by the participant during the computer assisted interview and/or the ECG documentation of AF or atrial flutter [16]. AF was adjudicated by at least two physicians with cardiology training and experience in ECG reading. In two individuals the information on AF was missing.

Biomarker determination

Routine laboratory parameters were measured from fasting blood samples by standardized methods for CRP, blood glucose, creatinine, fibrinogen and lipids at enrolment. For additional measurements, samples were aliquotted and stored at $-80°C$ immediately after blood draw. In EDTA plasma, we measured Copeptin (functional assay sensitivity <1 pmoL/L), CT proendothelin-1 (functional assay sensitivity 19 pmoL/L), MR-proADM (functional assay sensitivity 0.25 nmoL/L), MR-proANP (functional assay sensitivity <10 pmoL/L) (Kryptor Immunoassays, B.R.A.H.M.S, GmbH, Germany), myeloperoxidase (intra–/inter-assay coefficient of variation 6.2/8.6) (CardioMPO kit, Prognostix, USA), and serum Nt-proBNP (intra–/inter-assay coefficient of variation 2.6/1.5) (Elecsys proBNP II Roche Diagnostics, Germany) biomarkers using commercially available assays. Sensitive TnI ultra was measured using Dimension RxL TnI (Siemens Healthcare Diagnostics, Germany) with a detection limit of 6 pg/mL and an assay range of 0–50.000 pg/mL. Glutathione-peroxidase-1 activity was determined in washed red cells obtained from whole blood anticoagulated with EDTA. Glutathione-peroxidase-1 was measured as previously described using the Ransel test kit (Randox, UK). [17].

Statistical methods

Available case analysis was used. To give an impression of the representativeness of the sample of the underlying population we also provide the baseline characteristics weighted for the age and sex distribution of the general population (N = 210.867, ©Statistisches Bundesamt, Wiesbaden 2011). Skewed variables (|skewness|>1) including selected biomarkers were logarithmically transformed to achieve near normal distribution. Raw characteristics of the sample are given as mean and standard deviation for continuous variables, or median (25th and 75th percentile) for variables with a skewed distribution. Number and percent are shown for categorical variables. Characteristics are also shown weighted according to the age and sex distribution of the study population (N = 210,867, data of the German Federal Statistical Office, Wiesbaden, 2007). Sample quantiles were computed nonparametrically, except for those quantiles were the number of observations below the limit of detection did not permit this (CRP and TnI), in that case, a parametric estimate was used via Tobit regression after log-transformation using a t-distribution.

The panel of biomarkers was related to AF. In logistic regression models, biomarkers were tested for their association with AF per one standard deviation increase. Models were adjusted for age and sex as well as for age, sex and atrial fibrillation risk factors body mass index, systolic blood pressure, antihypertensive medication, and a history of cardiovascular disease. For these models the values CRP or TnI below the detection limit were substituted by the constant proposed by Richardson and Ciampi [18].

To understand the ranking of the biomarkers in their strength of association with AF, a classification tree was built for circulating markers that remained statistically significantly related to AF in multivariable-adjusted analyses. A tree is grown as follows: first the variable that best separates the data into two groups is used to split the data. Then this is repeated on each subgroup recursively until a stopping criterion is reached. The end result will be a model that is too complex and most likely overfits the data. To avoid this the tree is pruned using cross-validation [19].

We further assessed the area under the receiver operating characteristic curve and performed reclassification analyses [20] on models based on clinical variables of the Framingham risk score (age, age², sex, male sex*age², body mass index, systolic blood pressure, antihypertensive medication, congestive heart failure,

Table 1. Characteristics of the sample according to AF status.

Variable	Individuals without AF N = 4837	Individuals with AF N = 161
Age, years	55.2±10.9	64.9±8.3
Female sex, N (%)	2413 (49.9)	46 (28.6)
Current smoking, N (%)	941 (19.5)	18 (11.2)
Body mass index [kg/m²]	27.1±4.8	29.3±5.4
Height [m]	1.7±0.09	1.73±0.09
Systolic blood pressure [mmHg]	132.7±17.7	133.8±17.8
Diastolic blood pressure [mmHg]	83.2±9.4	82.4±11.1
Heart rate [bpm]	68.8±10.8	69.5±13.0
Total cholesterol [mg/dL]	223.9±41.2	211.0±44.0
HDL-cholesterol [mg/dL]	56.7±15.8	49.7±15.8
Diabetes, N (%)	353 (7.3)	21 (13.0)
Hypertension, N (%)	2445 (50.6)	118 (73.3)
Hypertension treatment, N (%)	1336 (27.6)	96 (59.6)
History of coronary artery disease, N (%)	192 (4)	34 (22.2)
History of myocardial infarction, N (%)	134 (2.8)	22 (13.8)
Prevalent heart failure, N (%)	887 (18.4)	78 (48.8)
Biomarkers		
Creatinine [mg/dL]	0.88 (0.79/0.97)	0.95 (0.83/1.06)
Glutathione-peroxidase-1 [U/gHb]	167.3±38.0	164.7±37.5
Myeloperoxidase [ng/mL]	299.3 (237.87/373.98)	323.24 (241.49/376.77)
C-reactive protein [mg/L]	1.6 (0.93*/3.2)	2.50 (1.37/4.93)
Fibrinogen [mg/dL]	345 (303/398)	404 (347/499)
MR-proADM [nmol/L]	0.46 (0.39/0.54)	0.60 (0.50/0.72)
MR-proANP [pmol/L]	65.2 (48.7/88.2)	134.6 (79.9/219.3)
Nt-proBNP [pg/mL]	60.21 (22. 72/118.21)	290.60 (90.44/977.73)
Copeptin [pmol/L]	2.75 (1.77/4.38)	3.87 (2.53/6.63)
CT-pro endothelin-1 [pmol/L]	58.7 (50.3/67.7)	69.9 (60.0/84.7)
TnI ultra [pg/mL]	5.3* (3.5*/8.0)	9.0 (6.0/15.0)

Provided are mean and standard deviation for continuous variables, or median (25th and 75th percentile) for variables with a skewed distribution (|skewness|>1). Number and percent are shown for categorical variables.
*Sample quantile estimated using parametric model.
Abbreviations: AF, atrial fibrillation; CT-pro-endothelin-1, C-terminal pro endothelin-1; HDL, high density lipoprotein; MR-proADM, mid-regional pro adrenomedullin; MR-proANP, midregional pro atrial natriuretic peptide; Nt-proBNP, N-terminal pro B-type natriuretic peptide; TnI ultra, sensitive troponin I ultra.

congestive heart failure*age) [21] and biomarkers associated with AF in multivariable-adjusted analyses to assess the additive discriminative ability of the biomarkers between AF individuals and the rest of the sample for the biomarkers separately and in combination. Summary statistics of net reclassification improvement and integrated discrimination improvement were calculated.

We assumed a threshold of $P<0.05$ as statistically significant. To account for multiple testing we performed a Bonferroni correction for the number of tests applied in each analysis.

Secondary analyses

In secondary analyses we performed logistic regression analyses for AF including left ventricular ejection fraction and serum creatinine as covariates. Further models were computed for those individuals with and without AF on the ECG at the time of blood draw separately.

For statistical calculations we used R software, Version 3.0.2 (R Development Core Team, 2009). R: A language and environment

for statistical computing. R Core Team, Vienna, Austria. URL http://www.R-project.org).

Results

The characteristics of the total sample and for individuals with AF are shown in **Table 1**. Whereas the mean age of individuals without AF was 55.2±10.9 years (49.9% female), participants with AF were about ten years older (64.9±8.3 years) and less likely to be female (28.6%). Data weighted for the age and sex distribution of the underlying population revealed similar results (**Table S1 in File S1**).

In individuals with AF classical risk factor burden was higher. Prevalent cardiovascular disease was also more frequent in AF with a history of coronary artery disease in about one fifth of the subgroup, myocardial infarction in approximately 14% compared to a prevalence of less than 5% in participants without AF. Nearly half of the patients with AF had prevalent heart failure. Creatinine concentrations were higher in AF individuals 0.95 mg/dL (0.83/1.06 mg/dL) compared to the non-AF individuals 0.88 mg/dL

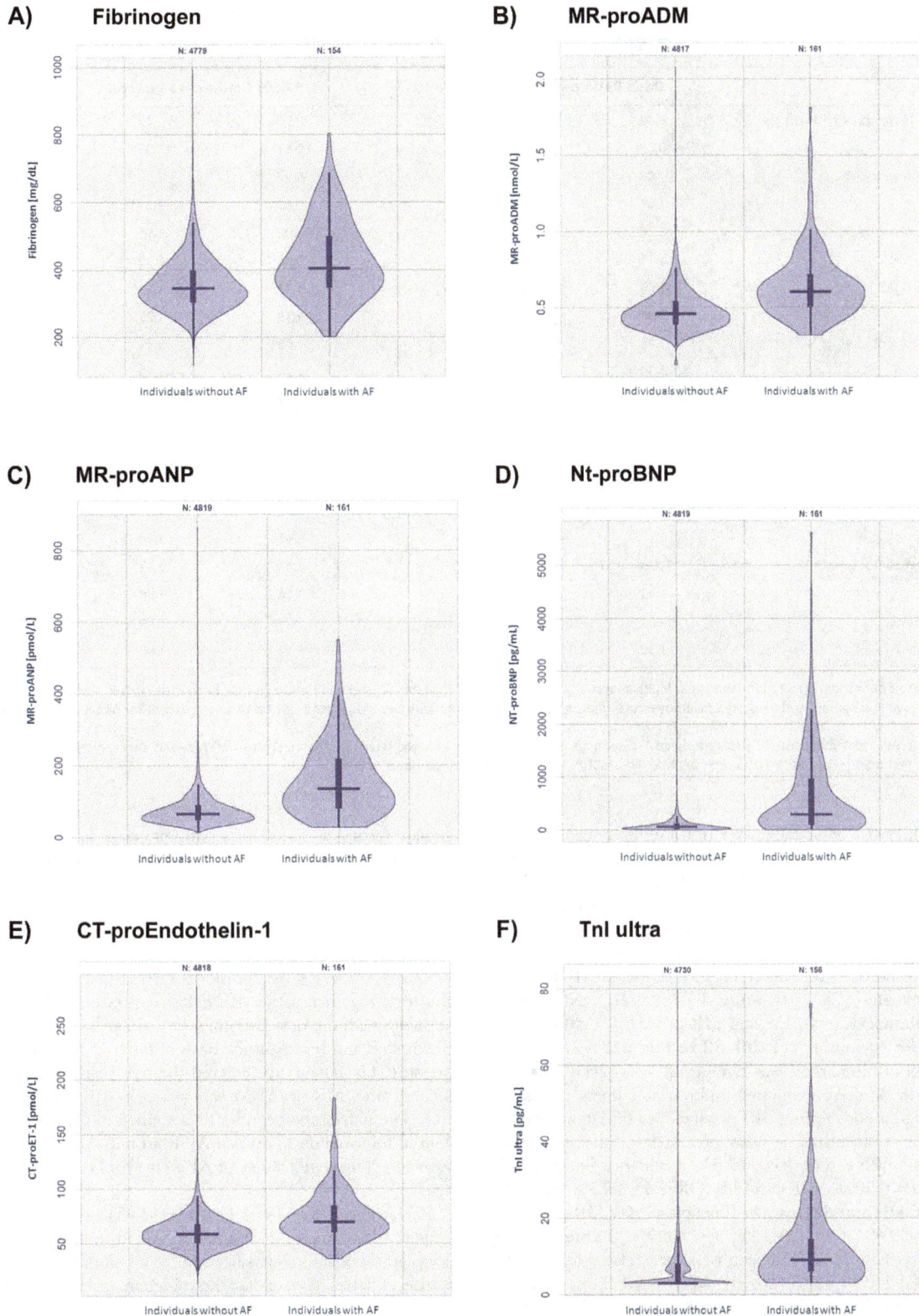

Figure 1. Violin plots of the distribution of circulating biomarkers in the total sample and in individuals with AF for markers that remained statistically significant in relation to AF in multivariable-adjusted models. For presentational reasons some outliers were removed from the plots. For MR-proADM values above 2.5 nmol/L (N = 2), Nt-proBNP values above 8000 pg/mL (N = 3), TnI ultra values above 80 pg/mL (N = 12) were excluded. Abbreviations: AF, atrial fibrillation; CT-proET, CT-pro endothelin-1; MR-proADM, mid-regional pro adrenomedullin; MR-proANP, midregional pro atrial natriuretic peptide; N-terminal pro B-type natriuretic peptide; TnI, troponin.

Table 2. Multivariable logistic regression models for biomarkers in relation to AF.

Variable	Odds Ratio per Standard Deviation	99.5% Confidence Interval		P Value*
Glutathione-peroxidase-1 [U/gHb]	0.88	0.70	1.12	1.00
	0.85	0.67	1.08	0.61
Myeloperoxidase [ng/mL]	1.09	0.87	1.36	1.00
	1.01	0.80	1.27	1.00
C-reactive protein [mg/L]	1.26	1.02	1.55	0.023
	1.11	0.88	1.39	1.00
Fibrinogen [mg/dL]	1.60	1.33	1.92	<0.0001
	1.44	1.19	1.75	<0.0001
MR-proADM [nmol/L]	1.86	1.48	2.34	<0.0001
	1.54	1.20	1.99	<0.0001
MR-proANP [pmol/L]	2.69	2.12	3.42	<0.0001
	2.45	1.91	3.14	<0.0001
Nt-proBNP [pg/mL]	3.36	2.52	4.49	<0.0001
	2.89	2.14	3.90	<0.0001
Copeptin [pmol/L]	1.27	1.00	1.61	0.049
	1.17	0.92	1.50	0.70
CT-pro endothelin-1 [pmol/L]	1.70	1.36	2.12	<0.0001
	1.43	1.14	1.80	0.00011
TnI ultra [pg/mL]	1.61	1.29	2.00	<0.0001
	1.50	1.19	1.90	<0.0001

*P values were Bonferroni corrected for ten tests. Multivariable-adjustment included age, sex (upper row) and age, sex, body mass index, systolic blood pressure, antihypertensive medication, and a history of cardiovascular disease (lower row). Biomarkers were logarithmically transformed except for glutathione-peroxidase-1 and fibrinogen.

Abbreviations: AF, atrial fibrillation; CT-pro-endothelin-1, C-terminal pro endothelin-1; TnI ultra, sensitive troponin I ultra; MR-proADM, mid-regional pro adrenomedullin; MR-proANP, midregional pro atrial natriuretic peptide; Nt-proBNP, N-terminal pro B-type natriuretic peptide.

(0.79/0.97 mg/dL). Most biomarker distributions appeared to be higher in AF. There seemed to be greater systemic inflammatory activity reflected by increased CRP and fibrinogen concentrations, whereas the distributions of glutathione-peroxidase-1 and myeloperoxidase largely overlapped with values in the overall cohort. All biomarkers of cardiovascular function were elevated.

Spearman partial correlation coefficients with AF revealed highest estimates for MR-proANP (r = 0.21), Nt-proBNP (r = 0.20), fibrinogen (r = 0.13), and MR-proADM (r = 0.12) after accounting for age and sex (**Table S2 in File S1**).

The panel of biomarkers was significantly associated with AF, P<0.0001. In Bonferroni-adjusted multivariable linear regression analyses greatest odds ratios [OR] per standard deviation increase in biomarker concentrations were observed for the natriuretic peptides Nt-proBNP (OR 2.89, 99.5% confidence interval [CI] 2.14–3.90; P<0.0001), MR-proANP (OR 2.45, 99.5% CI 1.91–3.14; P<0.0001) and the vascular function marker MR-proADM (OR 1.54, 99.5% CI 1.20–1.99; P<0.0001) (**Table 2**). The inflammatory biomarker fibrinogen remained related to AF (OR 1.44, 95% CI 1.19–1.75; P<0.0001) whereas CRP lost statistical significance, P = 1.00 in the multivariable model. Violin plots of the distribution of circulating biomarkers in the total sample and in individuals with AF for markers that retained statistical significance in multivariable-adjusted models are provided in **Figure 1**.

Associations were stronger in individuals in whom AF was present at the time of blood draw (**Table S3 in File S1**). Associations did not change markedly when adjusted for left ventricular ejection fraction and creatinine concentrations (**Table S4 in File S1**). Analyses stratified by heart failure status revealed

similar results in individuals without heart failure compared to participants with manifest disease (**Table S5 in File S1**).

In classification and regression tree analyses comparing the selection of clinical risk factors and biomarkers, which were significantly related to AF in multivariable-adjusted models, the natriuretic peptides Nt-proBNP and MR-proANP were the biomarkers selected by the model for the first two branchings of the tree, together with systolic blood pressure (**Figure 2**). The variables with the best discriminatory ability were selected first by the models and represent the basis of the tree. After systolic blood pressure, fibrinogen, age entered the tree besides MR-proANP a second time. MR-proADM was also selected to further split the tree. The natriuretic peptides thus seemed to provide the greatest gain in information to discern AF from non-AF participants. The strongest clinical indicators for AF were systolic blood pressure and age.

Reclassification analyses based on clinical risk factors and strongest biomarkers in relation to AF in multivariable analyses revealed significant reclassification for all biomarkers when added to the variables used in the Framingham risk model (**Table 3**). Greatest NRI and IDI was observed for the natriuretic peptides (NRI MR-proANP 0.599, IDI 0.088; NRI Nt-proBNP 0.545, IDI 0.095). Largest increases in the area under the curve (AUC) for the basic model 0.82 (99.3% CI 0.77–0.87) were observed for the addition of natriuretic peptides MR-proANP (AUC 0.85, 99.3% CI 0.80–0.90) or Nt-proBNP to the model (AUC 0.84, 99.3% CI 0.79–0.90). MR-proADM and TnI ultra were less strong and increased the AUC only to 0.83. All biomarkers combined resulted in a NRI of 0.665 (99.3% CI 0.441–0.888) with an IDI of more

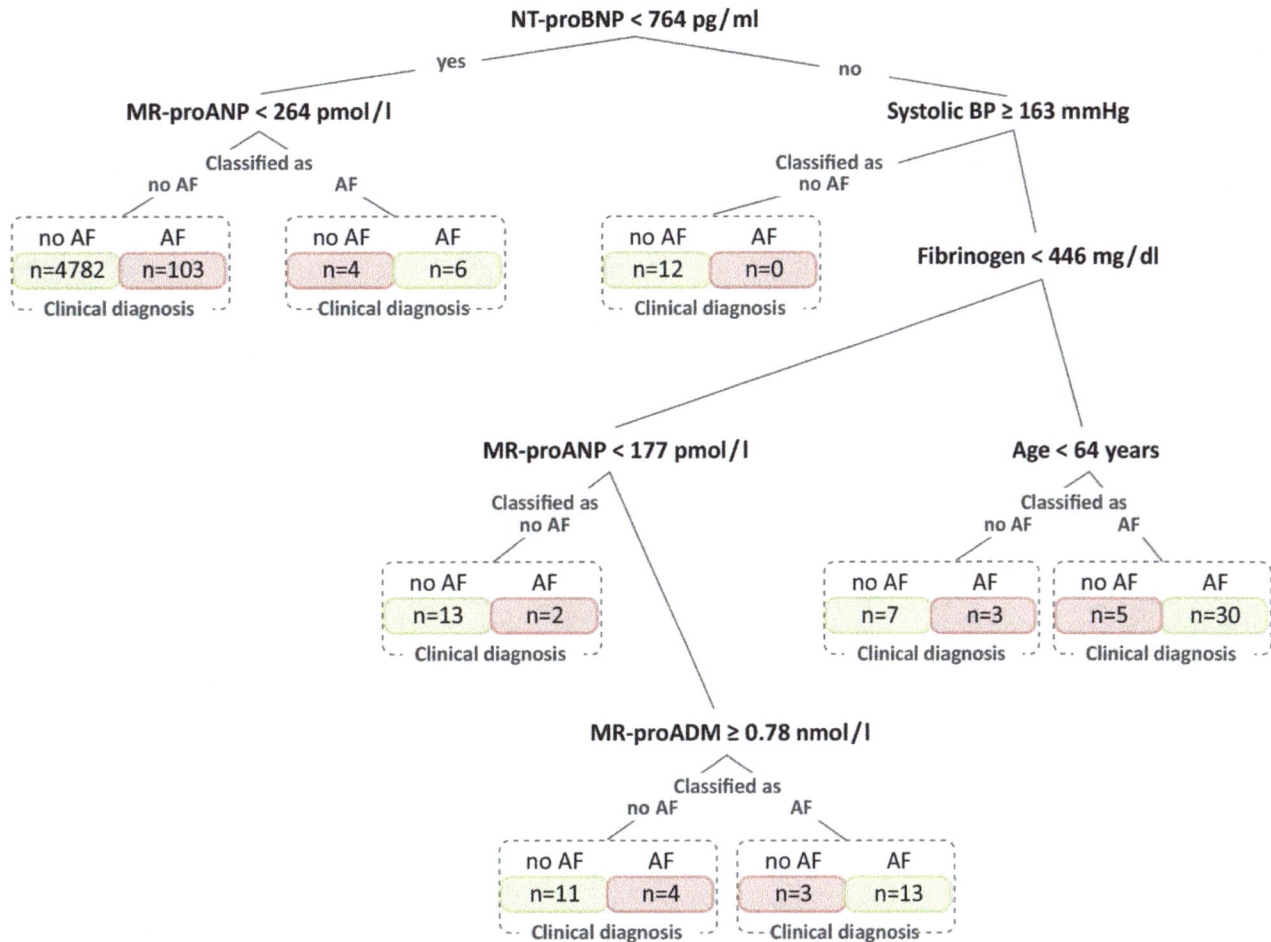

Figure 2. Regression tree for biomarkers that remained statistically significant in relation to AF in multivariable models. Provided are the mean that was selected for the split of the tree and the number of individuals for the respective branches of the regression tree. For every branch the classification of individuals according to the model and the correct, clinical diagnosis are shown. In red the number of participants misclassified by the statistical model is indicated. In two individuals the information on AF was missing. Abbreviations: AF, atrial fibrillation; BP, blood pressure; MR-proADM, mid-regional pro adrenomedullin; MR-proANP, midregional pro atrial natriuretic peptide; N-terminal pro B-type natriuretic peptide; TnI, troponin.

than 13% and an AUC of 0.86 (99.3% CI 0.80–0.91). The combination of all biomarkers provided more information than any of the biomarkers separately. R^2 reached 0.316 compared to 0.193 in a model containing the risk factors only.

Discussion

In our population-based sample, we identified biomarkers of cardiovascular function, MR-proADM and CT-pro endothelin, as novel correlates of AF. Natriuretic peptides were confirmed as strong predictors of AF. TnI ultra as an indicator of myocardial damage was also significantly related to AF. CRP lost statistical significance in relation to AF in multivariable-adjusted models whereas the pro-inflammatory and hemostatic biomarker fibrinogen remained significantly associated. No relevant association was observed for the examined indicators of oxidative stress. The increase in the AUC and net reclassification for biomarkers separately or combined was significant, but remained moderate.

As expected, natriuretic peptides were the strongest correlates of AF. However, we know that the additional value of B-type natriuretic peptide for reclassification in addition to clinical and electrocardiographic risk indicators may be modest [12]. More

novel biomarkers such as MR-proADM and CT-pro-endothelin have been in the focus of interest in cardiovascular disease because they reflect the activity of hormones central to vascular homeostasis [22,23]. In contrast to adrenomedullin and endothelin, the hormone precursors show higher analyte stability than their short-lived active hormones and more reliable assay characteristics [24,25].

Adrenomedullin exerts beneficial long-lasting vasodilatory and blood pressure lowering effects. It is expressed in endothelial cells but can also be found in the myocardium where adrenomedullin specific binding sites are expressed [26,27]. Whereas adrenomedullin has consistently been reported as a biomarker in a variety of diseases among them coronary artery disease and heart failure [28,29], little is known about the peptide in AF. In normal human cardiac tissue, the atria are the main site for positive inotropic effects of adrenomedullin measured by an increased force of contraction. Effects are blunted in ventricular myocardium and the failing heart [30]. During atrial stretch the adrenomedullin signaling cascade is down-regulated which may enhance susceptibility to AF [31]. In human cohorts MR-proADM appears to be less well suited to predict recurrence of AF [13] or incident AF events. [32] Whether MR-proADM is related to outcome in AF as

Table 3. Reclassification analysis for biomarkers significantly related to AF in multivariable-adjusted models.

	Odds Ratio per SD	P Value	NRI	P Value	IDI	P Value	Area Under the Curve	R²
Model with Framingham risk score variables	-	-	-	-	-	-	0.82 (0.77,0.87)	0.193
Fibrinogen	1.46 (1.21, 1.76)	<0.0001	0.345 (0.123, 0.566)	0.00020	0.023 (0.008, 0.038)	0.00031	0.82 (0.77,0.87)	0.213
MR-proADM	1.55 (1.21, 1.98)	<0.0001	0.212 (−0.005, 0.429)	0.060	0.014 (0.002, 0.027)	0.013	0.83 (0.78,0.87)	0.211
MR-proANP	2.53 (1.99, 3.22)	<0.0001	0.599 (0.382, 0.815)	<0.0001	0.088 (0.056, 0.120)	<0.0001	0.85 (0.80,0.90)	0.284
Nt-proBNP	3.04 (2.27, 4.07)	<0.0001	0.545 (0.328, 0.762)	<0.0001	0.095 (0.063, 0.127)	<0.0001	0.84 (0.79,0.90)	0.286
CT-pro endothelin-1	1.44 (1.15, 1.80)	<0.0001	0.158 (−0.059, 0.375)	0.35	0.014 (0.003, 0.026)	0.0070	0.82 (0.78,0.87)	0.209
TnI ultra	1.27 (1.11, 1.46)	<0.0001	0.500 (0.281, 0.720)	<0.0001	0.015 (0.004, 0.025)	0.00023	0.83 (0.79,0.88)	0.217
All biomarkers combined	-	-	**0.665 (0.441, 0.888)**	**<0.0001**	**0.125 (0.084, 0.166)**	**<0.0001**	**0.86 (0.81,0.91)**	**0.315**

The baseline model comprised Framingham risk score variables [21]: age, age², sex, male sex*age², body mass index, systolic blood pressure, antihypertensive medication, congestive heart failure, congestive heart failure*age. All biomarkers except for fibrinogen were logarithmically transformed for analyses. P values were Bonferroni corrected for seven tests.
R^2 is Nagelkerke R^2. Odds ratio, NRI, IDI and AUC are presented with 99.3% confidence interval in brackets.
Abbreviations: AF, atrial fibrillation; AUC, area under the curve; CRP, C-reactive Protein; CT-pro-endothelin-1, C-terminal pro endothelin-1; TnI ultra, sensitive troponin I ultra; IDI, integrated discrimination improvement; MR-proADM, mid-regional pro adrenomedullin; MR-proANP, midregional pro atrial natriuretic peptide; NRI, net reclassification improvement; Nt-proBNP, N-terminal pro B-type natriuretic peptide.

shown for congestive heart failure patients remains to be elucidated [29].

In contrast, endothelin-1 is one of the most potent vasocon-strictors, but also exerts hormone-like activities. Compensatory elevation of endothelin-1 activity can be measured in heart failure and AF [33]. More important than systemic endothelin may be the local endothelin production and auto- and paracrine effects in the atria in AF. In atrial tissue of patients with AF distinct gene expression patterns of the endothelin system can be demonstrated [34]. Changes seem to be pronounced in persistent AF compared to paroxysmal types of AF. Acute and chronic stretch response of the atria results in increased endothelin expression [31]. Atrial endothelin actions comprise the induction of natriuretic peptide secretion and increased mechanical and receptor-mediated transcriptional activation in cardiac myocytes [35]. The endothe-lin receptor antagonist bosentan attenuates transcription factor activity [31]. Whereas a small study that measured endothelin-1 did not show an association of the hormone with AF [36], systemic CT-pro-endothelin-1 elevation has been observed in cardiovascular disease and in patients with manifest AF compared to patients in sinus rhythm with a history of AF [13,23]. The origin of the measured circulating CT-pro-endothelin-1 is less clear. Endothe-lin-1 is most abundantly produced by vascular endothelium, but may also be a spill-over of cardiac myocyte or fibroblast endothelin-1 generation under the conditions of AF. [37].

For both vascular biomarkers we can extend recent findings of elevated MR-proADM and CT-pro-endothelin concentrations in patients with AF towards the general population [13].

Copeptin as a precursor of vasopressin only showed a borderline association with AF and lost statistical significance after risk factor adjustment similarly to recent publications [13,32].

Cardiac troponins are specific markers of myocardial injury. Tachyarrhythmias can be accompanied by elevated troponin despite the absence of coronary disease [38]. Minor troponin elevations are observed frequently in patients admitted with AF and may have prognostic importance [14]. Troponin T has been related to early recurrence of AF episodes in AF patients [13]. In our study in ambulatory individuals from the general population, TnI ultra was also significantly increased in AF compared to participants free of manifest disease although it was not selected among the strongest biomarkers in regression tree analyses. With the advent of more sensitive assays troponins will become increasingly common in biomarker panels assessing cardiovascular disease. More data will be accrued to understand the role of troponin elevations and outcome in AF. We will then get a better understanding of whether these biomarkers separately or in combination permit better risk prediction and may highlight pathways that can be addressed for therapeutic intervention.

Most of the strongest biomarkers in association with AF such as the natriuretic peptides, troponins and CT-pro-endothelin have also been related to heart failure [39–42]. Heart failure is an underlying disease in up to 50 percent of AF patients [43] and observed biomarker associations may be due to heart failure. However, despite a prevalence of almost 50 percent of heart failure in participants with AF in our cohort, association results did not markedly differ when analyses were stratified by heart failure status. To further elucidate the impact of heart failure on biomarker concentrations in AF larger cohorts or clinical AF cohorts might be necessary.

Despite sound experimental evidence on the central role of oxidative stress in AF genesis and perpetuation [44], we failed to show meaningful associations of circulating indicators of oxidative stress burden, i.e. glutathione-peroxidase-1 and myeloperoxidase. The missing correlation of systemically measured biomarkers is consistent with recent findings for different markers of oxidative stress myeloperoxidase and homocysteine [11,12]. One reason for the discrepancy may be the blood measurement that reflects systemic levels of biomarkers and may not adequately reflect the local milieu in the atria. Similarly, inflammatory activity is highly enhanced in atrial tissue, but systemic C-reactive protein is only mildly elevated and does not relevantly improve risk prediction of AF whereas the inflammatory and hemostatic biomarker fibrinogen ranges among the strongest correlates of AF [11,12].

Limitations

Owing to the nature of the study design we cannot exclude reverse causation with biomarker changes secondary to disease onset. Prospective studies are needed to understand the benefit of biomarker determination for AF risk prediction in addition to known risk factors of incident AF in the general population [12]. Among the strengths of the study are the comparatively large sample size and the availability of a broad spectrum of reliably measurable known and new biomarkers in a contemporary cohort. The direct clinical impact of our study is limited. Our results are hypothesis generating and may encourage future investigations into the pathophysiology and predictive value of biomarkers reflecting vascular function for risk stratification and opportunities for intervention. Whether the determination of biomarkers separately or in a panel combining the strongest biomarkers can improve clinical care and outcome needs to be shown.

In conclusion, besides the natriuretic peptides MR-proANP and Nt-proBNP and fibrinogen we identified novel candidate biomarkers reflecting vascular function, MR-proADM and C-terminal pro endothelin-1, and myocardial damage, TnI ultra, in relation to AF in the general population that may improve risk assessment in AF and merit prospective investigation in future studies.

Supporting Information

File S1 Supporting tables. Table S1. Characteristics of the sample according to AF status, weighted according to the age and sex distribution in the study population (N = 210,867). **Table S2.** Partial Spearman rank correlation coefficients for blood biomarkers and atrial fibrillation, adjusted for age and sex. **Table S3.** Logistic regression models for biomarkers in relation to history of AF in individuals with AF on the study ECG at the time of blood draw. **Table S4.** Logistic regression models for biomarkers in relation to AF adjusted for creatinine and left ventricular ejection fraction. **Table S5.** Age- and sex-adjusted logistic regression models for biomarkers in relation to AF stratified by heart failure status.

Acknowledgments

We thank the participants and dedicated study staff of the Gutenberg Health Study for their generous contribution of time and efforts. Thanks to Michael Schlüter for his careful review of the manuscript.

Author Contributions

Conceived and designed the experiments: RBS PSW SW FMO AS TZ JK KJL TM SB. Performed the experiments: RBS PSW SW CRS JK TZ. Analyzed the data: SW FMO AS TZ. Contributed reagents/materials/analysis tools: TZ JK. Wrote the paper: RBS PSW SW FMO AS CRS TM SB. Acquired funding: KJL TM SB.

References

1. Stefansdottir H, Aspelund T, Gudnason V, Arnar DO (2011) Trends in the incidence and prevalence of atrial fibrillation in Iceland and future projections. Europace 13: 1110–1117.

2. Holstenson E, Ringborg A, Lindgren P, Coste F, Diamand F, et al. (2011) Predictors of costs related to cardiovascular disease among patients with atrial fibrillation in five European countries. Europace 13: 23–30.

3. Wijffels MC, Kirchhof CJ, Dorland R, Allessie MA (1995) Atrial fibrillation begets atrial fibrillation. A study in awake chronically instrumented goats. Circulation 92: 1954–1968.

4. Matsukida K, Kisanuki A, Toyonaga K, Murayama T, Nakashima H, et al. (2001) Comparison of transthoracic Doppler echocardiography and natriuretic peptides in predicting mean pulmonary capillary wedge pressure in patients with chronic atrial fibrillation. J Am Soc Echocardiogr 14: 1080–1087.

5. Carnes CA, Chung MK, Nakayama T, Nakayama H, Baliga RS, et al. (2001) Ascorbate attenuates atrial pacing-induced peroxynitrite formation and electrical remodeling and decreases the incidence of postoperative atrial fibrillation. Circ Res 89: E32–E38.

6. Frustaci A, Chimenti C, Bellocci F, Morgante E, Russo MA, et al. (1997) Histological substrate of atrial biopsies in patients with lone atrial fibrillation. Circulation 96: 1180–1184.

7. Kim YM, Guzik TJ, Zhang YH, Zhang MH, Kattach H, et al. (2005) A myocardial Nox2 containing NAD(P)H oxidase contributes to oxidative stress in human atrial fibrillation. Circ Res 97: 629–636.

8. Tuinenburg AE, Brundel BJ, Van Gelder IC, Henning RH, van den Berg MP, et al. (1999) Gene expression of the natriuretic peptide system in atrial tissue of patients with paroxysmal and persistent atrial fibrillation. J Cardiovasc Electrophysiol 10: 827–835.

9. Aviles RJ, Martin DO, Apperson-Hansen C, Houghtaling PL, Rautaharju P, et al. (2003) Inflammation as a risk factor for atrial fibrillation. Circulation 108: 3006–3010.

10. Patton KK, Ellinor PT, Heckbert SR, Christenson RH, DeFilippi C, et al. (2009) N-terminal pro-B-type natriuretic peptide is a major predictor of the development of atrial fibrillation: the Cardiovascular Health Study. Circulation 120: 1768–1774.

11. Schnabel RB, Larson MG, Yamamoto JF, Kathiresan S, Rong J, et al. (2009) Relation of multiple inflammatory biomarkers to incident atrial fibrillation. Am J Cardiol 104: 92–96.

12. Schnabel RB, Larson MG, Yamamoto JF, Sullivan LM, Pencina MJ, et al. (2010) Relations of biomarkers of distinct pathophysiological pathways and atrial fibrillation incidence in the community. Circulation 121: 200–207.

13. Latini R, Masson S, Pirelli S, Barlera S, Pulitano G, et al. (2011) Circulating cardiovascular biomarkers in recurrent atrial fibrillation: data from the GISSI-atrial fibrillation trial. J Intern Med 269: 160–171.

14. van den Bos EJ, Constantinescu AA, van Domburg RT, Akin S, Jordaens LJ, et al. (2011) Minor elevations in troponin I are associated with mortality and adverse cardiac events in patients with atrial fibrillation. Eur Heart J 32: 611–617.

15. Rudolph V, Andrie RP, Rudolph TK, Friedrichs K, Klinke A, et al. (2010) Myeloperoxidase acts as a profibrotic mediator of atrial fibrillation. Nat Med 16: 470–474.

16. Camm AJ, Kirchhof P, Lip GY, Schotten U, Savelieva I, et al. (2010) Guidelines for the management of atrial fibrillation: the Task Force for the Management of Atrial Fibrillation of the European Society of Cardiology (ESC). Eur Heart J 31: 2369–2429.

17. Blankenberg S, Rupprecht HJ, Bickel C, Torzewski M, Hafner G, et al. (2003) Glutathione peroxidase 1 activity and cardiovascular events in patients with coronary artery disease. N Engl J Med 349: 1605–1613.

18. Richardson DB, Ciampi A (2003) Effects of exposure measurement error when an exposure variable is constrained by a lower limit. Am J Epidemiol 157: 355–363.

19. Hastie T, Tibshirani R, Friedman J (2009) The Elements of Statistical Learning: data mining, inference and prediction. New York: Springer.

20. Pencina MJ, D'Agostino RB Sr, D'Agostino RB Jr, Vasan RS (2008) Evaluating the added predictive ability of a new marker: from area under the ROC curve to reclassification and beyond. Stat Med 27: 157–172.

21. Schnabel RB, Aspelund T, Li G, Sullivan LM, Suchy-Dicey A, et al. (2010) Validation of an atrial fibrillation risk algorithm in whites and african americans. Arch Intern Med 170: 1909–1917.

22. Melander O, Newton-Cheh C, Almgren P, Hedblad B, Berglund G, et al. (2009) Novel and conventional biomarkers for prediction of incident cardiovascular events in the community. JAMA 302: 49–57.

23. Schnabel RB, Schulz A, Messow CM, Lubos E, Wild PS, et al. (2010) Multiple marker approach to risk stratification in patients with stable coronary artery disease. Eur Heart J 31: 3024–3031.

24. Morgenthaler NG, Struck J, Alonso C, Bergmann A (2005) Measurement of midregional proadrenomedullin in plasma with an immunoluminometric assay. Clin Chem 51: 1823–1829.

25. Papassotiriou J, Morgenthaler NG, Struck J, Alonso C, Bergmann A (2006) Immunoluminometric assay for measurement of the C-terminal endothelin-1 precursor fragment in human plasma. Clin Chem 52: 1144–1151.

26. Sugo S, Minamino N, Kangawa K, Miyamoto K, Kitamura K, et al. (1994) Endothelial cells actively synthesize and secrete adrenomedullin. Biochem Biophys Res Commun 201: 1160–1166.

27. Ichiki Y, Kitamura K, Kangawa K, Kawamoto M, Matsuo H, et al. (1994) Distribution and characterization of immunoreactive adrenomedullin in human tissue and plasma. FEBS Lett 338: 6–10.

28. Khan SQ, O'Brien RJ, Struck J, Quinn P, Morgenthaler N, et al. (2007) Prognostic value of midregional pro-adrenomedullin in patients with acute myocardial infarction: the LAMP (Leicester Acute Myocardial Infarction Peptide) study. J Am Coll Cardiol 49: 1525–1532.

29. Maisel A, Mueller C, Nowak R, Peacock WF, Landsberg JW, et al. (2010) Mid-region pro-hormone markers for diagnosis and prognosis in acute dyspnea: results from the BACH (Biomarkers in Acute Heart Failure) trial. J Am Coll Cardiol 55: 2062–2076.

30. Bisping E, Tenderich G, Barckhausen P, Stumme B, Bruns S, et al. (2007) Atrial myocardium is the predominant inotropic target of adrenomedullin in the human heart. Am J Physiol Heart Circ Physiol 293: H3001–H3007.

31. Kerkela R, Ilves M, Pikkarainen S, Tokola H, Ronkainen VP, et al. (2011) Key roles of endothelin-1 and p38 MAPK in the regulation of atrial stretch response. Am J Physiol Regul Integr Comp Physiol 300: R140–R149.

32. Smith JG, Newton-Cheh C, Almgren P, Struck J, Morgenthaler NG, et al. (2010) Assessment of conventional cardiovascular risk factors and multiple biomarkers for the prediction of incident heart failure and atrial fibrillation. J Am Coll Cardiol 56: 1712–1719.

33. Tuinenburg AE, van Veldhuisen DJ, Boomsma F, van den Berg MP, de Kam PJ, et al. (1998) Comparison of plasma neurohormones in congestive heart failure patients with atrial fibrillation versus patients with sinus rhythm. Am J Cardiol 81: 1207–1210.

34. Brundel BJ, van Gelder IC, Tuinenburg AE, Wietses M, van Veldhuisen DJ, et al. (2001) Endothelin system in human persistent and paroxysmal atrial fibrillation. J Cardiovasc Electrophysiol 12: 737–742.

35. Bruneau BG, Piazza LA, de Bold AJ (1997) BNP gene expression is specifically modulated by stretch and ET-1 in a new model of isolated rat atria. Am J Physiol 273: H2678–H2686.

36. Wozakowska-Kaplon B, Bartkowiak R, Janiszewska G, Grabowska U (2010) Does atrial fibrillation affect plasma endothelin level? Cardiol J 17: 471–476.

37. Kong P, Christia P, Frangogiannis NG (2014) The pathogenesis of cardiac fibrosis. Cell Mol Life Sci 71: 549–574.

38. Goette A, Bukowska A, Dobrev D, Pfeiffenberger J, Morawietz H, et al. (2009) Acute atrial tachyarrhythmia induces angiotensin II type 1 receptor-mediated oxidative stress and microvascular flow abnormalities in the ventricles. Eur Heart J 30: 1411–1420.

39. Maisel AS, Krishnaswamy P, Nowak RM, McCord J, Hollander JE, et al. (2002) Rapid measurement of B-type natriuretic peptide in the emergency diagnosis of heart failure. N Engl J Med 347: 161–167.

40. Velagaleti RS, Gona P, Larson MG, Wang TJ, Levy D, et al. (2010) Multimarker approach for the prediction of heart failure incidence in the community. Circulation 122: 1700–1706.

41. Bahrmann P, Bahrmann A, Hofner B, Christ M, Achenbach S, et al. (2014) Multiple biomarker strategy for improved diagnosis of acute heart failure in older patients presenting to the emergency department. Eur Heart J Acute Cardiovasc Care.

42. McKie PM, AbouEzzeddine OF, Scott CG, Mehta R, Rodeheffer RJ, et al. (2014) High-Sensitivity Troponin I and Amino-Terminal Pro-B-Type Natri-uretic Peptide Predict Heart Failure and Mortality in the General Population. Clin Chem.

43. Wang TJ, Larson MG, Levy D, Vasan RS, Leip EP, et al. (2003) Temporal relations of atrial fibrillation and congestive heart failure and their joint influence on mortality: the Framingham Heart Study. Circulation 107: 2920–2925.

44. Korantzopoulos P, Kolettis TM, Galaris D, Goudevenos JA (2007) The role of oxidative stress in the pathogenesis and perpetuation of atrial fibrillation. Int J Cardiol 115: 135–143.

26

Electrophysiological Changes Preceding the Onset of Atrial Fibrillation after Coronary Bypass Grafting Surgery

Feng Xiong[1,2], Yalin Yin[1], Bruno Dubé[1,3], Pierre Pagé[1,2,4], Alain Vinet[1,3]*

1 Research Center, Hôpital du Sacré-Cœur de Montréal, Université de Montréal, Montréal, Canada, 2 Montréal Heart Institute, Université de Montréal, Montréal, Canada, 3 Biomedical Engineering Institute, Université de Montréal, Montréal, Canada, 4 Department of Surgery, Université de Montréal, Montréal, Canada

Abstract

Background: The incidence of Post-CABG atrial fibrillation (AF) lies between 25% and 40%. It worsens morbidity and raises post-operative costs. Detection of incoming AF soon enough for prophylactic intervention would be helpful. The study is to investigate the electrophysiological changes preceding the onset of AF and their relationship to the preoperative risk.

Methods and Results: Patients were recorded continuously for the first four days after coronary artery bypass grafting surgery (CABG) with three unipolar electrodes sutured to the atria (AEG). The patients experiencing an AF lasting more than 10 minutes were selected and the two hours before the onset were analyzed. Four variables were found to show significant changes in the two hours prior to the first prolonged AF: increasing rate of premature atrial activation, increasing incidence of short transient arrhythmias, acceleration of heart rate, and rise of low frequency content of heart rate. The main contrast was between the first and last hour before AF onset. Preoperative risk was not predictive of the onset time of AF and did not correlate with the amplitude of changes prior to AF.

Conclusions: Post-CABG AF were preceded by electrophysiological changes occurring in the last hour before the onset of the arrhythmia, whereas none of these changes was found to occur in all AF patients. The risk was a weighted sum of factors related to the density of premature activations and the state of atrial substrate reflected by the sinus rhythm and its frequency content prior to AF. Preoperative risk score seems unhelpful in setting a detection threshold for the AF onset.

Editor: Xiongwen Chen, Temple University, United States of America

Funding: This study was supported by grants from: Natural Sciences and Engineering Research Council of Canada (NSERC: 121654 http://www.nserc-crsng.gc.ca); the Mathematics of Information Technology and Complex Systems, Canada (Mitacs, R13584 http://www.mitacs.ca). The funders had no role in study design, data collection and analysis, decision to publish, or preparation of the manuscript.

Competing Interests: The authors have declared that no competing interests exist.

* Email: alain.vinet@umontreal.ca

Introduction

Coronary artery bypass graft surgery (CABG) is performed to relieve angina, bypass atherosclerotic narrowing and improve blood supply to coronary circulation [1–5]. Currently about 500,000 CABG operations are carried out each year in United States. The incidence of post-CABG atrial fibrillation (AF) has been reported to be in the range of 25% to 40%, most often occurring in the second or third post CABG surgery day [6–8]. Postoperative AF is associated with worse morbidity, as well as longer and more expensive intensive-care hospitalization [9–14]. In the United States, the cost for intensive care for postoperative AF is substantial, with estimated annual expenditures exceeding 1 billion dollars [13,14]. Prediction of incoming AF after CABG soon enough to allow for prophylactic intervention would thus be helpful and cost-effective [2,3,12,13].

The fundamental mechanisms responsible for AF, especially for post-surgery patients, is still not well understood [2,3,12]. Electrical properties, such as heterogeneous spatial distribution of excitability and repolarization, may play an important role in the generation and perpetuation of the arrhythmia [15–17]. Many cardiac pathological changes may occur following CABG surgery [18]. These can enhance the heterogeneous spatial distribution of excitability and repolarization, thereby facilitating the occurrence of AF [19–23]. Studies to identify pre-, peri-, and postoperative risk factors have led to different and even controversial results [24–28]. Part of these discrepancies might originate from patients choice. The present study considers patients who did not have an AF diagnosis prior to surgery. It is based on the analysis of continuous post-operative recording of atrial electrograms to identify electrophysiological changes that might precede the AF onset, complemented by investigation of preoperative risk factors.

Material and Methods

Study Group

Patients admitted for CABG surgery from 1999 to 2004 at Hôpital du Sacré-Coeur de Montréal (HSC) and Institut de Cardiologie de Montréal (ICM) were screened. The protocol was approved by the Ethics Committee of Hôpital du Sacré-Coeur de Montréal (CE-95-11-69). Written consent was obtained from all patients. To document the process, the consent forms were kept in separate research files. Exclusion criteria were: not in sinus rhythm at admission, taking class I or III antiarrhythmic drugs or digoxin, having a prior history of AF, having congestive heart failure, receiving hemodialysis, or having a permanent pacemaker. A total of 137 patients were selected, 108 from HSC and 29 from ICM. The pre- and peri-operative available data were: age, sex, left ventricular ejection fraction (LVEF, insufficient if LVEF<60%), diagnosis of hypertension (HT), diabetes, chronic obstructive pulmonary disease (COPD), history of stroke, prior myocardial infarct (MI), serum creatinine level, preoperative use of beta-blocker, calcium channel inhibitor or vasopressor/inotrope, number of vessels at CABG surgery, beating heart or extra-corporal circulation used during CABG, duration of extracorpo-real circulation, duration of aortic clamp time. Patients who experienced an episode of AF lasting for more than 10 minutes in the first 4 post-operative days were classified as AF patients, and the others as Non-AF patients. 41 patients were classified as AF patients. Table 1 gives the distribution of the baseline character-istics in AF and Non-AF groups and the p values of the univariate logistic regression.

Preoperative Risk Factor

The distribution of the first sustained AF duration time was very inhomogeneous, ranging from 10 to 3732 minutes with a median of 353 minutes. Some of the Non-AF patients had short transient supraventricular arrhythmias, lasting from several seconds to 2 or 3 minutes with a maximum duration of 5 minutes. Association between preoperative data and AF was investigated by logistic regression. The effects of clinical variables and premature atrial activations on AF onset time was studied by Cox regression [29].

Variables Extracted from AEG in AF and Non-AF Patients

The recording device was a modified (class III) three-channel Holter digital recorder (Burdick, model 6632). Three unipolar electrodes (ETHICON model TPW40) were sutured on the atria epicardium and connected to the positive poles of the Holter by wires fixed on the patient's thoracic wall. Three negative poles were connected together to serve as a reference electrode positioned on the lateral side of the thigh with an adhesive skin solid gel electrode. In the most common setup, two electrodes were sutured on the right atrium and one on the left atrium. The sampling rate was 500 Hz per channel.

The main goal of this paper is to analyze changes that may occur before the onset of post-operative AF and, as such, the

Table 1. Demographic and surgical data.

Group	AF	Non-AF	p
Number (n, %)	41 (29.93%)	96 (70.07%)	
Age (years, mean±std)	68.54±7.40	62.42±9.19	<0.001
Sex (n, % among men/women)			0.939
Men	31 (29.8%)	73 (70.2%)	
Women	10 (30.3%)	23 (69.7%)	
LVEF (n, %)	7 (17.07%)	11 (11.46%)	0.197
Stroke (n, %)	4 (9.75%)	4 (4.16%)	0.222
MI (n, %)	23 (56.09%)	39 (40.62%)	0.007
COPD (n, %)	4 (9.75%)	10 (10.42%)	0.827
Hypertension (n, %)	30 (73.17%)	56 (58.33%)	0.072
Serum Creatinine (mean±std, mmol/L)	101.08±38.170	89.29±28.793	0.031
Diabetes (n, %)	13 (31.71%)	31 (32.29%)	0.575
Mean Number of Vessels of CABG surgery (Mean)	2.63	2.63	0.727
Beating Heart vs. Extracorporeal Circulation (n, %)	4 (9.75%)	10 (10.42%)	0.820
Extracorporeal Circulation Duration (minutes, mean±Std,)	71.07±38.89	66.27±34.54	0.528
Cross-clamp Duration (minutes, mean±Std)	44.05±26.09	42.94±25.66	0.682
Preop. Treatment (n, %)			
Beta-Blockers	28 (68.29%)	77 (80.21%)	0.474
Calcium Channel Blockers	11 (26.83%)	23 (23.96%)	0.444
Vasopressor/Inotropes	2 (4.87%)	3 (3.13%)	0.640

LVEF: left ventricular ejection fraction;
MI: prior myocardial infarct;
COPD: chronic obstructive pulmonary disease;
n is the number of the specified type of patients;
% represents the percentage among the AF or Non-AF group if not specified.

analysis of changes were firstly restricted to the group of patients having experience a prolonged (≥ 10 min) AF. To avoid the potential effects of anti-arrhythmic medications started after the AF onset, only the first sustained AF for each AF patient was considered and the two hours recordings before the onset were analyzed. 29 patients had analyzable three channels recordings and were selected for AEG analysis.

To verify the results obtained from AF patients, a control group of Non-AF patients was formed. Each AF patient was matched with two Non-AF patients, resulting in a group of 58 Non-AF patients. The priority order of matching criteria was preoperative risk score, date of surgery and gender. The criterion of risk score was intended to get the same distribution of preoperative risk in both groups. The criterion of date of surgery was aimed at bringing homogeneity in the surgery and post-surgery handling. The sex criterion was to reduce the differences that may be associated to gender. For Non-AF patients, the two hours corresponding to the same post-operative time than the matched AF patient were selected for analysis. Variables showing significant temporal changes among AF patients were analyzed using the matched 2 hours AEG recording of the Non-AF patients.

AEG records both local atrial activation (A) and far field ventricular activation (V) (see Figure 1). Since atrial activations are produced by the travelling of activation front close to the electrodes, they are not simultaneously throughout the recording channels. The order in which the channels activate provides information on the origin of the activation that can be used to separate normal sinus from abnormal activations. The atrial period of activation (AA: difference between the times of the first activation in consecutive beats), the intra-atrial conduction time (CTA: time between the first and last A within a beat) and the atrio-ventricular conduction time (CTAV: time elapsed from the last A to the following V within a beat) were computed for each beat.

Times of atrial (A) and ventricular (V) electrical activations were detected by using a dedicated method [30]. Atrial and ventricular activations of different channels belonging to the same beat were grouped together, and classified as normal sinus beats, premature atrial activation (PAA), premature ventricular activation (PVA), and episodes of ventricular or atrial arrhythmia (see detailed definition below). The detection and classification were finally validated using in-house software.

PAA were defined by two criteria: either the atrial firing order was different from that of normal sinus beats, or AA was less than 70% of the mean AA of normal sinus beats in the preceding five minutes. Rate of PAA (R_{PAA}) in a reference period (e.g. 5 minutes) was calculated as the number of PAA divided by the duration of the reference period, excluding intervals of atrial and ventricular arrhythmias. An episode of arrhythmia was considered to occur when there were more than 3 consecutive atrial or ventricular ectopic beats. In this case, the first ectopic beat was kept as a PAA or PVA, while the others were joined in an episode of arrhythmia.

The two-hour recordings were partitioned in 5 minutes intervals. All events different from normal sinus beats were excluded, as well as the first sinus beat immediately following a PAA or an episode of arrhythmia. The remaining normal sinus beats in each interval were used to calculate the mean AA (AAMean), its standard deviation (AAstd), the root mean square of differences between the successive AAs (rMSSD), the proportion of successive beats with a difference>50 ms (pNN50), mean intra-atrial (CTAMean) and atrio-ventricular conduction time (CTAVMean), and correlation between AA, CTA and CTAV time series, referred as CorrAA_AV, CorrAA_CTA, and CorrAV_CTA respectively. The spectral analysis of the AA was used to study the cardiac autonomic nervous system [31–37]. For each interval of 5 minutes, AA time series of normal sinus beats were extracted and detrended with a cubic spline. The detrended series were then resampled by interpolation with a fixed time step of 0.25 second. Successive windows of 512 points were considered, with a

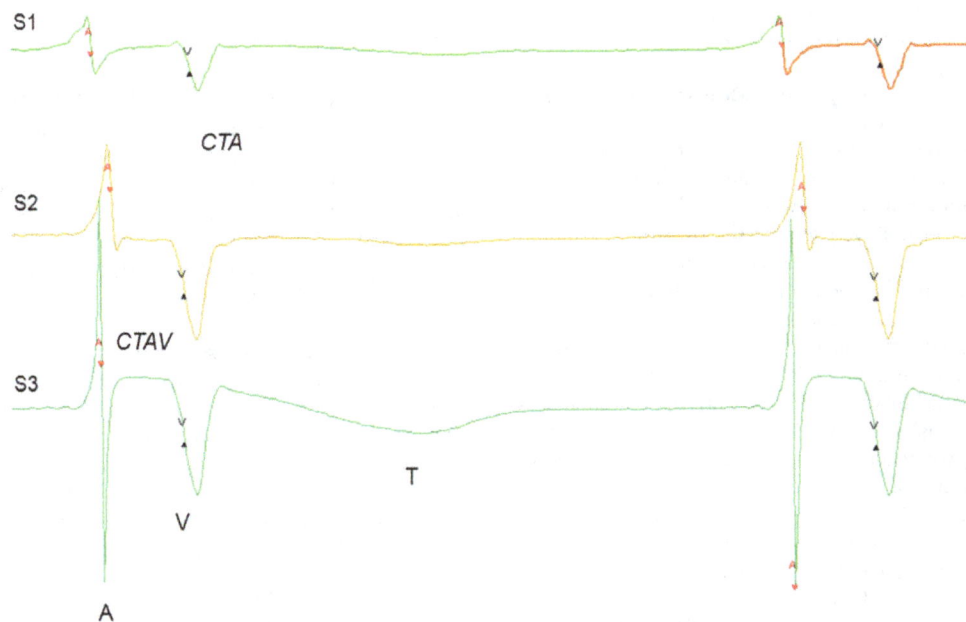

Figure 1. An example of recorded atrial electrogram (AEG): three channels (S1: superolateral right atrium. S2: inferior right atrium; S3: superior left atrium.) AEG in 2 consecutive normal sinus beats. The atrial (A) and ventricular (V) activations are indicated, as well as the ventricular T wave (T). AA, CTA and CTAV are also indicated.

256 points overlap. Results of the windows within each five minutes interval were averaged. Each time series of 512 points was convoluted with a Hamming window. Yule-Walker auto regression method was used to compute the power spectrum of the resulting time series. Following common rules in heart rate variability (*HRV*) analysis [35,37–39], power spectrum contents of the low (*LF*: 0.04–0.15 Hz) and high (*HF*: 0.15–0.40 Hz) frequencies components were calculated, as well as *LFPortion* (*LF/(LF+HF)*), *HFPortion* (*HF/(LF+HF)*), *LF/HF* and *HF/LF* Ratios. For some analysis, time partitions from 10 to 60 minutes were also considered. In these cases, the values assigned to each interval were the mean of 5 minutes intervals enclosed in each period.

An alternative method was developed to normalize data for each patient. For *AA*, *CTA* and *CTAV*, each data point was replaced by its position ($\in\{0,1\}$) in the cumulative distribution of values obtained for each patient during the two hours, and then the mean position was calculated for each 5 minutes interval. For *PAA* rate, arrhythmia duration, *AA* standard deviation, *LF*, *HF*, *LF* Portion and *HF* Portion, *LF/HF* and *HF/LF* ratio, *CTA*, *CTAMean*, *CTAStd*, *CTAV*, *CTAVStd*, *CorrAA_AV*, *CorrAA_CTA*, *CorrAV_CTA*, the values were obtained for each five minutes interval, and position was allocated with respect to the set of 24 values obtained from the two hours. The rule to compute values for >5 minutes partitions was the same as for 5 minutes data. In the sequel, these are designated as position data.

Cluster analysis was also use to compare the time course of different variables among patients. Pearson's correlation coefficient was used as similarity measure. If a patient temporal pattern of change was significantly ($p \leq 0.5$) correlated with the mean profile of an existing cluster, it was added to the cluster [40].

Results

Preoperative Risk Factor Analysis

It might be conjectured that the nature and amplitude of the changes needed to trigger an AF episode depend on the level of pre- and peri-operative risk. The data described in Table 1, available for 137 patients, were used to produce a preoperative risk score via logistic regression.

Preoperative Risk Score by Multivariate Logistic Regression Analysis. The study group had more men than women (104 vs. 33), but the proportion of AF patients among men or women was similar (29.8% vs. 30.3%). Analyses were performed using univariate and forward conditional multivariate logistic regression. For multivariate analysis, the model entry and retention criteria were set at $p<0.1$ and $p<0.15$. The final logistic models were evaluated using the Hosmer-Lemeshow goodness-of-fit test [41]. Both unweighted and weighted versions were tried, the latter to alleviate the men vs. women disproportion by multiplying women contribution to the likelihood function by the men to women ratio. Since there were only minor differences between the two types of models (same choice of variables, slight changes in parameters values and significance), only the results of the weighted versions are reported.

As seen in Table 2, four variables were identified as potential predictors by univariate logistic regression: age ($p<0.001$), prior myocardial infarct ($p = 0.007$), level of serum creatinine ($p = 0.03$), hypertension ($p = 0.072$). Three of these were kept in the multivariate model: 1) Age ($\beta = 0.101$; $p<0.001$); 2) Myocardial Infarct ($\beta = 0.711$; $p = 0.036$); 3) Serum Creatinine ($\beta = 0.012$; $p = 0.025$). Hypertension was not included because it was correlated with age. The sensitivity and specificity, calculated from the optimal threshold established from the ROC operating

curve built with the risk score, were 60.98% and 79.17% respectively. The low sensitivity, especially in the men group, was a consequence of the wide distribution of the preoperative risk scores among AF patients (Figure 2).

Cox Regression of Preoperative Risk Factor vs. Time of AF Occurrence. Cox regression was used to investigate the effect of the preoperative score upon the AF onset time. Figure 3 shows the survival curves of AF patients for three groups defined by the preoperative risk score: 1) ≤ 0.2 (11 AF patients); 2) $0.2 < P \leq 0.4$ (8 AF patients); 3) >0.4 (22 AF patients). AF started to occur in the second day, with a strong incidence in the second and third day. The higher and lower risk groups evolved together, illustrating the absence of relation between the time of AF onset and the preoperative risk, which was confirmed by its non-significance in the Cox regression ($\beta = 0.696$, $p = 0.45$) and the weak, non-significant correlation between the two variables ($r = -0.107$, $p = 0.54$). This suggests that the preoperative variables can, to a certain extent, predict who will get AF, but not the time when AF will occur.

Preoperative Risk Factor Analysis vs. Premature Atrial Activation (PAA)

PAA are known to be associated to the occurrence of AF [42–45]. For the 29 patients with complete 2-hours available data, the AF episode was found to be triggered by a PAA, which most often originated from the left atrium (26/29 patients). However, the total number of PAA during the two hours varied widely among patients. It had a long-tail distribution with $[n_{PAA,min}, n_{PAA,median}, n_{PAA,mean}, n_{PAA,max}] = [3,84,556,4539]$ and four patients with $n_{PAA} \geq 1400$. It can be hypothesized that the higher risk patients might either be more prone to produce PAA or more vulnerable to PAA. Cox regression of the number of PAA experienced before AF vs. preoperative risk was not significant ($\beta = 1.363$, $p = 0.173$). Figure 4 shows the evolution of the cumulative number of PAA before AF in three groups with increasing preoperative risk: ≤ 0.3, 9 patients, [0.3–0.5], 10 patients, >0.5, 10 patients). The three intertwined curves suggest that the preoperative risk score has no relationship with the number of PAA before onset of AF, as confirmed by Cox's regression.

Time Evolving Analysis of Variables Extracted from AEG

The two-hours preceding AF onset were analyzed as described in the section of "Variables Extracted from AEG in AF and Non-AF Patients". In addition to *PAA* rate and transient arrhythmia duration time, the variables related to the normal atrial activations were included: *AAMean*, *AAstd*, *rMSSD*, *pNN50*, *LF*, *HF*, *LFPortion*, *HFPortion*, *LF/HF*, *HF/LF*, *CTAMean*, *CTAStd*, *CTAVMean*, *CTAVStd*, *CorrAA_AV*, *CorrAA_CTA*, and *CorrAV_CTA*.

ANOVA and Post-hoc Analysis of Time Variables (Raw Data and Position Data) Before AF Onset. Time evolution of each variable was analyzed using repeated measure ANOVA [46]. Multivariate normality test of repeated measures was done for each variable using the Shapiro-Wilk test [47]. Non-normality was diagnosed except for *LFPortion* and *HFPortion*. Logarithm transformation of variables was performed to improve the normality distribution, except for *PAA* rate and arrhythmia duration which had some zero values. Upon repeated measures ANOVA, seven variables were diagnosed to have significant ($p<0.05$) time effects: *PAA* rate (R_{PAA}), transient atrial arrhythmia duration (*ArrhyDuration*), mean of sinus atrial activation interval (*AAMean*), low frequency portion of AA time series (*LFPortion*), high frequency portion of AA time series (*HFPortion*), low to high frequency ratio (*LF/HF*), and high to low frequency ratio (*HF/LF*).

Table 2. Beta values and significance of the variables in the logistic regression univariate and multivariate models.

		Univariate	Multivariate
Age	β	0.0847	0.101
	p	<0.001	<0.001
MI	β	0.8331	0.711
	p	0.0077	0.036
Serum Creatinine	β	0.0123	0.012
	p	0.0317	0.025
HT	β	0.6318	
	p	0.072	

MI(prior myocardial infarct);
HT (hypertension),

The same variables were significant for the analysis of position data, but most often with higher significance level (Table 3). The pairs (*LFPortion, HFPortion*) and (*LF/HF, HF/LF*) are redundant, but may have slightly different p values upon logarithm transformation. Post–hoc analysis of orthogonal contrasts detected a significant difference between the first and the second hour for R_{PAA}, arrhythmia duration and *AAMean*, while only the contrasts involving the last 30 minutes were significant for *LFPortion, HFPortion, LF/HF, HF/LF*.

Figure 5 shows the average R_{PAA} temporal evolution (panel A), as well as the most common patterns of change during the last hour identified by cluster analysis (panel B). The last hour data was chosen because the contrast analysis showed that significant changes occurred in this time period. R_{PAA} mean profile suggested a continuous increase starting around 50 minutes before AF. However, the sustained increasing trend was not present in the

cluster analysis results. The subgroup with the highest patient number rather demonstrated a modest increase in the last 30 minutes before AF. Similar analysis was repeated for *AAMean*. *AAMean* suggests a gradual and sustained acceleration of atrial rate, which was in fact presents in 15 patients (Figure 6). The phenomenon whereby the trend exhibited by the mean values can be found only in a subgroup patients was also found for the variables *ArrhyDuration, LFPortion, HFPortion, LF/HF* and *HF/LF*.

Sympathetic stimulation is known to decrease AA and might change *LFPortion* [48–53], which suggests that *AAMean* could be somewhat correlated to *LFPortion*, at least for patients with an accelerating or decelerating trend in sinus heart rate. However, the correlation coefficients between *AAMean* and *LFPortion* in the last hour before AF were widely distributed, ranging from −0.4 to 0.7. It was very low even for some of the patients with a marked decreasing AA time trend. It means that each variable can bring specific information since coordinated changes of all the variables were rare.

Analysis of Variables in Non-AF Control Patients. The variables extracted from AEG showing significant temporal changes before AF onset were analyzed in Non-AF patients by the similar methods discussed above. Repeated measurement ANOVA analysis was applied to the raw data and logarithmic transformed data. In contrast to the AF group, there was no significant time effect in the two hour time series of the variables as *PAA* rate, *ArrhyDuration, AAMean, LFPortion, HFPortion, LF/HF, and HF/LF* (Table 4). As aforementioned, the AF group post-hoc analysis showed that significant contrasts existed among one or more periods like [120 60] vs. [60 0], [60 30] vs. [30 0], [30 15] vs. [15 0], or [10 5] vs. [5 0]. None of them was found to be significant in the Non-AF control group. Figure 7 illustrates the time evolution of *PAA, AA, ArrhyDuration* and *LFPortion*, which did not show any obvious increasing or decreasing trend in the Non-AF group.

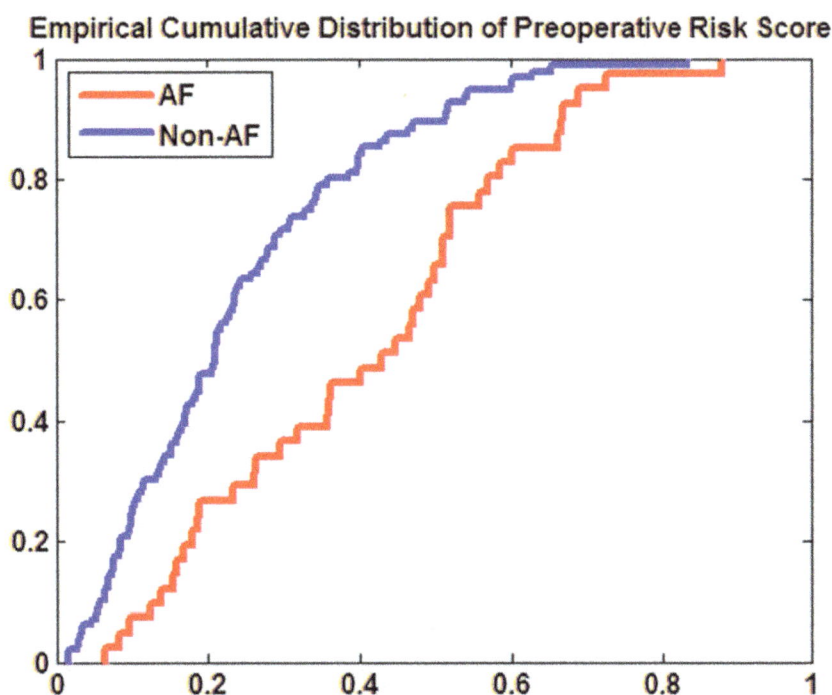

Empirical Cumulative Distribution of Preoperative Risk Score

Figure 2. The empirical CDF (cumulative distribution function) of preoperative risk score of AF and Non-AF groups.

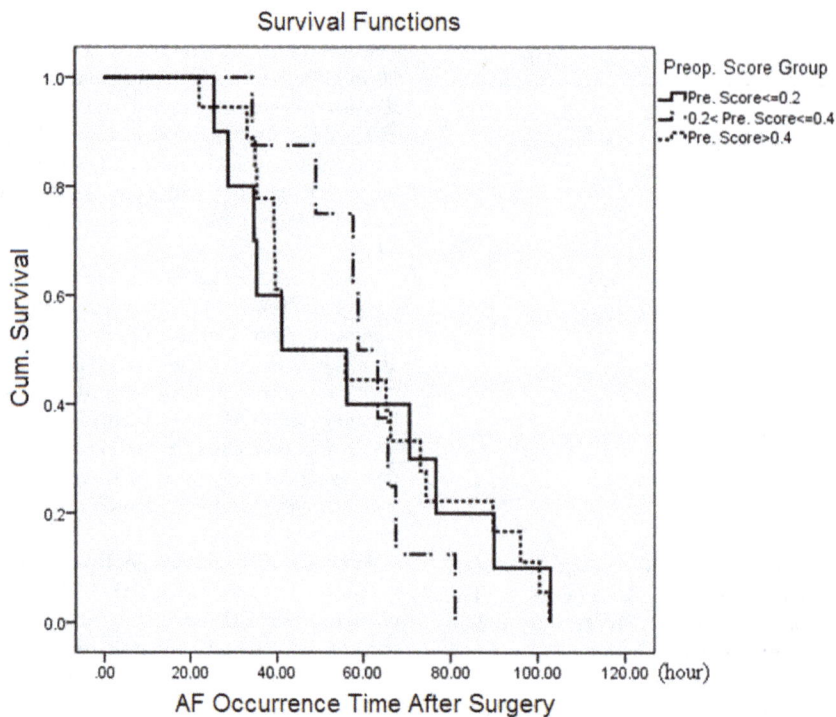

Figure 3. Survival curves as a function post-operative time of AF onset. The survival curves of three groups AF patients defined by their preoperative risk score: 1) ≤0.2; 2) 0.2<P≤0.4; 3)>0.4.

The same variables were also analyzed by two-way ANOVA (within: Time, between: AF vs. Non-AF group, Table 5). As expected for the lack of time effect in the Non-AF group, there was significant (or close to significance for *AAMean*) group*time interactions when either the two hours or the last hour before AF were considered. However, all variables, except *AAmean*, also showed a significant group effect. This group effect was also present in the first hour, except for *ArrhyDuration*. Since the

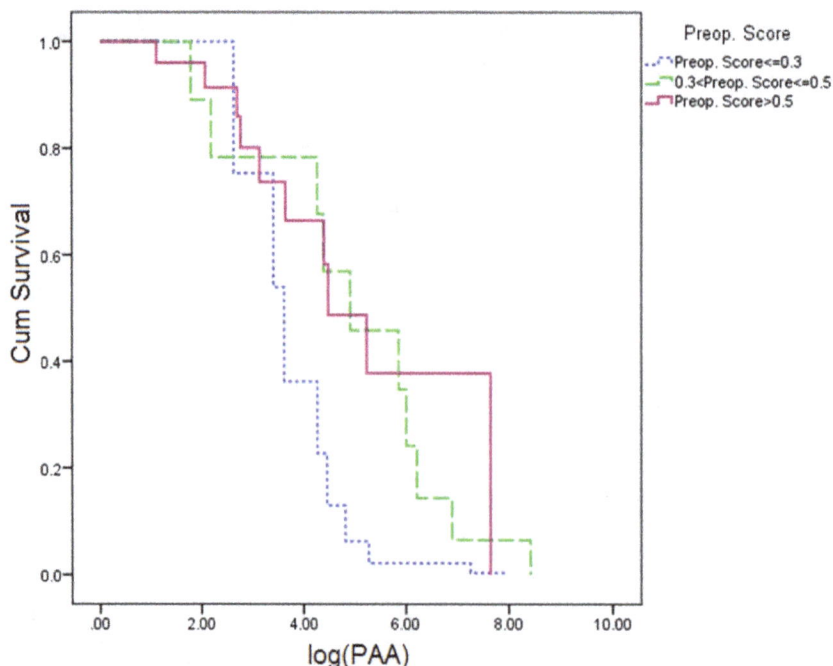

Figure 4. Survival curves as a function of the logarithm of the total number of PAA experienced before AF onset in 3 groups defined by their preoperative score ≤0.3, [0.3–0.5], and >0.5.

Table 3. ANOVA and contrast analysis of the raw and position data of variables with significant time-effects in 2-pre AF hours.

		Time	[120 60] vs. [60 0]	[60 30] vs. [30 0]	[30 15] vs. [15 0]	[10 5] vs. [5 0]
raw	RPAA	0.035	0.019 ↑			
	ArrhyDuration	0.03	0.016 ↑			0.01 ↑
	AAMean*	0.005	0.012 ↓	0.025 ↓	0.051 ↓	
	LFPortion*	0.005	0.004 ↑		0.035 ↑	0.032 ↑
	HFPortion*	0.005			0.002 ↓	0.001 ↓
	LF/HF*	0.028			0.003 ↑	0.001 ↑
	HF/LF*	0.028			0.003 ↓	0.001 ↓
Position	RPAA*	0.001	0.030 ↑			0.002 ↑
	ArrhyDuration*	0.001	0.034 ↑			0.002 ↑
	AAMean*	0.005	0.023 ↓	0.052 ↓	0.017 ↓	
	LFPortion*	0.043	0.049 ↑		0.026 ↑	0.005 ↑
	HFPortion*	0.018			0.008 ↓	<0.001 ↓
	LF/HF*	0.037			0.016 ↑	0.005 ↑
	HF/LF*	0.045		0.049 ↓	0.036 ↓	0.001 ↓

The upward and downward arrows stand respectively for the increasing and decreasing trend from one period to the next. "Time" column is the time effect significance in the two hours ANOVA analysis. The contrast analysis over the two time periods is listed subsequently. "0" is corresponding to the onset of AF. Variables with asterisk were log transformed.

group effect compares the mean values of all time intervals, it was more meaningful to the first hour period in which time effect was absent for most variables.

Taken together, the results of the one-way and two-way ANOVA can be summarized as follows:

- in the AF group, *PAA* rate, *ArrhyDuration* and the low frequency content of *AA* variation tended to increase between the first and the second hour, while remaining constant in Non-AF patients;
- Except for *ArrhyDuration*, mean *PAA* rate and the low frequency content indices were higher in the AF group in the first hour. This suggests a higher level of dysfunctional

autonomic neural balance and of atrial ectopic beats for AF patients that are further enhanced before AF onset. *AAMean* was shown to decrease before AF in about half of the patients (Figure 6). Figure 7B may suggest that *AAMean* was lower of Non-AF group in the first hour, but the high variance made this difference not statistically significant for raw or log-transform data.

Discrimination of Trigger and Non-Trigger Period. In an alternative approach, the capacity of variables to discriminate the closest time period to AF onset (triggering period) from others (non-triggering periods) was assessed by forward conditional stepwise logistic regression. The analysis was repeated for both

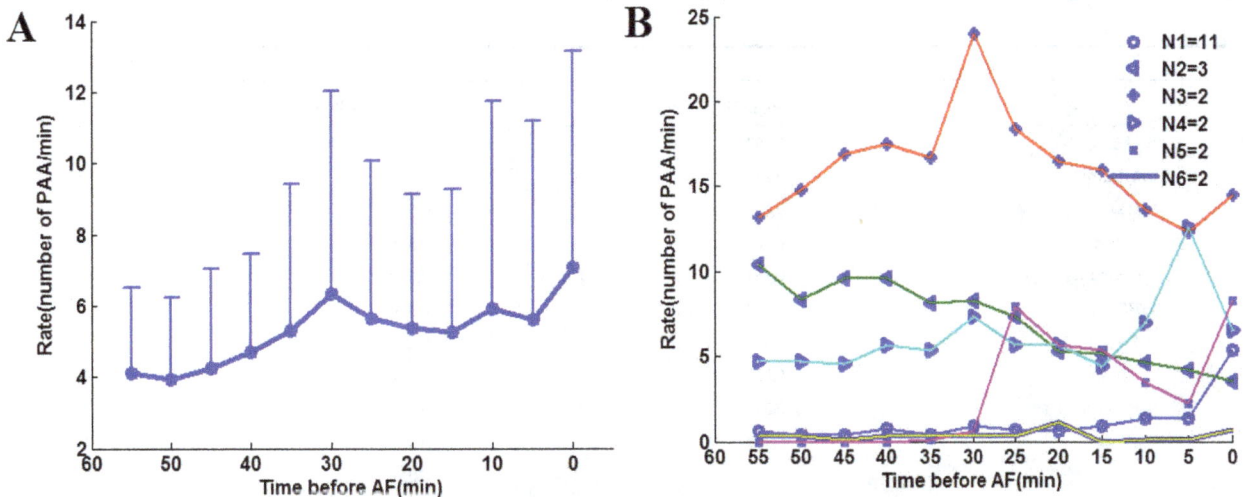

Figure 5. R_{PAA} temporal evolution and the patterns of change. (A) Mean value and standard deviation of PAA rate within each 5 minutes in the last hour before AF; (B) Mean patterns associated to the clusters obtained by the analysis of the five minutes time series. The number of patients corresponding to each pattern is indicated in the legend. Only the patterns with more than one patient are shown. The abscissa is the time before the onset of AF (minutes).

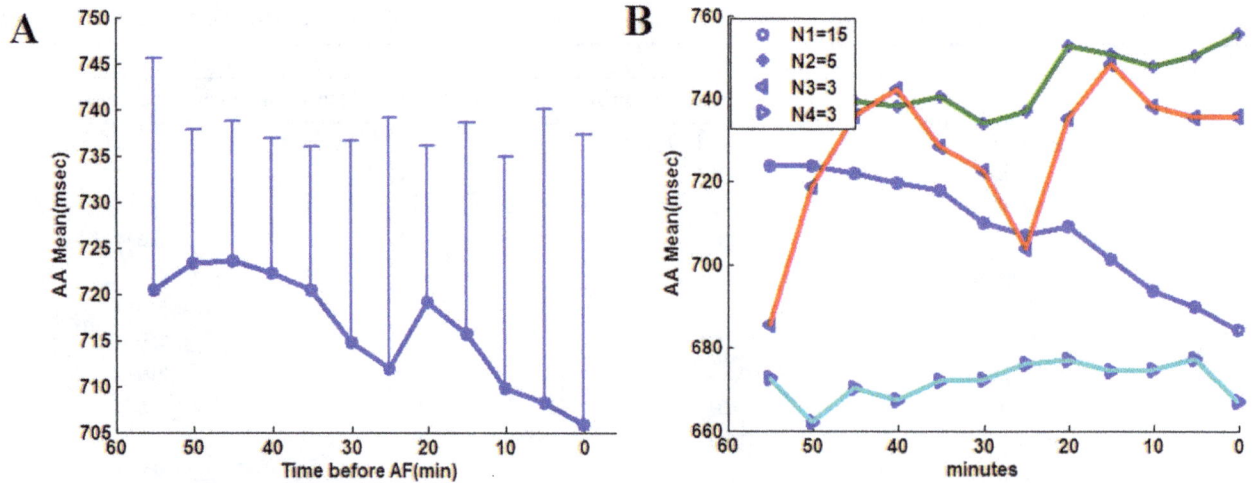

Figure 6. Temporal evolution and patter of changes of *AAMean* **A: The trend of mean value of variables** *AAMean.* B: Profiles obtained by cluster analysis.

raw and position data dividing the 2 pre-AF hours in equal time periods of 5, 10, 15, 20, 30 and 60 minutes.

Scores of the logistic model were used to build ROC curves and select the optimal cut-off point. The discrimination was much better using position data than raw data, even though the same variables were selected. The results obtained by position data are shown in Figure 8. Panel A gives the variables kept in the model for each time partition, the color code indicating whether higher (red) or lower values (green) were predictors of the triggering period. Four variables as R_{PAA}, *ArrhyDuration*, *AAMean* and *LFPortion* were more often present and should bring independent information. These were among the variables identified by Anova to have a significant time effect. The presence of *AAMean* and *LFPortion* confirms, as aforementioned, that they bring independent information. The sensitivity and specificity (correct classification of the trigger and non-trigger intervals respectively)

remained between 65% and 85% for all time partitions. Globally, the results suggested that AF incidence tends to be preceded by an increased number of PAA and transient arrhythmia episodes, on a background of accelerated sinus rhythm and a relative increase of its low frequency fluctuations. However, these changes did not occur simultaneously in all patients.

For 5 minutes interval partitioned data, the four variables were entered in the multivariate model in the following order: *RPAA, LFPortion, Arrhythmia Duration, AAMean.* Details of the univariate analysis are given in Table S1. Figure 9 shows the ROC curves associated with the successive models: I,R_{PAA}; II, *LFPortion*+R_{PAA}; III, *LFPortion* +R_{PAA}+*ArrhyDuration*; IV, *LFPortion*+ R_{PAA}+*ArrhyDuration*+*AAMean*. It is evident that the predictor R_{PAA} plays the most important role, achieving around 65% sensitivity and specificity. Then the other two predictors *LFPortion* and *ArrhyDuration* made some sensitivity

Table 4. ANOVA analysis of time effect of the Non-AF patient variables data, which were significant in 2-pre AF hours in AF patient group.

		Original Data	Logarithmic Data
raw	RPAA	0.194	N/A
	ArrhyDuration	0.283	N/A
	AAMean	0.403	0.541
	LFPortion	0.364	0.354
	HFPortion	0.364	0.438
	LF/HF	0.438	0.360
	HF/LF	0.438	0.360
Position	RPAA	0.329	0.402
	ArrhyDuration	0.235	0.267
	AAMean	0.330	0.866
	LFPortion	0.299	0.067
	HFPortion	0.299	0.407
	LF/HF	0.299	0.067
	HF/LF	0.299	0.407

N/A: not applicable.

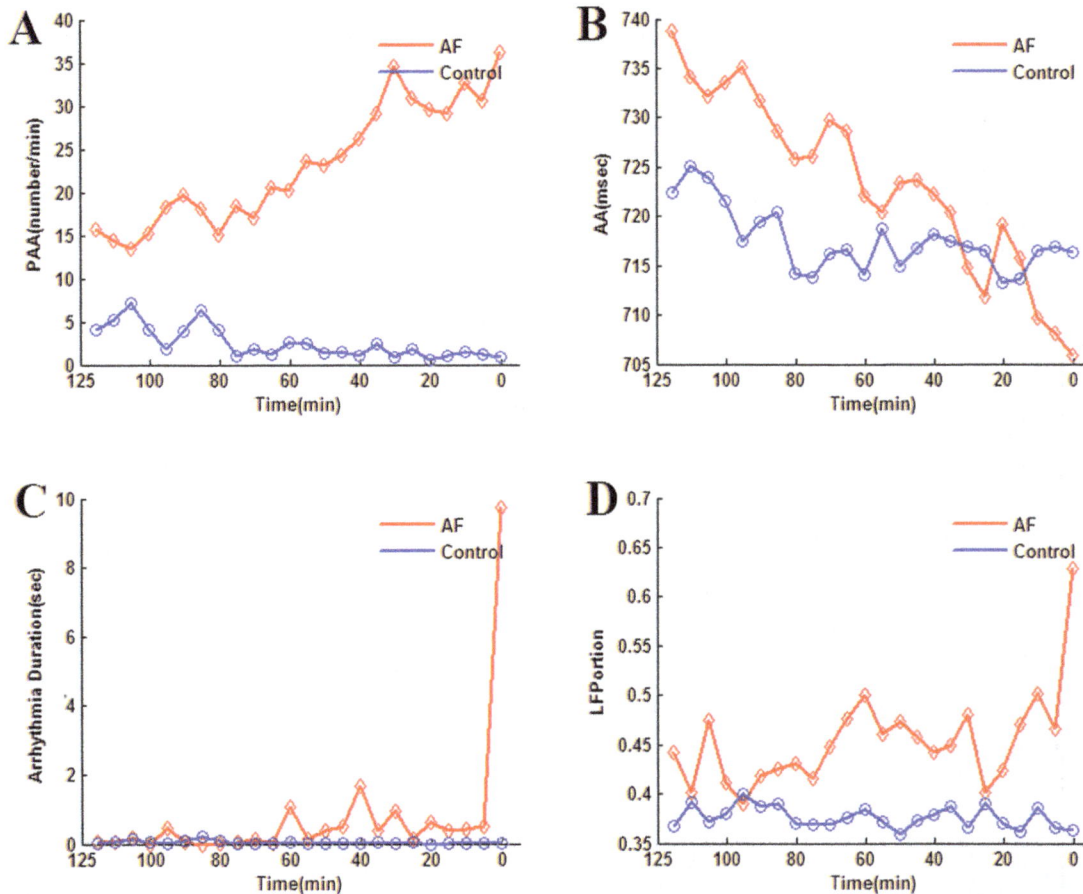

Figure 7. Mean value of *PAA* rate (A), *AA* (B), Arrhythmia duration (C), and *LFPortion* (D) within each 5 minutes for the 2 hours of Control (Non-AF) and AF groups.

improvements. The predictor of *AAMean*, finally introduced in the model, further improved the prediction, to reach a sensitivity of 71% and a specificity of 86%.

Preoperative Risk Score vs. Postoperative Evolving Risk

It was assumed that patients with a higher preoperative score need less change to develop AF. Correlation analysis was done to check the relation between the preoperative risk score and the score of the last interval, the mean score of all time intervals, the difference between the score of the last interval and the mean score of all other intervals (Table S2). None of them was found even close to be significant. The preoperative score did not seem to be related to the dynamic changes preceding the onset of AF.

Discussion

The mechanisms of the incidence of post-CABG AF are complex and still controversial. The present project is based on the analysis of multichannel epicardial electrograms to investigate electrophysiological changes preceding AF onset and their relationship to the preoperative risk factors. The main findings of the study are: The post-CABG AF was preceded by electrophysiological changes in the last hour before the onset of arrhythmia. The causes appear to be multifactorial, mainly involving increasing rate of premature atrial activation, short transient arrhythmias, accelerating heart rate, and rising low

frequency content of heart rate. None of the above changes was found to occur in all AF patients.

Preoperative Risk Factors

Diverse post-CABG AF risk factors have been identified, but results among different studies were often inconsistent, sometimes even controversial [54] [55] [56] [10,18,25,57–61]. Beyond the fact that the mechanisms of AF occurrence are complex and multi-factorial, this might result from the fact that most studies were observational and retrospective, with different inclusion criteria.

For our study population, age appeared as the most important pre-operative predictor, the mean age of AF patients being around 6 years older than Non-AF patients (Men: 67 vs. 61 years, women: 75 vs. 68 years old). Similar results were reported by several other studies [55,62–66]. The association could be attributable to age-related structural changes in the atrium such as dilation and fibrosis. These structural changes could influence the electrophys-iological properties of atrial myocardium, such as prolonging atrial conduction times, increasing atrial stiffening, and splitting of atrial excitation wave in the pectinated trabecula [67,68]. It has also been suggested that surgical trauma to sympathovagal fibers originating from the deep or superficial cardiac plexus during surgery may enhance age related pro-AF effect [62].

There are controversial reports about the effect of sex on postoperative AF [59,69,70]. There were around 3 times more men than women in our sample (104 vs. 33), but the incidence of AF was almost the same in the two groups. This explains why sex

Table 5. Two-way ANOVA analysis of time effect, and group effect between AF and Non-AF Patients.

		Group (AF vs. Non-AF)			Time			Group*Time		
		2 hrs.	1st hr	2nd hr	2 hrs.	1st hr	2nd hr	2 hrs.	1st hr	2nd hr
Original Data	RPAA	0.000	0.009	0.000	0.008	0.710	0.042	0.000	0.160	0.021
	ArrhyDuration	<0.001	0.329	0.000	0.478	0.915	0.437	<0.001	0.329	<0.001
	AAMean	0.847	0.702	0.998	0.001	0.045	0.070	0.072	0.773	0.080
	LFPortion	0.001	0.034	<0.001	<0.001	0.129	<0.001	<0.001	0.007	<0.001
	HFPortion	0.001	0.034	<0.001	<0.001	0.129	<0.001	<0.001	0.007	<0.001
	LF/HF	<0.001	<0.001	<0.001	<0.001	0.011	<0.001	<0.001	<0.001	<0.001
	HF/LF	0.272	0.058	0.754	0.124	0.491	0.118	0.030	0.275	0.062
Logarithmic Transform	AAMean	0.747	0.619	0.887	0.136	0.066	0.538	0.289	0.525	0.090
	LFPortion	0.144	0.717	0.011	0.018	0.085	0.004	<0.001	0.001	<0.001
	HFPortion	<0.001	0.002	<0.001	<0.001	0.027	<0.001	<0.001	<0.001	<0.001
	LF/HF	0.009	0.154	<0.001	<0.001	0.264	<0.001	<0.001	0.025	<0.001
	HF/LF	0.009	0.154	<0.001	<0.001	0.264	<0.001	<0.001	0.025	<0.001

RPAA, ArrhyDuration are not applicable to logarithmic transformation.

did not show up as a predictor in the current study. Women were on average older, but the age difference between AF and Non-AF patients was the same in the male and female groups. Sex did not appear in the multivariate logistic regression, even when an extra sex*age variable was added. This concurs with the conclusion of Auer et al. who indicated that sex was not an independent risk factor, but contradicts Zaman et al. who reached the inverse conclusion [55,59,71].

Hypertension is associated with left ventricular hypertrophy, which may impair ventricular filling, induce left atrial enlargement, slow down atrial conduction velocity, and increase cardiac tissue fibrosis and dispersion of atrial refractoriness. All these structural and electrophysiological changes predispose to AF [72–74]. Hypertensive patients in the current study had indeed a 78% increased risk of AF, an effect close to significance in univariate analysis. However, it did not appear as a predictor in the multivariate logistic model because the effect of hypertension was largely confounded by age, which contradicts the conclusion of Svedjeholm et al. [66].

Renal function impairment often induces an elevation of serum creatinine level [54]. The link between preoperative renal function and postoperative AF has been investigated in some studies. Patients with higher level of serum creatinine were more prone to postoperative AF [75,76]. In our sample, this was found in the subgroup older than 60 years, whereas the relation was even reversed for younger patients. The result is difficult to explain, and may reflect the limited size of our study population.

Following MI, the injured heart tissue conducts electrical impulses more slowly, which can promote reentry following a PVC and retrograde conduction to the atria that may trigger AF [77]. In our sample, AF was not found to be triggered by PVC. Inversely, AF can often complicate MI acute myocardial infarction by reducing heart pump function [78]. In our study population, the age confounding effect was to some extent present for prior myocardial infarct (MI), but MI was still a predictor in the final multivariate model.

Time Evolving Risk Factors

Different studies have investigated the dynamics of cardiac electrical recordings in the last two hours, one hour, thirty minutes, or even several minutes before the onset of post-CABG AF [79–81]. Some variables were found to have significant differences between the first and second hour before AF, or within the second hour, but never during the first hour. This suggests that the two hours before AF onset provided an appropriate time frame to analyze the evolving changes.

Globally, there was an R_{PAA} increase in the last hour before AF onset. This is in agreement with the observations that atrial ectopic beats tend to be more frequent before the start of paroxysmal or postoperative AF [82–84]. However, analysis of the temporal R_{PAA} evolution showed a sustained increasing trend was present only in a subgroup, which indicates that increasing PAA rate is not an absolute prerequisite to AF occurrence. Most patients also experienced an increased number of transient arrhythmia episodes. In contrast to R_{PAA}, this was mainly restricted to the last 10 or 5 minutes before AF. In general, the arrhythmias were short and last less than 1 minute, such that longer duration of arrhythmia in a time period was most often resulting from the presence of multiple bursts. Even though arrhythmia durations were correlated with R_{PAA} in the final period, both of them were predictors to discriminate trigger from non-trigger time periods.

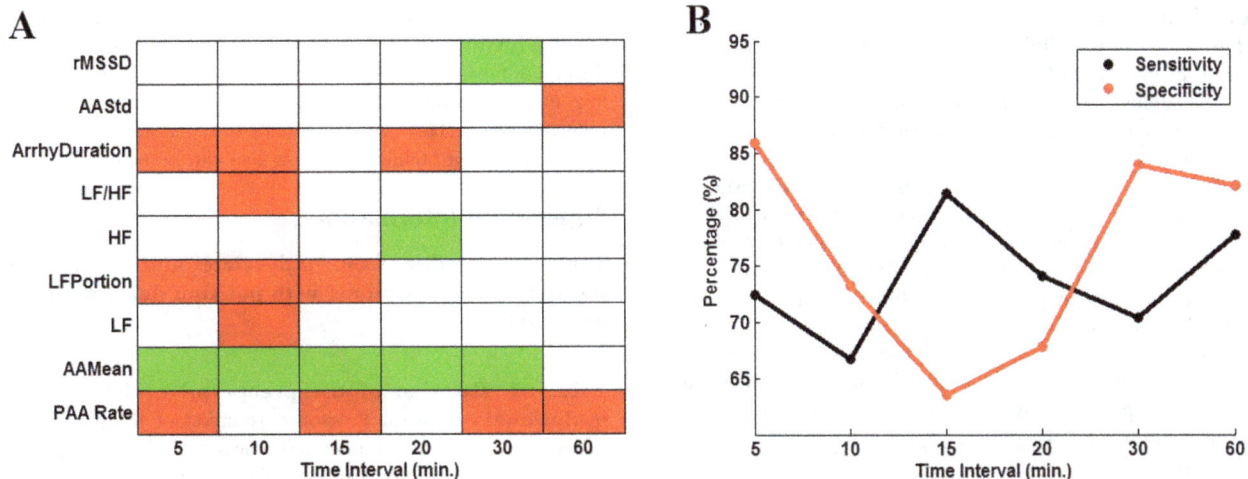

Figure 8. Results of logistic regression to discriminate trigger and non-trigger period. A) Results of the forward stepwise logistic regression using position data. Sign of estimated coefficient of predictors in the logistic model (red: positive coefficient, green: negative coefficient) for different partitions of 2 hours intervals before AF. B) Sensitivity (red, % of correct classification of the last interval) and specificity (black) of each model with cutting point calculated from the ROC curve.

The gradually accelerated heart rate during the last pre-AF hour coincides with previous observations that faster heart rate postoperative patients were at higher risk to develop AF [48,85–87]. However, cluster analysis (Figure 6 B) revealed that this accelerating trend was only present in a subgroup of AF patients, the others having either a decreasing trend or constant heart rate. We would rather conclude, as Hogue et al., that there is no unique pattern wholly predictive of impending AF [88].

The LF and HF power spectral components of the heart rate variability are often considered to be a marker of sympathetic and/or parasympathetic modulation, although this point of view remains somewhat disputable [39]. Heterogeneous electrophysiological properties could be due to autonomic innervations [88], while their possible implication in postoperative AF is complex,

sometimes even controversial [13,48,64,86,89]. It was reported that either vagal or sympathetic nerve stimulation, can decrease the atrial refractory period in a spatially heterogeneous way, thereby facilitating the occurrence of AF [90–94]. The difference between vagal and sympathetic stimulations might lie in the more spatially heterogeneous effect of vagal nerve activation. It has been put forward that elevated norepinephrine levels suggest sympathetic activation, while some other studies rather suggested divergent autonomic conditions to occur before arrhythmia onset, either heightened sympathetic or parasympathetic tone, or even dysfunctional autonomic heart rate control [13,48,64,86,89]. In both raw data and position data, we found an increasing trend of mean *LFPortion* in the last 30 minutes, reaching a peak in the last 10 minutes before AF. The increase of *LFPortion* might be ascribed to an augmentation of the sympathetic and/or decrease of the parasympathetic tone. However, the weak correlations between *AAMean* and *LFPortion* trend indicated that the evolving changes of these variables were not generally coordinated.

Position data always had higher level of statistical significance and classification accuracy. This comes from the huge variations of mean level and amplitude of changes observed for every variable among the patients. The normalization, based on the distribution of the values within each patient, removes the scale difference. It suggests that a relative threshold, adapted to the state of the patient, can be a better predictor of impending AF.

Preoperative Risk Factors vs. Time Delay, PAA and Time Evolving Risk Scores

It might be hypothesized that AF patients with higher preoperative risks should develop AF sooner and with less PAA. It might also be conjectured that the time evolving score could be higher from the beginning or need less change to trigger AF. None of these hypotheses were supported by the data analysis. The preoperative score appeared to be a static risk measure, relatively good to classify Non-AF patients (around 80%), but not for AF patients (around 60%). The preoperative risk score was not found to be significantly related to the dynamic electrophysiological changes prior to AF.

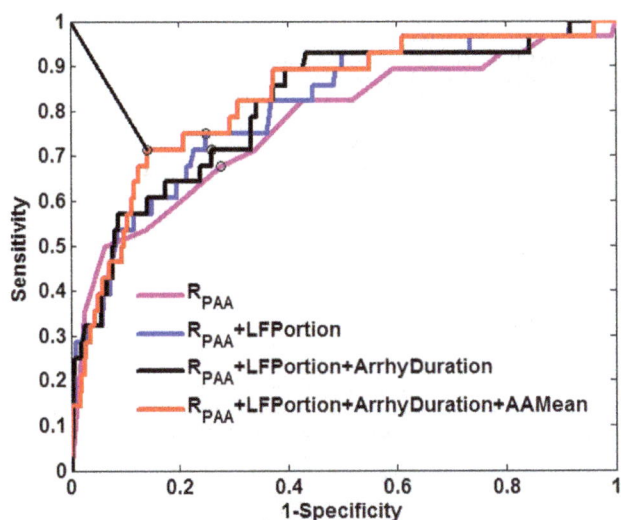

Figure 9. ROC curves of the scores obtained by stepwise logistic regression. ROC curves for the logistic regression models with successive inclusion of the variables: *RPAA, LFPortion, Arrhythmia Duration, AAMean*. The circles indicated the best cut off points for each model.

Study Limitation

The results of our study can only be considered as indicative because of the relatively small sample size owing to the limited data availability. The performance of both the preoperative and time evolving model should be evaluated with independent and larger population of patients.

Accordingly, the future study needs to use fewer criteria to exclude patients during the screening process, so that the predicting method could be improved to be useful for a larger set of postoperative patients. Other variables might also be considered in next step, such as activation waveform, whose change has been reported to precede the onset of AF [19,80]. Moreover, the monitoring of blood pressure could be useful, particularly in association with heart rhythm whose fluctuations could be a response to vascular events that must certainly occur after an open-heart surgery.

Conclusion

Our results show that post-CABG AF is preceded by epicardial electrocardiographic changes occurring in the last hour before the onset of arrhythmia, which is a prerequisite for monitoring and provide enough time for prophylactic intervention. Giving that none of these changes was found to occur in all AF patients, the predictive score should be a weighted sum of factors related to the potential triggers of AF, such as PAA, to the state of the tissue in which they occur, as well as the heart rate and the frequency content of its fluctuation. The better performance of position data suggests that detection threshold must be adapted to the state of each patient. Measures of preoperative risk factors do not seem to be helpful in setting threshold. The relative invariance of the data during the first hour before AF suggest that data could be normalized using the distribution of values collected during an initial reference period. Ideally, the reference period could be at the end of the first day since the incidence of AF appears to be very low in this period and the patients parameters appear to be relatively stable. However, it remains to be verified whether and when the relative stability of the indices can be reached.

Supporting Information

Table S1 p-value from univariate and multivariate logistic regression model with position data and 5 minutes partition.

Table S2 Relation of the preoperative risk with the evolutionary scores. Pearson correlation of the preoperative risk, with the score of last interval (I), the mean score of all intervals (II), and the difference the score of the last interval and the mean of other intervals (III) for time partitions of 5, 10, 20, 30, 60 minutes. The values in parentheses are the two tailed significance values.

Acknowledgments

The authors thank Dr. R. A. Nadeau and V. Jacquemet for editorial comments.

Author Contributions

Conceived and designed the experiments: PP AV. Performed the experiments: YY. Analyzed the data: FX BD AV. Contributed reagents/materials/analysis tools: FX BD. Wrote the paper: FX AV.

References

1. Sohn GH, Shin DH, Byun KM, Han HJ, Cho SJ, et al. (2009) The incidence and predictors of postoperative atrial fibrillation after noncardiothoracic surgery. Korean Circ J 39: 100–104.

2. Ryu JK (2009) Postoperative atrial fibrillation after noncardiothoracic surgery: is it different from after cardiothoracic surgery? Korean Circ J 39: 93–94.

3. Rossi P, Bianchi S, Barretta A, Della Scala A, Kornet L, et al. (2009) Post-operative atrial fibrillation management by selective epicardial vagal fat pad stimulation. Journal of Interventional Cardiac Electrophysiology 24: 37–45.

4. Jongnarangsin K, Oral H (2009) Postoperative atrial fibrillation. Cardiol Clin 27: 69–78, viii.

5. Nattel S (2011) From guidelines to bench: implications of unresolved clinical issues for basic investigations of atrial fibrillation mechanisms. Can J Cardiol 27: 19–26.

6. Echahidi N, Mohty D, Pibarot P, Despres JP, O'Hara G, et al. (2007) Obesity and metabolic syndrome are independent risk factors for atrial fibrillation after coronary artery bypass graft surgery. Circulation 116: I213–219.

7. Creswell LL, Damiano RJ Jr (2001) Postoperative atrial fibrillation: an old problem crying for new solutions. J Thorac Cardiovasc Surg 121: 638–641.

8. Hakala T, Hedman A, Turpeinen A, Kettunen R, Vuolteenaho O, et al. (2002) Prediction of atrial fibrillation after coronary artery bypass grafting by measuring atrial peptide levels and preoperative atrial dimensions. Eur J Cardiothorac Surg 22: 939–943.

9. Filardo G, Hamilton C, Hamman B, Hebeler RF Jr, Adams J, et al. (2010) New-onset postoperative atrial fibrillation and long-term survival after aortic valve replacement surgery. Ann Thorac Surg 90: 474–479.

10. El-Chami MF, Kilgo P, Thourani V, Lattouf OM, Delurgio DB, et al. (2010) New-onset atrial fibrillation predicts long-term mortality after coronary artery bypass graft. J Am Coll Cardiol 55: 1370–1376.

11. Contreras AE, Ferrero Guadagnoli A, Brenna EJ, Pogonza P, Coppa LA, et al. (2010) Atrial fibrillation in postoperative cardiac surgery. Prevalence and hospitalized period. Medicina (B Aires) 70: 339–342.

12. Bramer S, van Straten AHM, Hamad MAS, Berreklouw E, Martens EJ, et al. (2010) The Impact of New-Onset Postoperative Atrial Fibrillation on Mortality After Coronary Artery Bypass Grafting. Annals of Thoracic Surgery 90: 443–450.

13. Hogue CW Jr, Creswell LL, Gutterman DD, Fleisher LA (2005) Epidemiology, mechanisms, and risks: American College of Chest Physicians guidelines for the prevention and management of postoperative atrial fibrillation after cardiac surgery. Chest 128: 9S–16S.

14. Maisel WH, Rawn JD, Stevenson WG (2001) Atrial fibrillation after cardiac surgery. Ann Intern Med 135: 1061–1073.

15. Janse MJ (2007) Focus, reentry, or "focal" reentry? Am J Physiol Heart Circ Physiol 292: H2561–2562.

16. Moe GK, Abildskov JA (1959) Atrial fibrillation as a self-sustaining arrhythmia independent of focal discharge. Am Heart J 58: 59–70.

17. Moe GK, Rheinboldt WC, Abildskov JA (1964) A Computer Model of Atrial Fibrillation. Am Heart J 67: 200–220.

18. Hogue CW Jr, Hyder ML (2000) Atrial fibrillation after cardiac operation: risks, mechanisms, and treatment. Ann Thorac Surg 69: 300–306.

19. Nadeau R, Cardinal R, Armour JA, Kus T, Richer LP, et al. (2007) Cervical vagosympathetic and mediastinal nerves activation effects on atrial arrhythmia formation. Anadolu Kardiyol Derg 7 Suppl 1: 34–36.

20. Page P, Andrew Armour J, Yin Y, Vermeulen M, Nadeau R, et al. (2006) Differential effects of cervical vagosympathetic and mediastinal nerve activation on atrial arrhythmia formation in dogs. Auton Neurosci 128: 9–18.

21. Oliveira M, da Silva MN, Timoteo AT, Feliciano J, Sousa L, et al. (2009) Inducibility of atrial fibrillation during electrophysiologic evaluation is associated with increased dispersion of atrial refractoriness. Int J Cardiol 136: 130–135.

22. Li Z, Hertervig E, Carlson J, Johansson C, Olsson SB, et al. (2002) Dispersion of refractoriness in patients with paroxysmal atrial fibrillation. Evaluation with simultaneous endocardial recordings from both atria. J Electrocardiol 35: 227–234.

23. Fynn SP, Todd DM, Hobbs WJ, Armstrong KL, Fitzpatrick AP, et al. (2003) Effect of amiodarone on dispersion of atrial refractoriness and cycle length in patients with atrial fibrillation. J Cardiovasc Electrophysiol 14: 485–491.

24. Zhu DW (2010) Race: another risk factor for postoperative atrial fibrillation? Heart Rhythm 7: 1464–1465.

25. Silva RG, Lima GG, Laranjeira A, Costa AR, Pereira E, et al. (2004) Risk factors, morbidity, and mortality associated with atrial fibrillation in the postoperative period of cardiac surgery. Arq Bras Cardiol 83: 105–110; 199–104.

26. Motsinger AA, Donahue BS, Brown NJ, Roden DM, Ritchie MD (2006) Risk factor interactions and genetic effects associated with post-operative atrial fibrillation. Pac Symp Biocomput: 584–595.

27. Arias MA, Sanchez-Gila J (2006) Obesity as a risk factor for developing postoperative atrial fibrillation. Chest 129: 828; author reply 828–829.

28. Mueller XM, Tevaearai HT, Ruchat P, Stumpe F, Von Segesser LK (2002) Atrial fibrillation and minimally invasive coronary artery bypass grafting: risk factor analysis. World J Surg 26: 639–642.

29. David W, Hosmer SL (1999) Applied survival analysis: regression modeling of time to event data. John Wiley & Sons, Inc.

30. Dube B, Vinet A, Xiong F, Yin Y, LeBlanc AR, et al. (2009) Automatic detection and classification of human epicardial atrial unipolar electrograms. Physiol Meas 30: 1303–1325.

31. Pichon A, Roulaud M, Antoine-Jonville S, de Bisschop C, Denjean A (2006) Spectral analysis of heart rate variability: interchangeability between autoregressive analysis and fast Fourier transform. J Electrocardiol 39: 31–37.

32. Grimaldi D, Pierangeli G, Barletta G, Terlizzi R, Plazzi G, et al. (2010) Spectral analysis of heart rate variability reveals an enhanced sympathetic activity in narcolepsy with cataplexy. Clin Neurophysiol 121: 1142–1147.

33. Fagard RH, Pardaens K, Staessen JA, Thijs L (1998) Power spectral analysis of heart rate variability by autoregressive modelling and fast Fourier transform: a comparative study. Acta Cardiol 53: 211–218.

34. Chemla D, Young J, Badilini F, Maison-Blanche P, Affres H, et al. (2005) Comparison of fast Fourier transform and autoregressive spectral analysis for the study of heart rate variability in diabetic patients. Int J Cardiol 104: 307–313.

35. Singh D, Vinod K, Saxena SC (2004) Sampling frequency of the RR interval time series for spectral analysis of heart rate variability. J Med Eng Technol 28: 263–272.

36. Persson PB (1997) Spectrum analysis of cardiovascular time series. Am J Physiol 273: R1201–1210.

37. Kamath MV, Fallen EL (1993) Power spectral analysis of heart rate variability: a noninvasive signature of cardiac autonomic function. Crit Rev Biomed Eng 21: 245–311.

38. Lippman N, Stein KM, Lerman BB (1994) Comparison of methods for removal of ectopy in measurement of heart rate variability. Am J Physiol 267: H411–418.

39. Task Force ES (1996) Heart rate variability. Standards of measurement, physiological interpretation, and clinical use. Task Force of the European Society of Cardiology and the North American Society of Pacing and Electrophysiology. Eur Heart J 17: 354–381.

40. Brian S, Everitt SL, Leese M, Stahl D (2011) Cluster Analysis. John Wiley & Sons, Ltd.

41. David B, Hosmer SL (2000) Applied Logistic Regression. John Wiley & Sons, Inc.

42. Frost L, Christiansen EH, Molgaard H, Jacobsen CJ, Allermand H, et al. (1995) Premature atrial beat eliciting atrial fibrillation after coronary artery bypass grafting. J Electrocardiol 28: 297–305.

43. Ashar MS, Pennington J, Callans DJ, Marchlinski FE (2000) Localization of arrhythmogenic triggers of atrial fibrillation. J Cardiovasc Electrophysiol 11: 1300–1305.

44. Taylor AD, Groen JG, Thorn SL, Lewis CT, Marshall AJ (2002) New insights into onset mechanisms of atrial fibrillation and flutter after coronary artery bypass graft surgery. Heart 88: 499–504.

45. Hsu LF, Jais P, Keane D, Wharton JM, Deisenhofer I, et al. (2004) Atrial fibrillation originating from persistent left superior vena cava. Circulation 109: 828–832.

46. Davis CS (2002) Statistical Methods for the Analysis of Repeated Measurements: Springer.

47. Shapiro SS, Wilk MB (1965) An Analysis of Variance Test for Normality Complete Samples. Biometrika 52: 591–611.

48. Amar D, Zhang H, Miodownik S, Kadish AH (2003) Competing autonomic mechanisms precede the onset of postoperative atrial fibrillation. J Am Coll Cardiol 42: 1262–1268.

49. Pomeranz B, Macaulay RJ, Caudill MA, Kutz I, Adam D, et al. (1985) Assessment of autonomic function in humans by heart rate spectral analysis. Am J Physiol 248: H151–153.

50. Haïssaguerre M, Jaïs P, Shah DC, Takahashi A, Hocini M, et al. (1998) Spontaneous Initiation of Atrial Fibrillation by Ectopic Beats Originating in the Pulmonary Veins. New England Journal of Medicine 339: 659–666.

51. Cheung DW (1981) Electrical activity of the pulmonary vein and its interaction with the right atrium in the guinea-pig. J Physiol 314: 445–456.

52. Katra RP, Laurita KR (2005) Cellular mechanism of calcium-mediated triggered activity in the heart. Circ Res 96: 535–542.

53. Curran J, Hinton MJ, Rios E, Bers DM, Shannon TR (2007) Beta-adrenergic enhancement of sarcoplasmic reticulum calcium leak in cardiac myocytes is mediated by calcium/calmodulin-dependent protein kinase. Circ Res 100: 391–398.

54. Mathew JP, Fontes ML, Tudor IC, Ramsay J, Duke P, et al. (2004) A multicenter risk index for atrial fibrillation after cardiac surgery. JAMA 291: 1720–1729.

55. Zaman AG, Archbold RA, Helft G, Paul EA, Curzen NP, et al. (2000) Atrial fibrillation after coronary artery bypass surgery: a model for preoperative risk stratification. Circulation 101: 1403–1408.

56. Amar D, Shi W, Hogue CW Jr, Zhang H, Passman RS, et al. (2004) Clinical prediction rule for atrial fibrillation after coronary artery bypass grafting. J Am Coll Cardiol 44: 1248–1253.

57. Raman T, Roistacher N, Liu J, Zhang H, Shi W, et al. (2011) Preoperative left atrial dysfunction and risk of postoperative atrial fibrillation complicating thoracic surgery. J Thorac Cardiovasc Surg.

58. Tran CT, Schmidt TA, Christensen JB, Kjeldsen K (2009) Atrial Na, K-ATPase increase and potassium dysregulation accentuate the risk of postoperative atrial fibrillation. Cardiology 114: 1–7.

59. Auer J, Weber T, Berent R, Ng CK, Lamm G, et al. (2005) Risk factors of postoperative atrial fibrillation after cardiac surgery. J Card Surg 20: 425–431.

60. Shah DC, Haissaguerre M, Jais P (2001) Toward a mechanism-based understanding of atrial fibrillation. J Cardiovasc Electrophysiol 12: 600–601.

61. Aranki SF, Shaw DP, Adams DH, Rizzo RJ, Couper GS, et al. (1996) Predictors of atrial fibrillation after coronary artery surgery. Current trends and impact on hospital resources. Circulation 94: 390–397.

62. Amar D, Zhang H, Leung DH, Roistacher N, Kadish AH (2002) Older age is the strongest predictor of postoperative atrial fibrillation. Anesthesiology 96: 352–356.

63. Amar D (2002) Postoperative atrial fibrillation. Heart Dis 4: 117–123.

64. Budeus M, Hennersdorf M, Rohlen S, Schnitzler S, Felix O, et al. (2006) Prediction of atrial fibrillation after coronary artery bypass grafting: the role of chemoreflex-sensitivity and P wave signal averaged ECG. Int J Cardiol 106: 67–74.

65. Haghjoo M, Basiri H, Salek M, Sadr-Ameli MA, Kargar F, et al. (2008) Predictors of postoperative atrial fibrillation after coronary artery bypass graft surgery. Indian Pacing Electrophysiol J 8: 94–101.

66. Svedjeholm R, Hakanson E (2000) Predictors of atrial fibrillation in patients undergoing surgery for ischemic heart disease. Scand Cardiovasc J 34: 516–521.

67. Spach MS, Dolber PC (1986) Relating extracellular potentials and their derivatives to anisotropic propagation at a microscopic level in human cardiac muscle. Evidence for electrical uncoupling of side-to-side fiber connections with increasing age. Circ Res 58: 356–371.

68. Davies MJ, Pomerance A (1972) Pathology of atrial fibrillation in man. Br Heart J 34: 520–525.

69. Bernet F, Baykut D, Reineke D, Matt P, Zerkowski HR (2006) Impact of female gender on the early outcome in off-pump coronary artery bypass surgery. Eur J Med Res 11: 114–118.

70. Kalavrouziotis D, Buth KJ, Ali IS (2007) The impact of new-onset atrial fibrillation on in-hospital mortality following cardiac surgery. Chest 131: 833–839.

71. Auer J, Weber T, Berent R, Ng CK, Lamm G, et al. (2005) Postoperative atrial fibrillation independently predicts prolongation of hospital stay after cardiac surgery. J Cardiovasc Surg (Torino) 46: 583–588.

72. Reich DL, Bennett-Guerrero E, Bodian CA, Hossain S, Winfree W, et al. (2002) Intraoperative tachycardia and hypertension are independently associated with adverse outcome in noncardiac surgery of long duration. Anesth Analg 95: 273–277, table of contents.

73. Almassi GH, Sommers T, Moritz TE, Shroyer AL, London MJ, et al. (1999) Stroke in cardiac surgical patients: determinants and outcome. Ann Thorac Surg 68: 391–397; discussion 397–398.

74. Healey JS, Connolly SJ (2003) Atrial fibrillation: hypertension as a causative agent, risk factor for complications, and potential therapeutic target. Am J Cardiol 91: 9G–14G.

75. Radmehr H, Forouzannia SK, Bakhshandeh AR, Sanatkar M (2011) Relation between preoperative mild increased in serum creatinine level and early outcomes after coronary artery bypass grafting. Acta Med Iran 49: 89–92.

76. Najafi M, Goodarzynejad H, Karimi A, Ghiasi A, Soltaninia H, et al. (2009) Is preoperative serum creatinine a reliable indicator of outcome in patients undergoing coronary artery bypass surgery? J Thorac Cardiovasc Surg 137: 304–308.

77. Nilsson KR Jr, Al-Khatib SM, Zhou Y, Pieper K, White HD, et al. (2010) Atrial fibrillation management strategies and early mortality after myocardial infarction: results from the Valsartan in Acute Myocardial Infarction (VALIANT) Trial. Heart 96: 838–842.

78. Schmitt J, Duray G, Gersh BJ, Hohnloser SH (2009) Atrial fibrillation in acute myocardial infarction: a systematic review of the incidence, clinical features and prognostic implications. Eur Heart J 30: 1038–1045.

79. Poli S, Barbaro V, Bartolini P, Calcagnini G, Censi F (2003) Prediction of atrial fibrillation from surface ECG: review of methods and algorithms. Ann Ist Super Sanita 39: 195–203.

80. Pichlmaier AM, Lang V, Harringer W, Heublein B, Schaldach M, et al. (1998) Prediction of the onset of atrial fibrillation after cardiac surgery using the monophasic action potential. Heart 80: 467–472.

81. Zimmermann M, Kalusche D (2001) Fluctuation in autonomic tone is a major determinant of sustained atrial arrhythmias in patients with focal ectopy originating from the pulmonary veins. J Cardiovasc Electrophysiol 12: 285–291.

82. Pellman J, Lyon RC, Sheikh F (2010) Extracellular matrix remodeling in atrial fibrosis: mechanisms and implications in atrial fibrillation. J Mol Cell Cardiol 48: 461–467.

83. Tan AY, Zimetbaum P (2010) Atrial Fibrillation and Atrial Fibrosis. J Cardiovasc Pharmacol.

84. Waktare JE, Hnatkova K, Sopher SM, Murgatroyd FD, Guo X, et al. (2001) The role of atrial ectopics in initiating paroxysmal atrial fibrillation. Eur Heart J 22: 333–339.

85. Vikman S, Makikallio TH, Yli-Mayry S, Pikkujamsa S, Koivisto AM, et al. (1999) Altered complexity and correlation properties of R-R interval dynamics before the spontaneous onset of paroxysmal atrial fibrillation. Circulation 100: 2079–2084.

86. Dimmer C, Tavernier R, Gjorgov N, Van Nooten G, Clement DL, et al. (1998) Variations of autonomic tone preceding onset of atrial fibrillation after coronary artery bypass grafting. Am J Cardiol 82: 22–25.

87. Dimmer C, Szili-Torok T, Tavernier R, Verstraten T, Jordaens LJ (2003) Initiating mechanisms of paroxysmal atrial fibrillation. Europace 5: 1–9.

88. Hogue CW Jr, Domitrovich PP, Stein PK, Despotis GD, Re L, et al. (1998) RR interval dynamics before atrial fibrillation in patients after coronary artery bypass graft surgery. Circulation 98: 429–434.

89. Lu Z, Scherlag BJ, Lin J, Niu G, Fung KM, et al. (2008) Atrial fibrillation begets atrial fibrillation: autonomic mechanism for atrial electrical remodeling induced by short-term rapid atrial pacing. Circ Arrhythm Electrophysiol 1: 184–192.

90. Olgin JE, Sih HJ, Hanish S, Jayachandran JV, Wu J, et al. (1998) Heterogeneous atrial denervation creates substrate for sustained atrial fibrillation. Circulation 98: 2608–2614.

91. Lo LW, Chiou CW, Lin YJ, Lee SH, Chen SA (2011) Neural mechanism of atrial fibrillation: insight from global high density frequency mapping. J Cardiovasc Electrophysiol 22: 1049–1056.

92. Comtois P, Nattel S (2011) Impact of tissue geometry on simulated cholinergic atrial fibrillation: a modeling study. Chaos 21: 013108.

93. Katsouras G, Sakabe M, Comtois P, Maguy A, Burstein B, et al. (2009) Differences in atrial fibrillation properties under vagal nerve stimulation versus atrial tachycardia remodeling. Heart Rhythm 6: 1465–1472.

94. Oliveira M, Silva MN, Geraldes V, Postolache G, Xavier R, et al. (2010) Effects of vagal stimulation on induction and termination of atrial fibrillation in an in vivo rabbit heart model. Rev Port Cardiol 29: 375–389.

27

The Comparison between Robotic and Manual Ablations in the Treatment of Atrial Fibrillation: A Systematic Review and Meta-Analysis

Wenli Zhang[1], Nan Jia[2], Jinzi Su[3], Jinxiu Lin[3], Feng Peng[3]*, Wenquan Niu[4,5]*

1 Department of Cardiology, Fuzhou General Hospital of Nanjing Command, PLA, Fujian Medical University, Fuzhou, Fujian, China, **2** Department of Cardiology, The Fourth People's Hospital of Shenzhen, Shenzhen, Guangdong, China, **3** Department of Cardiology, The First Affiliated Hospital of Fujian Medical University, Fuzhou, Fujian, China, **4** State Key Laboratory of Medical Genomics, Ruijin Hospital, Shanghai Jiao Tong University School of Medicine, Shanghai, China, **5** Shanghai Institute of Hypertension, Ruijin Hospital, Shanghai Jiao Tong University School of Medicine, Shanghai, China

Abstract

Objective: To examine in what aspects and to what extent robotic ablation is superior over manual ablation, we sought to design a meta-analysis to compare clinical outcomes between the two ablations in the treatment of atrial fibrillation.

Methods and Results: A literature search was conducted of PubMed and EMBASE databases before December 1, 2013. Data were extracted independently and in duplicate from 8 clinical articles and 792 patients. Effect estimates were expressed as weighted mean difference (WMD) or odds ratio (OR) and the accompanied 95% confidence interval (95% CI). Pooling the results of all qualified trials found significant reductions in fluoroscopic time (minutes) (WMD; 95% CI; P: -8.9; -12.54 to -5.26; <0.0005) and dose-area product ($Gy \times cm^2$) (WMD; 95% CI; P: -1065.66; -1714.36 to -416.96; 0.001) for robotic ablation relative to manual ablation, with evident heterogeneity (P<0.0005) and a low probability of publication bias. In subgroup analysis, great improvement of fluoroscopic time in patients with robotic ablation was consistently presented in both randomized and nonrandomized clinical trials, particularly in the former (WMD; 95% CI; P: -12.61; -15.13 to -10.09; <0.0005). Success rate of catheter ablation was relatively higher in patients with robotic ablation than with manual ablation (OR; 95% CI; P: 3.45; 0.24 to 49.0; 0.36), the difference yet exhibiting no statistical significance.

Conclusions: This study confirmed and extended previous observations by quantifying great reductions of fluoroscopic time and dose-area product in patients referred for robotic ablation than for manual ablation in the treatment of atrial fibrillation, especially in randomized clinical trials.

Editor: Larisa G. Tereshchenko, Johns Hopkins University SOM, United States of America

Funding: Funding provided by Shanghai Rising Star Program (11QA1405500). The funders had no role in study design, data collection and analysis, decision to publish, or preparation of the manuscript.

Competing Interests: The authors have declared that no competing interests exist.

* E-mail: pengfeng@medmail.com.cn (FP); niuwenquan_shcn@163.com (WN)

Introduction

Treating atrial fibrillation via catheter ablation has long been established as a safe and effective strategy [1]. Recent years have witnessed extraordinary innovation in catheter ablation from conventional manual approach to the robotic-guided navigation system [2,3]. Nonetheless, the benefits of robotic ablation over manual ablation are currently subject to an ongoing debate [4]. For example, in a relatively large clinical trial by Thomas et al [5], early use of robotic ablation led to a significant reduction of fluoroscopic time compared with manual ablation, whereas there was no material difference between the two ablations in another clinical trial by Rillig et al [6]. However, it should be noted that the majority of these clinical trials have been seriously underpowered, and some are even nonrandomized. In this context, a meta-analysis represents a powerful statistical methodology for synthesizing research evidence across independent trials [7]. Given the accumulation of data, we sought to design a meta-analysis to compare procedure outcomes between robotic and manual ablations in terms of fluoroscopic time, total procedure duration, radiofrequency time and dose-area product, as well as the success rates of catheter ablation and its major complications in the treatment of atrial fibrillation.

Methods

We undertook this meta-analysis of clinical trials in conformity with the guidelines put forth by the Preferred Reporting Items for Systematic Reviews and Meta-analyses (PRISMA) statement (Checklist S1) [8].

Search Strategy

A literature search was conducted of PubMed and EMBASE databases covering the period from the earliest possible year to December 1, 2013, with search terms including "ablation", "robotic", or "navigation", annexed with "atrial fibrillation" or "arrhythmias". In addition, this search was complemented with the perusal of the bibliographies of retrieved original reports and review articles to identify additional eligible articles. Search results were restricted to English-language and clinical trials.

Trial Selection

Two investigators (F.P. and W.N.) independently read the titles and abstracts to assess their eligibility, and they retrieved the full texts of potentially eligible articles. When necessary, we emailed the corresponding authors to avoid the double counting of study groups involved in more than one clinical trial. Where more than one publication of a clinical trial existed, we extracted data from the most recent or complete publication.

Eligibility Criteria

For inclusion, trials had to involve patients needing catheter ablation treatment for atrial fibrillation and compare the changes of either fluoroscopic time, total procedure time, radiofrequency time or dose-area product between robotic and manual ablations. Trials were excluded if they were cross-over trials or conference abstracts or proceedings, case reports or series, editorials, narrative reviews, or non-English articles.

Data Extraction

Two investigators (F.P. and W.N.) independently extracted data using a standardized Excel template (Microsoft Corp, Redmond, WA). Disagreements were settled by consensus.

For each article, the following data were summarized: the first author's surname, year of publication, ethnicity of study patients, sample size of each treatment, fluoroscopic time (minutes), total procedure time (minutes), radiofrequency time (minutes), dose-area product ($Gy \times cm^2$), the success rate of catheter ablation, and major complication rate between two ablations, as well as the characteristics of trial patients including age, gender, body mass index, atrial fibrillation duration (years), left atrium size (mm), the percentages of paroxysmal atrial fibrillation, left ventricular ejection fraction (LVEF), coronary artery disease (CAD), hypertension and diabetes.

Total procedure time was defined as the time from venous puncture until sheath withdrawal. Radiofrequency time, also known as ablation time, was defined as the time from the first to the last ablation. The success of catheter ablation was defined as complete pulmonary vein isolation, which was confirmed by the disappearance of all pulmonary vein potentials or the dissociation of pulmonary vein potentials from left atrial activity. Major complications referred to adverse events causing either temporary or permanent change in health status requiring intervention.

Diagnosis of hypertension was based on the presence of elevated systolic (≥ 140 mmHg) and/or diastolic (≥ 90 mmHg) blood pressure, or current use of antihypertensive medications. Diabetes was defined as fasting plasma glucose levels ≥ 7.0 mmol/L or non-fasting plasma glucose levels ≥ 11.0 mmol/L, or taking hypoglycemic drugs or receiving parenteral insulin therapy.

Statistical Analysis

For a certain clinical outcome, where data from three or more independent trials were available, a meta-analysis was done. Quantitative outcomes were summarized and compared by weighted mean difference (WMD) with 95% confidence interval (95% CI) between robotic and manual ablations. Categorical variables were compared between the two groups by weighted odds ratio (OR) and its corresponding 95% CI. For each study, weight was calculated as the reciprocal of the variance of the estimated intervention effect. The random-effects model using the DerSimonian & Laird method [9] was employed irrespective of

the existence of heterogeneity. Heterogeneity across studies was examined with the inconsistency index (I^2) test, which ranges from 0 to 100% and is defined as the percentage of the observed variability that is due to heterogeneity rather than chance. Given the limited power of I^2 test for a small number of studies, we considered the presence of heterogeneity at 10% level of significance.

Predefined subgroup analysis was conducted a priori according to study design (randomized and nonrandomized clinical trials). Sensitivity analysis was performed to assess the contribution of individual trials to pooled effect estimates by sequentially omitting each trial one at a time and computing differential estimates for remaining trials. Meta-regression analysis was carried out to evaluate the extent to which different trial-level variables including all characteristics of trial patients as mentioned above explained the heterogeneity of different effect estimates between robotic and manual ablations.

Begg's funnel plot was constructed for assessment of publication bias. The asymmetry of this plot was assessed by Egger's regression test and then corrected by the trim and fill method with the adjusted effect estimates and number of studies. Also considering the small number of studies involved in this meta-analysis, we considered the presence of publication bias at 10% level of significance for Egger's regression test [10]. Statistical analyses were completed with the use of STATA software (StataCorp, College Station, TX, version 11.2 for Windows).

Results

Eligible Trials

The characteristics of study patients involved in all qualified trials are summarized in Table 1 and Table 2. The primary search for clinical trials comparing the procedure outcomes between robotic and manual ablations yielded 114 potentially relevant articles published in English language. Figure 1 illustrates a flow diagram schematizing the process of excluding articles with specific reasons. Consequently, 8 articles met our selection criteria and were published from the year 2009 to 2013 [2,5,6,11-15]. Two of 8 qualified articles recorded outcomes with more than one bipolar voltage of radiofrequency ablation [11,13], resulting in a total of 10 trials in the final analysis.

All 10 qualified trials were conducted in Caucasian populations, and four of them were on a randomized design [2,11,12]. There were respectively total 375 and 417 patients assigned to the robotic ablation and manual ablation procedures in atrial fibrillation treatment. Patients with robotic ablation (mean age: 59.0 years) were younger than those with manual ablation (61.2 years, P = 0.03), and there were no distribution differences for gender and body mass index between the two procedures. The average values of atrial fibrillation duration (6.57 years versus 5.8 years) and left atrium size (43.5 mm versus 42.06 mm) were slightly larger in patients with robotic ablation than with manual ablation group. The percentages of paroxysmal atrial fibrillation, LVEF, CAD, hypertension and diabetes were comparable between the two procedures.

Overall and Subgroup Analyses

Overall effect estimates for fluoroscopic time, total procedure time, radiofrequency time, and dose-area product, as well as the corresponding subgroup analyses by study design are presented in Figure 2. Pooling the results of all qualified trials observed significant reductions in fluoroscopic time (minutes) (WMD; 95% CI; P: -8.9; -12.54 to -5.26; <0.0005) and dose-area product ($Gy \times cm^2$) (-1065.66; -1714.36 to -416.96; 0.001) for robotic

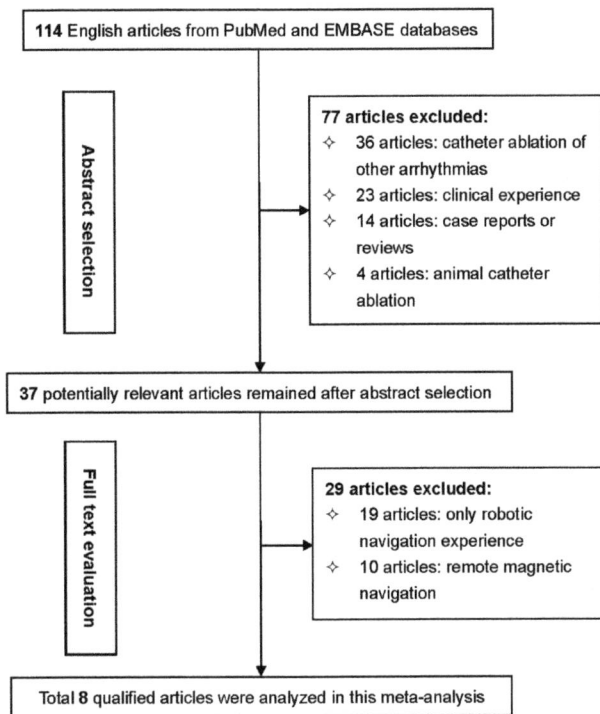

Figure 1. Flow diagram of search strategy and study selection.

ablation compared with manual ablation, accompanying strong evidence of heterogeneity for both estimates (P<0.0005) and low probability of publication bias as estimated by the Begg's and Egger's tests and the visual inspection of funnel plots based on the trim and fill method (Figure 3). The differences in the magnitude of total procedure time and radiofrequency time were matched between robotic and manual ablations with the presence of heterogeneity (Figure 2) and the absence of publication bias (Figure 3).

In subgroup analyses, great improvement of fluoroscopic time in patients with robotic ablation was consistently seen in both randomized and nonrandomized clinical trials, particularly in the former (WMD; 95% CI; P: -12.61; -15.13 to -10.09; <0.0005). Moreover, there was no indication of heterogeneity ($I^2 = 0.0\%$; P = 0.574) and publication bias (data not shown) for randomized clinical trials. As for dose-area product, significant difference was only noticed in randomized trials (-1192.0; -1461.82 to -922.18), which involved only one trial.

Success Rates and Major Complications

Success rate of catheter ablation was relatively higher in patients with robotic ablation than with manual ablation (OR; 95% CI; P: 3.45; 0.24 to 49.0; 0.36), the difference yet exhibiting no statistical significance (Figure 4). Similarly for major complications, robotic ablation approach was associated with slightly high rate compared with manual ablation approach (1.41; 0.38 to 5.21; 0.606), and still the difference was nonsignificant.

Sensitivity Analyses

Overall, there was not an individual trial influencing the overall effect estimates significantly. After removing each trial and calculating the overall estimates for the remaining trials, the significance of the WMD or OR remained materially unchanged (data not shown).

Table 1. Baseline characteristics of study patients in qualified studies.

Author (year)	Country	Random	Number	Age (year)	Gender (Male)	AF duration (year)	BMI (kg/m²)	LA size (mm)
Malcolme-Lawes et al (2013) (30 W)	UK	Yes	10/10	59.3/64.6	NA	3.28/3.48	NA	42.7/38
Malcolme-Lawes et al (2013) (60 W)	UK	Yes	10/10	60.6/64.6	NA	4.99/3.48	NA	42.5/38
Thomas et al (2012)	Germany	No	25/61	60/62	0.64/0.8	4.9/5.5	NA	41/42
Rillig et al (2012)	Germany	No	50/20	60/66.5	0.58/0.75	NA	26.7/26.9	47.5/47.5
Duncan et al (2012)	UK	Yes	21/23	53/55	0.62/0.61	6.83/6.67	NA	NA
Tilz et al (2010) (20 W)	Germany	No	10/25	58/61	0.6/0.56	8.3/8.5	26/25	44/44
Tilz et al (2010) (30 W)	Germany	No	4/25	59/61	0.75/0.56	13/8.5	28/25	48/44
Steven et al (2010)	Germany	Yes	30/30	62/61	0.67/0.47	7/6	NA	40/39
Kautzner et al (2009)	Czech	No	22/16	55/55	0.73/0.81	NA	NA	NA
Di Biase et al (2009)	USA	No	193/197	63/61	0.75/0.74	4.25/4.25	30/30	42.3/44

Table 2. Baseline characteristics of study patients in qualified studies.

Paroxysmal AF (%)	LVEF (%)	CAD (%)	Hypertension (%)	Diabetes (%)	Freedom from AF (%)	Major complications (%)
100/100	56.2/52	9.1/11.1	27.3/55.6	0/22.2	50/60	10/0
100/100	56.4/52	11.1/11.1	33.3/55.6	11.1/22.2	80/60	0/0
76/52	NA	28/16	72/62	NA	NA	4/5
58/60	NA	14/5	62/75	8/10	NA	NA
100/100	NA	NA	NA	NA	NA	NA
NA	NA	NA	60/72	NA	NA	NA
NA	NA	NA	75/72	NA	NA	NA
100/100	68/67	13/7	73/80	NA	73/77	NA
100/100	NA	NA	NA	NA	NA	NA
66/69	58/57	22/21	65/50	8/9	100/68	2/1

Abbreviations: AF, atrial fibrillation; BMI, body mass index; LA, left atrium; LVEF, left ventricular ejection fraction; CAD, coronary artery disease; NA, not available. Data are expressed as mean values or percentages unless otherwise indicated between robotic and manual ablations.

Meta-Regression Analyses

A set of meta-regression analyses were conducted accordingly to explore the extent to which trial-level variables account for heterogeneity among the effect estimates. Unfortunately, none of the examined trial-level confounders contributed to the changes of effect estimates between the robotic ablation and manual ablation approaches (data not shown). It is widely accepted that meta-regression analysis, albeit enabling continuous variables to be

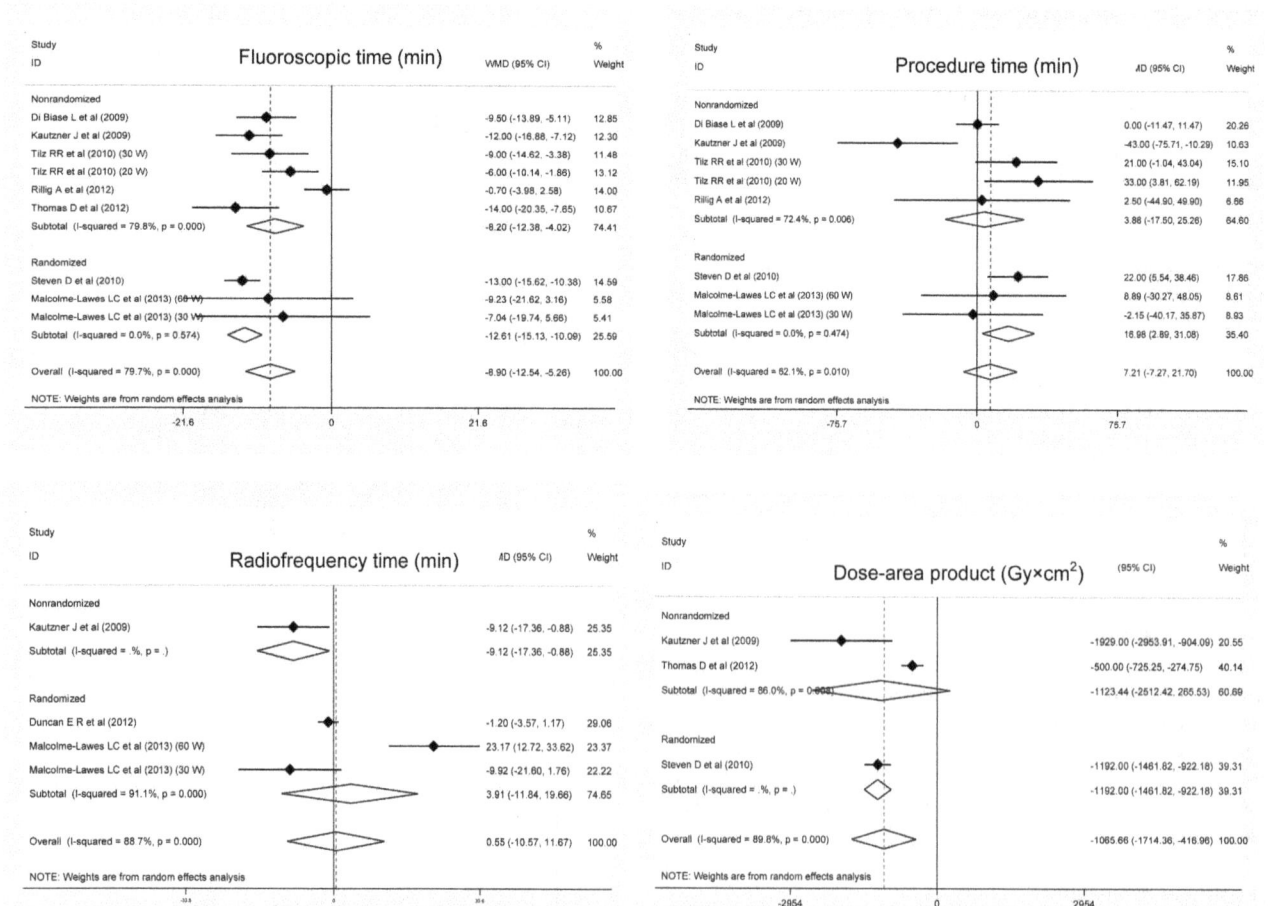

Figure 2. Forest plots of changes of fluoroscopic time, total procedure time, radiofrequency time, dose-area product for the comparison of robotic ablation with manual ablation.

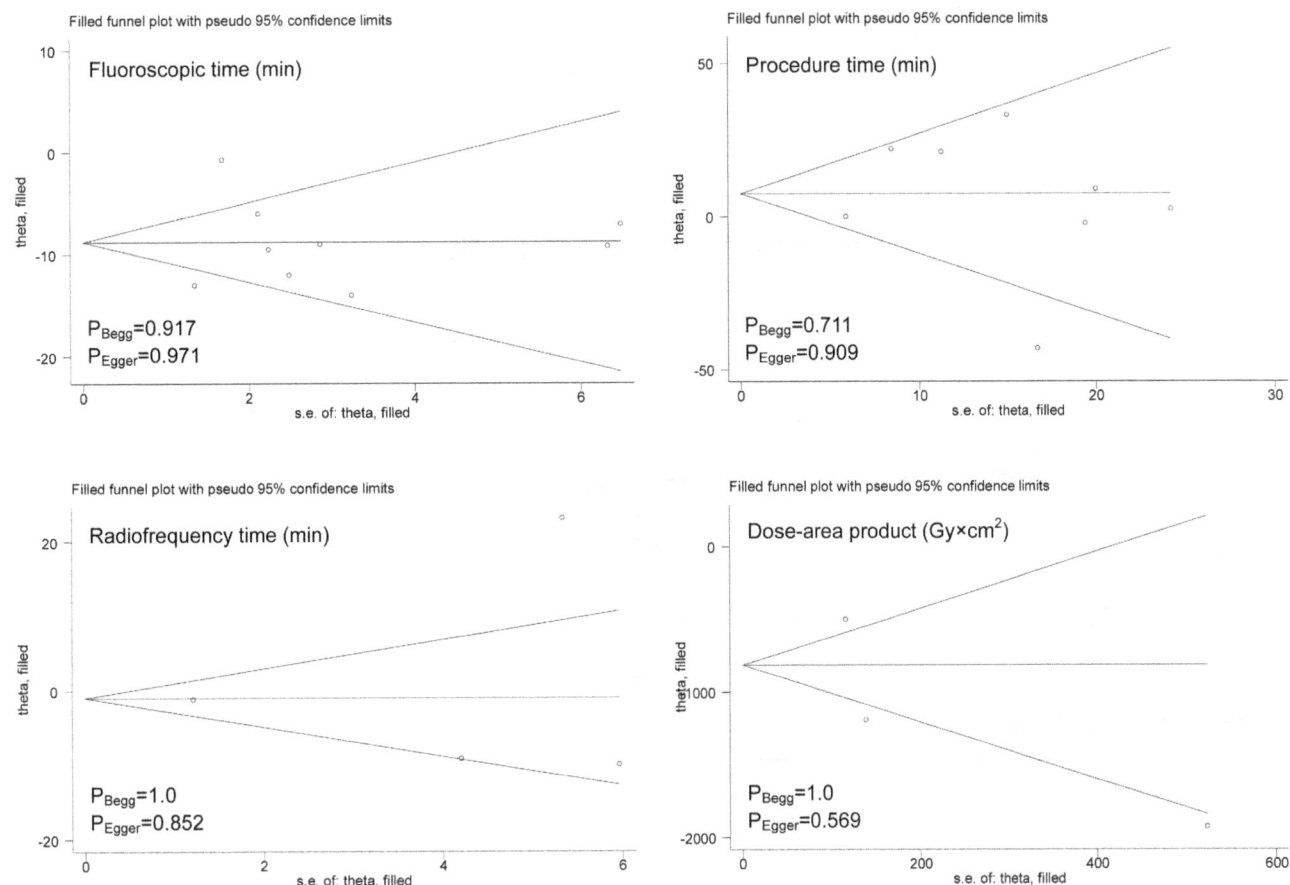

Figure 3. Filled funnel plots of fluoroscopic time, total procedure time, radiofrequency time, dose-area product for the comparison of robotic ablation with manual ablation.

considered, does not have the methodological rigor of a properly designed study that is intended to test the effect of these covariates formally.

Discussion

To the authors' knowledge, this is to date the first meta-analysis synthesizing data on the comparison of robotic ablation with manual ablation based on 8 clinical articles and 792 patients for the treatment of atrial fibrillation. The principal finding of this study was the greater reductions of both fluoroscopic time and dose-area product in patients with robotic ablation than with manual ablation, especially in randomized clinical trials. However, caution is urged about the interpretation of these comparisons due to the evident heterogeneity. Moreover, although the success rate of catheter ablation was relatively high by using robotic ablation, significance was not reached likely due to the lack of statistical power or the initial learning stage of this novel technique.

The application of robotic ablation in clinical routine is still in its infancy, and the benefits of this novel technique for catheter ablation in treating atrial fibrillation are unquestionable [16], including excellent catheter stability and accuracy of its movement, reduced fluoroscopic time, catheter contact monitoring, improved comfort of the operator during the procedure as they can sit most of the time unexposed to radiation and a very short learning curve potentially allowing for more complicated procedures [17]. Various attempts to summarize the existing evidence have been made in recent years, but always in the context of a

narrative review of the literature [17-19]. This therefore prompts us to quantitatively assess the superiority of the robotic ablation over the manual ablation in the form of a meta-analysis. Despite approximate 9 minutes in fluoroscopic time were averagely saved in patients with robotic ablation relative to with manual ablation in our findings, total procedure duration remained similar between the two procedures, which is likely attributable to the longer patient prepping time for robotic ablation. This is also understandable because the findings of most enrolled trials were based on the initial experience of robotic ablation systems. More importantly, shorter fluoroscopic time to scattered x-ray is beneficial not only to the operator's health during a long interventional career and but also to the patients themselves [20], as partly reflected by the reduced dose-area product in our overall analyses. However, this potential benefit might be balanced out by the high costs, increasing the burden of patients. Nevertheless, we believe that with the accumulation of practical evidence, procedures will be greatly improved by using the robotic ablation systems.

However, a note of caution should be added because since heterogeneity in our principle findings might potentially limit the interpretation of the pooled effect estimates. Of note, study design might be a potential source of heterogeneity between trials in the subgroup analyses of this meta-analysis because heterogeneity between trials totally disappeared for fluoroscopic time after restricting analysis to randomized clinical trials. To further account for the contribution of examined trial-level continuous

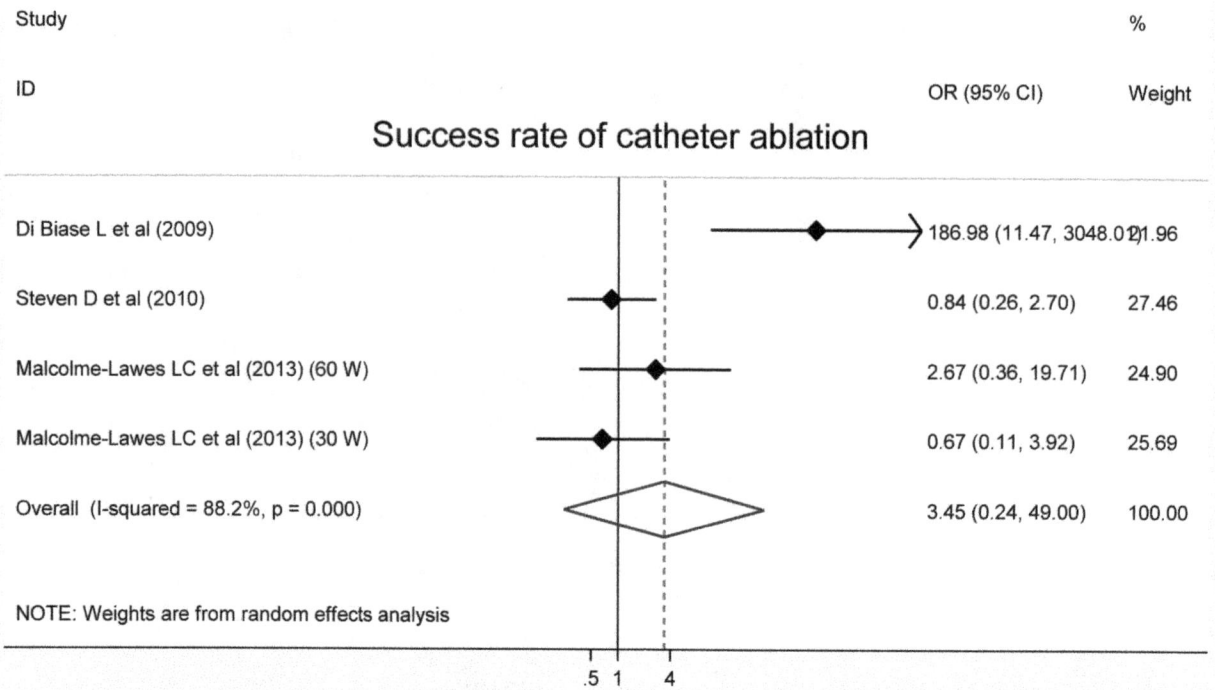

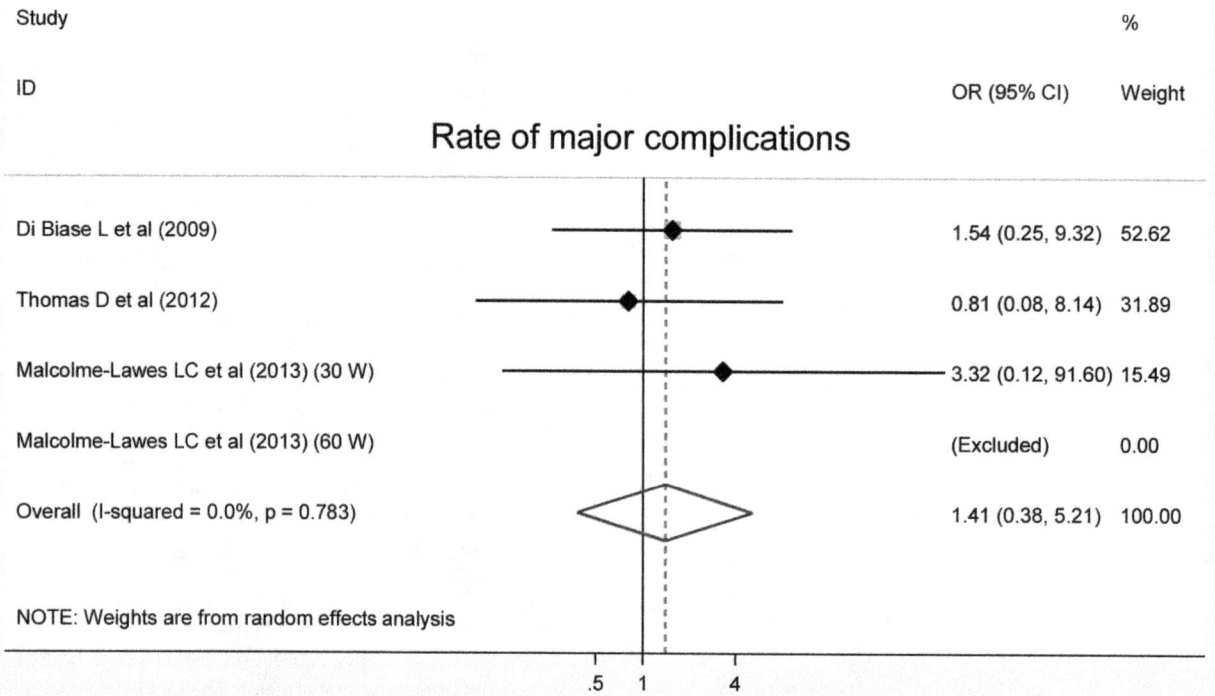

Figure 4. Forest plots of changes of the successful procedure of catheter ablation and the incidence of major complications for the comparison of robotic ablation with manual ablation.

moderators to the overall heterogeneity, we undertook a set of meta-regression analyses, but unfortunately we failed to tease out any contributory factors. It should be noted, however, this meta-regression analysis involves trials of limited sample size, rendering it underpowered to detect a small or moderate effect, and definitively there is a need for further large trials.

Despite the clear strengths of this meta-analysis including the low probability of publication bias, and the robustness of statistical analyses, interpretation of our findings, however, should be viewed in light of several limitations. First, six of ten qualified trials were performed on a nonrandomized design, raising the potential existence of potential biases. On the other hand, although randomized trials can minimize bias and are regarded as the gold standard for quantifying effect estimates, they may not be reflective of patients treated in general clinical practice [21]. Second, there was strong evidence of heterogeneity in a majority of our overall and subgroup analyses, limiting the interpretation of pooled effect estimates. Third, the total sample size of this meta-analysis was not large enough to draw a firm conclusion, such that our findings need to be validated in a large, well-designed clinical trial, and fortunately the ongoing prospective international man-and-machine trial by Rillig et al is designed to fully address the superiority of robotic ablation over manual ablation [22]. Fourth, the fact that study patients were all Caucasians limited the generalizability of our findings, necessitating the future validation

in other ethnics. Last but not the least, as with all meta-analyses, despite the low probability of publication bias reported in this meta-analysis, selection bias cannot be completely excluded, since we merely identified articles from the English journals and published trials.

In summary, this study confirmed and extended previous observations by quantifying the great reductions of fluoroscopic time and dose-area product in patients with robotic ablation than with manual ablation, especially in randomized clinical trials. For practical reasons, with the accumulation of data from large randomized clinical trials, successful validation of our findings will revolutionize the current clinical practice and healthcare system by bringing great benefits to doctors and patients alike in the near future.

Author Contributions

Conceived and designed the experiments: WN FP. Performed the experiments: WZ FP NJ. Analyzed the data: WN FP. Contributed reagents/materials/analysis tools: WZ NJ JS JL. Wrote the paper: WN FP.

References

1. Verma A, Sanders P, Macle L, Deisenhofer I, Morillo CA, et al. (2012) Substrate and Trigger Ablation for Reduction of Atrial Fibrillation Trial-Part II (STAR AF II): design and rationale. Am Heart J 164: 1-6 e6.

2. Steven D, Servatius H, Rostock T, Hoffmann B, Drewitz I, et al. (2010) Reduced fluoroscopy during atrial fibrillation ablation: benefits of robotic guided navigation. J Cardiovasc Electrophysiol 21: 6-12.

3. Nolker G, Gutleben KJ, Muntean B, Vogt J, Horstkotte D, et al. (2012) Novel robotic catheter manipulation system integrated with remote magnetic navigation for fully remote ablation of atrial tachyarrhythmias: a two-centre evaluation. Europace 14: 1715-1718.

4. Smilowitz NR, Weisz G (2012) Robotic-assisted angioplasty: current status and future possibilities. Curr Cardiol Rep 14: 642-646.

5. Thomas D, Scholz EP, Schweizer PA, Katus HA, Becker R (2012) Initial experience with robotic navigation for catheter ablation of paroxysmal and persistent atrial fibrillation. J Electrocardiol 45: 95-101.

6. Rillig A, Meyerfeldt U, Tilz RR, Talazko J, Arya A, et al. (2012) Incidence and long-term follow-up of silent cerebral lesions after pulmonary vein isolation using a remote robotic navigation system as compared with manual ablation. Circ Arrhythm Electrophysiol 5: 15-21.

7. Dagres N, Varounis C, Flevari P, Piorkowski C, Bode K, et al. (2009) Mortality after catheter ablation for atrial fibrillation compared with antiarrhythmic drug therapy. A meta-analysis of randomized trials. Am Heart J 158: 15-20.

8. Moher D, Liberati A, Tetzlaff J, Altman DG (2009) Preferred reporting items for systematic reviews and meta-analyses: the PRISMA statement. Ann Intern Med 151: 264-269, W264.

9. DerSimonian R, Kacker R (2007) Random-effects model for meta-analysis of clinical trials: an update. Contemp Clin Trials 28: 105-114.

10. Bowden J, Tierney JF, Copas AJ, Burdett S (2011) Quantifying, displaying and accounting for heterogeneity in the meta-analysis of RCTs using standard and generalised Q statistics. BMC Med Res Methodol 11: 41.

11. Malcolme-Lawes LC, Lim PB, Koa-Wing M, Whinnett ZI, Jamil-Copley S, et al. (2013) Robotic assistance and general anaesthesia improve catheter stability and increase signal attenuation during atrial fibrillation ablation. Europace 15: 41-47.

12. Duncan ER, Finlay M, Page SP, Hunter R, Goromonzi F, et al. (2012) Improved electrogram attenuation during ablation of paroxysmal atrial fibrillation with the Hansen robotic system. Pacing Clin Electrophysiol 35: 730-738.

13. Tilz RR, Chun KR, Metzner A, Burchard A, Wissner E, et al. (2010) Unexpected high incidence of esophageal injury following pulmonary vein isolation using robotic navigation. J Cardiovasc Electrophysiol 21: 853-858.

14. Kautzner J, Peichl P, Cihak R, Wichterle D, Mlcochova H (2009) Early experience with robotic navigation for catheter ablation of paroxysmal atrial fibrillation. Pacing Clin Electrophysiol 32 Suppl 1: S163-166.

15. Di Biase L, Wang Y, Horton R, Gallinghouse GJ, Mohanty P, et al. (2009) Ablation of atrial fibrillation utilizing robotic catheter navigation in comparison to manual navigation and ablation: single-center experience. J Cardiovasc Electrophysiol 20: 1328-1335.

16. Willems S, Steven D, Servatius H, Hoffmann BA, Drewitz I, et al. (2010) Persistence of pulmonary vein isolation after robotic remote-navigated ablation for atrial fibrillation and its relation to clinical outcome. J Cardiovasc Electrophysiol 21: 1079-1084.

17. Jan P, Jan Š (2012) Robot-assisted navigation in atrial fibrillation ablation—Of any benefits? Cor et Vasa 54: e408-413.

18. Nazarian S (2010) New technologies and therapies for cardiac arrhythmias. Minerva Cardioangiol 58: 731-740.

19. Bai R, L DIB, Valderrabano M, Lorgat F, Mlcochova H, et al. (2012) Worldwide experience with the robotic navigation system in catheter ablation of atrial fibrillation: methodology, efficacy and safety. J Cardiovasc Electrophysiol 23: 820-826.

20. Picano E, Vano E (2011) The radiation issue in cardiology: the time for action is now. Cardiovasc Ultrasound 9: 35.

21. Piccini JP, Berger JS, O'Connor CM (2009) Amiodarone for the prevention of sudden cardiac death: a meta-analysis of randomized controlled trials. Eur Heart J 30: 1245-1253.

22. Rillig A, Schmidt B, Steven D, Meyerfeldt U, L DIB, et al. (2013) Study design of the man and machine trial: a prospective international controlled noninferiority trial comparing manual with robotic catheter ablation for treatment of atrial fibrillation. J Cardiovasc Electrophysiol 24: 40-46.

28

Three-Dimensional Computer Model of the Right Atrium Including the Sinoatrial and Atrioventricular Nodes Predicts Classical Nodal Behaviours

Jue Li, Shin Inada, Jurgen E. Schneider, Henggui Zhang, Halina Dobrzynski, Mark R. Boyett*

Institute of Cardiovascular Sciences, University of Manchester, Core Technology Facility, Manchester, United Kingdom

Abstract

The aim of the study was to develop a three-dimensional (3D) anatomically-detailed model of the rabbit right atrium containing the sinoatrial and atrioventricular nodes to study the electrophysiology of the nodes. A model was generated based on 3D images of a rabbit heart (atria and part of ventricles), obtained using high-resolution magnetic resonance imaging. Segmentation was carried out semi-manually. A 3D right atrium array model (~3.16 million elements), including eighteen objects, was constructed. For description of cellular electrophysiology, the Rogers-modified FitzHugh-Nagumo model was further modified to allow control of the major characteristics of the action potential with relatively low computational resource requirements. Model parameters were chosen to simulate the action potentials in the sinoatrial node, atrial muscle, inferior nodal extension and penetrating bundle. The block zone was simulated as passive tissue. The sinoatrial node, crista terminalis, main branch and roof bundle were considered as anisotropic. We have simulated normal and abnormal electrophysiology of the two nodes. In accordance with experimental findings: (i) during sinus rhythm, conduction occurs down the interatrial septum and into the atrioventricular node via the fast pathway (conduction down the crista terminalis and into the atrioventricular node via the slow pathway is slower); (ii) during atrial fibrillation, the sinoatrial node is protected from overdrive by its long refractory period; and (iii) during atrial fibrillation, the atrioventricular node reduces the frequency of action potentials reaching the ventricles. The model is able to simulate ventricular echo beats. In summary, a 3D anatomical model of the right atrium containing the cardiac conduction system is able to simulate a wide range of classical nodal behaviours.

Editor: Alexander V. Panfilov, Gent University, Belgium

Funding: This study is financially supported by a programme grant from the British Heart Foundation (RG/11/18/29257). Jurgen E. Schneider is a BHF Senior Basic Science Research Fellow (FS/11/50/29038). The funders had no role in study design, data collection and analysis, decision to publish, or preparation of the manuscript.

Competing Interests: The authors have declared that no competing interests exist.

* Email: mark.boyett@manchester.ac.uk

Introduction

Accurate simulation of the generation and propagation of cardiac electrical activity requires detailed anatomical and electrophysiological models. A variety of heart anatomical models (human and animal) have been generated by various investigators. David et al. [1] generated a boundary-conforming mesh of the human atria comprised entirely of hexahedral elements. Bernus et al. [2] developed a human ventricular model, which reproduces geometry and fibre orientation in the right and left ventricles of the human heart. Several whole human heart models have been generated [3–5]. Aslanidi et al. [6] integrated a three-dimensional (3D) model of the human sinoatrial node (SAN) [7] into a 3D model of the whole atria dissected from the Visible Human dataset [8]. Apart from human heart models, a number of animal heart models have been generated. Nielsen et al. [9] developed a mathematical representation of the ventricular geometry and fibre orientation for the dog. Vetter and McCulloch [10] developed a 3D finite element model of rabbit ventricular geometry with fibre orientation. However, none of these models includes both the sinoatrial and atrioventricular (AVN) nodes. We have previously generated 3D anatomically-detailed models of the isolated SAN and isolated AVN of the rabbit [11,12]. More recently, we have generated a 3D anatomically-detailed model of the rabbit heart, including the conduction system, using micro-CT [13], although at present the model is unsuitable for electrophysiological simulation. In this study, a 3D anatomically-detailed model of the right atrium of the rabbit heart, including the SAN and AVN and suitable for electrophysiological simulations, was generated based on magnetic resonance (MR) imaging.

There are two groups of electrophysiological models for simulation of the cardiac action potential. One comprises biophysically-detailed (ionic) models, and another comprises mathematical caricature (simplified) models. Based on patch clamp etc., a large number of biophysically-detailed models of the action potential in single cells from different regions of the heart have been developed [14]. For example, such models have been developed for: human atrial [15,16] and ventricular [17–22] muscle; dog atrial [23,24] and ventricular [25–28] muscle; sheep Purkinje fibres [29,30]; rabbit SAN [31–38], AVN [39], Purkinje

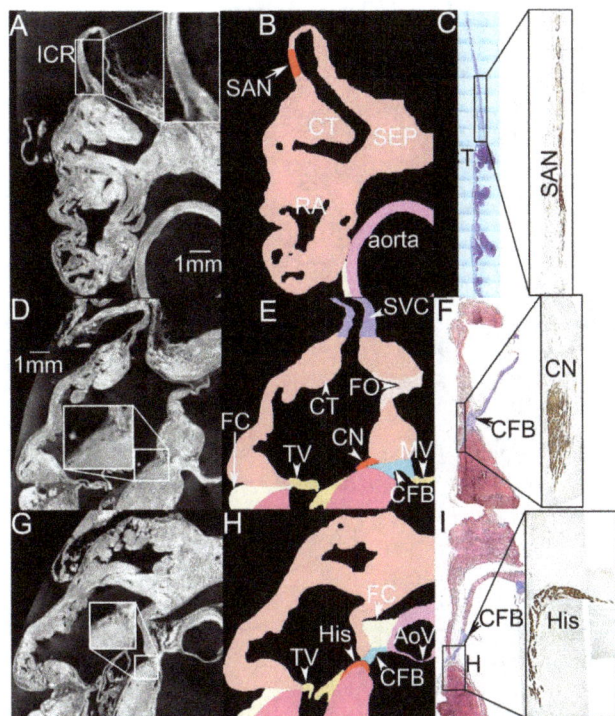

Figure 1. Identification of the SAN and AVN by comparing the MR images with Masson's trichrome stained and neurofilament-immunolabelled sections from the intercaval region and triangle of Koch region. A, D and G, MR images including the intercaval region (A), the compact node (part of the AVN; D) and the His bundle (G). Nodal regions are enlarged (boxes). B, E and H, corresponding segmented model sections including the SAN (B) and AVN (E and H). Different segmented structures are shown in different colours. C, F and I, sections through the SAN (C) and AVN (F and I) stained with Masson's trichrome and labelled for neurofilament (inset boxes). Masson's trichrome stains myocytes red and connective tissue blue. The neurofilament-positive (brown) cells are nodal. AoV, aortic valve; CFB, central fibrous body; CN, compact AVN; CT, crista terminalis; FC, outer fatty and connective tissue; FO, fossa ovalis; His, His bundle; ICR, intercaval region; MV, mitral valve; RA, right atrium; RV, right ventricle; SEP, interatrial septum; SVC, superior vena cava; TV, tricuspid valve.

fibres [40] and atrial [41–43] and ventricular [40,44,45] muscle; guinea-pig ventricular muscle [46–51]; and mouse SAN [52] and ventricular muscle [53]. Caricature models of the action potential include the cellular automaton model, coupled map lattices [54], lattices of coupled ordinary differential equations [55], FitzHugh-Nagumo models [56] and the Fenton-Karma model [57]. Action potential propagation through the heart can be simulated using caricature models as well as biophysically-detailed models. To investigate complex electrophysiological behaviour in the complex anatomical structure of the heart, the use of a set of caricature models is computationally more effective compared to the use of a set of biophysically-detailed models, as they enable testable predictions about heart electrophysiological behaviour to be made with relatively low computational resource.

The purpose of this study was to create a platform with an anatomically-detailed model of rabbit right atrium and a set of caricature action potential models to investigate nodal electrophysiology in health and disease. A 3D anatomically-detailed model of the rabbit right atrium with multiple objects, including the cardiac conduction system (SAN and AVN), was generated.

This model can be used for education and research. The propagation of the action potential through the right atrium during sinus rhythm, atrial fibrillation and AVN reentry was simulated using this anatomically-detailed right atrium model, together with a set of Rogers-modified FitzHugh-Nagumo models as well as a cellular automaton model.

Methods

Ethics Statement

New Zealand White rabbits (1.5–2.5 kg) were sacrificed humanely according to the United Kingdom Animals (Scientific Procedures) Act 1986; in addition, the investigation conformed with the Guide for the Care and Use of Laboratory Animals published by the US National Institutes of Health (NIH Publication No. 85–23, revised 1996). The rabbits were humanely sacrificed by injection of an overdose of sodium pentobarbital into the central ear vein (an approved Schedule 1 method). The heart was removed after confirmation of death of the rabbit.

Development of a 3D anatomically-detailed model of the right atrium of the rabbit including the SAN and AVN

Our aim was the reconstruction of the right atrium, and the right atrium retained its shape by retaining other structures. The atria and a part of the ventricles were dissected for imaging. 3D images were obtained using high-resolution MR imaging carried out on a 11.7 T Bruker MR system (Bruker Medical, Ettlingen, Germany) at the University of Oxford. The voxel size after reconstruction was 26.4 μm×26.4 μm×24.4 μm (anisotropic). To form a convenient platform for numerical simulations, the anisotropic images were transformed into isotropic images with a voxel size of 30 μm×30 μm×30 μm and also 60 μm×60 μm×60 μm. MATLAB (version 7; The Math Works, Inc., Matick, MA, USA) was used to analyse the data: the anisotropic images were imported into the workspace of MATLAB and transformed into isotropic 3D images (voxel size, 30 μm×30 μm×30 μm; Figure S1A) using cubic interpolation.

The superior vena cava (SVC), crista terminalis (CT) and tricuspid valve (TV) could be recognised (Figure S1A). The 3D images were rotated to be in the normal anatomical orientation (x: right-left; y: ventral-dorsal; z: caudal-cranial) for segmentation. The right atrium structure was extracted based on the global threshold; the resulting binary images are shown in Figure S1B. Isosurface rendering was used to display the overall structure of the 3D model for visualisation (Figure S1C). Figure S1D shows the 3D model after segmentation, which is discussed below.

Segmentation was carried out semi-manually by analysing the MR imaging data from three directions (along x, y and z axes). First, the best orientation for segmentation was chosen. Secondly, the object of interest was extracted from the structure every 5~10 images. Thirdly, interpolation was carried out to obtain the 3D object. Finally, the object was combined with other objects to produce a 3D multiple-object model. Eighteen objects were segmented in this study. The right atrial wall, crista terminalis, main branch (a thick muscle bundle projecting from the crista terminalis towards the atrial appendage), roof bundle (a thick muscle bundle projecting from the interatrial septum towards the atrial appendage), a small part of the right ventricle, the aorta with the aortic valve, the coronary sinus, the tricuspid valve, part of the mitral valve and the fossa ovalis were easy to recognise in the MR images and were segmented as described above.

The SAN and AVN were identified by comparing the MR images with Masson's trichrome stained and neurofilament-immunolabelled sections from the intercaval region (cut perpen-

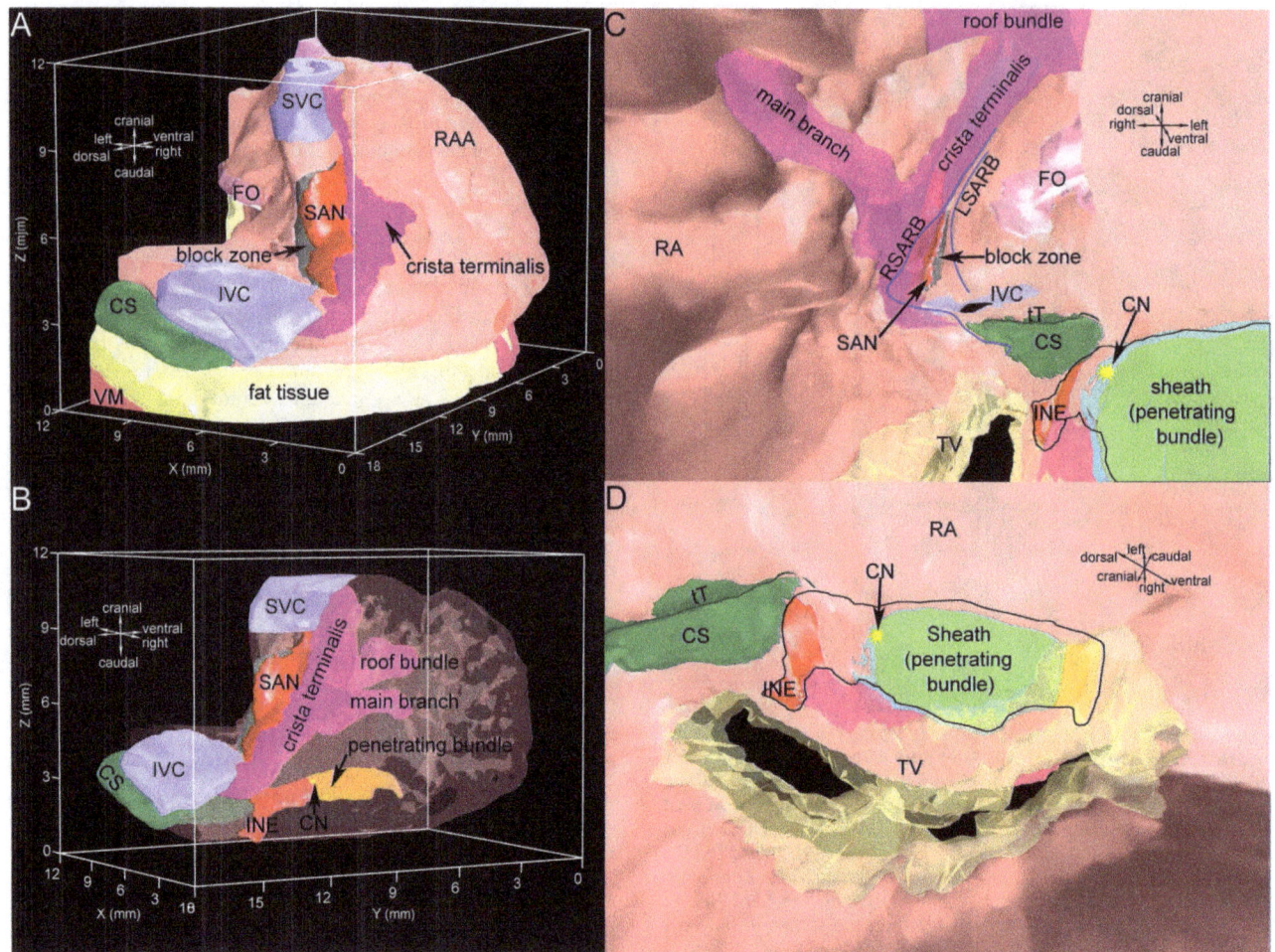

Figure 2. 3D model of the rabbit right atrium including the SAN and AVN. A, dorsal oblique view of the model. B, model with transparent atrium to reveal internal structures. C, internal ventral view of the model. D, internal cranial right view of the model. Different segmented structures are shown in different colours. CN, compact node; CS, coronary sinus; INE, inferior nodal extension; IVC, inferior vena cava; FO, fossa ovalis; LSARB, left sinoatrial ring bundle; RAA, right atrial appendage; RSARB, right sinoatrial ring bundle; SVC, superior vena cava; tT, tendon of Todaro; TV, tricuspid valve.

dicular to the crista terminalis [11]) and triangle of Koch (cut roughly perpendicular to septal leaflet of tricuspid valve [12]), as well as our previous 3D SAN and AVN models [11,12,58]. Neurofilament is a neuronal cytoskeletal protein that is exclusively expressed in the cardiac conduction system of the rabbit. The SAN and AVN can be recognised because they express neurofilament (brown label), whereas the surrounding atrial tissue does not (Figure 1C, F, I). To segment the SAN, MR images (Figure 1A) and Masson's trichrome stained (Figure 1C, left) and neurofilament-immunolabelled sections (Figure 1C, right) with the same features were compared. In the enlarged image within Figure 1A, it is possible to distinguish the SAN from the surrounding atrial tissue. To determine the extent of the SAN, the distance between the crista terminalis and the SAN centre and the length of the SAN centre as seen in Masson's trichrome stained and neurofilament-immunolabelled sections were measured (Figure 1C). Then the SAN was segmented accordingly. The result is shown in Figure 1B. The SAN periphery was not included in this model due to its complexity [59].

Figure 1D-F shows images through the compact part of the AVN. Once again, a MR image (Figure 1D) was compared with Masson's trichrome stained (Figure 1F, left) and neurofilament-

immunolabelled (Figure 1F, right) sections with the same features. The neurofilament-positive (brown) cells in Figure 1F are AVN cells. In the enlarged image within Figure 1D, the AVN can be easily distinguished from the surrounding atrial muscle. The central fibrous body, stained blue with Masson's trichrome (Figure 1F, left), can be distinguished from the surrounding atrial muscle in the MR images by comparing Figure 1D with Figure 1F. Figure 1E shows a section from the segmented multiple-object model based on Figure 1D. Figure 1G-I shows comparable images through the His bundle; an analogous method was used to segment it (Figure 1H). The location of the tendon of Todaro and the right and left sinoatrial ring bundles were determined by comparing the MR images and Masson's trichrome stained sections of a similar region. It is well known that there is a conduction block zone from the SAN towards the interatrial septum [60]. It was not possible to detect the block zone in either MR images or tissue sections. Hence, the block zone was segmented according to previously published activation maps of the rabbit SAN [61].

Finally, a 3D right atrium volume model with ~3.16 million elements and eighteen objects was constructed (Model S1). The objects are the right atrial wall, the crista terminalis, the main branch, the roof bundle, the SAN, the AVN (inferior nodal extension and penetrating bundle), part of the right ventricle, the aorta with the aortic valve, the superior vena cava, the inferior vena cava, the coronary sinus, the tricuspid valve, part of the mitral valve, the fossa ovalis, the central fibrous body, the block zone, and the outer fatty and connective tissue. The isosurface rendering technique was used to visualise the 3D volume model. The tendon of Todaro and the right and left sinoatrial ring bundles were highlighted using spline lines. Figure 2 shows various views of the 3D volume model. Figure 2A shows a dorsal oblique view of the model. The outer shape of the right atrium can be seen. The atrial muscle is shown in pink. The right atrial appendage can be easily recognised. The SAN (red) is located on the dorsal side within the intercaval region (the region between the superior vena cava and inferior vena cava). The crista terminalis (purple) is located on the right side of the SAN and the block zone (grey) is located on the left side of the SAN. The coronary sinus (green) runs under the inferior vena cava (blue), approximately perpendicular to the inferior vena cava. Figure 2B shows the model with transparent atrium to reveal internal structures. The ventricles, valves and central fibrous body were removed to reveal the AVN. The main branch (purple), roof bundle (purple) and AVN (inferior nodal extension, red; penetrating bundle, orange) can be seen through the transparent right atrium. Figure 2C is an internal ventral view. The tricuspid valve (yellow) and connective tissue sheath (blue) surrounding the penetrating bundle (orange) are transparent. The tendon of Todaro (green line) and the right and left sinoatrial ring bundles (dark blue lines) can be seen. The fossa ovalis (pink) is located on the left side of the left sinoatrial ring bundle. The SAN is surrounded by the right and left sinoatrial ring bundles. The three big muscle bundles (crista terminalis, main branch and roof bundle; purple) are clearly seen. The main branch branches from the crista terminalis. The roof bundle is analogous to a roof beam connecting the interatrial septum with the right atrial free wall. Figure 2D shows an internal cranial right view. The area surrounded by a thin black line is the AVN. Part of the inferior nodal extension (red) is covered by a thin layer of atrial tissue (pink). The penetrating bundle is covered by a connective tissue sheath (transparent blue). The ventral end of the penetrating bundle lies underneath the tricuspid valve (transparent yellow). The bright yellow stars in Figure 2B, C, D mark the position of the compact AVN.

Simulation of the electrophysiological behaviour of the rabbit right atrium

Simulation domain. For numerical simulation, a simulation domain (Model S2) was defined to exclude some objects which are electrically inexcitable: aorta and aortic valve, tricuspid valve, mitral valve, central fibrous body and the fatty and connective tissue. Because the model did not include Purkinje fibres, the ventricle was not included in the simulation domain. It is not possible to separate the superior and inferior vena cava from the right atrium (Figure 1A, D) and, therefore, they were treated as excitable tissue with the same properties as atrial muscle. There are cardiac myocytes in the coronary sinus area [62] and again it was treated as excitable tissue with the same properties as atrial muscle. Cardiac myocyte orientation is important for the propagation of the action potential. It was not possible to detect myocyte orientation from the MR imaging data. However, it is reasonable to assume that cardiac myocytes run longitudinally along the muscle bundles of the atria. The pectinate muscle bundles within the right atrial wall are complex and difficult to segment. Also it is not possible to infer myocyte orientation within the intercaval region and interatrial septum by segmenting muscle

bundles. Hence these parts of the atrial wall were defined as isotropic. Only three major muscle bundles (crista terminalis, main branch and roof bundle) were segmented and considered as anisotropic with myocytes running longitudinally along the muscle bundles. The SAN was simulated as an anisotropic material [60]. In summary, we have six zones (~1.6 million elements) with different properties: part of the atrial wall (isotropic atrial tissue), three major muscle bundles (anisotropic atrial muscle), SAN (anisotropic), inferior nodal extension and penetrating bundle (isotropic material) and the block zone (passive atrial tissue – non excitable).

Because the right atrial model has structural complexity and consists of ~1.6 million elements, instead of biophysically-detailed models, two caricature models of the action potential were used to simulate the action potential of the right atrium.

Electrophysiological models. The original FitzHugh-Nagumo model [56] was modified to simulate the spontaneous action potential of the SAN, which shows pacemaker behaviour:

$$\frac{\partial u}{\partial t} = \nabla \cdot \boldsymbol{D} \nabla u + c(u(u-\alpha)(1-u)-v); \quad \begin{cases} c = c_{1S} & \frac{\partial u}{\partial t} \geq 0 \\ c = c_{2S} & \frac{\partial u}{\partial t} < 0 \end{cases} \quad (1)$$

$$\frac{\partial v}{\partial t} = b(u-dv-0.1)$$

where u and v are the excitation variable and recovery variable, $\mathbf{n}$ is a vector normal to the boundary, $\boldsymbol{D}$ is the diffusion tensor, and α, b, c_{1S}, c_{2S}, and d are parameters that define the shape of the excitation variable u. The action potential V_m and the threshold potential V_{th} are normalised by:

$$u = \frac{V_m - V_r}{V_{os} - V_r}; \quad \alpha = \frac{V_{th} - V_r}{V_{os} - V_r} \quad (2)$$

where V_{os} is the overshoot potential and V_r is the resting potential.

The Rogers-modified FitzHugh-Nagumo model [63] is shown below:

$$\frac{\partial u}{\partial t} = \nabla \cdot \boldsymbol{D} \nabla u + c_1 u(u-\alpha)(1-u) - c_2 uv$$

$$\frac{\partial v}{\partial t} = b(u-dv) \quad (3)$$

with boundary condition

$$\frac{\partial u}{\partial \mathbf{n}} = 0$$

The first equation of the Rogers-modified FitzHugh-Nagumo model (above) was modified further to simulate the action potential of the atrial muscle, inferior nodal extension and penetrating bundle:

$$\frac{\partial u}{\partial t} = \nabla \cdot \boldsymbol{D} \nabla u + c[u(u-\alpha)(1-u)-uv]; \quad \begin{cases} c = c_{1A} & \frac{\partial u}{\partial t} \geq 0 \\ c = c_{2A} & \frac{\partial u}{\partial t} < 0 \end{cases} \quad (4)$$

In this equation, c_{1A} and c_{2A} are different from c_1 and c_2 of Equation 3.

The SAN periphery was not included in the 3D atrial model because of its complexity [11]. However, a border area of the SAN, 0.24 mm (4 elements) wide, was defined as an ideal SAN

Table 1. Parameters for the Fitzhugh-Nagumo model for the SAN, atrial muscle and AVN.

Parameters	SAN	Atrial muscle	Inferior nodal extension	Penetrating bundle
D	2	7	2	2
c_1	1	12.7	1.45	3.05
c_2	0.22	1.84	1	1
b	0.003	0.01	0.013	0.0048
d	3.5	2.475	2.5	2

periphery using Equation 1. Its property changes gradually as follows:

$$c_{1P} = c_{1S} + disSA \frac{(c_{1A} - c_{1S})}{0.24} \qquad (5)$$

where c_{1P} is c_{1S} in the SAN model (Equation 1). $disSA$ is the minimum distance between one SAN element and atrial elements.

The block zone was modelled as a passive tissue:

$$\frac{\partial u}{\partial t} = \nabla \cdot D\nabla u - \frac{u}{R_b} \qquad (6)$$

where R_b is resistivity. R_b was set to 0.5, which is sufficient to inhibit the action potential.

To define model parameters for SAN, atrial muscle, inferior nodal extension and penetrating bundle, a $50 \times 5 \times 5$ elements strand tissue model was used [64]. Stimulation was applied to the first three layers of elements ($3 \times 5 \times 5$). The conduction velocity was measured as the average conduction velocity calculated from the 10th element layer to the 40th element layer. Action potential duration was measured at 90% repolarization. A standard $S1$–$S2$ protocol was used to measure the refractory period. The spontaneous cycle length of the SAN (set by the modified Fitzhugh-Nagumo model) is 330 ms (corresponding to a heart rate of 182 beats/min). Table 1 lists the parameters for the SAN, atrial muscle, inferior nodal extension and penetrating bundle. Table 2 lists the conduction velocity, maximum upstroke velocity, action potential duration and refractory period of the SAN, atrial

muscle, inferior nodal extension and penetrating bundle from simulations and compares them to experimentally determined values. The data show that the majority of simulation results are within the range of experimental results. Figure 3 shows action potential waveforms from simulations (left) and experiment (right). The simulated action potential waveforms are a reasonable fit to the experimental waveforms.

The SAN and three major muscle bundles (crista terminalis, main branch and roof bundle) were considered as anisotropic. In the SAN, cells are reported to be oriented in different directions (forming a mesh) [11]. Experimental results suggest that the SAN is anisotropic, and the conduction velocities near the centre of SAN towards the SVC and IVC are faster than towards the crista terminalis and interatrial septum [65–67]. Hence it is reasonable to assume that most myocytes in the SAN run parallel to the crista terminalis. Let f denote the fibre orientation: $f = li + mj + nk$, where i, j and k are unit vectors of a Cartesian coordinate system; l, m and n are direction cosines, respectively. The properties of anisotropic fibres are introduced through an anisotropic diffusion tensor D_f in the fibre coordinate system:

$$D_f = \begin{pmatrix} D_l & 0 & 0 \\ 0 & D_t & 0 \\ 0 & 0 & D_t \end{pmatrix} \qquad (7)$$

where D_l is the diffusion in the fibre direction and D_t is the diffusion in the transverse direction. Then it is transformed to the global coordinate system as

Table 2. Measurements of conduction velocity, maximum upstroke velocity of the action potential, action potential duration and refractory period of the SAN, atrial muscle and AVN from the Fitzhugh-Nagumo model and experiment.

		SAN	Atrial muscle	Inferior nodal extension	Penetrating bundle
Conduction velocity (m/s)	simulation	0.0673	0.5333	0.0949	0.1413
	experiment	0.02–0.12 [65]	0.3–0.8 [81]	0.02–0.1 [82]	0.1–0.15
Maximum upstroke velocity (ms^{-1})	Simulation	0.124	1.583	0.1578	0.3755
	experiment	0.075–0.16 [83–88]	1.5±0.5 [89]	0.164 [39]	0.376 [39]
Action potential duration (ms)	Simulation	185	75.05	93.7	118.07
	experiment	107–151 [88,90,91]	77±5 [89]	97.2 [39]	117.5 [39]
Refractory period (ms)	Simulation	283	82	91	154
	experiment	166±30 [92]	68±11 [92] 81±5 [39]	91±10 [93] 91±12 [39] 100±9 [94]	–

The maximum upstroke velocity is expressed as $\frac{du}{dt}$, where u is the excitation variable and t is time. For the experimental data, $\frac{du}{dt} = \frac{dV_m/dt}{APA}$, where V_m is the membrane potential and APA is action potential amplitude.

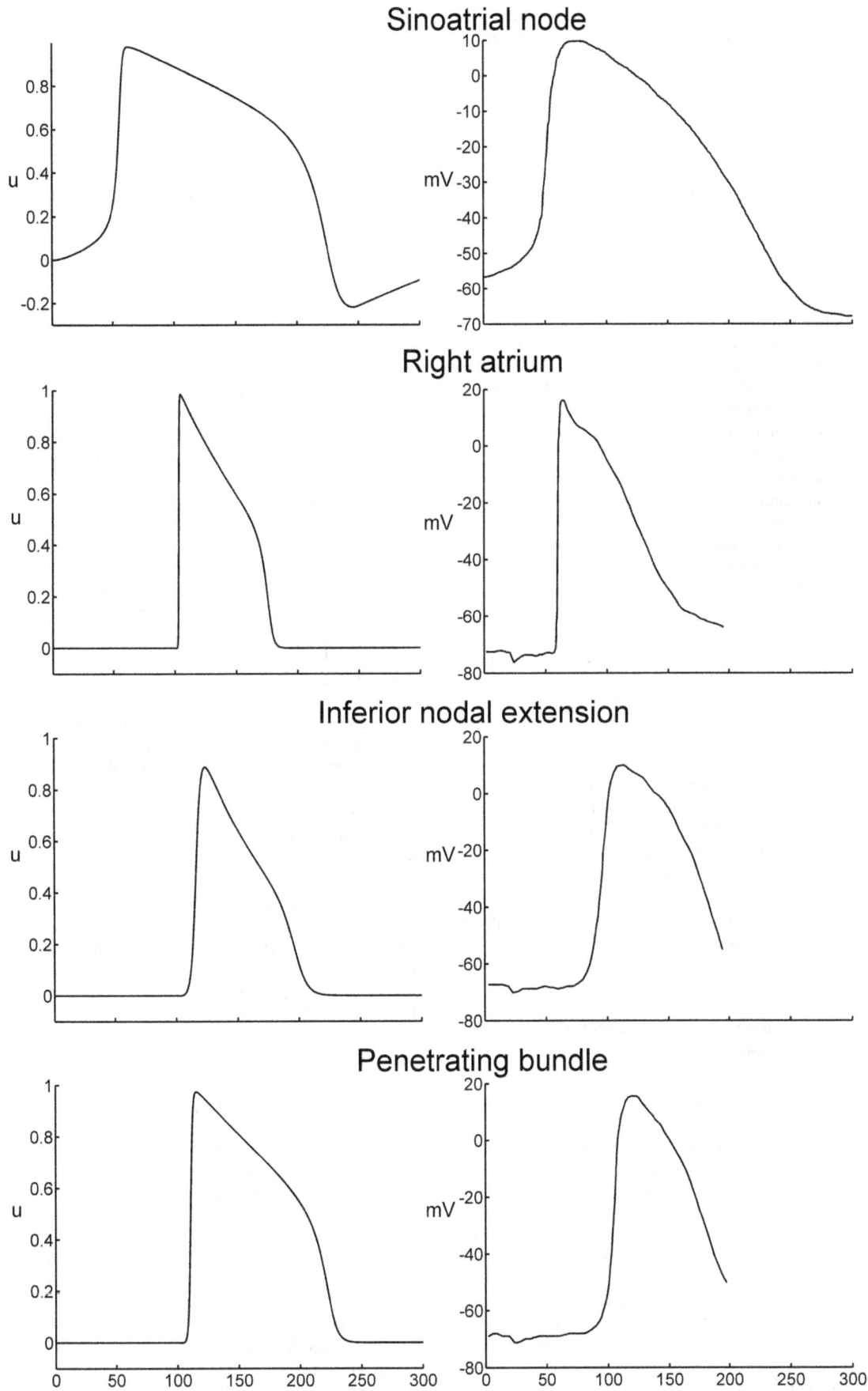

Sinoatrial node

Right atrium

Inferior nodal extension

Penetrating bundle

Figure 3. Comparison of action potential waveforms in the SAN, right atrium, inferior nodal extension and penetrating bundle in simulations (left) and experiment (right). Experimental recordings from Kodama et al. [95] (SAN) and de Carvalho and de Almeida [96].

$$\boldsymbol{D} = D_t \boldsymbol{I}_3 + (D_l - D_t) \begin{bmatrix} l \\ m \\ n \end{bmatrix} \begin{bmatrix} l & m & n \end{bmatrix} \qquad (8)$$

where $\boldsymbol{I_3}$ is the identity matrix. The diffusion anisotropy ratio was defined as 10 (D_l/D_t). This yields a $\sim$3.2 conduction velocity anisotropy ratio since conduction velocity is proportional to the square root of the diffusion [68].

Cellular automaton model. In the cellular automaton model, each node can be in one of three states: resting, excited or refractory. In the model, each node i has a variable (u_i), which signifies node state. When the node state is resting, u_i is set to 0. Once a node is excited, the node state is changed to 1. After that the node state is gradually decreased from 1 to 0. The speed of decrease determines the refractory period. The 'action potential' in the cellular automaton model is, therefore, characterised by the time at which the node is excited and at which it returns to the resting state, and the shape of the action potential can be considered triangular (Figure 4A). In the simulation program, if a node is in the resting state, the program checks at every time step whether one of its neighbours j is in the excited state. If so, an inner variable (e_i) called the excitation counter (corresponding to ionic current from each excited neighbouring myocyte) is increased at each time step. If the excitation counter exceeds a predefined threshold $(\theta \le \sum_j e_j)$, the node switches to the excited state $(u_i = 1)$. In the excited state, a node can excite its neighbours for predefined time steps (E_i) and then switches to the refractory state, where it again stays for a constant number of time steps (R_i). At the end of the refractory state, the node switches back into the resting state $(u_i = 0)$. Figure 4B shows a flow-chart of the program. Changes in conduction velocity and refractory period in different tissues (shown in Table 3) were introduced as discussed by Li et al. [12].

All simulations were carried out on a high-performance computing cluster which has 10 quad-processors nodes.

Results

Conduction of the action potential from the SAN to the AVN during sinus rhythm

The conduction of the action potential through the right atrium during sinus rhythm was simulated using the 3D anatomically-detailed right atrium model, together with a set of Rogers modified FitzHugh-Nagumo models. Figure 5 shows the activation sequence of the right atrium during sinus rhythm. The action potential was generated spontaneously in the centre of the SAN at 0 ms (Figure 5A, B). It spread preferentially in an oblique cranial direction (as a result of the orientation of nodal myocytes) and reached the crista terminalis first at $\sim$15 ms and then spread in a radial fashion to the rest of the right atrium (Figure 5A, B). It had to propagate around the block zone to reach the interatrial septum at $\sim$35 ms (Figure 5A, B). In the model, the action potential reached the rest of the right atrium in $\sim$50 ms (Figure 5A, B). Propagation from the SAN to the AVN is shown in Figure 6A, B: the action potential rapidly spread down the crista terminalis (Figure 6A) and it entered the AVN at the inferior nodal extension

$\sim$40 ms after it first entered the crista terminalis (Figure 6B) and $\sim$50 ms after its initiation in the SAN (Figure 5C). Meanwhile, the action potential also spread up the crista terminalis (Figure 6A) and down the interatrial septum and it entered the AVN via the compact node at the junction of the inferior nodal extension with the penetrating bundle again $\sim$40 ms after it first entered the crista terminalis (Figure 6B) and $\sim$50 ms after its initiation in the SAN (Figure 5C). This suggests that there are two principal pathways from the SAN to the AVN: one via the crista terminalis and the second via the interatrial septum. Although the action potential arrived at the AVN via both pathways at approximately the same time, the action potential arriving via the crista terminalis entered the atrioventricular conduction pathway at an upstream site, whereas the action potential arriving via the interatrial septum entered at a downstream site. Once the action potential from the crista terminalis had entered the AVN, it then began propagating along the inferior nodal extension towards the penetrating bundle (Figure 5D). Once the action potential from the interatrial septum had entered the AVN, the action potential propagated antero-gradely along the penetrating bundle (Figure 5D). However, it also propagated retrogradely along the inferior nodal extension (Figure 5D) and finally collided with the action potential coming from the opposite direction (Figure 5D). Figure 5E is a summary of the activation sequence from the SAN to the AVN. The simulation suggests that the most important pathway for the action potential from the SAN to the AVN is the interatrial septum; the pathway from the SAN to the AVN via the crista terminalis is secondary. The action potential propagated anterogradely along the penetrating bundle and it reached the bundle of His at $\sim$120 ms after its initiation in the SAN (Figure 5D).

Nodal activity during atrial fibrillation

In the model, an $S1$–$S2$ protocol was used to simulate an atrial fibrillation-like arrhythmia. The $S1$ 'stimulus' was a normal sinus rhythm beat initiated in the centre of SAN (Figure 7A; 39 ms). The activation time was counted from starting the simulation. The $S2$ stimulus was a premature planar stimulation applied to the superior vena cava (Figure 7B; 159 ms). Three reentrant circuits were observed (Movie S1, S2 and S3). The first reentrant circuit was located on the SVC and was a sustained reentrant circuit (Figure 7C; top). The second reentrant circuit was located on the IVC; it started at 495 ms and it did not stop by the end of the simulation at 1500 ms (Figure 7C; bottom). The third reentrant circuit was located on the atrial free wall and started at 780 ms and stopped at 1020 ms (Figure 7D). Figure S2 shows a set of snapshots of the action potential distribution on the epicardial surface during the atrial reentrant arrhythmia. Figure S3 shows a set of snapshots of the action potential distribution on the endocardial surface during the atrial reentrant arrhythmia.

Figure 7E shows the predicted behaviour of the SAN during atrial fibrillation. It shows action potentials recorded at different sites along a line perpendicular to the crista terminalis through the SAN: atrial muscle (e.g. site 1), SAN periphery (e.g. site 10), SAN centre (e.g. site 15), block zone (sites 16 and 17) and interatrial septum (sites 18 and 19). There is a high frequency of fibrillatory action potentials in the atrial muscle ($\sim$14 Hz; e.g. site 1), chaotic activity in the periphery of the SAN (site 10) and a slow frequency of the action potentials in the centre of the SAN ($\sim$6 Hz; e.g. site 15) as a result of alternating 2:1 and 3:1 SAN entrance block

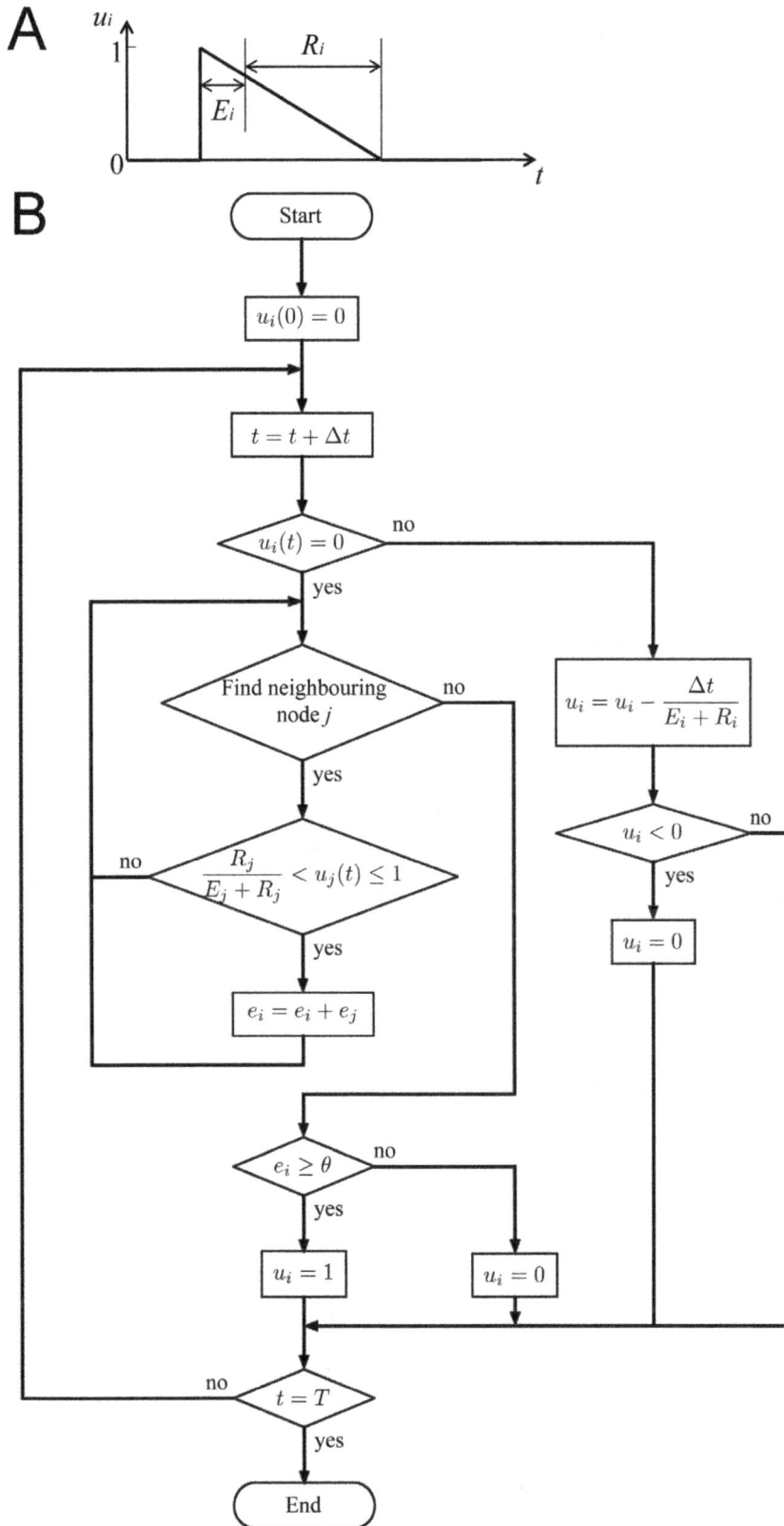

Figure 4. Cellular automaton model. A, time course of state (*u*) of node *i* in the cellular automaton model. If node *i* is excited the node state u_i is changed from 0 (resting) to 1 (excited). u_i then declines back to 0. B, program flow-chart of the cellular automaton model. E_i, the excited period; R_i, the refractory period. *t*, time; Δt, the time increment; *T*, the end time of simulation; e_i, the excitation counter; θ, the threshold.

Table 3. Measurements of conduction velocity and refractory period of atrial muscle and AVN from the cellular automaton model and experiment.

		Atrial muscle	Inferior nodal extension	Transitional zone	Penetrating bundle
Conduction velocity (m/s)	simulation	0.27–0.55	0.05–0.114	0.154	0.104
	experiment	0.3–0.8 [81]	0.02–0.1 [82]	0.35±0.17 [70]	0.1–0.15
Refractory period (ms)	simulation	81	94	134	154
	experiment	68±11 [92] 81±5 [39]	91±10 [93] 91±12 [39] 100±9 [94]	127±9 [39] 141±15 [93]	–

(compare action potentials in and around the periphery of the SAN at sites 9, 10 and 11). The model predicts that the SAN is protected against the high rate of fibrillatory action potentials and is not overdriven - this behaviour is due to the long refractory period of the SAN (Table 2).

Figure 8 shows the predicted behaviour of the AVN during atrial fibrillation. Figure 8A–E shows an internal view of the right atrium and atrial action potential propagation during atrial fibrillation. Action potential propagation during normal sinus rhythm (S1) is shown in Figure 8A. Figure 8B–E shows action potential propagation at different time points of the atrial

fibrillation. During atrial fibrillation, the action potential entered the AVN at different times through both pathways (fast and slow). Some reentrant action potentials reached the fast pathway and the compact node from the roof bundle and the interatrial septum (Figure 8B, D), whereas others reached the fast pathway from the area of inferior vena cava and coronary sinus (Figure 8C, E). Some reentrant action potentials were blocked (dashed lines in Figure 8B, D), because of the long refractory period of the penetrating bundle (Table 2). Figure 8F shows action potentials recorded at the atrioventricular junction axis: atrial muscle (sites 1–7), inferior nodal extension (sites 8–14) and penetrating bundle

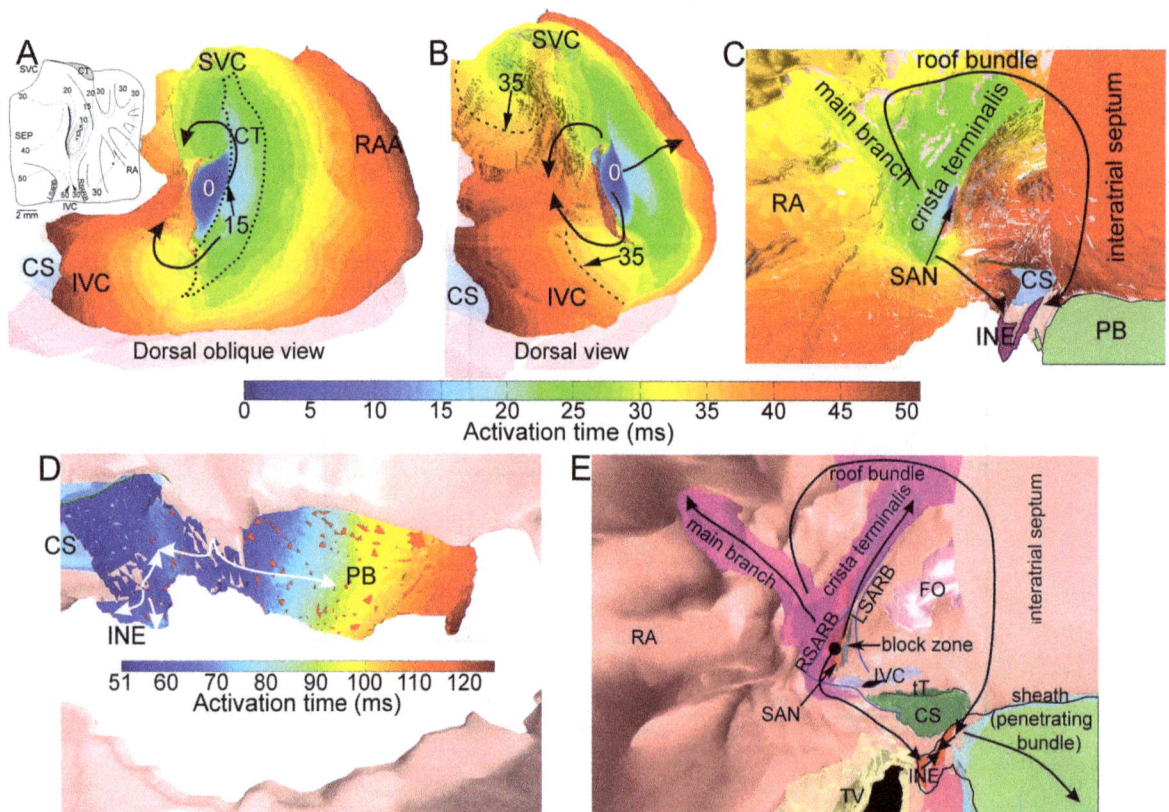

Figure 5. The sequence of right atrial activation during normal sinus rhythm in the 3D model of the rabbit right atrium. A–E, external (A, dorsal oblique view and B, dorsal view) and internal (C–E) views of the model. In A, the crista terminalis is outlined by a dotted line. In B, the dashed line is an example isochrone at 35 ms. In A to D, the activation sequence is shown by a colour scale and the arrows show the direction of action potential conduction. In E, different segmented structures are shown in different colours and the arrows summarise action potential conduction from the SAN to the AVN. CS, coronary sinus; INE, inferior nodal extension; IVC, inferior vena cava; FO, fossa ovalis; LSARB, left sinoatrial ring bundle; PB, penetrating bundle; RA, right atrium; RAA, right atrial appendage; RSARB, right sinoatrial ring bundle; SVC, superior vena cava; TV, tricuspid valve.

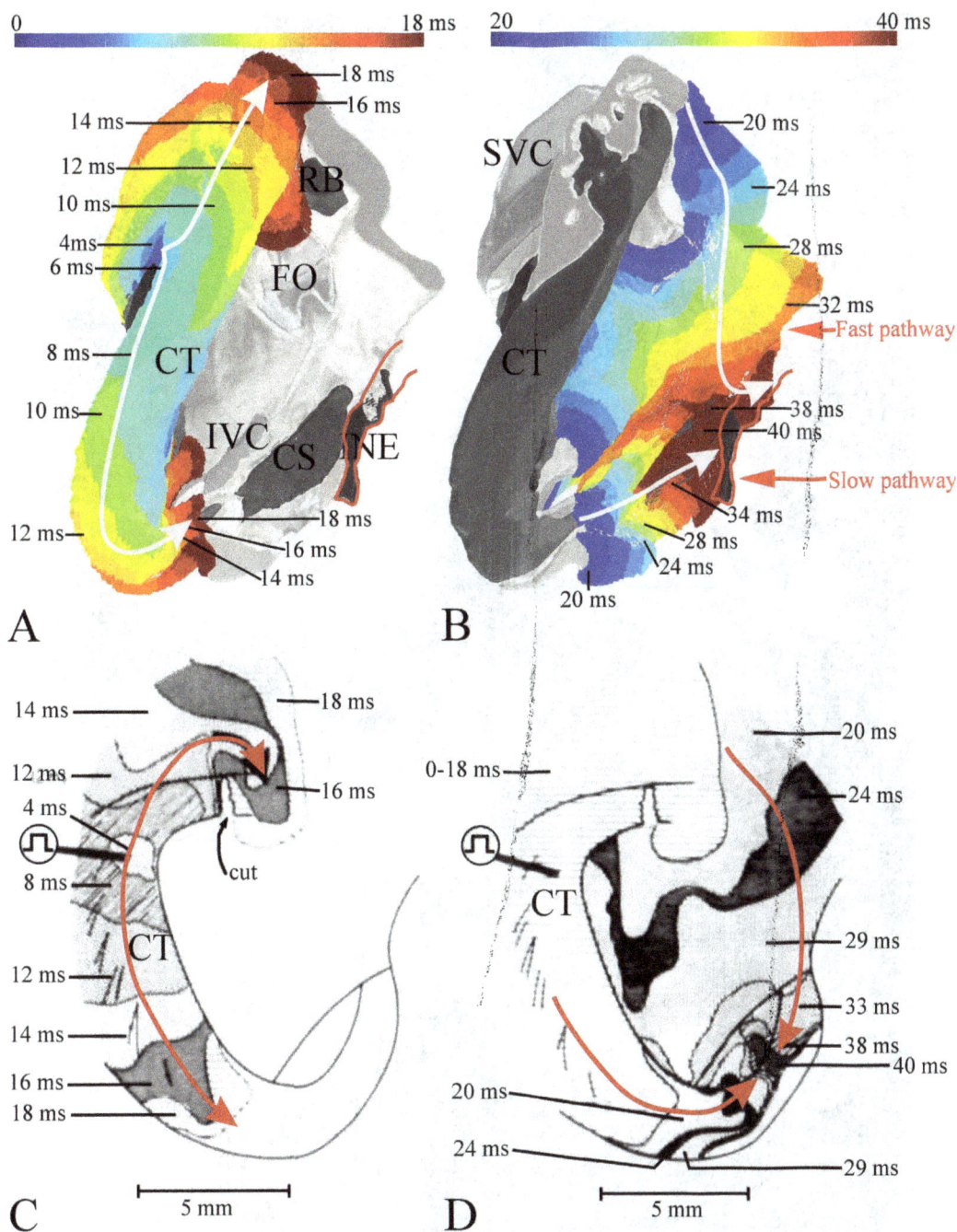

Figure 6. Action potential conduction from the SAN to the AVN. A and B, simulation of action potential conduction from the SAN to the AVN in the model of the right atrium during sinus rhythm (A, early times; B, later times). Internal right view of the model shown. Anatomical structures are shown in grey scale. The activation sequence is shown by a colour scale and the arrows show the direction of action potential conduction. Activation times are relative to the arrival of the action potential at the crista terminalis from the SAN. C and D, equivalent experimental data for the rabbit right atrium from Spach et al. [72]. In the experiment, the crista terminalis was stimulated close to the site where the action potential is expected to arrive first from the SAN. CN, compact node; CS, coronary sinus; CT, crista terminalis; FO, fossa ovalis; INE, inferior nodal extension; IVC, inferior vena cava; PB, penetrating bundle; RB, roof bundle; SVC, superior vena cava.

(sites 15–21). It shows the high frequency (~14 Hz) fibrillatory action potentials in the atrial muscle (sites 1–7), chaotic activity in some transitional regions of the AVN (e.g. site 15) and a low frequency (~5 Hz) of action potentials in the distal penetrating bundle (site 16), as the result of ~3:1 Wenckebach block (compare recordings at sites 15 and 16). The Wenckebach block is the result

of the long refractory period of the AVN (Table 2). In summary, the simulation shows that the high frequency fibrillatory activity is filtered by the AVN; this is important, because it prevents the ventricles from being paced too fast.

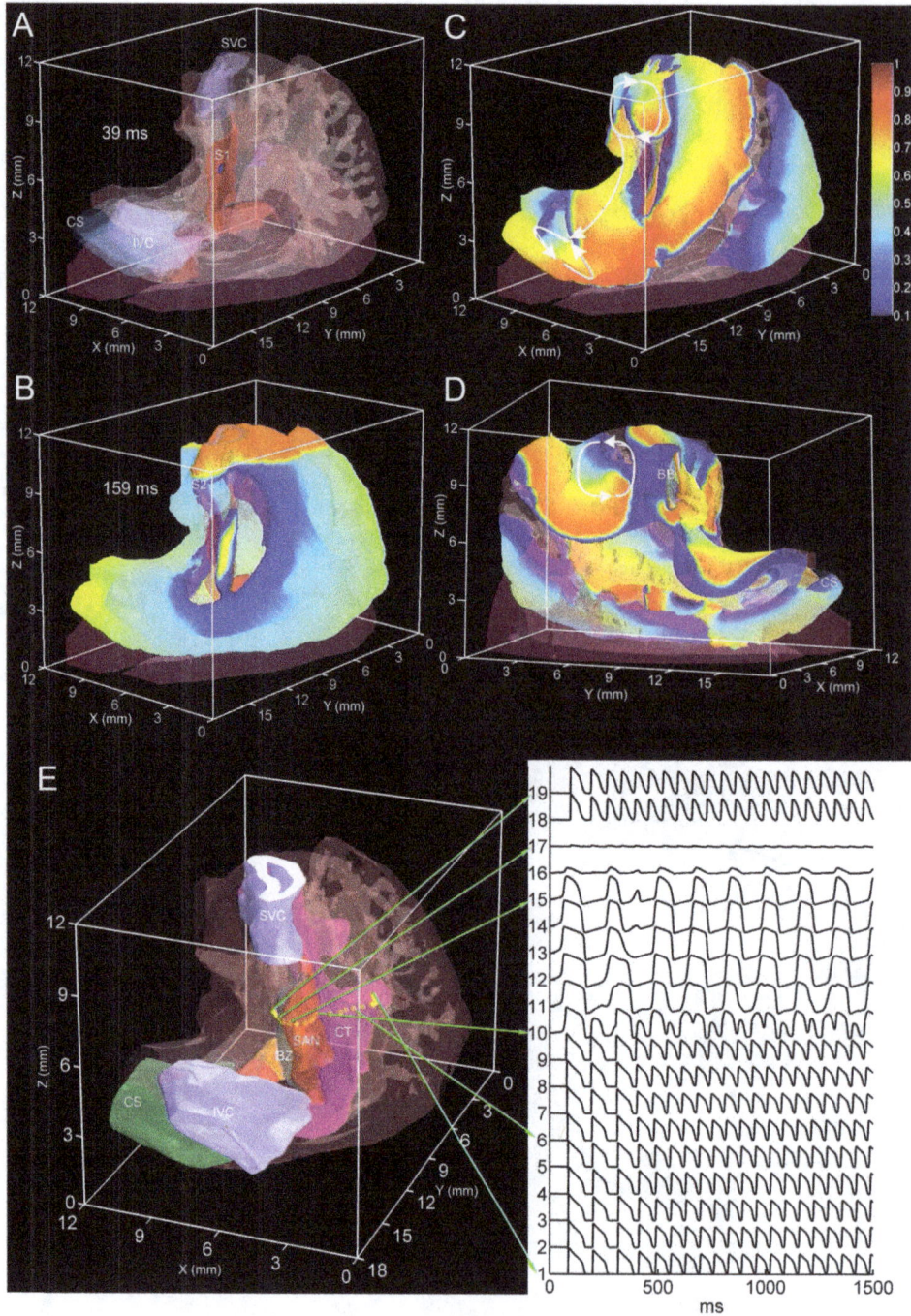

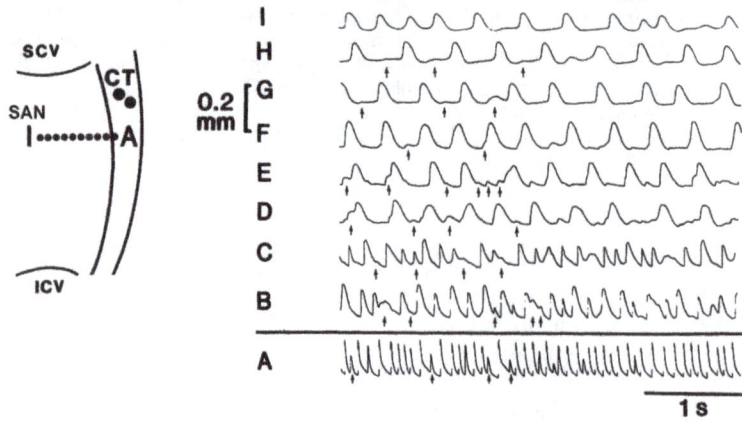

Figure 7. Behaviour of the SAN during atrial fibrillation. Panels A–E show external views (A–C and E, dorsal oblique view; D, ventral oblique view) of the model of the right atrium with transparent atrial muscle and different segmented structures shown in different colours. A–D, snapshots of the action potential distribution on the epicardial surface on initiation of an *S1* stimulus (A), on initiation of an *S2* stimulus, and at two times points after the induction of atrial fibrillation (C and D). The reentry loops are highlighted by arrows. E, right atrium model showing the location of the recording sites of the action potentials shown on the right. The sites lie along a line perpendicular to the crista terminalis through the SAN. Inset, experimental data showing the behaviour of the rabbit SAN during atrial fibrillation. Left, schematic diagram of the preparation showing the location of the recording sites of the action potentials on the right. The sites lie along a line perpendicular to the crista terminalis through the SAN. From Kirchhof et al. [75]. BB, bachmann bundle; BZ, block zone; CS, coronary sinus; CT, crista terminalis; IVC (or ICV), inferior vena cava; SVC (or SCV), superior vena cava.

Simulation of AVN reentry and a ventricular echo beat generated by premature ventricular stimulation

A premature ventricular action potential can elicit a ventricular echo beat as a result of retrograde conduction through the AVN followed by AVN reentry and anterograde conduction through the AVN [69]. This was investigated using the 3D anatomically-detailed right atrium model together with the cellular automaton model of the action potential (less computationally intensive than the Fitzhugh-Nagumo model). AVN reentry is dependent on the fast pathway (a transitional zone contacting the compact node) and the slow pathway (inferior nodal extension) into the AVN having different refractory periods; the refractory period of the fast pathway is longer than that of the slow pathway (Table 3) [39,70]. The model of the right atrium (Figure 2) does not have a transitional zone, because it was not detectable in the MR images. Therefore, a transitional zone (shown in green in Figure 9) was segmented based on our previous 3D rabbit AVN model [12]. To replicate ventricular activation, a *S1* stimulus was applied at the penetrating bundle of the AVN (Figure 9; 20 ms time point) and then a *S2* stimulus was applied with a short cycle length (Figure 9; 120 ms time point). The *S1* action potential was conducted retrogradely from the penetrating bundle to the atrium via both fast and slow pathways, i.e. by both the transitional zone and the inferior nodal extension (Figure 9; 70 ms time point). After applying the *S2* stimulus, conduction was blocked through the transitional zone (Figure 9; 200 ms time point), because of its long refractory period (Table 3). However, the refractory period of the inferior nodal extension is shorter (Table 3) and the action potential was conducted to the atrium via the inferior nodal extension (Figure 9; 230 ms time point). From the atrium, the action potential was then able to enter the transitional zone, because its refractory period had ended (Figure 9; 270 ms time point). From the transitional zone, the action potential was then conducted anterogradely to the penetrating bundle (Figure 9; 270 ms time point); in a heart, this would result in a ventricular echo beat.

Discussion

In this study, a 3D anatomically-detailed rabbit right atrium model including the two nodes was generated. Using this anatomical model together with mathematical caricature models of the action potential, we were able to replicate some known nodal electrophysiology: (i) the two routes of action potential conduction from the SAN into the AVN via the crista terminalis and interatrial septum; (ii) the dominance of the interatrial septum route over the crista terminalis route; (iii) little or no overdrive of the SAN during atrial fibrillation; (iv) reduction of action potential frequency by the AVN during atrial fibrillation; and (v) ventricular echo beats. The success of the simulations is a validation of the model. It also demonstrates that the phenomena can be explained on the basis of the elements incorporated in the model and in particular on anatomy, conduction velocities and refractory periods.

Comparison of model and experiments

Conduction of the action potential from the SAN to the AVN during sinus rhythm. In the simulation of sinus rhythm, the action potential from the SAN had to propagate around the block zone to reach the interatrial septum at ~35 ms (Figure 5A, B). A similar pattern is seen in experiments [60]. As an example, the inset in Figure 5A shows conduction from the leading pacemaker site in the rabbit SAN – the action potential spread preferentially in an oblique cranial direction, reaching the crista terminalis in 15–20 ms, and propagated around the block zone to reach the interatrial septum at 40–50 ms. In the model, the action potential reached the rest of the right atrium in ~50 ms (Figure 5A, B). There is little experimental data to compare this too. De Carvalho et al. [71] worked with a large right atrial preparation from the rabbit including both the SAN and AVN and the furthest reaches of the preparation were activated in 70–80 ms. The model suggests that there are two routes for the action potential from the SAN to the AVN: the crista terminalis and the interatrial septum (Figure 6A, B). This is consistent with experimental data from the rabbit from Spach et al. [72] shown in Figure 6C, D. In this experimental study, the crista terminalis was stimulated (at 0 ms) close to the leading pacemaker site in the SAN. As in the equivalent simulation (Figure 6A, B), the action potential rapidly spread down the crista terminalis and entered the AVN (inferior nodal extension) as well as up the crista terminalis and down the interatrial septum where it entered the AVN downstream of the inferior nodal extension. In the work of Spach et al. [72] the action potential entered the AVN at ~40 ms after stimulation of the crista terminalis (Figure 6C, D). In other work on the rabbit [71], the action potential entered the AVN at ~50 ms after its initiation in the sinus node. These timings are similar in the corresponding simulations (Figures 5C and 6A, B). Both in the human and animal models, it is well known that there are dual inputs into the AVN: the slow and fast pathways [73]. The slow pathway is the inferior nodal extension and the fast pathway is the transitional zone leading into the compact node [12]. The simulations show that the crista terminalis connects to the slow pathway, i.e. the inferior nodal extension, whereas the interatrial septum connects to the fast pathway, i.e. the region of the transitional zone and compact node (Figure 5E). The simulations suggest that the most important pathway for the action potential from the SAN to the AVN is the interatrial septum followed by the fast pathway; this is because the action potential enters the atrioventricular conduction axis at a more downstream site via this route (shortening the conduction time to the His bundle). This is consistent with what is known: both in the human and animal models, it is well known that the fast pathway is the primary pathway for atrioventricular conduction [73]. The slow pathway only operates if the fast pathway fails (for example, during premature stimulation when the fast pathway fails because of its long refractory period [39]). In the model, the action potential propagated anterogradely along the penetrating bundle and reached the bundle of His at ~120 ms (Figure 5D). This is less than an experimental value of 140 ms for the rabbit heart from De

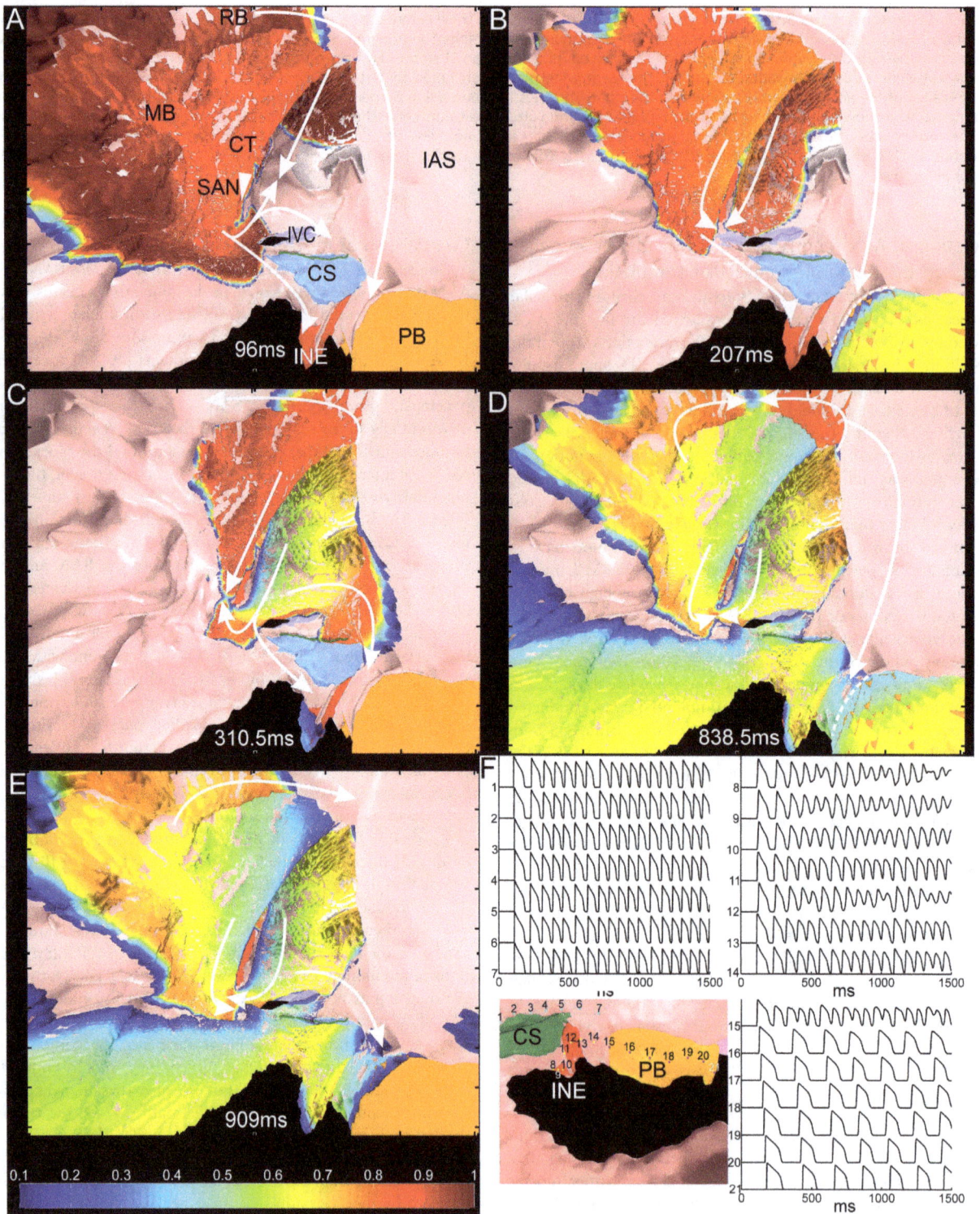

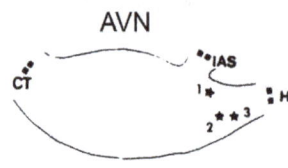

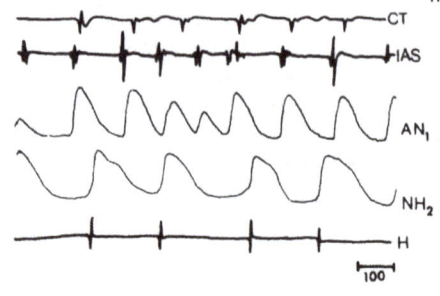

Figure 8. Behaviour of the AVN during atrial fibrillation. Panels A–E show a ventral internal view of the model of the right atrium with different segmented structures shown in different colours. A–E, snapshots of the action potential distribution on the endocardial surface during normal sinus rhythm (A) and at different times points after the induction of atrial fibrillation (B–E). The white arrows highlight wave propagation. The white dotted line in B and D indicates a line of conduction block. F, right atrium model showing the location of the recording sites of the action potentials shown above and on the right. Inset, experimental data showing the behaviour of the rabbit AVN during atrial fibrillation. Left, schematic diagram of the preparation showing the location of the recording sites of the electrograms and action potentials on the right. From Mazgalev et al. [80]. AN, atrionodal cell; CS, coronary sinus; CT, crista terminalis; IAS, interatrial septum; INE, inferior nodal extension; IVC, inferior vena cava; H, His bundle; MB, main branch; NH, nodal-His cell; PB, penetrating bundle; RB, roof bundle.

Carvalho et al. [71]. However, the PR interval is the time from atrial depolarization to the first activation of the ventricular conduction system and in the rabbit is 62 ms (Boyett, unpublished data). If the time from initiation of the action potential in the SAN to the arrival of the action potential in the atria is 15 ms (Figure 5A), then the time from the initiation of the action potential in the SAN to the first activation of the ventricular conduction system is ~80 ms. In summary, there is good agreement between model and experiment in terms of conduction of the action potential from the SAN to the AVN. The success of the simulations indicates that the principal factor determining the pattern of conduction from the SAN to the AVN is anatomy, in particular the arrangement of fast conducting atrial muscle bundles with longitudinally arranged myocytes, although the slow

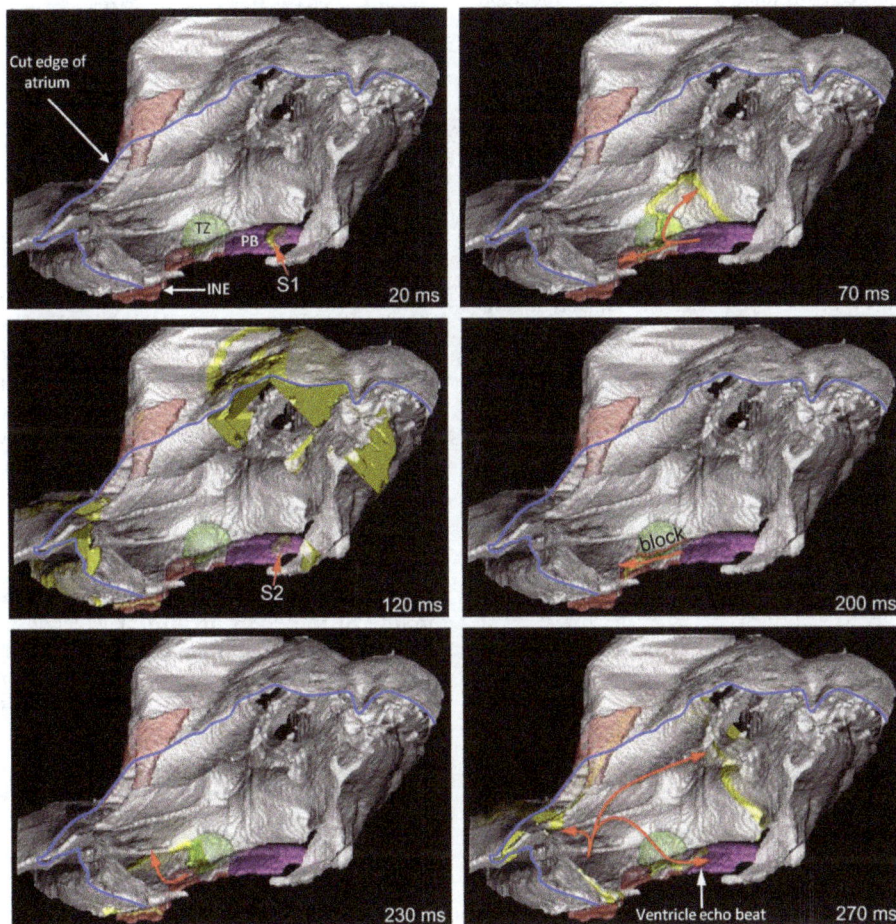

Figure 9. Simulation of a ventricular echo beat. A right view of the model of the right atrium is shown with one face of the right atrium removed (the blue line shows the cut edge of the right atrium). Different segmented structures are shown in different colours. The panels show snapshots of activation after S1–S2 stimulation of the penetrating bundle. The thick yellow lines show the advancing wavefront of activation. The arrows show the direction of action potential conduction. 20 ms, retrograde conduction of the action potential along the penetrating bundle following S1 stimulation. 70 ms, retrograde conduction of the action potential along the fast (transitional zone; green) and slow (inferior nodal extension, red) pathways out of the AVN following S1 stimulation. 120 ms, retrograde conduction of the action potential along the penetrating bundle following S2 stimulation. Note the action potential following S1 stimulation has reached the outer parts of the right atrium. 200 ms, block of conduction along the fast pathway (line of block, red dotted line) and retrograde conduction along the slow pathway following S2 stimulation. 230 ms, retrograde conduction out of the slow pathway and into the right atrium following S2 stimulation. 270 ms, retrograde conduction throughout the right atrium and reentry into the AVN – the action potential conducted anterogradely through the transitional zone to the penetrating bundle. It is this action potential that would result in a ventricular echo beat. INE, inferior nodal extension; PB, penetrating bundle; TZ, transitional zone.

conduction velocity of the inferior nodal extension is another contributory factor (working against the crista terminalis-slow pathway route).

From simulations, conduction velocities in the SAN were measured as 0.028 m/s in the transverse direction and 0.089 m/s in the longitudinal direction; conduction velocities in the crista terminalis were measured as 0.183 m/s in the transverse direction and 0.417 m/s in the longitudinal direction. The conduction velocity anisotropy ratio in the SAN (~3.16) is within the range of experimental results (1.9~4.1) from rabbit SAN preparations [65]. The conduction velocity anisotropy ratio in the crista terminalis (~2.28) is similar to that measured experimentally in rabbit crista terminalis preparations (1.7~4.1 depending on age [74]).

Nodal activity during atrial fibrillation. The rabbit heart has been widely used in the study of atrial fibrillation [75–78]. In the simulation of atrial fibrillation (Figure 7), the fibrillation frequency was 14 Hz in the atrial muscle. This is similar to that measured in the rabbit experimentally under baseline conditions (11.6 Hz [75]; 5.9–6.5 Hz [78]) and following vagal stimulation (12–13 Hz [78]). In the model, the arrhythmia was maintained by reentry located at the SVC and IVC. This is consistent with observations from patients with paroxysmal atrial fibrillation [79]. Kirchhof et al. [75] studied the SAN during atrial fibrillation in the rabbit and an example from their work is shown in the inset at the bottom of Figure 7; it shows action potentials recorded at different sites from the atrial muscle (site A), SAN periphery (e.g. site B) and SAN centre (e.g. site I). The behaviour is qualitatively similar to that predicted by the model: there is a high frequency of fibrillatory action potentials in the atrial muscle (site A), chaotic activity in the periphery of the SAN (e.g. site B) and a slow frequency of the action potentials in the centre of the SAN (e.g. site I) as a result of high degree (5:1) SAN entrance block (compare action potentials at sites A–D). Mazgalev et al. [80] studied the AVN during atrial fibrillation in the rabbit and an example from their work is shown in the inset at the bottom of Figure 8; it shows extracellular electrograms recorded from the crista terminalis (CT), interatrial septum (IAS) and His bundle (H) as well as intracellular action potentials recorded at upstream (site 1) and downstream (site 2) sites in the atrioventricular conduction axis. Again the behaviour is qualitatively similar to that predicted by the model: there is a high frequency of fibrillatory action potentials in the atrial muscle (CT and IAS), chaotic activity in a transitional region (site 1) and a slow frequency of action potentials downstream of this, including in the His bundle (corresponding to ~2:1 Wenckebach block). In summary, there is good agreement between model and experiment in terms of the behaviour of the nodes during atrial fibrillation. The success of the simulations can be attributed to the long refractory period of the nodal tissues.

AVN reentry and ventricular echo beats. A premature ventricular action potential can elicit a ventricular echo beat as a result of AVN reentry [69] and the model was able to successfully simulate this (Figure 9).

Limitations of the study

It was not possible to obtain fibre orientation from the MR images and only three major muscle bundles (crista terminalis, main branch and roof bundle) were segmented in order to introduce the well known anisotropic property of the bundles. The SAN was also assumed to be anisotropic in order to replicate the known anisotropic conduction in the SAN, whereas the rest of the right atrium was assumed to be isotropic. Although the success of the simulations demonstrates that the level of detail in the model is sufficient to explain the various behaviours, incorporation of fibre orientation throughout the right atrium model is expected to

improve the accuracy of simulations. Mathematical caricature models of the action potential were used to make computation more tractable. Once again, although the success of the simulations demonstrates that the level of detail in the models is sufficient to explain the various behaviours, use of biophysically-detailed models of the action potential is expected to improve the accuracy of simulations.

Supporting Information

Figure S1 3D segmentation. A, isotropic 3D MR images; B, converted 3D binary images; C, the 3D model before segmentation; D, the 3D model after segmentation. CT, crista terminalis; RA, right atrium; RV, right ventricle; SAN, sinoatrial node; SVC, superior vena cava; TV, tricuspid valve.

Figure S2 A set of snapshots of the action potential during the atrial reentrant arrhythmia viewed from the outside of the right atrium. The normal sinus rhythm beat (S1, 'stimulus') was initiated in the SAN at 39 ms. The action potential broke out from the SAN to the atrium at the crista terminalis (75 ms). In the opposite direction, the action potential was blocked in the block zone and propagated around the block zone to reach the interatrial septum at 90~117 ms. The S2 stimulus at the superior vena cava was delivered at 159 ms. The first reentry wave started on the superior vena cava near the top of the SAN (175.5 ms). The action potential propagated around the SAN (202.5 ms and 211.5 ms) due to the SAN's long refractory period. The second reentry wave started at a similar position and another SAN wave was initiated in the low part of the SAN (247.5 ms). These two waves moved towards each other and finally merged (267~301.5 ms). Then the third reentry wave started, while the wave in the SAN had not faded away (367 ms). Similar as the first reentry wave, the third wave did not stimulate the SAN due to the long refractory period the SAN.

Figure S3 A set of snapshots of the action potential during the atrial reentrant arrhythmia viewed from inside of the right atrium. The action potential propagated faster along the crista terminalis and the main branch than in the rest of the atrial wall (90 ms). The action potential propagated around the block zone to reach the interatrial septum. It then reached the compact node (fast pathway) and inferior nodal extension (slow pathway) (108 ms~120 ms) at same time. The first reentry wave propagated around the SAN to the interatrial septum due to the SAN's long refractory period (202.5 ms, 207 ms). The wave front reached the compact node (fast pathway) (220 ms) first. It then reached the inferior nodal extension (slow pathway) by passing below the coronary sinus (238.5 ms). The first reentrant wave failed to propagate along the penetrating bundle (277 ms, 300 ms) due to the long refractory period of the penetrating bundle. The second reentrant wave propagated to the interatrial septum earlier than the right atrial free wall (300 ms, 315 ms). The wave front reached the penetrating bundle earlier than the inferior nodal extension and propagated successfully along the penetrating bundle (375 ms).

Movie S1 Dorsal right view of first reentrant circuit located on the SVC and second reentrant circuit located on the IVC.

Movie S2 Dorsal left view of first reentrant circuit located on the SVC and second reentrant circuit located on the IVC.

Movie S3 Left oblique view of third reentrant circuit located on the atrial free wall.

Model S1 MATLAB workspace file (3D anatomically-detailed model). Resolution is 60 μm×60 μm×60 μm. The digits in the model signify different tissues: 1 – Outer fatty and connective tissue. 2 – Aortic valve. 3 – Tricuspid valve. 4 – Bicuspid (mitral) valve. 5 – Atrial muscle. 6 – Ventricular muscle. 7 – Coronary sinus. 8 – Fossa ovalis. 9 – Superior vena cava. 10 – Inferior vena cava. 11 – Inferior nodal extension. 12 – Central fibres body. 13 – Sinoatrial node. 14 – Crista terminalis. 15 – Roof bundle. 16 – Main brunch. 17 – Penetrating bundle. 18 – Block zone.

Model S2 MATLAB workspace file (3D array for simulations). Resolution is 60 μm×60 μm×60 μm. The digits

in the model (Array) signify different tissues: 1 – Atrial wall (isotropic). 2 – Inferior nodal extension (AVN, isotropic). 3 – Sinoatrial node (SAN, anisotropic). 4 – Crista terminalis (anisotropic). 5 – Roof bundle (anisotropic). 6 – Main brunch (anisotropic). 7 – Block zone (passive atrial tissue). 8 – Penetrating bundle (AVN, isotropic). Fibre orientations: (Alpha, Beta, Gamma). (2, 0, 0) in (Alpha, Beta, Gamma) indicate isotropic tissue.

Acknowledgments

We would like to acknowledge the assistance and insight of Dr. Mitsuru Yamamoto in the early part of this study.

Author Contributions

Conceived and designed the experiments: JL SI JES HZ HD MRB. Performed the experiments: JL SI JES HD. Analyzed the data: JL SI JES MRB. Contributed reagents/materials/analysis tools: JL SI JES HD MRB. Wrote the paper: JL SI MRB.

References

1. David MH (2000) A computer model of normal conduction in the human atria. Circ Res 87: e25–e36.
2. Bernus O, Verschelde H, Panfilov AV (2003) Reentry in an anatomical model of the human ventricles. Int J Bifurcation Chaos 13: 3693–3702.
3. Eifler WJ, Macchi E, Ritsema van Eck HJ, Horacek BM, Rautaharju PM (1981) Mechanism of generation of body surface electrocardiographic P-waves in normal, middle, and lower sinus rhythms. Circ Res 48: 168–182.
4. Lorange M, Gulrajani RM (1993) A computer heart model incorporating anisotropic propagation: I. Model construction and simulation of normal activation. J Electrocardiol 26: 245–261.
5. Sachse FB, Werner CD, Stenroos MH, Schulte RF, Zerfass P, et al. (2000) Modeling the anatomy of the human heart using the cryosection images of the visible female dataset. Proceedings of the Third Users Conference of the National Library of Medicine's Visible Human Project.
6. Aslanidi OV, Colman MA, Stott J, Dobrzynski H, Boyett MR, et al. (2011) 3D virtual human atria: A computational platform for studying clinical atrial fibrillation. Prog Biophys Mol Biol 107: 156–168.
7. Chandler N, Aslanidi O, Buckley D, Inada S, Birchall S, et al. (2011) Computer three-dimensional anatomical reconstruction of the human sinus node and a novel paranodal area. Anat Rec 294: 970–979.
8. Seemann G, Höper C, Sachse F, Dössel O, Holden A, et al. (2006) Heterogeneous three-dimensional anatomical and electrophysiological model of human atria. Phil Trans R Soc A 364: 1465–1481.
9. Nielsen PM, LeGrice IJ, Smaill BH, Hunter PJ (1991) Mathematical model of geometry and fibrous structure of the heart. Am J Physiol Heart Circ Physiol 29: H1365–H1378.
10. Vetter FJ, McCulloch AD (1998) Three-dimensional analysis of regional cardiac function: a model of rabbit ventricular anatomy. Prog Biophys Mol Biol 69: 157–183.
11. Dobrzynski H, Li J, Tellez J, Greener ID, Nikolski VP, et al. (2005) Computer three-dimensional reconstruction of the sinoatrial node. Circulation 111: 846–854.
12. Li J, Greener ID, Inada S, Nikolski VP, Yamamoto M, et al. (2008) Computer three-dimensional reconstruction of the atrioventricular node. Circ Res 102: 975–985.
13. Stephenson RS, Boyett MR, Hart G, Nikolaidou T, Cai X, et al. (2012) Contrast enhanced micro-computed tomography resolves the 3-dimensional morphology of the cardiac conduction system in mammalian hearts. PLoS ONE 7: e35299.
14. Boyett MR, Li J, Inada S, Dobrzynski H, Schneider JE, et al. (2005) Imaging the heart: computer 3-dimensional anatomic models of the heart. J Electrocardiol 38: 113–120.
15. Courtemanche M, Ramirez RJ, Nattel S (1998) Ionic mechanisms underlying human atrial action potential properties: insights from a mathematical model. Am J Physiol Heart Circ Physiol 275: H301–H321.
16. Nygren A, Fiset C, Firek L, Clark JW, Lindblad DS, et al. (1998) Mathematical model of an adult human atrial cell: the role of K⁺ currents in repolarization. Circ Res 82: 63–81.
17. Priebe L, Beuckelmann DJ (1998) Simulation study of cellular electric properties in heart failure. Circ Res 82: 1206–1223.
18. Bernus O, Wilders R, Zemlin CW, Verschelde H, Panfilov AV (2002) A computationally efficient electrophysiological model of human ventricular cells. Am J Physiol Heart Circ Physiol 282: H2296–H2308.
19. ten Tusscher KHWJ, Panfilov AV (2006) Alternans and spiral breakup in a human ventricular tissue model. Am J Physiol Heart Circ Physiol 291: H1088–H1100.
20. Iyer V, Mazhari R, Winslow RL (2004) A computational model of the human left-ventricular epicardial myocyte. Biophys J 87: 1507–1525.
21. Fink M, Noble D, Virag L, Varro A, Giles WR (2008) Contributions of HERG current to repolarization of the human ventricular action potential. Prog Biophys Mol Biol 96: 357–376.
22. Grandi E, Pasqualini FS, Bers DM (2010) A novel computational model of the human ventricular action potential and Ca transient. J Mol Cell Cardiol 48: 112–121.
23. Ramirez RJ, Nattel S, Courtemanche M (2000) Mathematical analysis of canine atrial action potentials: rate, regional factors, and electrical remodeling. Am J Physiol Heart Circ Physiol 279: H1767–H1785.
24. Kneller J, Zou R, Vigmond EJ, Wang Z, Leon LJ, et al. (2002) Cholinergic atrial fibrillation in a computer model of a two-dimensional sheet of canine atrial cells with realistic ionic properties. Circ Res 90: 73e–787.
25. Winslow RL, Rice J, Jafri S, Marbàn E, O'Rourke B (1999) Mechanisms of altered excitation-contraction coupling in canine tachycardia-induced heart failure, II: model studies. Circ Res 84: 571–586.
26. Hund TJ, Rudy Y (2004) Rate dependence and regulation of action potential and calcium transient in a canine cardiac ventricular cell model. Circulation 110: 3168–3174.
27. Benson AP, Aslanidi OV, Zhang H, Holden AV (2008) The canine virtual ventricular wall: A platform for dissecting pharmacological effects on propagation and arrhythmogenesis. Prog Biophys Mol Biol 96: 187–208.
28. Decker KF, Heijman J, Silva JR, Hund TJ, Rudy Y (2009) Properties and ionic mechanisms of action potential adaptation, restitution, and accommodation in canine epicardium. Am J Physiol Heart Circ Physiol 296: H1017–H1026.
29. McAllister RE, Noble D, Tsien RW (1975) Reconstruction of the electrical activity of cardiac Purkinje fibres. J Physiol 251: 1–59.
30. DiFrancesco D, Noble D (1985) A model of cardiac electrical activity incorporating ionic pumps and concentration changes. Philos Trans R Soc Lond B Biol Sci 307: 353–398.
31. Yanagihara K, Noma A, Irisawa H (1980) Reconstruction of sino-atrial node pacemaker potential based on the voltage clamp experiments. Jpn J Physiol 30: 841–857.
32. Demir SS, Clark JW, Murphey CR, Giles WR (1994) A mathematical model of a rabbit sinoatrial node cell. Am J Physiol Cell Physiol 266: C832–C852.
33. Dokos S, Celler B, Lovell N (1996) Ion currents underlying sinoatrial node pacemaker activity: a new single cell mathematical model. J Theor Biol 181: 245–272.
34. Demir SS, Clark JW, Giles WR (1999) Parasympathetic modulation of sinoatrial node pacemaker activity in rabbit heart: a unifying model. Am J Physiol Heart Circ Physiol 276: H2221–H2244.
35. Kurata Y, Hisatome I, Imanishi S, Shibamoto T (2002) Dynamical description of sinoatrial node pacemaking: improved mathematical model for primary pacemaker cell. Am J Physiol Heart Circ Physiol 283: H2074–H2101.
36. Zhang H, Holden AV, Kodama I, Honjo H, Lei M, et al. (2000) Mathematical models of action potentials in the periphery and center of the rabbit sinoatrial node. Am J Physiol Heart Circ Physiol 279: H397–H421.

37. Oehmen CS, Giles WR, Demir SS (2002) Mathematical model of the rapidly activating delayed rectifier potassium current I_{Kr} in rabbit sinoatrial node. J Cardiovasc Electrophysiol 13: 1131–1140.

38. Wilders R, Jongsma HJ, van Ginneken AC (1991) Pacemaker activity of the rabbit sinoatrial node. A comparison of mathematical models. Biophys J 60: 1202–1216.

39. Inada S, Hancox JC, Zhang H, Boyett MR (2009) One-dimensional mathematical model of the atrioventricular node including atrio-nodal, nodal, and nodal-his cells. Biophys J 97: 2117–2127.

40. Aslanidi OV, Sleiman RN, Boyett MR, Hancox JC, Zhang H (2010) Ionic mechanisms for electrical heterogeneity between rabbit Purkinje fiber and ventricular cells. Biophys J 98: 2420–2431.

41. Hilgemann DW, Noble D (1987) Excitation-contraction coupling and extracellular calcium transients in rabbit atrium: reconstruction of basic cellular mechanisms. Proc Biol Sci 230: 163–205.

42. Lindblad DS, Murphey CR, Clark JW, Giles WR (1996) A model of the action potential and underlying membrane currents in a rabbit atrial cell. Am J Physiol Heart Circ Physiol 271: H1666–H1696.

43. Aslanidi OV, Boyett MR., Dobrzynski H, Li J, Zhang H (2009) Mechanisms of transition from normal to reentrant electrical activity in a model of rabbit atrial tissue: interaction of tissue heterogeneity and anisotropy. Biophys J 96: 798–817.

44. Shannon TR, Wang F, Puglisi J, Weber C, Bers DM (2004) A mathematical treatment of integrated Ca dynamics within the ventricular myocyte. Biophys J 87: 3351–3371.

45. Puglisi JL, Bers DM (2001) LabHEART: an interactive computer model of rabbit ventricular myocyte ion channels and Ca transport. Am J Physiol Cell Physiol 281: C2049–C2060.

46. Noble D, Kohl P, Noble P, Varghese A (1998) Improved guinea-pig ventricular cell model incorporating a diadic space, I_{Kr} and I_{Ks}, and length- and tension-dependent processes. Can J Cardiol: 123–134.

47. Beeler GW, Reuter H (1977) Reconstruction of the action potential of ventricular myocardial fibres. J Physiol 268: 177–210.

48. Luo CH, Rudy Y (1994) A dynamic model of the cardiac ventricular action potential. I. Simulations of ionic currents and concentration changes. Circ Res 74: 1071–1096.

49. Zeng J, Laurita KR, Rosenbaum DS, Rudy Y (1995) Two components of the delayed rectifier K^+ current in ventricular myocytes of the guinea pig type: theoretical formulation and their role in repolarization. Circ Res 77: 140–152.

50. Shaw RM, Rudy Y (1997) Electrophysiologic effects of acute myocardial ischemia: a theoretical study of altered cell excitability and action potential duration. Cardiovasc Res 35: 256–272.

51. Viswanathan PC, Shaw RM, Rudy Y (1999) Effects of I_{Kr} and I_{Ks} heterogeneity on action potential duration and its rate dependence: a simulation study. Circulation 99: 2466–2474.

52. Kharche S, Yu J, Lei M, Zhang H (2011) A mathematical model of action potentials of mouse sinoatrial node cells with molecular bases. Am J Physiol Heart Circ Physiol 301: H945–H963.

53. Bondarenko VE, Szigeti GP, Bett GCL, Kim SJ, Rasmusson RL (2004) Computer model of action potential of mouse ventricular myocytes. Am J Physiol Heart Circ Physiol 287: H1378–H1403.

54. Holden AV, Zhang H (1993) Modelling propagation and re-entry in anisotropic and smoothly heterogeneous cardiac tissue. J Chem Soc, Faraday Trans 89: 2833–2837.

55. Winslow RL, Varghese A, Noble D, Adlakha C, Hoythya A (1993) Generation and propagation of ectopic beats induced by spatially localized Na-K pump inhibition in atrial network models. Proc Biol Sci 254: 55–61.

56. FitzHugh R (1961) Impulses and physiological states in theoretical models of nerve membrane. Biophys J 1: 445–466.

57. Fenton F, Karma A (1998) Vortex dynamics in three-dimensional continuous myocardium with fiber rotation: Filament instability and fibrillation. Chaos: An Interdisciplinary Journal of Nonlinear Science 8: 20–47.

58. Li J, Schneider JE, Yamamoto M, Greener ID, Dobrzynski H, et al. (2005) A detailed 3D model of the rabbit right atrium including the sinoatrial node, atrioventricular node, surrounding blood vessels and valves. Computers in Cardiology 32: 603–606.

59. Li J, Dobrzynski H, Greener ID, Nikolski VP, Yamamoto M, et al. (2004) Development of 3-D anatomically-detailed mathematical models of the sinoatrial and atrioventricular nodes. Computers in Cardiology 31: 89–92.

60. Boyett MR, Honjo H, Kodama I (2000) The sinoatrial node, a heterogeneous pacemaker structure. Cardiovasc Res 47: 658–687.

61. Bleeker WK, Mackaay AJ, Masson-Pevet M, Bouman LN, Becker AE (1980) Functional and morphological organization of the rabbit sinus node. Circ Res 46: 11–22.

62. Coakley JB, King TS (1959) Cardiac muscle relations of the coronary sinus, the oblique vein of the left atrium and the left precaval vein in mammals. J Anat 93: 30–35.

63. Rogers JM, McCulloch AD (1994) A collocation-Galerkin finite element model of cardiac action potential propagation. IEEE Trans Biomed Eng 41: 743–757.

64. Li J, Inada S, Dobrzynski H, Zhang H, Boyett MR (2009) A modified FitzHugh-Nagumo model that allows control of action potential duration and refractory period. Computers in Cardiology 36: 65–68.

65. Fedorov VV, Hucker WJ, Dobrzynski H, Rosenshtraukh LV, Efimov IR (2006) Postganglionic nerve stimulation induces temporal inhibition of excitability in rabbit sinoatrial node. Am J Physiol Heart Circ Physiol 291: H612–H623.

66. Yamamoto M, Honjo H, Niwa R, Kodama I (1998) Low-frequency extracellular potentials recorded from the sinoatrial node. Cardiovasc Res 39: 360–372.

67. Boyett MR, Honjo H, Yamamoto M, Nikmaram MR, Niwa R, et al. (1999) Downward gradient in action potential duration along conduction path in and around the sinoatrial node. Am J Physiol Heart Circ Physiol 276: H686–H698.

68. Clayton RH (2009) Influence of cardiac tissue anisotropy on re-entrant activation in computational models of ventricular fibrillation. Physica D: Nonlinear Phenomena 238: 951–961.

69. Toshida N, Hirao K, Yamamoto N, Tanaka M, Suzuki F, et al. (2001) Ventricular echo beats and retrograde atrioventricular nodal exits in the dog heart: multiplicity in their electrophysiologic and anatomic characteristics. J Cardiovasc Electrophysiol 12: 1256–1264.

70. Nikolski VP, Jones SA, Lancaster MK, Boyett MR, Efimov IR (2003) Cx43 and dual-pathway electrophysiology of the atrioventricular node and atrioventricular nodal reentry. Circ Res 92: 469–475.

71. de Carvalho AP, de Mello WC, Hoffman BF (1959) Electrophysiological evidence for specialized fiber types in rabbit atrium. Am J Physiol 196: 483–488.

72. Spach MS, Lieberman M, Scott JG, Barr RC, Johnson EA, et al. (1971) Excitation sequences of the atrial septum and the AV node in isolated hearts of the dog and rabbit. Circ Res 29: 156–172.

73. Mazgalev TN, Tchou PJ (2000) Atrial-AV nodal electrophysiology: a view from the millennium. Wiley-Blackwell.

74. Litchenberg WH, Norman LW, Holwell AK, Martin KL, Hewett KW, et al. (2000) The rate and anisotropy of impulse propagation in the postnatal terminal crest are correlated with remodeling of Cx43 gap junction pattern. Cardiovasc Res 45: 379–387.

75. Kirchhof CJ, Allessie MA (1992) Sinus node automaticity during atrial fibrillation in isolated rabbit hearts. Circulation 86: 263–271.

76. Xiao J, Zhang H, Liang D, Liu Y, Zhao H, et al. (2010) Taxol, a microtubule stabilizer, prevents atrial fibrillation in in vitro atrial fibrillation models using rabbit hearts. Med Sci Monit 16: BR353–BR360.

77. Li H, Scherlag BJ, Kem DC, Zillner C, Male S, et al. (2014) The propensity for inducing atrial fibrillation: a comparative study on old versus young rabbits. Journal of Aging Research 2014: 684918.

78. Oliveira M, da Silva MN, Geraldes V, Xavier R, Laranjo S, et al. (2011) Acute vagal modulation of electrophysiology of the atrial and pulmonary veins increases vulnerability to atrial fibrillation. Exp Physiol 96: 125–133.

79. Che X, Qu B, Wu L, Hu X, Yu J, et al. (2003) The initial study on the origin and reentrant mechanism of paroxysmal atrial fibrillation arising from right atrium with non-contact mapping system. Chinese Journal of Cardiac Pacing and Electrophysiology 17: 22–26.

80. Mazgalev T, Dreifus LS, Bianchi J, Michelson EL (1982) Atrioventricular nodal conduction during atrial fibrillation in rabbit heart. Am J Physiol 243: H754–H760.

81. Fozzard HA (1991) The heart and cardiovascular system: scientific foundations. New York: Raven Press, c1991.

82. Efimov IR, Nikolski VP, Rothenberg F, Greener ID, Li J, et al. (2004) Structure-function relationship in the AV junction. Anat Rec 280A: 952–965.

83. Nakayama T, Kurachi Y, Noma A, Irisawa H (1984) Action potential and membrane currents of single pacemaker cells of the rabbit heart. Pflugers Arch 402: 248–257.

84. Denyer JC, Brown HF (1990) Rabbit sino-atrial node cells: isolation and electrophysiological properties. J Physiol 428: 405–424.

85. van Ginneken AC, Giles W (1991) Voltage clamp measurements of the hyperpolarization-activated inward current I_f in single cells from rabbit sino-atrial node. J Physiol 434: 57–83.

86. Ono K, Ito H (1995) Role of rapidly activating delayed rectifier K^+ current in sinoatrial node pacemaker activity. Am J Physiol Heart Circ Physiol 269: H453–H462.

87. Verheijck EE, van Ginneken ACG, Bourier J, Bouman LN (1995) Effects of delayed rectifier current blockade by E-4031 on impulse generation in single sinoatrial nodal myocytes of the rabbit. Circ Res 76: 607–615.

88. Wilders R, Verheijck EE, Kumar R, Goolsby WN, van Ginneken AC, et al. (1996) Model clamp and its application to synchronization of rabbit sinoatrial node cells. Am J Physiol Heart Circ Physiol 271: H2168–H2182.

89. Yamashita T, Nakajima T, Hazama H, Hamada E, Murakawa Y, et al. (1995) Regional differences in transient outward current density and inhomogeneities of repolarization in rabbit right atrium. Circulation 92: 3061–3069.

90. Wu J, Schuessler RB, Rodefeld MD, Saffitz JE, Boineau JP (2001) Morphological and membrane characteristics of spider and spindle cells isolated from rabbit sinus node. Am J Physiol Heart Circ Physiol 280: H1232–H1240.

91. Lei M, Cooper PJ, Camelliti P, Kohl P (2002) Role of the 293b-sensitive, slowly activating delayed rectifier potassium current, i_{Ks}, in pacemaker activity of rabbit isolated sino-atrial node cells. Cardiovasc Res 53: 68–79.

92. Kerr CR, Prystowsky EN, Browning DJ, Strauss HC (1980) Characterization of refractoriness in the sinus node of the rabbit. Circ Res 47: 742–756.

93. Reid MC, Billette J, Khalife K, Tadros R (2003) Role of compact node and posterior extension in direction-dependent changes in atrioventricular nodal function in rabbit. J Cardiovasc Electrophysiol 14: 1342–1350.

94. Lin IJ, Billette JACQ, Medkour DJAM, Reid MC, Tremblay MAUR, et al. (2001) Properties and substrate of slow pathway exposed with a compact node targeted fast pathway ablation in rabbit atrioventricular node. J Cardiovasc Electrophysiol 12: 479–486.

Permissions

The contributors of this book come from diverse backgrounds, making this book a truly international effort. This book will bring forth new frontiers with its revolutionizing research information and detailed analysis of the nascent developments around the world.

We would like to thank all the contributing authors for lending their expertise to make the book truly unique. They have played a crucial role in the development of this book. Without their invaluable contributions this book wouldn't have been possible. They have made vital efforts to compile up to date information on the varied aspects of this subject to make this book a valuable addition to the collection of many professionals and students.

This book was conceptualized with the vision of imparting up-to-date information and advanced data in this field. To ensure the same, a matchless editorial board was set up. Every individual on the board went through rigorous rounds of assessment to prove their worth. After which they invested a large part of their time researching and compiling the most relevant data for our readers.

The editorial board has been involved in producing this book since its inception. They have spent rigorous hours researching and exploring the diverse topics which have resulted in the successful publishing of this book. They have passed on their knowledge of decades through this book. To expedite this challenging task, the publisher supported the team at every step. A small team of assistant editors was also appointed to further simplify the editing procedure and attain best results for the readers.

Apart from the editorial board, the designing team has also invested a significant amount of their time in understanding the subject and creating the most relevant covers. They scrutinized every image to scout for the most suitable representation of the subject and create an appropriate cover for the book.

The publishing team has been an ardent support to the editorial, designing and production team. Their endless efforts to recruit the best for this project, has resulted in the accomplishment of this book. They are a veteran in the field of academics and their pool of knowledge is as vast as their experience in printing. Their expertise and guidance has proved useful at every step. Their uncompromising quality standards have made this book an exceptional effort. Their encouragement from time to time has been an inspiration for everyone.

The publisher and the editorial board hope that this book will prove to be a valuable piece of knowledge for researchers, students, practitioners and scholars across the globe.

Contributors

Tamara T. Koopmann, Michiel E. Adriaens, Roos F. Marsman, Margriet L. Westerveld, Elisabeth M. Lodder and Connie R. Bezzina
Department of Experimental Cardiology, Heart Failure Research Centre, Academic Medical Center, Amsterdam, The Netherlands

Perry D. Moerland
Bioinformatics Laboratory, Department of Clinical Epidemiology, Biostatistics and Bioinformatics, Academic Medical Center, Amsterdam, The Netherlands

Cristobal dos Remedios and Sean Lal
Muscle Research Unit, Department of Anatomy, Bosch Institute, The University of Sydney, Sydney, Australia

Taifang Zhang
Department of Medicine, University of Miami School of Medicine, Miami, Florida, United States of America

Christine Q. Simmons and Alfred L. George, Jr.
5 Division of Genetic Medicine, Department of Medicine, Vanderbilt University, Nashville, Tennessee, United States of America

Istvan Baczko and Andras Varro
Department of Pharmacology and Pharmacotherapy, Faculty of Medicine, University of Szeged, Szeged, Hungary

Nanette H. Bishopric
Department of Medicine, University of Miami School of Medicine, Miami, Florida, United States of America
Department of Molecular and Cellular Pharmacology, University of Miami School of Medicine, Miami, Florida, United States of America

Hui-Shan Wang, Zeng-Wei Wang and Zong-Tao Yin
Department of Cardiovascular Surgery, Shenyang Northern Hospital, Shenyang, Liaoning Province, China

Alfonso Bueno-Orovio and Blanca Rodriguez
Department of Computer Science, Computational Biology Group, University of Oxford, Oxford, United Kingdom

Ben M. Hanson
Department of Mechanical Engineering, University College London, London, United Kingdom,

Jaswinder S. Gill
Guy's and St. Thomas' Hospital, London, United Kingdom

Peter Taggart
The Neurocardiology Research Unit, University College Hospital, London, United Kingdom

Efstratios I. Charitos, Ulrich Stierle, Bernhard Graf, Hans-Hinrich Sievers and Thorsten Hanke
Department of Cardiac and Thoracic Vascular Surgery, University of Luebeck, Luebeck, Germany

Paul D. Ziegler
Medtronic Inc., Minneapolis, Minnesota, United States of America

Derek R. Robinson
Department of Mathematics, School of Mathematical and Physical Sciences, University of Sussex, Brighton, United Kingdom

Junxia Xu
Department of Geratology, Fuzhou General Hospital of Nanjing Command, PLA, Fuzhou, Fujian, China

Department of Geratology, Fozhou General Hospital, Fujian Medical University, Fuzhou, Fujian, China

Yingqun Huang, Hongbin Cai, Jinxiu Lin and Feng Peng
Department of Cardiology, The First Affiliated Hospital of Fujian Medical University, Fuzhou, Fujian, China

Yue Qi
Department of Epidemiology, Capital Medical University Affiliated Beijing An Zhen Hospital, Beijing Institute of Heart, Lung and Blood Vessel Diseases, Beijing, China

Nan Jia
Department of Cardiology, The Fourth People's Hospital of Shenzhen, Shenzhen, Guangdong, China

Weifeng Shen
Department of Cardiology, Ruijin Hospital, Shanghai Jiao Tong University School of Medicine, Shanghai, China

Wenquan Niu
Department of Human Genetics and Biostatistics, Institute of Cardiovascular Disease, Dalian Medical University, Dalian, Liaoning, China
Center for Evidence-Based Medicine, Institute of Cardiovascular Disease, Dalian Medical University, Dalian, Liaoning, China
State Key Laboratory of Medical Genomics, Ruijin Hospital, Shanghai Jiao Tong University School of Medicine, Shanghai, China

Paolo Verdecchia
Department of Medicine, Hospital of Assisi, Assisi, Italy

Fabio Angeli
Cardiology and Cardiovascular Pathophysiology, University Hospital of Perugia, Perugia, Italy,

Gregory Y. H. Lip
University of Birmingham Centre for Cardiovascular Sciences, City Hospital, Birmingham, United Kingdom

Gianpaolo Reboldi
Department of Medicine, University of Perugia, Perugia, Italy

Judith Kooiman, Bas Spaans, Koen A. J. van Beers, Jonna R. Bank, Wilke R. van de Peppel, Frederikus A. Klok and Menno V. Huisman
Department of Thrombosis and Hemostasis, Leiden University Medical Center, Leiden, The Netherlands

Nienke van Rein
Department of Thrombosis and Hemostasis, Leiden University Medical Center, Leiden, The Netherlands
Einthoven Laboratory of Experimental Vascular Medicine, Leiden University Medical Center, Leiden, The Netherlands

Antonio Iglesias del Sol
Department of Internal Medicine, Rijnland Hospital, Leiderdorp, The Netherlands

Suzanne C. Cannegieter
Department of Clinical Epidemiology, Leiden University Medical Center, Leiden, The Netherlands

Ton J. Rabelink
Department of Nephrology, Leiden University Medical Center, Leiden, The Netherlands

Gregory Y. H. Lip
Haemostasis, Thrombosis, and Vascular Biology Unit, University of Birmingham Centre for Cardiovascular Sciences, City Hospital, Birmingham, United Kingdom

Kai Friedrichs, Lisa Remane, Martin Mollenhauer, Volker Rudolph, Tanja K. Rudolph, Thorben Ravekes, Stephan Baldus and Anna Klinke
Heart Center, University of Cologne, Cologne, Germany
Cologne Cardiovascular Research Center, University of Cologne, Cologne, Germany

Florian Deuschl and Matti Adam
Department of General and Interventional Cardiology, University Heart Center Hamburg, Hamburg, Germany

Georg Nickenig, René P. Andrié, Florian Stöckigt and Jan W. Schrickel
Department of Medicine-Cardiology, University Hospital of Bonn, Bonn, Germany

Stephan Willems
Department of Electrophysiology, University Heart Center Hamburg, Hamburg, Germany

Yiguo Sun, Matthew D. Hills, Willy G. Ye, Xiaoling Tong and Donglin Bai
Department of Physiology and Pharmacology, The University of Western Ontario, London, Ontario, Canada

Giovanni Targher and Giacomo Zoppini
Division of Endocrinology, Diabetes and Metabolism, Department of Medicine, University and Azienda Ospedaliera Universitaria Integrata of Verona, Verona, Italy

Filippo Valbusa
Division of General Medicine, "Sacro Cuore" Hospital of Negrar, Verona, Italy

Stefano Bonapace and Enrico Barbieri
Division of Cardiology, "Sacro Cuore" Hospital of Negrar, Verona, Italy

Lorenzo Bertolini and Luciano Zenari
Diabetes Unit, "Sacro Cuore" Hospital of Negrar, Verona, Italy

Stefano Rodella
Division of Radiology, "Sacro Cuore" Hospital of Negrar, Verona, Italy

William Mantovani
Section of Hygiene and Preventive, Environmental and Occupational Medicine, Department of Public Health and Community Medicine, University of Verona, Verona, Italy
Department of Prevention, Public Health Trust, Trento, Italy

Christopher D. Byrne
Nutrition and Metabolism, Faculty of Medicine, University of Southampton, Southampton, United Kingdom
Southampton National Institute for Health Research Biomedical Research Centre, University Hospital Southampton, Southampton, United Kingdom

Aldo Casaleggio
Institute of Biophysics, National Research Council, Genova, Italy

Michael L. Hines
Dept. of Neurobiology, Yale University School of Medicine, New Haven, Connecticut, United States of America

Michele Migliore
Institute of Biophysics, National Research Council, Palermo, Italy

Shuang Li, Baoxin Liu, Dachun Xu and Yawei Xu
Department of Cardiology, Shanghai Tenth People's Hospital, Tongji University School of Medicine, Shanghai, China

Luciane Cruz Lopes
Pharmaceutical Sciences Postgraduate Course, University of Sorocaba, Sao Paulo, Brazil

Frederick A. Spencer
Department of Medicine, Division of Cardiology, McMaster University, Hamilton, Ontario, Canada

Ignacio Neumann
Internal Medicine Department, School of Medicine, Pontificia Universidad Catolica de Chile, Santiago, Chile
Department of Clinical Epidemiology and Biostatistics, McMaster University, Hamilton, Ontario, Canada

Matthew Ventresca, Gordon Guyatt and Qi Zhou
Department of Clinical Epidemiology and Biostatistics, McMaster University, Hamilton, Ontario, Canada

Shanil Ebrahim
Department of Clinical Epidemiology and Biostatistics, McMaster University, Hamilton, Ontario, Canada
Department of Anesthesia, McMaster University, Hamilton, Ontario, Canada
Stanford Prevention Research Center, Stanford University, Stanford, California, United States of America

Neera Bhatnagar
Health Sciences Library McMaster University, Hamilton, Ontario, Canada

Sam Schulman
Department of Clinical Epidemiology and Biostatistics, McMaster University, Hamilton, Ontario, Canada
Department of Medicine, McMaster University, Hamilton, Ontario, Canada

John Eikelboom
Department of Medicine, Division of Hematology and Thromboembolism, McMaster University, Hamilton, Ontario, Canada

Thomas A. Dewland and Gregory M. Marcus
Department of Internal Medicine, Division of Cardiology, Electrophysiology Section, University of California San Francisco, San Francisco, California, United States of America

David V. Glidden
Department of Epidemiology and Biostatistics, University of California San Francisco, San Francisco, California, United States of America

Karl Frontzek
Institute of Neuropathology, University Hospital Zurich, Zurich, Switzerland
Department of Neurology, University Hospital Basel, Basel, Switzerland

Felix Fluri
Department of Neurology, University Hospital Basel, Basel, Switzerland
Department of Neurology, University Hospital Zurich, Zurich, Switzerland

Mira Katan
Department of Neurology, University Hospital Zurich, Zurich, Switzerland

Jakob Siemerkus
University Hospital of Psychiatry, Zurich, Switzerland

Beat Müller
Medical University Clinic, Cantonal Hospital Aarau, Aarau, Switzerland

Achim Gass
Department of Neurology, University Hospital Mannheim, Mannheim, Germany

Mirjam Christ-Crain
Department of Endocrinology, University Hospital Basel, Basel, Switzerland

Mikko Taina, Miika Korhonen, Mika Haataja, Antti Muuronen, Otso Arponen, Petri Sipola and Ritva Vanninen
Department of Clinical Radiology, Kuopio University Hospital, Kuopio, Finland
Unit of Radiology, Institute of Clinical Medicine, University of Eastern Finland, Kuopio, Finland

Marja Hedman
Department of Clinical Radiology, Kuopio University Hospital, Kuopio, Finland
Heart Center, Kuopio University Hospital, Kuopio, Finland

Pekka Jäkälä
NeuroCenter, Kuopio University Hospital, Kuopio, Finland
Unit of Neurology, Institute of Clinical Medicine, University of Eastern Finland, Kuopio, Finland

Pirjo Mustonen
Department of Cardiology, Keski-Suomi Central Hospital, Jyväskylä, Finland

Michael Nagler
Division of Haematology and Central Haematology Laboratory, Luzerner Kantonsspital, Lucerne, and Department of Haematology and Central Haematology Laboratory, Inselspital University Hospital, Berne, Switzerland

Lucas M. Bachmann
medignition Inc., Zug, Switzerland

Pirmin Schmid and Pascale Raddatz Müller
Division of Haematology and Central Haematology Laboratory, Luzerner Kantonsspital, Lucerne, Switzerland,

Walter A. Wuillemin
Division of Haematology and Central Haematology Laboratory, Luzerner Kantonsspital, 6000 Lucerne, and University of Berne, Berne, Switzerland

Anand N. Ganesan, Anthony Brooks, Darius Chapman, Dennis H. Lau, Kurt C. Roberts-Thomson and Prashanthan Sanders
Centre for Heart Rhythm Disorders (CHRD), South Australian Health and Medical Research Institute (SAHMRI), University of Adelaide and Royal Adelaide Hospital, Adelaide, Australia

Ali Gharaviri
Department of Physiology, Maastricht University Medical Center, Maastricht, The Netherlands

Pawel Kuklik
Department of Physiology, Maastricht University Medical Center, Maastricht, The Netherlands
Department of Cardiology, Electrophysiology, University Heart Center, Hamburg, Germany

Kyoung-Im Cho, Tae-Joon Cha, Su-Jin Lee, In-Kyeung Shim, Jung-Ho Heo, Hyun-Su Kim and Jae-Woo Lee
Cardiovascular Research Institute, Department of Internal Medicine, Kosin University College of Medicine, Busan, South Korea

Sung Joon Kim and Yin Hua Zhang
Department of Physiology, Seoul National University College of Medicine, Seoul, South Korea

Kyoung-Lyoung Kim
Department of Molecular Biology, Kosin University College of Medicine, Busan, South Korea

Jae Yoo
College of Pharmacy, The Ohio State University, Columbus, Ohio, United States of America

Ingrid M. Bonilla and Victor P. Long, III
College of Pharmacy, The Ohio State University, Columbus, Ohio, United States of America
Dorothy M. Davis Heart and Lung Research Institute, The Ohio State University Wexner Medical Center, Columbus, Ohio, United States of America

Patrick Wright, Andriy Belevych, Qing Lou, Philip F. Binkley, Vadim V. Fedorov, Sandor Györke, Paulus M. L. Janssen, Ahmet Kilic and Peter J. Mohler
Dorothy M. Davis Heart and Lung Research Institute, The Ohio State University Wexner Medical Center, Columbus, Ohio, United States of America

Cynthia A. Carnes
College of Pharmacy, The Ohio State University, Columbus, Ohio, United States of America
College of Veterinary Medicine, The Ohio State University, Columbus, Ohio, United States of America

Pedro Vargas-Pinto
College of Veterinary Medicine, The Ohio State University, Columbus, Ohio, United States of America

Kent Mowrey
St Jude Medical, Sylmar, California, United States of America

Yoshinobu Wakisaka, Junya Kuroda and Tetsuro Ago
Department of Medicine and Clinical Science, Graduate School of Medical Sciences, Kyushu University, Fukuoka, Japan

Ryu Matsuo
Department of Medicine and Clinical Science, Graduate School of Medical Sciences, Kyushu University, Fukuoka, Japan
Department of Health Care Administration and Management, Graduate School of Medical Sciences, Kyushu University, Fukuoka, Japan

Takanari Kitazono and Jun Hata
Department of Medicine and Clinical Science, Graduate School of Medical Sciences, Kyushu University, Fukuoka, Japan
Center for Cohort Studies, Graduate School of Medical Sciences, Kyushu University, Fukuoka, Japan

Masahiro Kamouchi and Haruhisa Fukuda
Department of Health Care Administration and Management, Graduate School of Medical Sciences, Kyushu University, Fukuoka, Japan
Center for Cohort Studies, Graduate School of Medical Sciences, Kyushu University, Fukuoka, Japan

Li-hui Zheng, Ling-min Wu, Yan Yao, Wen-sheng Chen, Jing-ru Bao, Wen Huang, Rui Shi, Kui-jun Zhang and Shu Zhang
State Key Laboratory of Cardiovascular Disease, Clinical EP Lab and Arrhythmia Center, Fuwai Hospital, National Center for Cardiovascular Diseases, Chinese Academy of Medical Sciences and Peking Union Medical College, Beijing, China

Joshua Wallace, Spiros C. Denaxas, Anoop D. Shah and Harry Hemingway
Farr Institute of Health Informatics Research, University College London, London, United Kingdom, and Clinical Epidemiology, Department of Epidemiology and Public Health, University College London, London, United Kingdom

Katherine I. Morley
Farr Institute of Health Informatics Research, University College London, London, United Kingdom, and Clinical Epidemiology, Department of Epidemiology and Public Health, University College London, London, United Kingdom
Institute of Psychiatry, Psychology and Neuroscience, King's College London, London, United Kingdom
Melbourne School of Global and Population Health, The University of Melbourne, Melbourne, Australia

Ross J. Hunter, Adam D. Timmis and Richard J. Schilling
Barts NIHR Biomedical Research Unit, Queen Mary University London, London, United Kingdom

Riyaz S. Patel
Farr Institute of Health Informatics Research, University College London, London, United Kingdom, and Clinical Epidemiology, Department of Epidemiology and Public Health, University College London, London, United Kingdom

The Heart Hospital, University College London NHS Trust, London, United Kingdom

Pablo Perel
Farr Institute of Health Informatics Research, University College London, London, United Kingdom, and Clinical Epidemiology, Department of Epidemiology and Public Health, University College London, London, United Kingdom
London School of Hygiene and Tropical Medicine, London, United Kingdom

Alvaro Alonso, Faye L. Lopez and Aaron R. Folsom
Division of Epidemiology and Community Health, School of Public Health, University of Minnesota, Minneapolis, Minnesota, United States of America

Paul N. Jensen and Susan R. Heckbert
Department of Epidemiology, School of Public Health, University of Washington, Seattle, Washington, United States of America

Lin Y. Chen
Cardiovascular Division, Department of Medicine, University of Minnesota Medical School, Minneapolis, Minnesota, United States of America

Bruce M. Psaty
Cardiovascular Health Research Unit, Departments of Medicine, Epidemiology, and Health Services, University of Washington, Seattle, Washington, United States of America
Group Health Research Institute, Group Health Cooperative, Seattle, Washington, United States of America

Renate B. Schnabel, Sandra Wilde, Francisco M. Ojeda, Tanja Zeller, Christoph R. Sinning and Stefan Blankenberg
Department of General and Interventional Cardiology, University Heart Center Hamburg-Eppendorf, Germany

Andreas Schulz and Thomas Munzel
Department of Medicine 2, University Medical Center of the Johannes Gutenberg-University Mainz, Germany

Philipp S. Wild
Department of Medicine 2, University Medical Center of the Johannes Gutenberg-University Mainz, Germany
Center of Thrombosis and Hemostasis University Medical Center of the Johannes Gutenberg-University Mainz, Germany

Jan Kunde
BRAHMS GmbH, Hennigsdorf/Germany

Karl J. Lackner
Institute of Clinical Chemistry and Laboratory Medicine, University Medical Center of the Johannes Gutenberg- University Mainz, Germany

Yalin Yin
Research Center, Hôpital du Sacré-Coeur de Montré al, Université de Montré al, Montréal, Canada

Feng Xiong
Research Center, Hôpital du Sacré-Coeur de Montré al, Université de Montré al, Montréal, Canada
Montréal Heart Institute, Université de Montréal, Montréal, Canada

Pierre Pagé
Research Center, Hôpital du Sacré-Coeur de Montré al, Université de Montré al, Montréal, Canada
Montréal Heart Institute, Université de Montréal, Montréal, Canada
Department of Surgery, Université de Montréal, Montréal, Canada

Bruno Dubé and Alain Vinet
Research Center, Hôpital du Sacré-Coeur de Montré al, Université de Montré al, Montréal, Canada
Biomedical Engineering Institute, Université de Montréal, Montréal, Canada

Wenli Zhang
Department of Cardiology, Fuzhou General Hospital of Nanjing Command, PLA, Fujian Medical University, Fuzhou, Fujian, China

Nan Jia
Department of Cardiology, The Fourth People's Hospital of Shenzhen, Shenzhen, Guangdong, China

Jinzi Su, Jinxiu Lin and Feng Peng
Department of Cardiology, The First Affiliated Hospital of Fujian Medical University, Fuzhou, Fujian, China

Wenquan Niu
State Key Laboratory of Medical Genomics, Ruijin Hospital, Shanghai Jiao Tong University School of Medicine, Shanghai, China
Shanghai Institute of Hypertension, Ruijin Hospital, Shanghai Jiao Tong University School of Medicine, Shanghai, China

Jue Li, Shin Inada, Jurgen E. Schneider, Henggui Zhang, Halina Dobrzynski and Mark R. Boyett
Institute of Cardiovascular Sciences, University of Manchester, Core Technology Facility, Manchester, United Kingdom

Index